OCULAR ONCOLOGY

OCULAR ONCOLOGY

edited by

DANIEL M. ALBERT
ARTHUR POLANS

University of Wisconsin Medical School
Madison, Wisconsin, U.S.A.

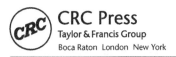

CRC Press
Taylor & Francis Group
Boca Raton London New York

CRC Press is an imprint of the
Taylor & Francis Group, an **informa** business

First published 2003 by Marcel Dekker, Inc.

Published 2019 by CRC Press
Taylor & Francis Group
6000 Broken Sound Parkway NW, Suite 300
Boca Raton, FL 33487-2742

© 2003 by Taylor & Francis Group, LLC
CRC Press is an imprint of Taylor & Francis Group, an Informa business

First issued in paperback 2019

No claim to original U.S. Government works

ISBN 13: 978-0-367-44667-3 (pbk)
ISBN 13: 978-0-8247-4016-0 (hbk)

Visit the Taylor & Francis Web site at
http://www.taylorandfrancis.com

and the CRC Press Web site at
http://www.crcpress.com

Although great care has been taken to provide accurate and current information, neither the author(s) nor the publisher, nor anyone else associated with this publication, shall be liable for any loss, damage, or liability directly or indirectly caused or alleged to be caused by this book. The material contained herein is not intended to provide specific advice or recommendations for any specific situation.

Library of Congress Cataloging-in-Publication Data
A catalog record for this book is available from the Library of Congress

To the scientists and clinicians who have labored and continue to labor to determine the causes, pathogenesis, and effective treatments of eye tumors.

Preface

Ocular tumors are unique among the diseases of the eye, threatening both sight and life. Prior texts in oncology and ophthalmology have focused primarily on providing physicians with information about the treatment of eye tumors. *Ocular Oncology* differs in that it is our objective to present a comprehensive account of the most current basic and clinical science related to eye tumors, and to offer new ideas about innovative treatments derived from recent genetic, biochemical, and immunological studies. In addition, this book discusses the current status of clinical trials in ocular oncology, as well as provides an up-to-date review of risk and prognostic factors associated with eye tumors. Finally, current findings are presented from studies of animal models and their use to assess the efficacy of novel treatment modalities with potential for human treatment.

Ocular Oncology focuses on uveal melanoma and retinoblastoma, the principal tumors originating in the eyes of adults and children, respectively. Although considered uncommon diseases, we need to acknowledge that rare and uncommon diseases often provide insights into fundamental biological processes and advance the development of innovative treatments of more prevalent diseases. There is perhaps no better example in science than retinoblastoma, a rare childhood ocular tumor with an incidence of only 300 to 400 cases per year in the United States. Studies of retinoblastoma, however, funded by the National Eye Institute, led to the identification of the first tumor suppressor gene. Prior to these studies, cancer was considered solely a "gain of function" phenomenon; studies of retinoblastoma instigated a fundamental change in thinking and scientific approach. In addition, studies of retinoblastoma led to the identification of further genes and pathways involved in one of the most fundamental processes in biology, namely the molecular control of cellular growth. Likewise, while much attention has been focused recently on anti-angiogenic strategies for the treatment of solid tumors, new studies of uveal melanoma have revealed a form of non-endothelial-based tumor microcirculation, owing to the dedifferentiation of tumor cells, that may compromise anti-angiogenic treatments. The relevance of such an alternative circulatory pathway during the growth and progression of other types of cancer is now an active area of investigation, instigated by studies of a rare eye tumor.

What is evident from recent technological advances, encompassed in new cytogenetic methods and the use of DNA chip arrays, is that ocular tumors, like eye diseases such as retinitis pigmentosa, are really a composite of different sentinel mutations that lead to the alteration of very different cellular pathways. Ultimately, the phenotype is unrestricted growth, a fairly limited description that likely undervalues the variety of causes leading to an eye tumor. This diversity and the ensuing complexity at a molecular level eventually will require methods of diagnosis and treatment that are tailored on a more individual level.

We would like to thank all of the contributors who thoughtfully considered the complexities of their particular scientific subdiscipline of ocular oncology, who fairly presented the controversies and candidly acknowledged the limitations of our knowledge, and who speculated boldly on what we need to accomplish before we can hope to successfully treat or prevent eye tumors and their metastases.

Daniel M. Albert
Arthur S. Polans

Contents

Contents

Contributors

David H. Abramson, M.D., F.A.C.S. Department of Ophthalmology, New York Presbyterian Hospital, New York, New York, U.S.A.

Daniel M. Albert, M.D., M.S. Department of Ophthalmology and Visual Sciences, University of Wisconsin, Madison, Wisconsin, U.S.A.

Isabelle Audo, M.D., Ph.D. Laboratoire de Physiopathologie Cellulaire et Moléculaire de la Rétine, Hôpital Saint Antoine, Paris, France

James J. Augsburger, M.D. Department of Ophthalmology, University of Cincinnati College of Medicine; Department of Ophthalmology, The University Hospital; Division of Ophthalmology, Department of Surgery, Cincinnati Children's Hospital Medical Center; and Division of Ophthalmology, Department of Surgery, Veteran's Affairs Medical Center, Cincinnati, Ohio, U.S.A.

H. Culver Boldt, M.D. Department of Ophthalmology, University of Iowa, Iowa City, Iowa, U.S.A.

Jacobus J. Bosch, M.D. Department of Ophthalmology, Harvard Medical School and Schepens Eye Research Institute, Boston, Massachusetts, U.S.A.

Vivette D. Brown, Ph.D. Division of Cancer Informatics, University Health Network, Toronto, Ontario, Canada

Helen S. L. Chan, M.D. Department of Pediatrics, University of Toronto, Toronto, Ontario, Canada

Emily Y. Chew, M.D. Division of Epidemiology and Clinical Research, National Eye Institute/National Institutes of Health, Bethesda, Maryland, U.S.A.

Soesiawati R. Darjatmoko Department of Ophthalmology and Visual Sciences, University of Wisconsin, Madison, Wisconsin, U.S.A.

Marie Diener-West, Ph.D.   Department of Biostatistics, Johns Hopkins Bloomberg School of Public Health, Baltimore, Maryland, U.S.A.

Stefan Dithmar, M.D.   Department of Ophthalmology, University of Heidelberg, Heidelberg, Germany

Robert Folberg, M.D.   Department of Pathology, University of Illinois at Chicago, Chicago, Illinois, U.S.A.

Brenda L. Gallie, M.D.   Departments of Ophthalmology, Molecular and Medical Genetics, and Medical Biophysics, University of Toronto, Toronto, Ontario, Canada

Dan S. Gombos, M.D.   Department of Ophthalmology, M. D. Anderson Hospital, Houston, Texas, U.S.A.

Hans E. Grossniklaus, M.D.   Department of Ophthalmology, Emory University, Atlanta, Georgia, U.S.A.

J. William Harbour, M.D.   Departments of Ophthalmology and Visual Sciences, Cell Biology and Physiology, and Molecular Oncology, Washington University School of Medicine, St. Louis, Missouri, U.S.A.

Brandy C. Hayden   Department of Ophthalmology, Bascom Palmer Eye Institute/ University of Miami School of Medicine, Miami, Florida, U.S.A.

Dan-Ning Hu, M.D.   Department of Ophthalmology, The New York Eye and Ear Infirmary and New York Medical College, New York, New York, U.S.A.

Bruce R. Ksander, Ph.D.   Department of Ophthalmology, Harvard Medical School and Schepens Eye Research Institute, Boston, Massachusetts, U.S.A.

Ian W. McLean, M.D.   Division of Ophthalmic Pathology, Armed Forces Institute of Pathology, Washington, D.C., U.S.A.

Steven A. McCormick, M.D.   Departments of Pathology, Ophthalmology, and Otorhinolaryngology, The New York Eye and Ear Infirmary and New York Medical College, New York, New York, U.S.A.

William F. Mieler, M.D.   Department of Ophthalmology, Baylor College of Medicine, Houston, Texas, U.S.A.

Claudia Scala Moy, Ph.D.   Division of Extramural Research, National Institutes of Health/National Institute of Neurological Disorders and Stroke, Bethesda, Maryland, U.S.A.

Timothy G. Murray, M.D.   Department of Ophthalmology, Bascom Palmer Eye Institute/University of Miami School of Medicine, Miami, Florida, U.S.A.

Robert W. Nickells, Ph.D. Department of Ophthalmology and Visual Sciences, University of Wisconsin, Madison, Wisconsin, U.S.A.

Jerry Y. Niederkorn, Ph.D. Department of Ophthalmology, University of Texas Southwestern Medical Center, Dallas, Texas, U.S.A.

Joan M. O'Brien, M.D. Department of Ophthalmology, University of California–San Francisco, San Francisco, California, U.S.A.

Jacob Pe'er, M.D. Department of Ophthalmology, Hadassah-Hebrew University Hospital, Jerusalem, Israel

Diane Puccetti, M.D. Department of Pediatric Hematology/Oncology, University of Wisconsin Children's Hospital, Madison, Wisconsin, U.S.A.

Ian G. Rennie, F.R.C.S. Department of Ophthalmology, University of Sheffield, Sheffield, England

José Sahel, M.D. Laboratoire de Physiopathologie Cellulaire et Moléculaire de la Rétine, Hôpital Saint Antoine, Paris, France

Amy C. Schefler, M.D. Department of Ophthalmology, New York Presbyterian Hospital, New York, New York, U.S.A.

Cassandra L. Schlamp, Ph.D. Department of Ophthalmology and Visual Sciences, University of Wisconsin, Madison, Wisconsin, U.S.A.

Carol L. Shields, M.D. Ocular Oncology Service, Wills Eye Hospital, and Department of Ophthalmology, Thomas Jefferson University, Philadelphia, Pennsylvania, U.S.A.

Jerry A. Shields, M.D. Ocular Oncology Service, Wills Eye Hospital, and Department of Ophthalmology, Thomas Jefferson University, Philadelphia, Pennsylvania, U.S.A.

Karen Sisley, Ph.D. Academic Unit of Ophthalmology and Orthoptics, University of Sheffield, Sheffield, England

Paul R. van Ginkel, Ph.D. Department of Ophthalmology and Visual Sciences, University of Wisconsin, Madison, Wisconsin, U.S.A.

Kurtis R. Van Quill Department of Ophthalmology, University of California–San Francisco, San Francisco, California, U.S.A

Jolene J. Windle, Ph.D. Department of Human Genetics, Virginia Commonwealth University, Richmond, Virginia, U.S.A.

1

Clinical Overview of Uveal Melanoma: Introduction to Tumors of the Eye

J. WILLIAM HARBOUR

Washington University School of Medicine, St. Louis, Missouri, U.S.A.

I. INTRODUCTION

A. Background

Melanoma of the uveal tract is the most common primary intraocular cancer in humans and accounts for about 12% of all melanomas [1]. Over 90% of uveal melanomas arise from the ciliary body and/or choroid and are referred to as posterior uveal melanomas; whereas about 5–8% of uveal melanomas arise in the iris [2]. Iris melanomas are generally much smaller, have a better prognosis, and are managed somewhat differently than posterior uveal melanomas.

B. Epidemiology/Demographics

Uveal melanoma occurs in about 5–7 persons per million persons annually (1200–1700 new cases per year) in the United States [1,3]. Uveal melanomas can arise from pre-existing uveal nevi or de novo. Based on earlier prevalence estimates for choroidal nevi (3.1% in persons over 30 years old), it was calculated that about 1 in 4000–5000 nevi transform into melanomas [4]. However, more recent studies, including a prospective analysis from our group, suggest that the prevalence of choroidal nevi may be as high as 18% in Caucasian populations, which would indicate that the proportion of nevi that convert to melanomas may be even smaller than previously assumed.

1

There is now convincing evidence that solar ultraviolet (UV) light plays an etiological role in cutaneous melanoma through induction of DNA damage in dermal melanocytes [5]. However, the relationship between uveal melanoma and UV irradiation remains controversial. Several studies found a link between uveal melanoma and increased UV exposure, sensitivity to UV light, ancestry from northern latitudes, light skin color, residence at lower latitudes, sunlamp use, and a history of intense sunlight exposure [6–9]. Light iris color has also been linked to uveal melanoma [6,9,10]. However, other studies have failed to support an association between uveal melanoma and UV exposure [1,11]. If there is an etiological link between UV light and uveal melanoma, it is probably much weaker than that for cutaneous melanoma.

Uveal melanoma has been linked to a variety of occupational and environmental factors, such as indoor working conditions, exposure to chemicals, and radiofrequency radiation [6,10,12,13], but the epidemiological significance of these associations has not been established.

C. Clinical Genetics

Uveal melanoma is usually a nonheritable, sporadic tumor. In fact, the world literature contains only a few families in which uveal melanomas were documented in more than two members in a bona fide Mendelian inheritance pattern [14–16]. There is little evidence for a hereditary uveal melanoma syndrome, which might include such features as the development of melanoma at an early age, bilateral ocular tumors, or predisposition to other second primary cancers [15]. Aside from rare patients with the familial atypical nevus-melanoma syndrome, there is a weak association between uveal and cutaneous melanoma. The systemic disorder most commonly linked to uveal melanoma is oculo(dermal) melanocytosis [17]. Uveal melanoma has also been reported in association with neurofibromatosis type 1 (NF1), but there does not appear to be a predisposition to uveal melanoma among NF1 patients, and we have shown that NF1 mutations are rare in uveal melanoma. The lack of hereditary pattern or association with an inherited condition has greatly hampered the search for causative genes in uveal melanoma, since genetic linkage analysis is not possible. This situation stands in contrast to retinoblastoma, where the hereditary pattern led to discovery of the first tumor suppressor gene [18,19]. Efforts to identify causative genes in uveal melanoma will rely on other approaches, such as the study of cytogenetic changes and mutations in known cancer genes [20,21].

II. DIAGNOSIS

A. Clinical Features

The clinical appearance, size, and location of uveal melanomas are highly variable (Fig. 1). Many other lesions can simulate uveal melanoma [22]. However, clinical examination and ancillary testing can accurately diagnose most uveal melanomas. Iris melanomas usually present as a variably pigmented, elevated mass that replaces the iris stroma (Fig. 1). The color of the tumor can vary from light tan to dark

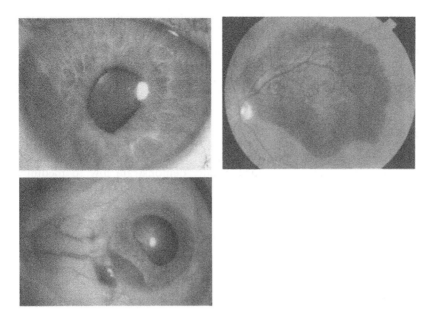

Figure 1 Uveal melanoma can involve the iris (top, left), choroid (top, right), and/or ciliary body (bottom).

brown, and intrinsic tumor vessels can often be identified in lightly pigmented tumors. Distortion and contraction of the iris stroma may lead to pupillary peaking or ectropion uveae. Shedding of tumor cells onto the iris surface and into the anterior chamber angle can lead to satellite lesions, hyperpigmentation of the trabecular meshwork, and secondary glaucoma. Lenticular touch may lead to focal cataract formation. About 6.5% of small iris melanocytic lesions will grow over a 5-year period; the clinical features most predictive of growth and malignancy include increased size and thickness, pigment shedding, secondary glaucoma, intrinsic tumor vessels, and visual changes [23].

Posterior uveal melanomas can involve the ciliary body, choroid, or both (Fig. 1). Tumors involving the ciliary body and/or peripheral choroid tend to grow to a larger size before detection, whereas tumors in the posterior pole tend to be detected when they are smaller, due to earlier visual changes. Posterior uveal melanomas can vary in color from light tan to dark brown. They are usually dome- or mushroom-shaped, which indicates that the tumor has broken through Bruch's membrane (mostly in tumors ⩾5 mm thick). Exudative retinal detachment is often present. Subretinal or vitreous hemorrhage may occur, especially in larger tumors. Choroidal neovascularization may occur in chronic, dormant lesions [24]. Small melanocytic lesions under 2.5–3 mm in thickness are often followed for evidence of growth prior to treatment, since many of these lesions will prove to be dormant. In a group of patients with small tumors that were observed in the Collaborative Ocular Melanoma Study (COMS), 31% of the tumors grew within 5 years [25], which is similar to the 26–36% growth rate reported in earlier retrospective studies [26,27]. Clinical features associated with growth of small choroidal melanocytic lesions include increased thickness and diameter, subretinal fluid, orange lipofuscin pigment overlying the tumor, juxtapapillary location, visual changes, internal quiet zone on B-scan ultrasonography, and hot spots on fluorescein angiography [25–27]. Features associated with lower risk for lesion growth include drusen and retinal pigment epithelial atrophic changes around the tumor [25].

B. Diagnostic Modalities

For posterior uveal melanoma, ultrasonography is generally the most useful ancillary diagnostic test. Uveal melanomas usually demonstrate low to medium internal reflectivity on standardized A-scan ultrasonography (Fig. 2). B-scan mode demonstrates the overall shape and topography of the tumor (Fig. 2). These features usually allow melanomas to be distinguished from simulating lesions such as choroidal metastases, which tend to have high irregular reflectivity, and choroidal hemangiomas, which usually demonstrate high and relatively uniform reflectivity [2]. The recent development of high-frequency (20- to 50-MHz) ultrasound units for examining the anterior segment have aided greatly in determining the size, location, extent, internal characteristics, and growth of iris and ciliary body lesions (Fig. 2) [28].

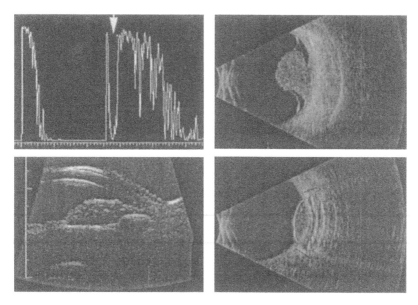

Figure 2   Ultrasonography can be very helpful in diagnosing uveal melanoma. Low internal reflectivity within the tumor on A scan (arrow) is characteristic of melanoma (top, left). Tumor topography, such as the mushroom shape, can be seen using B-scan ultrasonography (top, right). Iris melanomas can be evaluated with high-frequency anterior segment ultrasonography (bottom, left). Intraoperative ultrasonography is extremely useful for localizing radioactive plaques (bottom, right). The white line indicates the tumor and the black lines indicate the edges of the plaque, demonstrating excellent localization of the plaque over the tumor.

Fluorescein angiography can be useful but is not diagnostic in the evaluation of choroidal melanoma [29]. In particular, fluorescein angiography can help to distinguish between a melanoma, which often has intrinsic hyperfluorescence and vascularity, and a hemorrhagic lesion such as a ruptured retinal arterial macroaneurysm or peripheral choroidal neovascularization, which generally blocks fluorescence. Indocyanine green (ICG) angiography can be useful in detecting choroidal neovascularization and ruling out a choroidal hemangioma, which usually displays a characteristic late "washout" of dye [30]. Magnetic resonance imaging (MRI) is occasionally useful for distinguishing between uveal melanoma and other lesions [31]. MRI is most useful when performed with surface coils and fat suppression to maximize the sensitivity for evaluating intraocular masses. Melanomas characteristically demonstrate hyperintensity compared to vitreous on T1 weighting and hypointensity on T2 weighting [32].

The COMS reported a diagnostic accuracy rate of 99.7% for posterior uveal melanomas using the noninvasive techniques described above [33]. This high accuracy rate is due in part to the collective experience gained in the clinical evaluation of intraocular tumors but also to the fact that tumors with atypical features were excluded from the COMS for the specific purposes of the study. Therefore, the COMS results do not account for a significant proportion of melanomas (approximately 10% in our institution) with atypical features that can only be diagnosed with certainty by tissue biopsy. Intraocular fine-needle aspiration biopsy is most commonly used for tumors with atypical clinical features in which the biopsy will determine treatment. Fine-needle biopsy can be performed by transscleral, transvitreous, or transcorneal approaches, depending on the size and location of the tumor. When performed by an experienced surgeon and interpreted by an experienced ocular cytopathologist, intraocular biopsy yields a high percentage of positive cytopathological diagnoses, is relatively safe, and poses an extremely small risk of extraocular tumor dissemination [34,35].

III. TREATMENTS

A. Observation

Although there is general agreement among ocular oncologists that most uveal melanomas should be treated to minimize the risk of metastatic disease, there has never been a clinical study proving that treatment improves survival. Ethical and practical concerns will probably preclude such a trial from ever being performed. However, the rationale for treating uveal melanomas is based on several well-established observations, including the following. Patients who undergo enucleation or plaque radiotherapy for small melanomas have a much lower risk of metastasis than those with large melanomas [36,37], suggesting that treatment may prevent the further accumulation of risk that accompanies tumor enlargement. Conversely, local tumor recurrence following plaque radiotherapy greatly increases the risk of metastasis [9,38], suggesting that successful radiotherapy significantly reduces the risk of metastasis, as opposed to unsuccessful radiotherapy. Nevertheless, there are circumstances where observation is appropriate, as in patients with small indeterminate lesions that may be dormant or in those who may have a limited life expectancy.

B. Enucleation

Enucleation, or surgical removal of the eye, was the primary form of treatment for many years and is still the best option in many patients. Contemporary indications for enucleation include (1) large tumor size, (2) tumor invasion of the optic nerve head, (3) lack of access to other treatment options, (4) inability to return for follow-up, and (5) patient choice. Macular tumor location is a relative indication for enucleation, since radiotherapy in this location will usually result in poor vision. However, quality-of-life studies are needed to determine whether patients with macular tumors are more satisfied with enucleation or radiotherapy. Although pre-enucleation radiotherapy reduces the viability and replicative capacity of uveal melanoma cells [38–40], the COMS recently determined that external-beam radiotherapy prior to enucleation does not improve the survival of patients with large uveal melanomas (thickness greater than 10 mm or diameter greater than 16 mm) [41], confirming earlier retrospective studies [42,43].

In the 1970s, Zimmerman and colleagues raised the possibility that enucleation may hasten the development of metastatic disease, possibly by disseminating tumor emboli [44]. The "Zimmerman hypothesis" was based on certain statistical assumptions that are now questioned, but there is still evidence from animal models that enucleation may promote metastatic disease. Primary tumors that produce angiostatin, an inhibitor of endothelial cell proliferation, may suppress the vascularization and growth of metastatic deposits; therefore, removal of the primary tumor may allow metastases to grow [45]. Since some uveal melanomas produce angiostatin and appear to suppress metastasis in animal models [46], further work is needed to investigate this mechanism in humans and to determine whether angiostatin therapy may be beneficial in uveal melanoma patients at high risk for metastasis.

C. Radiotherapy

Conventional external-beam radiotherapy is not often used for uveal melanoma, because the high radiation doses required to treat this radioresistant tumor would lead to severe ocular and periocular complications. Brachytherapy allows much higher radiation doses to be delivered locally with acceptable complications. Although ocular brachytherapy for intraocular tumors had been attempted earlier in the twentieth century, it was not until the 1970s that interest in brachytherapy intensified as a result of the Zimmerman hypothesis (see above). Typically, ocular brachytherapy involves attaching radioactive seeds to a lead or gold "plaque" that is sewn to the sclera overlying the tumor. Currently, iodine 125 (^{125}I) is the most common radioisotope used in the United States [47], whereas ruthenium 106 (^{106}Ru) is commonly used in Europe [48]. Other isotopes, such as palladium 103 (^{103}Pd), have also been used [49]. Typically, 80–100 Gy is delivered to the tumor apex over 4–5 days, with a 2-mm plaque margin around the tumor base [47]. While the dosimetric characteristics of ^{125}I allow treatment of tumors up to 10–12 mm in thickness, ^{106}Ru has much weaker penetration and can be used only to treat tumors up to about 5 mm in thickness [48]. This fact has probably contributed to the more rapid development of other treatment modalities in Europe, such as local resection and stereotactic radiosurgery (see below).

In a prospective, multicenter trial conducted by the COMS to compare enucleation versus ^{125}I radiotherapy for medium-sized tumors (2.5 to 8 mm in thickness, diameter no greater than 16 mm), no significant difference in survival was identified [50], confirming previous impressions from retrospective studies [51]. An initial quality-of-life study from several COMS centers showed that patients undergoing radiotherapy scored higher on vitality and mental components of the Medical Outcome Study Short Form than patients treated by enucleation, but no other significant differences in quality of life were detected [52]. Additional outcomes studies of patient subgroups (e.g., tumor location and size, patient age and health status) are needed to guide the optimal treatment choice for a given patient.

Many uveal melanomas do not meet the COMS criteria for plaque radiotherapy but may nevertheless benefit from this treatment. In many centers, larger tumors up to about 18 mm in diameter and 10–12 mm in thickness are often treated with plaque radiotherapy with acceptable results, albeit with higher radiation complication rates. Some centers have been reluctant to treat juxtapapillary tumors with plaque therapy, due to a higher risk of local recurrence and metastasis. However, the success rate for treating these tumors appears to be improved by using notched plaques, intraoperative ultrasound to guide plaque placement, and adjuvant transpupillary thermotherapy (Fig. 3) [53–56]. In addition, selected iris melanomas appear to respond favorably to plaque radiotherapy [57,58]. Further prospective, controlled studies will be needed to determine the indications for plaque therapy other than those addressed in the COMS.

Complications of plaque radiotherapy include radiation complications (e.g., cataract, retinopathy, papillopathy, and neovascular glaucoma) and local tumor recurrence, which is a strong risk factor for metastatic disease [38,59,60]. The incidence of radiation complications are dose-dependent and begin to increase sharply over about 40 Gy [61], which is below the minimum threshold thought to be necessary for local tumor control. Therefore, pharmacological interventions that render the tumor more radiosensitive could greatly improve visual and ocular outcomes after plaque therapy. Local tumor relapse, which may occur in up to 15% of patients, is most common in posterior tumors near the optic nerve and macula [62–64]. One explanation for these local failures in posterior tumors may be inaccurate plaque placement due to limited surgical access and obstruction by extraocular muscles, optic nerve sheath, and other structures. Recent studies have shown that intraoperative ultrasonography is very helpful for localizing plaques accurately and identifying plaques that are tilted away from the sclera (Fig. 2) [54,65]. Preliminary studies have further shown that routine use of intraoperative ultrasonography may reduce the rate of local tumor recurrence [56].

Charged particle therapy, usually from a proton beam or helium ion source, is a means of delivering highly focused radiation to treat uveal melanomas. The indications and complications are similar to those for plaque radiotherapy except that anterior segment complications and neovascular glaucoma are more common with charged particles [62]. Reported rates of local tumor recurrence are lower for charged particles than plaque radiotherapy (especially for juxtapapillary tumors) [38,59,62], but results with plaque therapy may be substantially improved by the use

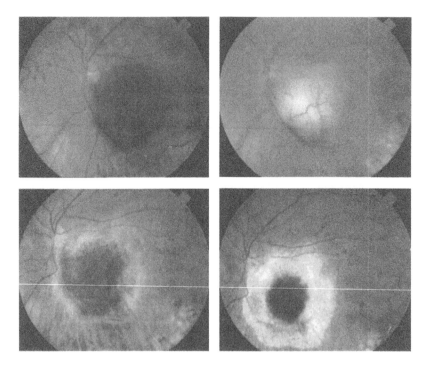

Figure 3 Plaque radiotherapy and transpupillary thermotherapy have a synergistic effect on uveal melanoma regression. A juxtapapillary tumor did not shrink significantly at 12 months following plaque radiotherapy (top, left). Therefore, adjunctive transpupillary thermotherapy was applied (top, right). Within 6 weeks, the tumor began to respond (bottom, left), and after 6 months the tumor was markedly regressed (bottom, right). Local control has been maintained on long-term follow-up. The retinal hemorrhages are due to a branch retinal vein occlusion.

of intraoperative ultrasonography for plaque localization and adjuvant laser thermotherapy (see above) [54–56]. In addition, charged particle therapy is more expensive than plaque therapy and is available at only a limited number of centers. Therefore, the situations where charged particle therapy is clearly preferable to plaque therapy remain unclear. Stereotactic radiosurgery is another modality that allows a radiation source to be focused from an external source in order to minimize radiation complications to the eye and periocular tissues [65]. Most experience with this technique had been in Europe, and it remains unclear what role it will have in the treatment armamentarium.

D. Local Resection

Iridocyclectomy is widely performed for melanomas involving the iris and ciliary body [66]. Cyclochoroidectomy is occasionally used in some centers for more posterior tumors [67]. Complications may include retinal detachment, proliferative vitreoretinopathy, intraocular hemorrhage, and local tumor recurrence, for which prophylactic scleral buckling, vitrectomy, hypotensive anesthesia, and postoperative plaque radiotherapy, respectively, have been advocated [68]. However, these interventions carry their own risks and must be weighed against potential benefits compared to other treatments such as plaque radiotherapy. Melanoma-containing eyes that were enucleated as part of the COMS demonstrated frequent invasion of local structures such as the retina, vitreous, and blood vessels [33], suggesting that tumor cells may often be left in the eye following local resection. On the other hand, most of the melanomas in this study were large, advanced tumors that may not have been candidates for local resection.

A matched-group, retrospective study by Augsburger and colleagues comparing local resection to cobalt-60 (^{60}Co) plaque radiotherapy found no significant difference in survival between the two treatments [69]. Interestingly, local resection was associated with a much higher risk of vision loss (<20/200) immediately following treatment, but the risk leveled off after about 1 year. In contrast, plaque therapy resulted in a slower but relentless loss of vision. The visual survival curves appeared to cross at about 7 years posttreatment, suggesting that the rate of long-term visual loss may actually be higher in the radiated patients. Based on these findings, the authors suggested that the optimal indications for local resection may include younger patient age, anterior tumor location, greater tumor thickness, and smaller tumor base.

In the absence of a prospective, randomized clinical trial to examine patient outcomes after local resection, ocular oncologists will continue to be guided by their training experience, familiarity, and skill with this challenging surgical technique as well as the availability of alternative treatments. ^{125}I plaque radiotherapy would appear to provide superior visual potential and local control in many situations, but ^{125}I is not uniformly available. Where only ^{106}Ru is available, combining local resection with plaque therapy may be a reasonable approach to avoid enucleation. A well-designed clinical study is needed to determine the optimal surgical technique and the appropriate indications for local resection.

E. Transpupillary Thermotherapy

Hyperthermia acts synergistically with radiation to induce regression of tumors [70]. Various techniques have been used for ocular hyperthermia, including microwaves, localized current field, ferromagnetic seeds, and ultrasound [71–74]. More recently, Oosterhuis and colleagues introduced "transpupillary thermotherapy" (TTT) as a less invasive and more convenient technique for delivering heat to intraocular tumors [75]. The Oosterhuis group established the current parameters for TTT, including 810-nm infrared diode laser, a large spot size (2–3 mm), 1-min exposures, and low energy, with the goal of creating a light-gray discoloration of the tumor at the end of each application. For uveal melanoma, TTT is usually administered via a slit-lamp attachment, but it can also be delivered through the operating microscope or indirect ophthalmoscope. Using this technique, TTT increases the temperature of the tumor above 45°C but below the threshold for photocoagulation; it can cause tumor necrosis to a depth of 3.9 mm [75].

The Oosterhuis group has advocated the use of TTT in conjunction with plaque therapy [55]. Nevertheless, it has been adopted in the United States largely as primary therapy for small melanomas [76–78]. Although early reports from United States centers have been favorable, these results must be interpreted with the following cautions in mind. First, TTT can cause significant vision-threatening complications such as macular traction, retinal vascular occlusion, macular edema, macular pucker, retinal or vitreous hemorrhage, and visual field defects [77,78]. Therefore, it remains unclear whether visual outcomes following TTT are superior (or even equivalent) to plaque therapy. Second, although the available data from the literature indicate a low local recurrence rate for TTT, these reports included very short follow-up. With longer observation, most centers are now seeing more local recurrences with TTT. Since local recurrence is a risk factor for metastasis after plaque radiotherapy [38], incomplete treatment with TTT may not have a neutral effect on survival. Third, many of the tumors treated with TTT that have been reported in the literature were very small with little or no documented growth [76–78], raising the question of whether some of these lesions may actually have been nevi. Further, if these studies used indications for treatment that differed substantially from those generally accepted for plaque therapy and other modalities, comparisons will be difficult to make between TTT and these other modalities. Thus, the role of TTT as primary therapy for uveal melanomas must be viewed with caution until there is a well-designed prospective study that provides treatment guidelines and meaningful estimates of visual outcome, local control, and metastatic risk.

Despite these reservations, TTT may still be appropriate in some situations (e.g., in patients that cannot undergo surgery), and TTT is likely to play an important role as an adjunct to plaque radiotherapy. TTT following plaque therapy causes melanomas to regress more rapidly and completely [55,79], indicating a possible synergistic interaction (Fig. 3). Combination therapy may be particularly useful in tumors with a high risk of local recurrence, such as juxtapapillary tumors. Radioresistant tumors are often responsive to plaque radiotherapy when combined with TTT (Fig. 3) [55]. Limited areas of local tumor recurrence often can be treated successfully with TTT, thereby avoiding enucleation. Although attitudes toward TTT continue to vary widely, the appropriate role of this modality will remain unclear until a properly designed clinical study is performed.

IV. PROGNOSIS AND SURVIVAL

Metastasis occurs in a substantial proportion of patients with uveal melanoma. In a metanalysis of patients enucleated for uveal melanoma, 5-year mortality rates were 16% for small tumors, 32% for medium-size tumors, and 53% for large tumors, with most mortality due to metastatic disease [36]. The most common metastatic sites include liver (87–93%), lung (24–46%), bone (16–29%), and skin (11–17%) [80,81]. The median time from ocular diagnosis to metastasis is about 2 years [82]. Median survival following clinical detection of metastasis is about 5–9 months [81–83]. Patients diagnosed with metastatic disease during routine screening examinations have a longer survival than those who become symptomatic prior to detection [82], supporting the practice of periodic systemic screening. Based on estimates of growth rates of metastatic tumors, an interval of 4–6 months has been suggested for systemic screening, although many centers perform this testing on an annual basis [84].

Numerous treatments have been proposed for metastatic uveal melanoma, including systemic chemotherapy, hepatic intra-arterial chemotherapy, chemoembolization, interferon, cytotoxic immunotherapy, and surgical resection [85–90]. Even though these therapies are rarely curative, they may reduce the growth rate of metastatic tumors and prolong survival [82,84]. Accurate prediction of metastatic risk may allow appropriate patients to be identified for prophylactic systemic therapy. Clinical risk factors for metastasis include advanced age, male gender, larger tumor size, anterior location, and extrascleral extension [91–95]. Pathological risk factors for metastasis include epithelioid cell type, nuclear and nucleolar pleomorphism, and intratumoral vascular patterns [86,92,95–98]. Nonrandom cytogenetic abnormalities have also been linked to metastasis and poor survival, including loss of chromosome 3, loss of chromosome 6q, and gain of chromosome 8q [99–102]. Further studies are needed to determine how clinical, pathological and molecular characteristics of a tumor can be combined to provide highly accurate prognostic information.

V. UNANSWERED QUESTIONS

Despite significant advances in the diagnosis and treatment of uveal melanoma over the past decades, many important questions remain unanswered. When should small melanocytic lesions be treated? The consensus has been to observe small, indeterminate lesions for growth prior to treatment, but this response raises other questions. What is the appropriate definition of a small, indeterminate lesion? Most ocular oncologists consider lesions over 2.5–3 mm in thickness to be highly suspicious for melanomas. The COMS initially defined tumors up to 3.0 mm in thickness to be small tumors to be observed, but this definition was later changed arbitrarily to 2.5 mm [103]. More objective data are still needed to identify which small tumors are melanomas that should be promptly treated. Does observation until growth is documented increase the risk of metastasis? Augsburger and Vrabec found no difference in mortality in a case-matched, retrospective survival study comparing patients who were promptly treated versus those who were treated only after tumor growth was documented [104]. In contrast, Shields and colleagues determined from a retrospective study that documented growth was a risk factor for metastasis in small melanocytic choroidal tumors ⩽ 3 mm in thickness [105]. These contradictory results, and the other unanswered questions discussed above, point out the need for a prospective, randomized study of small tumors to compare prompt treatment versus observation.

VI. FUTURE ADVANCES

Future advances in diagnosis, prognosis, and treatment may improve survival in uveal melanoma patients. Current diagnostic techniques are highly accurate in differentiating melanoma from simulating lesions [33], but future advances in imaging and molecular diagnostic techniques may yield therapeutic and prognostic information that could allow management to be customized for individual patients. High-resolution ultrasonographic and angiographic imaging techniques, such as confocal ICG angiography, may allow the delineation of histological characteristics and vascular patterns within the tumor [106]. Noninvasive molecular imaging may allow the expression of cancer genes to be monitored [107]. Minimally invasive fine-needle aspiration biopsy can yield sufficient tumor material for molecular and genetic testing [108]. For example, a small biopsy specimen could be screened using microsatellite markers, gene expression microarray analysis, and other techniques to examine genetic abnormalities known to have prognostic significance [109]. Current metastatic screening with liver function studies and conventional imaging modalities have a relatively low sensitivity for detecting metastasis, but new molecular diagnostic techniques may allow the detection of early micrometastasis at a stage where systemic intervention would be more effective. One such technique utilizes the reverse transcriptase polymerase chain reaction to detect melanocyte-specific genes in patient serum [110].

Effective treatment for metastatic uveal melanoma is one of the most recalcitrant and challenging areas for research. Most experimental approaches focus on immune modulation, such as interferon therapy [86], cytotoxic T-cell immunotherapy [89], and vaccination [111]. In light of animals studies linking angiostatin production by the primary tumor with suppression of metastasis [46], further studies are needed to test the efficacy of angiostatin or other antiangiogenic agents in metastatic disease. Some investigators are searching for molecular characteristics of melanoma cells that account for their profound chemoresistance. Melanoma cells express transport proteins that lead to multidrug resistance by pumping chemotherapeutic agents out of the cell, and expression of these genes has been linked to poor survival [112,113]. Agents that block these proteins could render melanoma cells more sensitive to chemotherapy. Radioresistance in melanoma cells may be may be due in part to defective signaling in the p53 pathway [114], suggesting that reactivation of p53 may render melanomas more radiosensitive. As our molecular understanding of uveal melanoma increases, molecular phenotyping of individual tumors may allow therapy to be individualized for each patient [115].

Looking into the future, a patient diagnosed with a uveal melanoma may undergo a series of noninvasive and/or minimally invasive studies to generate an array of clinical, pathological, and molecular data that indicate the optimal therapy for the intraocular tumor, the risk of metastatic disease, and other prognostic and therapeutic information. The intraocular tumor will then be treated, and prophylactic systemic therapy may be initiated if the metastatic risk is high. Vision loss from plaque radiotherapy may be significantly reduced by the use of adjunctive molecular agents that render the melanoma more radiosensitive, thereby allowing lower radiation doses to be used. The patient subsequently will be screened at regular intervals using sensitive molecular assays for micrometastasis. Metastatic disease will be detected much earlier than by conventional screening, allowing systemic therapy to be more effective. Molecular phenotyping may indicate the optimal of combination of immunotherapy and highly selective molecular agents for systemic treatment.

REFERENCES

1. Egan KM, Seddon JM, Glynn RJ, Gragoudas ES, Albert DM. Epidemiologic aspects of uveal melanoma. Surv Ophthalmol 32:239–251, 1988.
2. Char DH. *Clinical Ocular Oncology*. Philadelphia: Lippincott-Raven, 1997.

3. Ganley JP, Comstock GW. Benign nevi and malignant melanomas of the choroid. Am J Ophthalmol 76:19–25, 1973.
4. de Gruijl FR. Skin cancer and solar UV radiation. Eur J Cancer 35:2003–2009, 1999.
5. Holly EA, Aston DA, Ahn DK, Smith AH. Intraocular melanoma linked to occupations and chemical exposures. Epidemiology 7:55–61, 1996.
6. Margo CE, Mulla Z, Billiris K. Incidence of surgically treated uveal melanoma by race and ethnicity. Ophthalmology 105:1087–1090, 1998.
7. Seddon JM, Gragoudas ES, Glynn RJ, et al. Host factors, UV radiation, and risk of uveal melanoma. A case-control study. Arch Ophthalmol 108:1274–1280, 1990.
8. Tucker MA, Shields JA, Hartge P, et al. Sunlight exposure as risk factor for intraocular malignant melanoma. N Engl J Med 313:789–792, 1985.
9. Gallagher RP, Elwood JM, Rootman J, et al. Risk factors for ocular melanoma: Western Canada Melanoma Study. J Natl Cancer Inst 74:775–778, 1985.
10. Scotto J, Fraumeni JF Jr, Lee JA. Melanomas of the eye and other noncutaneous sites: epidemiologic aspects. J Natl Cancer Inst 56:489–491, 1976.
11. Lutz JM, Cree IA, Foss AJ. Risk factors for intraocular melanoma and occupational exposure. Br J Ophthalmol 83:1190–1193, 1999.
12. Stang A, Anastassiou G, Ahrens W, et al. The possible role of radiofrequency radiation in the development of uveal melanoma. Epidemiology 12:7–12, 2001.
13. Canning CR, Hungerford J. Familial uveal melanoma. Br J Ophthalmol 72:241–243, 1988.
14. Singh AD, Shields CL, De Potter P, et al. Familial uveal melanoma. Clinical observations on 56 patients. Arch Ophthalmol 114:392–399, 1996.
15. Young LH, Egan KM, Walsh SM, Gragoudas ES. Familial uveal melanoma. Am J Ophthalmol 117:516–520, 1994.
16. Singh AD, De Potter P, Fijal BA, et al. Lifetime prevalence of uveal melanoma in white patients with oculo(dermal) melanocytosis. Ophthalmology 105:195–198, 1998.
17. Friend SH, Bernards R, Rogelj S, et al. A human DNA segment with properties of the gene that predisposes to retinoblastoma and osteosarcoma. Nature 323:643–646, 1986.
18. Fung YK, Murphree AL, T'Ang A, et al. Structural evidence for the authenticity of the human retinoblastoma gene. Science 236:1657–1661, 1987.
19. Brantley MA Jr, Harbour JW. Deregulation of the Rb and p53 pathways in uveal melanoma. Am J Pathol 157:1795–1801, 2000.
20. Sisley K, Cottam DW, Rennie IG, et al. Non-random abnormalities of chromosomes 3, 6, and 8 associated with posterior uveal melanoma. Genes Chromosomes Cancer 5:197–200, 1992.
21. Shields JA, Augsburger JJ, Brown GC, Stephens RF. The differential diagnosis of posterior uveal melanoma. Ophthalmology 87:518–522, 1980.
22. Harbour JW, Augsburger JJ, Eagle RC Jr. Initial management and follow-up of melanocytic iris tumors. Ophthalmology 102:1987–1993, 1995.
23. Callanan DG, Lewis ML, Byrne SF, Gass JD. Choroidal neovascularization associated with choroidal nevi. Arch Ophthalmol 111:789–794, 1993.
24. COMS. Factors predictive of growth and treatment of small choroidal melanoma: COMS Report No. 5. The Collaborative Ocular Melanoma Study Group. Arch Ophthalmol 115:1537–1544, 1997.
25. Augsburger JJ, Schroeder RP, Territo C, Gamel JW, Shields JA. Clinical parameters predictive of enlargement of melanocytic choroidal lesions. Br J Ophthalmol 73:911–917, 1989.
26. Butler P, Char DH, Zarbin M, Kroll S. Natural history of indeterminate pigmented choroidal tumors. Ophthalmology 101:710–716, 1994.
27. Pavlin CJ, McWhae JA, McGowan HD, Foster FS. Ultrasound biomicroscopy of anterior segment tumors. Ophthalmology 99:1220–1228, 1992.

28. Meyer K, Augsburger JJ. Independent diagnostic value of fluorescein angiography in the evaluation of intraocular tumors. Graefes Arch Clin Exp Ophthalmol 237:489–494, 1999.

29. Arevalo JF, Shields CL, Shields JA, Hykin PG, De Potter P. Circumscribed choroidal hemangioma: Characteristic features with indocyanine green videoangiography. Ophthalmology 107:344–350, 2000.

30. Mihara F, Gupta KL, Joslyn JN, Haik BG. Intraocular hemorrhage and mimicking lesions: Role of gradient-echo and contrast-enhanced MRI. Clin Imaging 17:171–175, 1993.

31. De Potter P, Flanders AE, Shields JA, et al. The role of fat-suppression technique and gadopentetate dimeglumine in magnetic resonance imaging evaluation of intraocular tumors and simulating lesions. Arch Ophthalmol 112:340–348, 1994.

32. COMS. Histopathologic characteristics of uveal melanomas in eyes enucleated from the Collaborative Ocular Melanoma Study. COMS report no. 6. Am J Ophthalmol 125:745–766, 1998.

33. Augsburger JJ, Shields JA, Folberg R, et al. Fine needle aspiration biopsy in the diagnosis of intraocular cancer. Cytologic-histologic correlations. Ophthalmology 92:39–49, 1985.

34. Shields JA, Shields CL, Ehya H, Eagle RJ, De PP. Fine-needle aspiration biopsy of suspected intraocular tumors. The 1992 Urwick Lecture. Ophthalmology 100:1677–1684, 1993.

35. Diener-West M, Hawkins BS, Markowitz JA, Schachat AP. A review of mortality from choroidal melanoma. II. A meta-analysis of 5-year mortality rates following enucleation, 1966 through 1988. Arch Ophthalmol 110:245–250, 1992.

36. Donoso LA, Augsburger JJ, Shields JA, Greenberg RA, Gamel J. Metastatic uveal melanoma. Correlation between survival time and cytomorphometry of primary tumors. Arch Ophthalmol 104:76–78, 1986.

37. Seregard S. Long-term survival after ruthenium plaque radiotherapy for uveal melanoma. A meta-analysis of studies including 1,066 patients. Acta Ophthalmol Scand 77:414–417, 1999.

38. Harbour JW, Char DH, Kroll S, Quivey JM, Castro J. Metastatic risk for distinct patterns of postirradiation local recurrence of posterior uveal melanoma. Ophthalmology 104:1785–1792, 1997.

39. Kenneally CZ, Farber MG, Smith ME, Devineni R. In vitro melanoma cell growth after preenucleation radiation therapy. Arch Ophthalmol 106:223–224, 1988.

40. Rousseau AP, Deschenes J, Pelletier G, Tremblay M, Larochelle-Belland M. Effect of pre-enucleation radiotherapy on the viability of human choroidal melanoma cells. Can J Ophthalmol 24:10–14, 1989.

41. COMS. The Collaborative Ocular Melanoma Study (COMS) randomized trial of pre-enucleation radiation of large choroidal melanoma II: Initial mortality findings. COMS report no. 10. Am J Ophthalmol 125:779–796, 1998.

42. Augsburger JJ, Lauritzen K, Gamel JW, Lowry JC, Brady LW. Matched group study of preenucleation radiotherapy versus enucleation alone for primary malignant melanoma of the choroid and ciliary body. Am J Clin Oncol 13:382–387, 1990.

43. Char DH, Phillips TL, Andejeski Y, Crawford JB, Kroll S. Failure of preenucleation radiation to decrease uveal melanoma mortality. Am J Ophthalmol 106:21–26, 1988.

44. Zimmerman LE, McLean IW, Foster WD. Does enucleation of the eye containing a malignant melanoma prevent or accelerate the dissemination of tumour cells. Br J Ophthalmol 62:420–425, 1978.

45. O'Reilly MS, Holmgren L, Shing Y, et al. Angiostatin: A novel angiogenesis inhibitor that mediates the suppression of metastases by a Lewis lung carcinoma. Cell 79:315–328, 1994.

46. Apte RS, Niederkorn JY, Mayhew E, Alizadeh H. Angiostatin produced by certain primary uveal melanoma cell lines impedes the development of liver metastases. Arch Ophthalmol 119:1805–1809, 2001.

47. Robertson DM, Earle J, Anderson JA. Preliminary observations regarding the use of iodine-125 in the management of choroidal melanoma. Trans Ophthalmol Soc UK 103:155–160, 1983.

48. Lommatzsch PK, Werschnik C, Schuster E. Long-term follow-up of Ru-106/Rh-106 brachytherapy for posterior uveal melanoma. Graefes Arch Clin Exp Ophthalmol 238:129–137, 2000.

49. Finger PT, Berson A, Szechter A. Palladium-103 plaque radiotherapy for choroidal melanoma: Results of a 7-year study. Ophthalmology 106:606–613, 1999.

50. Diener-West M, Earle JD, Fine SL, et al. The COMS randomized trial of iodine 125 brachytherapy for choroidal melanoma, III: Initial mortality findings. COMS Report No. 18. Arch Ophthalmol 119:969–982, 2001.

51. Augsburger JJ, Schneider S, Freire J, Brady LW. Survival following enucleation versus plaque radiotherapy in statistically matched subgroups of patients with choroidal melanomas: Results in patients treated between 1980 and 1987. Graefes Arch Clin Exp Ophthalmol 237:558–567, 1999.

52. Cruickshanks KJ, Fryback DG, Nondahl DM, et al. Treatment choice and quality of life in patients with choroidal melanoma. Arch Ophthalmol 117:461–467, 1999.

53. De Potter P, Shields CL, Shields JA, Cater JR, Brady LW. Plaque radiotherapy for juxtapapillary choroidal melanoma. Visual acuity and survival outcome. Arch Ophthalmol 114:1357–1365, 1996.

54. Harbour JW, Murray TG, Byrne SF, et al. Intraoperative echographic localization of iodine 125 episcleral radioactive plaques for posterior uveal melanoma. Retina 16:129–134, 1996.

55. Oosterhuis JA, Journee-de Korver HG, Keunen JE. Transpupillary thermotherapy: Results in 50 patients with choroidal melanoma. Arch Ophthalmol 116:157–162, 1998.

56. Tabandeh H, Chaudhry NA, Murray TG, et al. Intraoperative echographic localization of iodine-125 episcleral plaque for brachytherapy of choroidal melanoma. Am J Ophthalmol 129:199–204, 2000.

57. Finger PT. Plaque radiation therapy for malignant melanoma of the iris and ciliary body. Am J Ophthalmol 132:328–335, 2001.

58. Shields CL, Shields JA, De Potter P, et al. Treatment of non-resectable malignant iris tumours with custom designed plaque radiotherapy. Br J Ophthalmol 79:306–312, 1995.

59. Gragoudas ES, Egan KM, Seddon JM, Walsh SM, Munzenrider JE. Intraocular recurrence of uveal melanoma after proton beam irradiation. Ophthalmology 99:760–766, 1992.

60. Vrabec TR, Augsburger JJ, Gamel JW, et al. Impact of local tumor relapse on patient survival after cobalt 60 plaque radiotherapy. Ophthalmology 98:984–988, 1991.

61. Parsons JT, Bova FJ, Mendenhall WM, Million RR, Fitzgerald CR. Response of the normal eye to high dose radiotherapy. Oncology (Huntingt) 10:837–847, 1996.

62. Char DH, Quivey JM, Castro JR, Kroll S, Phillips T. Helium ions versus iodine 125 brachytherapy in the management of uveal melanoma. A prospective, randomized, dynamically balanced trial. Ophthalmology 100:1547–1554, 1993.

63. Karlsson UL, Augsburger JJ, Shields JA, et al. Recurrence of posterior uveal melanoma after ^{60}Co episcleral plaque therapy. Ophthalmology 96:382–388, 1989.

64. Packer S, Stoller S, Lesser ML, Mandel FS, Finger PT. Long-term results of iodine 125 irradiation of uveal melanoma. Ophthalmology 99:767–773, 1992.

65. Mueller AJ, Talies S, Schaller UC, et al. Stereotactic radiosurgery of large uveal melanomas with the gamma-knife. Ophthalmology 107:1381–1387, 2000.

66. Williams DF, Mieler WF, Lewandowski M, Greenberg M. Echographic verification of radioactive plaque position in the treatment of melanomas. Arch Ophthalmol 106:1623–1624, 1988.

67. Char DH, Miller T, Crawford JB. Uveal tumour resection. Br J Ophthalmol 85:1213–1219, 2001.

68. Foulds WS, Damato BE, Burton RL. Local resection versus enucleation in the management of choroidal melanoma. Eye 1:676–679, 1987.

69. Damato B. *Ocular Tumors: Diagnosis and Treatment.* Oxford, UK: Butterworth-Heinemann, 2000.

70. Augsburger JJ, Lauritzen K, Gamel JW, et al. Matched group study of surgical resection versus cobalt-60 plaque radiotherapy for primary choroidal or ciliary body melanoma. Ophthalm Surg 21:682–688, 1990.

71. Leeper D. *Molecular and Cellular Mechanism of Hyperthermia Alone or Combined with Other Modalities.* Overgaard J, ed. London: Taylor & Francis, 1985.

72. Coleman DJ, Lizzi FL, Burgess SE, et al. Ultrasonic hyperthermia and radiation in the management of intraocular malignant melanoma. Am J Ophthalmol 101:635–642, 1986.

73. Liggett PE, Ma C, Astrahan M, et al. Combined localized current field hyperthermia and irradiation for intracular tumors. Ophthalmology 98:1830–1835, 1991.

74. Mieler WF, Jaffe GJ, Steeves RA. Ferromagnetic hyperthermia and iodine 125 brachytherapy in the treatment of choroidal melanoma in a rabbit model. Arch Ophthalmol 107:1524–1528, 1989.

75. Swift PS, Stauffer PR, Fries PD, et al. Microwave hyperthermia for choroidal melanoma in rabbits. Invest Ophthalmol Vis Sci 31:1754–1760, 1990.

76. Oosterhuis JA, Journee-de Korver HG, Kakebeeke-Kemme HM, Bleeker JC. Transpupillary thermotherapy in choroidal melanomas. Arch Ophthalmol 113:315–321, 1995.

77. Godfrey DG, Waldron RG, Capone A Jr. Transpupillary thermotherapy for small choroidal melanoma. Am J Ophthalmol 128:88–93, 1999.

78. Robertson DM, Buettner H, Bennett SR. Transpupillary thermotherapy as primary treatment for small choroidal melanomas. Arch Ophthalmol 117:1512–1519, 1999.

79. Shields CL, Shields JA, Cater J, et al. Transpupillary thermotherapy for choroidal melanoma: Tumor control and visual results in 100 consecutive cases. Ophthalmology 105:581–590, 1998.

80. Augsburger JJ, Mullen D, Kleineidam M. Planned combined I-125 plaque irradiation and indirect ophthalmoscope laser therapy for choroidal malignant melanoma. Ophthalm Surg 24:76–81, 1993.

81. COMS. Assessment of metastatic disease status at death in 435 patients with large choroidal melanoma in the Collaborative Ocular Melanoma Study (COMS): COMS report no. 15. Arch Ophthalmol 119:670–676, 2001.

82. Kath R, Hayungs J, Bornfeld N, et al. Prognosis and treatment of disseminated uveal melanoma. Cancer 72:2219–2223, 1993.

83. Gragoudas ES, Egan KM, Seddon JM, et al. Survival of patients with metastases from uveal melanoma. Ophthalmology 98:383–389, 1991.

84. Eskelin S, Pyrhonen S, Summanen P, Hahka-Kemppinen M, Kivela T. Tumor doubling times in metastatic malignant melanoma of the uvea: tumor progression before and after treatment. Ophthalmology 107:1443–1449, 2000.

85. Aoyama T, Mastrangelo MJ, Berd D et al. Protracted survival after resection of metastatic uveal melanoma. Cancer 89:1561–1568, 2000.

86. Dithmar S, Rusciano D, Lynn MJ, et al. Neoadjuvant interferon alfa-2b treatment in a murine model for metastatic ocular melanoma: A preliminary study. Arch Ophthalmol 118:1085–1089, 2000.

87. Egerer G, Lehnert T, Max R, et al. Pilot study of hepatic intraarterial fotemustine chemotherapy for liver metastases from uveal melanoma: A single-center experience with seven patients. Int J Clin Oncol 6:25–28, 2001.
88. Fournier GA, Albert DM, Arrigg CA, et al. Resection of solitary metastasis. Approach to palliative treatment of hepatic involvement with choroidal melanoma. Arch Ophthalmol 102:80–82, 1984.
89. Sutmuller RP, Schurmans LR, van Duivenvoorde LM, et al. Adoptive T cell immunotherapy of human uveal melanoma targeting gp100. J Immunol 165:7308–7315, 2000.
90. Woll E, Bedikian A, Legha SS. Uveal melanoma: Natural history and treatment options for metastatic disease. Melanoma Res 9:575–581, 1999.
91. Augsburger JJ, Gamel JW. Clinical prognostic factors in patients with posterior uveal malignant melanoma. Cancer 66:1596–1600, 1990.
92. McLean IW, Foster WD, Zimmerman LE. Prognostic factors in small malignant melanomas of choroid and ciliary body. Arch Ophthalmol 95:48–58, 1977.
93. Nowakowski VA, Ivery G, Castro JR, et al. Uveal melanoma: Development of metastases after helium ion irradiation. Radiology 178:277–280, 1991.
94. Sato T, Babazono A, Shields JA, et al. Time to systemic metastases in patients with posterior uveal melanoma. Cancer Invest 15:98–105, 1997.
95. Seddon JM, Albert DM, Lavin PT, Robinson N. A prognostic factor study of disease-free interval and survival following enucleation for uveal melanoma. Arch Ophthalmol 101:1894–1899, 1983.
96. Folberg R, Pe'er J, Gruman LM, et al. The morphologic characteristics of tumor blood vessels as a marker of tumor progression in primary human uveal melanoma: A matched case-control study. Hum Pathol 23:1298–1305, 1992.
97. Gamel JW, McLean IW, Foster WD, Zimmerman LE. Uveal melanomas: Correlation of cytologic features with prognosis. Cancer 41:1897–1901, 1978.
98. Seddon JM, Polivogianis L, Hsieh CC, et al. Death from uveal melanoma. Number of epithelioid cells and inverse SD of nucleolar area as prognostic factors. Arch Ophthalmol 105:801–806, 1987.
99. Aalto Y, Eriksson L, Seregard S, Larsson O, Knuutila S. Concomitant loss of chromosome 3 and whole arm losses and gains of chromosome 1, 6, or 8 in metastasizing primary uveal melanoma. Invest Ophthalmol Vis Sci 42:313–317, 2001.
100. Prescher G, Bornfeld N, Hirche H, et al. Prognostic implications of monosomy 3 in uveal melanoma. Lancet 347:1222–1225, 1996.
101. Sisley K, Rennie IG, Parsons MA, et al. Abnormalities of chromosomes 3 and 8 in posterior uveal melanoma correlate with prognosis. Genes Chromosomes Cancer 19:22–28, 1997.
102. White VA, Chambers JD, Courtright PD, Chang WY, Horsman DE. Correlation of cytogenetic abnormalities with the outcome of patients with uveal melanoma. Cancer 83:354–359, 1998.
103. Hawkins BS, Schachat AP. *Collaborative Ocular Melanoma Study*. Ryan SJ, ed. St. Louis: Mosby, 2001.
104. Augsburger JJ, Vrabec TR. Impact of delayed treatment in growing posterior uveal melanomas. Arch Ophthalmol 111:1382–1386, 1993.
105. Shields GL, Shields JA, Kiratli H, De Potter P, Cater JR. Risk factors for growth and metastasis of small choroidal melanocytic lesions. Ophthalmology 102:1351–1361, 1995.
106. Mueller AJ, Folberg R, Freeman WR, et al. Evaluation of the human choroidal melanoma rabbit model for studying microcirculation patterns with confocal ICG and histology. Exp Eye Res 68:671–678, 1999.
107. Larson SM. Molecular imaging in oncology: The diagnostic imaging "revolution." Clin Cancer Res 6:2125, 2000.

108. Sisley K, Nichols C, Parsons MA, et al. Clinical applications of chromosome analysis, from fine needle aspiration biopsies, of posterior uveal melanomas. Eye 12:203–207, 1998.

109. Parrella P, Sidransky D, Merbs SL. Allelotype of posterior uveal melanoma: implications for a bifurcated tumor progression pathway. Cancer Res 59:3032–3037, 1999.

110. Tobal K, Sherman LS, Foss AJ, Lightman SL. Detection of melanocytes from uveal melanoma in peripheral blood using the polymerase chain reaction. Invest Ophthalmol Vis Sci 34:2622–2625, 1993.

111. Berd D, Sato T, Cohn H, Maguire HC Jr, Mastrangelo MJ. Treatment of metastatic melanoma with autologous, hapten-modified melanoma vaccine: regression of pulmonary metastases. Int J Cancer 94:531–539, 2001.

112. Berger W, Hauptmann E, Elbling L, et al. Possible role of the multidrug resistance-associated protein (MRP) in chemoresistance of human melanoma cells. Int J Cancer 71:108–115, 1997.

113. Dunne BM, McNamara M, Clynes M, et al. MDR1 expression is associated with adverse survival in melanoma of the uveal tract. Hum Pathol 29:594–598, 1998.

114. Satyamoorthy K, Chehab NH, Waterman MJ, et al. Aberrant regulation and function of wild-type p53 in radioresistant melanoma cells. Cell Growth Differ 11:467–474, 2000.

115. Satherley K, de Souza L, Neale MH, et al. Relationship between expression of topoisomerase II isoforms and chemosensitivity in choroidal melanoma. J Pathol 192:174–181, 2000.

2

Clinical Overview: Retinoblastoma

JERRY A. SHIELDS and CAROL L. SHIELDS

Wills Eye Hospital and Thomas Jefferson University, Philadelphia, Pennsylvania, U.S.A.

Retinoblastoma is the most common and most important malignant intraocular tumor of childhood. It is important for the ophthalmologist to make a prompt and accurate diagnosis and to refer the patient to an ocular oncologist and/or other specialists for appropriate treatment. This chapter considers general aspects and clinical features of retinoblastoma. For completeness, it briefly alludes to pathology and management of retinoblastoma, but these are discussed in greater detail in other chapters. The subject of retinoblastoma is also covered in more detail in the authors' textbooks on the subject of intraocular tumors [1–3].

I. GENERAL CONSIDERATIONS

Retinoblastoma is second to uveal melanoma as the most common primary intraocular malignancy in humans. In parts of the world where uveal melanoma is rare, such as Africa and Asia, retinoblastoma is the most common primary malignant intraocular tumor. Although estimates vary, it occurs with a frequency of approximately 1 in 15,000 to 1 in 23,000 live births [4]. Approximately 6% of newly diagnosed retinoblastoma cases are familial and 94% are sporadic. All patients with familial retinoblastoma are at risk to pass the predisposition for the development of the tumor to their offspring. The details of the genetics of retinoblastoma are discussed in Chap. 3.

There is no apparent predisposition of retinoblastoma for race or sex and no predilection for the right or left eye. The tumor occurs bilaterally in 25–35% of cases. In the multicentric or bilateral cases, the average number of tumors per eye is five, with a random distribution between the two eyes. The tumor is diagnosed at an average age of 18 months, with the bilateral cases being recognized at an average age of about 12 months and the unilateral cases at 23 months. In rare instances, the tumor is first recognized at birth, in the teens, or even in adulthood [1,5].

II. CLINICAL FEATURES

The clinical features of retinoblastoma vary with the stage of the disease at the time of diagnosis.

A. Early Signs

1. Strabismus

When retinoblastoma arises in the foveal region, it can cause loss of central fixation, which can lead to strabismus, either exotropia or esotropia. Although most children with strabismus do not have retinoblastoma, it is important that every child with this finding have a comprehensive fundus examination to exclude the possibility of retinoblastoma or other organic cause for visual loss [1].

2. Leukocoria

As retinoblastoma grows, it eventually causes leukocoria (white pupillary reflex). When the tumor is small, the leukocoria may be apparent only in certain fields of gaze. When the tumor is large enough to fill more than one-third of the globe, the white reflex becomes apparent in all fields of gaze (Fig. 1) [1].

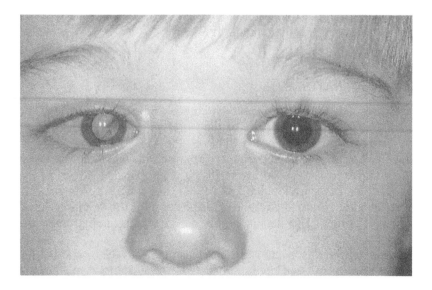

Figure 1   Leukocoria in a child with retinoblastoma.

B. Growth Patterns

1.   Intraretinal Lesions

Retinoblastoma begins as a transparent lesion in the sensory retina. As it enlarges, it becomes opaque white (Fig. 2). With further tumor enlargement, dilated tortuous retinal arteries and veins develop to supply and drain the tumor (Fig. 3). Some untreated retinoblastomas show foci of chalk-like calcification that has been likened to cottage cheese (Fig. 4). More characteristically, retinoblastoma is larger at the time of presentation and it assumes either an endophytic or an exophytic growth pattern. Such larger tumors almost always cause leukocoria.

2.   Endophytic Growth Pattern

Some retinoblastomas are associated with seeding of tumor cells into the overlying vitreous. Such an endophytic growth pattern is characterized by a white hazy mass over which no retinal vessels can be visualized (Fig. 5). Because of their friable nature, endophytic tumors can eventually seed the entire vitreous cavity and simulate endophthalmitis. An endophytic retinoblastoma can also seed into the anterior chamber and produce multiple nodules at the pupillary margin. With time, the cells may settle into the inferior portion of the anterior chamber angle and resemble a hypopyon [1].

3.   Exophyic Growth Pattern

An exophytic retinoblastoma is one that grows from the retina outward into the subretinal space. In contrast to an endophytic tumor, the retinal vessels are apparent with ophthalmoscopy. Such tumors produce a progressive retinal detachment, with the retina often displaced anteriorly behind the clear lens and a white mass

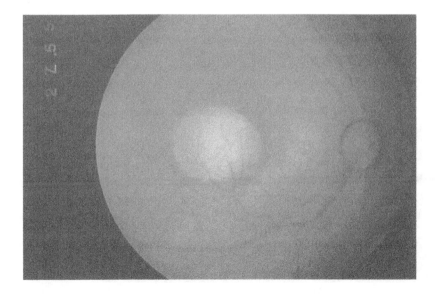

Figure 2   Small retinoblastoma showing white color of tumor.

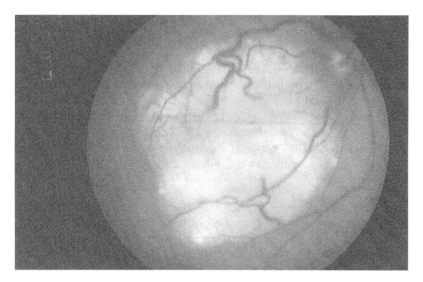

Figure 3 Retinoblastoma with dilated, tortuous retinal blood vessels.

immediately behind the detached retina (Fig. 6). An exophytic retinoblastoma can clinically resemble Coats disease or other forms of exudative retinal detachment [1].

4. Diffuse Infiltrating Growth Pattern

Diffuse infiltrating retinoblastoma is a less common form of retinoblastoma, characterized by a relatively flat infiltration of the retina by tumor cells [6,7]. Because an obvious mass is not present, there is often a delay in diagnosis and sometimes

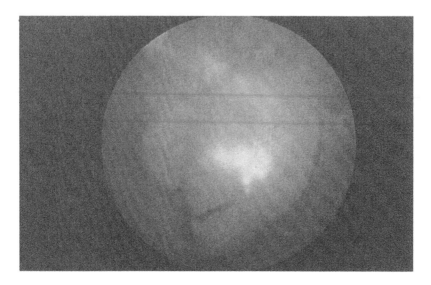

Figure 4 Retinoblastoma with foci of calcification.

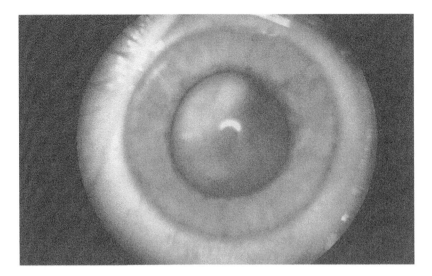

Figure 5 Endophytic retinoblastoma.

misdirected intraocular surgery [8]. Therefore, diffuse retinoblastoma is usually recognized clinically at an older age than typical cases of retinoblastoma. These lesions frequently produce vitreous and anterior chamber seeding, which may cause diagnostic confusion with intraocular inflammation (Fig. 7). Fortunately, almost all reported cases of diffuse infiltrating retinoblastoma have been unilateral sporadic cases with a negative family history. Because of the extensive intraocular seeding in most instances, enucleation has been considered to be the best management.

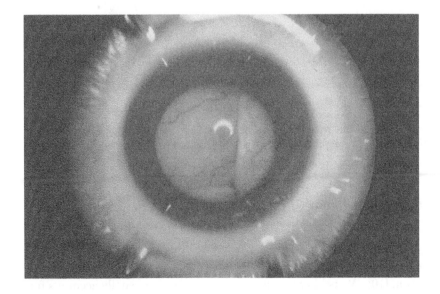

Figure 6 Exophytic retinoblastoma.

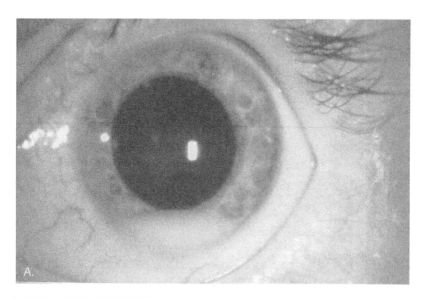

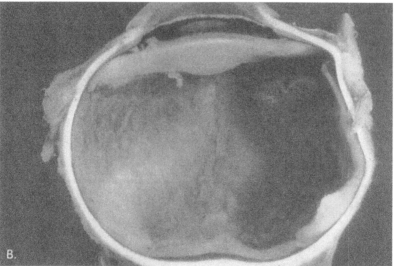

Figure 7 Spontaneous pseudohypopyon secondary to diffuse infiltrating retinoblastoma. A. Anterior segment, showing white pseudohypopyon. B. Section of enucleated eye through main calotte, showing flat diffuse retinoblastoma with not elevated mass and no calcification.

C. Advanced Presentations

1. Neovascular Glaucoma

Iris neovascularization (rubeosis iridis) occurs in 17% of all children with retinoblastoma [9] and in about 50% of eyes with advanced retinoblastoma that require enucleation [10]. We believe that iris neovascularization usually accounts for the acquired heterochromia iridis that characterizes some cases of retinoblastoma.

Any infant with unexplained acquired heterochromia should be evaluated for possible retinoblastoma. Spontaneous bleeding form these vessels may cause a hyphema [11].

2. Orbital Cellulitis

Some necrotic retinoblastomas produce severe secondary periocular inflammation, resulting in a clinical appearance of preseptal cellulitis or endophthalmitis [12,13]. Computed tomography (CT) in such cases can reveal a large calcified intraocular mass with periocular soft tissue density suggesting extraocular extension of retinoblastoma.. However, these advanced cases usually do not have evidence of extraocular extension after enucleation of the affected eye. The periocular inflammation seen with appears to be secondary to necrosis within the tumor and not secondary to extraocular extension of the tumor.

3. Extraocular Extension

Although some retinoblastomas can exhibit extension into the optic nerve, it is usually a microscopic observation found on histopathological study of the eye following enucleation. However, it neglected cases, or when the parents or guardians refuse treatment, the tumor can eventually break out of the eye and exhibit massive orbital and extraorbital extension (Fig. 8). Such an advanced presentation is rare in countries with advanced medical care, but it is common in third-world countries where advanced medical care is not readily available.

D. Other Clinical Variations

1. Trilateral Retinoblastoma

In recent years it has been recognized that some children with the familial form of retinoblastoma can also develop a pinealoblastoma [14,15]. The pineal tumor has many similarities to retinoblastoma from embryological, pathological, and immunological standpoints. The pineal tumor is best detected with high quality CT or magnetic resonance imaging (MRI). The prognosis for life is guarded. Most children who die from retinoblastoma have some degree of intracranial involvement, usually secondary to direct spread through the optic nerve or subarachnoid space. It is quite likely that some earlier reported cases of presumed brain metastasis probably represented pinealoblastoma or other parasellar neoplasms ("trilateral retinoblastoma") that were misdiagnosed as metastatic retinoblastoma before the entity of trilateral retinoblastoma was recognized.

2. Retinocytoma

Recent evidence has accumulated to support the existence of an uncommon benign variant of retinoblastoma that has been termed *retinoma* [16] or *retinocytoma* [17]. We believe that the term *retinoma* is too general, since it could be interpreted to mean any tumor of the retina. Although no terminology is perfect, there is a stronger argument for using either the term *retinocytoma* or *spontaneously arrested retinoblastoma* to define this condition [1]. A retinocytoma carries the same genetic implications as an active retinoblastoma [16].

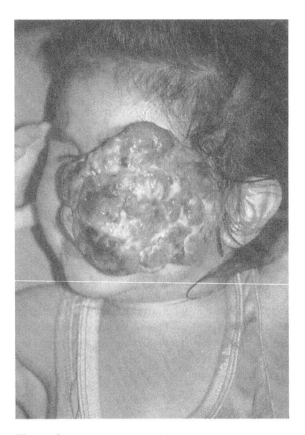

Figure 8   Advanced retinoblastoma with massive extraocular extension.

3. Spontaneously Regressed Retinoblastoma

Complete spontaneous necrosis leading to regression and a "cure" is a well-known phenomenon that is said to occur more frequently in neuroblastoma and retinoblastoma than with other malignant neoplasms [1]. It is characterized by a severe inflammatory reaction in the eye, sometimes followed by the development of phthisis bulbi. In cases of spontaneous regression of a smaller retinoblastoma, the eye may retain useful vision. (Fig. 9) It is not certain whether such tumor regression occurs secondary to vascular ischemia to the tumor or whether more complex immunopathologic mechanisms play a role. In any child with a phthisical eye of uncertain cause, the diagnosis of spontaneously regressed retinoblastoma should be considered. Spontaneously regressed retinoblastoma carries the same genetic implications as an active retinoblastoma.

III. DIFFERENTIAL DIAGNOSIS

There are a number of conditions that can simulate retinoblastoma, either by causing a small white fundus lesion or by producing leukocoria. In a series of 500 consecutive

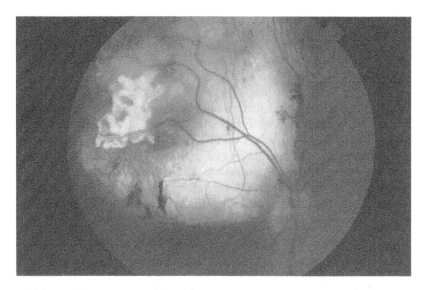

Figure 9 Spontaneously regressed retinoblastoma in an eye with useful vision. The margin of the regressed tumor barely spares the foveola.

patients referred with the diagnosis of possible retinoblastoma, 288 proved on subsequent evaluation to have retinoblastoma and 212 proved to have simulating lesions [18–20].

A. Other Intraocular Tumors

Other tumors are known to sometime simulate retinoblastomas. These include astrocytic hamartoma, medulloepithelioma, combined hamartoma, retinal capillary hemangioma, and sometimes amelanotic choroidal melanoma [18–20].

B. Other Nontumorous Conditions

In the above series, the conditions most often referred for suspected retinoblastoma were persistent hyperplastic primary vitreous (28%) Coats disease (16%) [21], and ocular toxocariasis (16%) [22]. Other nonneoplastic conditions included retinopathy of prematurity, retinopathy of prematurity, dominant exudative vitreoretinopathy, endogenous endophthalmitis, congenital cataract, congenital toxoplasmosis, chorioretinal coloboma, myelinated nerve fibers, and scar tissue secondary to surgical trauma [18–20].

IV. DIAGNOSTIC APPROACHES

A patient with suspected retinoblastoma should have a detailed history taken and receive general medical evaluation, external ocular examination, slit-lamp biomicroscopy, and indirect ophthalmoscopy to substantiate the diagnosis. In addition, certain ancillary studies—such as fluorescein angiography, ultrasonography, CT, and MRI—can assist in the diagnosis.

A. Fluorescein Angiography

Fluorescein angiography can provide diagnostic and therapeutic information in selected children with discreet retinoblastoma [3,24]. Very small intraretinal tumors show only minimally dilated feeding vessels in the arterial phase, mild hypervascularity in the venous phase, and mild late staining of the mass (Fig. 10). Slightly larger intraretinal tumors show more intense hypervascularity and late staining. Moderate-sized tumors usually demonstrate markedly dilated feeding arteries and draining veins. Such tumors also show numerous fine capillary ramifications on the tumor surface.

B. Ultrasonography

Retinoblastomas have ultrasonographic features that usually help to differentiate them from the pseudoretinoblastomas [3]. A-scan typically shows constant high internal echoes within the tumor and rapid attenuation of the normal orbital pattern. There is frequently an anechoic area in the basal portion of the tumor nearest the sclera. B-scan ultrasonography characteristically shows a rounded or irregular intraocular mass with numerous highly reflective echoes within the lesion. A characteristic feature of B scan is attenuation or absence of the normal soft tissue echoes in the orbit directly behind the tumor (Fig. 11). This occurs as a result of

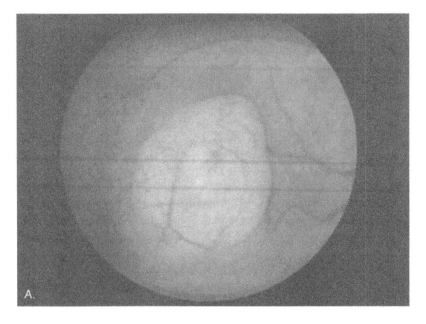

Figure 10 Fluorescein angiography of retinoblastoma. A. Clinical appearance of tumor. B. Arterial phase, showing two feeding arteries. C. Late angiogram showing continued hyperfluorescence of the mass.

attenuation and reflection of the sound by the calcification within the mass. These reflective focal echoes within the tumor persist after the soft tissues echoes of the eye have disappeared when the sensitivity of the ultrasound machine is lowered. Ultrasonography can be used to document tumor regression following radiotherapy.

C. Computed Tomography

Although both ultrasonography and CT can detect calcium in retinoblastoma, CT has the advantage over ultrasound in that it is better able to delineate extraocular

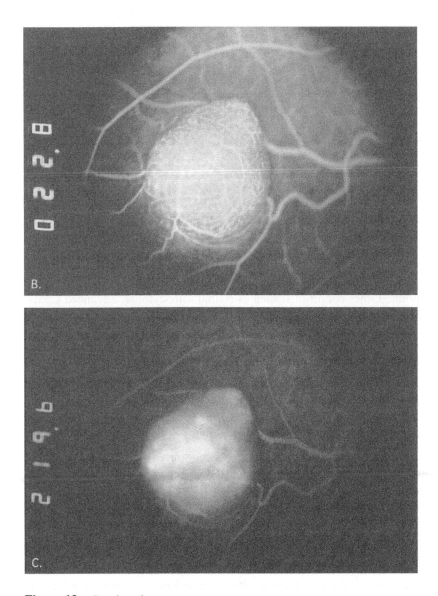

Figure 10 Continued.

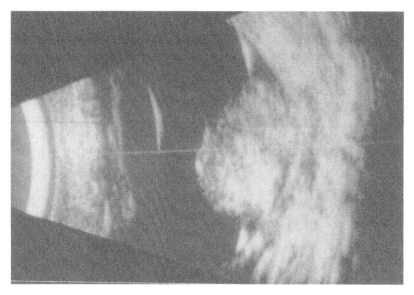

Figure 11   B-scan ultrasonography of retinoblastoma showing mass with calcification.

extension of tumor and to detect the presence of an associated pinealoblastoma (trilateral retinoblastoma).

With CT, retinoblastoma typically appears as an intraocular mass with foci of calcification within the tumor in greater than 80% of tumors [3] (Fig. 12). The presence of intraocular calcification with CT is suggestive of retinoblastoma but is not pathognomonic. Other conditions, such as retinal astrocytoma, advanced Coats disease, retinal angiomatosis, and ocular toxocariasis, can occasionally produce intraocular calcification or even ossification that can lead to misdiagnosis with ultrasonography or CT. Therefore, all of the clinical findings should be taken into account in making the diagnosis of retinoblastoma.

D. Magnetic Resonance Imaging

MRI may be of some diagnostic assistance in the evaluation of a child with suspected retinoblastoma [25]. A retinoblastoma is moderately hyperintense to vitreous on T1 weighted images and becomes hypointense in T2-weighted images. Areas of calcification are often accentuated on T2-weighted images. Some authorities have reported that associated hemorrhage and exudation appears markedly different from retinoblastoma tissue on T2-weighted images. Thus, MRI has potential value in evaluating patients prior to treatment and in monitoring their response to therapy by helping to differentiate between active tumor, hemorrhage, and exudation. However, more studies will be necessary to determine the value and limitations of MRI in the evaluation of children with suspected retinoblastoma.

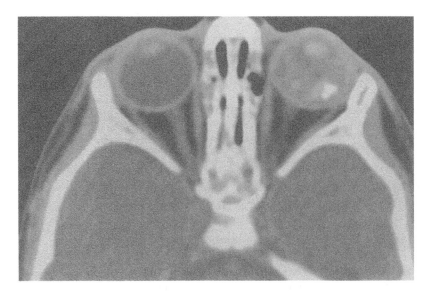

Figure 12 Computed tomography of retinoblastoma showing calcified intraocular mass.

V. PATHOLOGY

In most cases, retinoblastoma can be readily recognized in the sectioned eye by its typical appearance (Fig. 13). It is a chalky white, friable tumor with dense foci of calcification. An endophytic retinoblastoma usually produces seeding into the vitreous cavity An exophytic tumor tends to push the retina anteriorly and to occupy the subretinal space. Some tumors have both endophytic and exophytic components and others appear to be totally calcified as a result of marked necrosis [1]. The histopathological features of retinoblastoma are discussed in Chap. 9.

VI. MANAGEMENT

The management of retinoblastoma can be complex, and it is impossible to establish firm rules regarding treatment [26,27]. Each case must be individualized according to the entire clinical situation. Proper management necessitates the ability to use the various instruments, familiarity with the disease, and above all, experience in dealing with such problems [4]. There are several options available for the treatment of retinoblastoma, and the method selected should depend on the size and extent of the tumor(s), whether there is unilateral or bilateral involvement, and the patient's systemic status. The methods that we currently advocate include enucleation, external-beam irradiation, scleral plaque irradiation, photocoagulation, cryotherapy, chemotherapy, chemothermotherapy, and chemoreduction. In many cases it may be necessary to employ various combinations of treatment to achieve a satisfactory result [26–44]. These therapeutic modalities are considered in more detail in Chap. 8.

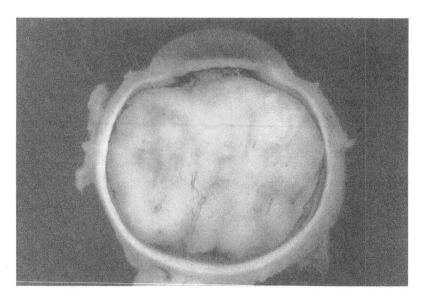

Figure 13 Grossly sectioned eye showing white retinoblastoma filling the interior of the eye. The massive white tumor correlates with the leukocoria seen clinically.

REFERENCES

1. Shields JA, Shields CL. Retinoblastoma: Clinical and pathologic features. In: Shields JA, Shields CL, eds. Intraocular Tumors. A Text and Atlas. Philadelphia: Saunders, 1992, pp 305–332.
2. Shields JA, Shields CL. Diagnostic approaches to retinoblastoma. In: Shields JA, Shields CL, eds. Intraocular Tumors. A Text and Atlas. Philadelphia: Saunders, 1992, pp 363–376.
3. Shields JA, Shields CL. Management and prognosis of retinoblastoma. In Shields JA, Shields CL, eds. Intraocular Tumors. A Text and Atlas. Philadelphia: Saunders, 1992, pp 377–391.
4. Saunders BM, Draper GJ, Kingston JE. Retinoblastoma in Great Britain 1969–1980, Br J Ophthalmol 72:576–583, 1988.
5. Shields CL, Shields JA, Shah P. Retinoblastoma in older children. Ophthalmology 98:395–399, 1991.
6. Nicholson DH, Norton EW. Diffuse infiltrating retinoblastoma. Trans Am Ophthalmol Soc 78:265–289, 1980.
7. Shields JA, Shields CL, Eagle RC, Blair CJ. Spontaneous pseudohypopyon secondary to diffuse infiltrating retinoblastoma. Arch Ophthalmol 106:1301–1302, 1988.
8. Shields CL, Honavar S, Shields JA, Demirci H, Meadows AT. Vitrectomy in eyes with unsuspected retinoblastoma. Ophthalmology 107:2250–2255, 2000.
9. Shields CL, Shields JA, Shields MB, et al. Prevalence and mechanisms of secondary intraocular pressure elevation in eyes with intraocular tumors. Ophthalmology 94:839–846, 1987.
10. Walton DS, Grant WM. Retinoblastoma and iris neovascularization. Am J Ophthalmol 65:598–599, 1968.

11. Shields JA, Shields CL, Materin M. Diffuse infiltrating retinoblastoma presenting as a total hyphema. J Ped Ophthalmol Strabism 37:311–312, 2000. Manifesting as orbital cellulitis. Am J Ophthalmol 112:442–449, 1991.

12. Stafford WR, Yanoff M, Parnell B. Retinoblastoma initially misdiagnosed as primary ocular inflammation. Arch Ophthalmol 82:771–773, 1969.

13. Shields JA, Shields CL, Suvarnamani C, Schroeder RP, DePotter P. Retinoblastoma manifesting as orbital cellulitis. Am J Ophthalmol 112:442–449, 1991.

14. Zimmerman LE, Burns RP, Wankum G, et al. Trilateral retinoblastoma: Ectopic intracranial retinoblastoma associated with bilateral retilnoblastoma. J Pediatr Ophthalmol Strab 19:310–315, 1982.

15. De Potter P, Shields CL, Shields JA. Clinical variations of trilateral retinoblastoma. A report of 13 cases. J Pediatr Ophthalmol Strabismus 31:26–31, 1994.

16. Gallie BL, Ellsworth RM, Abramson DH, Phillips RA. Retinoma: Spontaneous regression of retinoblastoma or benign manifestation of a mutation? Br J Cancer 45:513–521, 1982.

17. Margo C, Hidayat A, Kopelman J, Zimmerman LE. Retinocytoma: A benign variant of retinoblastoma. Arch Ophthalmol 101:1519–1531, 1983.

18. Shields JA, Shields CL. Differential diagnosis of retinoblastoma. In: Shields JA, Shields CL. Intraocular Tumors. A Text and Atlas. Philadelphia: Saunders, 1992, pp 341–362.

19. Shields JA, Parsons HM, Shields CL, Shah P. Lesions simulating retinoblastoma. J Pediatr Ophthalmol Strabismus 28:338–340, 1991.

20. Shields JA, Shields CL, Parsons HM. Review: Differential diagnosis of retinoblastoma. Retina 11:232–243, 1991.

21. Shields JA, Shields CL, Honavar S, Demirci H. Coats' disease. Clinical variations and complication of Coats' disease in 150 cases. The 2000 Sanford Gifford Memorial Lecture. Am J Ophthalmol 131:561–571, 2001.

22. Shields JA. Ocular toxocariasis. A review. Surv Ophthalmol 28:361–381, 1984.

23. Shields JA, Shields CL, Eagle RC Jr, Barrett J, De Potter P. Endogenous endophthalmitis simulating retinoblastoma. A report of six cases. The 1993 Seslen Lecture. Retina 15:213–219, 1995.

24. Shields JA, Sanborn GE, Augsburger JJ, Orlock D, Donoso LA. Fluorescein angiography of retinoblastoma. Retina 2:206–214, 1982.

25. DePotter P, Shields JA, Shields CL. Tumors and pseudotumors of the retina. In: DePotter P, Shields JA, Shields CL, eds. MRI of the Eye and Orbit. Philadelphia: Lippincott, 1995, pp 93–94.

26. Shields JA. Misconceptions and techniques in the management of retinoblastoma. The 1992 Paul Henkind Memorial Lecture. Retina 12:320–330, 1992.

27. Shields JA, Shields CL, Donoso LA, Lieb WE. Changing concepts in the management of retinoblastoma. Ophthalm Surg 21:72–76, 1990.

28. Shields JA, Shields CL, De Potter P. Enucleation technique for children with retinoblastoma. J Pediatr Ophthalmol Strabismus 29:213–215, 1992.

29. De Potter P, Shields CL, Shields JA, Singh AD. Use of the orbital hydroxyapatite implant in the pediatric population. Arch Ophthalmol 112:208–212, 1994.

30. Shields JA, Shields CL, Sivalingam V. Decreasing frequency of enucleation in patients with retinoblastoma. Am J Ophthalmol 108:185–188, 1989.

31. Shields JA, Giblin ME, Shields CL, Markoe AM, Karlsson U, Brady LW, Amendola BE, Woodleigh R. Episcleral plaque radiotherapy for retinoblastoma. Ophthalmology 96:530–537, 1989.

32. Shields CL, Shields JA, Minelli S, DePotter P, Hernandez JC, Cater J, Brady LW. Regression of retinoblastoma after plaque radiotherapy. Am J Ophthalmol 115:181–187, 1993.

33. Shields JA, Shields CL, De Potter P, Hernandez JC, Brady LW. Plaque radiotherapy for residual or recurrent retinoblastoma in 91 cases. J Pediatr Ophthalmol Strabismus 31:242–245, 1994.

34. Shields JA, Parsons H, Shields CL, Giblin, ME. The role of cryotherapy in the management of retinoblastoma. Am J Ophthalmol 108:260–264, 1989.

35. Shields JA, Parsons H, Shields CL, Giblin, ME. The role of photocoagulation in the management of retinoblastoma. Arch Ophthalmol 108:205–208, 1990.

36. Shields CL, Shields JA, Kiratli H, De Potter P. Treatment of retinoblastoma with indirect ophthalmoscope laser photocoagulation. J Pediatr Ophthalmol Strabismus 32:317–322, 1995.

37. White L. Chemotherapy in retinoblastoma: current status and future directions. Am J Pediatr Hematol Oncol 13:189–201, 1991.

38. Shields CL, Shields JA, De Potter P. New treatment modalities for retinoblastoma. Curr Opin Ophthalmol 7:20–26, 1996.

39. Shields CL, De Potter P, Himmelstein B, Shields JA, Meadows AT, Maris J. Chemoreduction in the initial management of intraocular retinoblastoma. Arch Ophthalmol 114:1330–1338, 1996.

40. Gallie BL, Budning A, DeBoer G, et al. Chemotherapy with focal therapy can cure intraocular retinoblastoma without radiotherapy. Arch Ophthalmol 114;1321–1328, 1996.

41. Murphree AL, Villablanca JG, Deegan WF, Sato JK, Malogolowkin M, Fisher A, Parker RK, Reed KE, Gomer CJ. Chemotherapy plus focal treatment in the management of intraocular retinoblastoma. Arch Ophthalmol 114:1348–1356, 1996.

42. Shields CL, Shields JA, De Potter P, Himmelstein B, Meadows AT. The effect of chemoreduction on retinoblastoma-induced retinal detachment. J Pediatr Ophthalmol Strabismus 34:165–169, 1997.

43. Shields CL, Shields JA, Needle M, De Potter P, Kheterpal S, Hamada A, Meadows AT. Combined chemoreduction and adjuvant treatment for intraocular retinoblastoma. Ophthalmology 104:2101–2111, 1997.

44. Shields JA, Shields CL, De Potter P, Needle M. Bilateral macular retinoblastoma managed by chemoreduction and chemothermotherapy. Arch Ophthalmol 114:1426, 1996.

3

Epidemiology of Uveal Melanoma: Patient Characteristics, Risk Factors, and Predisposing Elements

MARIE DIENER-WEST

Johns Hopkins Bloomberg School of Public Health, Baltimore, Maryland, U.S.A.

CLAUDIA SCALA MOY

National Institutes of Health/National Institute of Neurological Disorders and Stroke, Bethesda, Maryland, U.S.A.

Uveal melanoma is a rare disease but is the most common primary intraocular tumor and has a high potential for metastasis. The study of factors that determine the occurrence and distribution of this disease is critical in the understanding of its possible prevention. Previous knowledge of the epidemiology of uveal melanoma has been reviewed extensively [1–4], and we recommend these excellent readings. In the present chapter, we discuss the challenges associated with the epidemiologic study of uveal melanoma, review the current knowledge of its incidence and possible risk factors for diagnosis in light of new evidence, and outline future directions for epidemiologic research.

I. CHALLENGES ASSOCIATED WITH THE EPIDEMIOLOGIC STUDY OF UVEAL MELANOMA

Most of the current understanding of the epidemiology of uveal melanoma is based on surveys or registry data from many populations and on small observational studies in series of patients followed within clinical settings. The comparability of findings from these studies and generalizability to other populations are limited by differences in study design and inconsistencies in the methods of disease classification, completeness of case ascertainment, and assessment of risk.

Definition and classification of uveal melanoma cases is central to any descriptive or analytic study. In developed countries, where access to state-of-the-art diagnostic tools is readily available, the accuracy of diagnosis is considered to be quite high [5,6]. However, considerable variability in inclusion criteria across published series complicates comparison. For example, some studies use "eye cancer" as a proxy for uveal melanoma in adults; this may be reasonable in the context of published series documenting that at least 70% of ocular neoplasms in adults comprise melanoma cell types [7]. Tumor stage and shape (usually inferred from basal dimension and/or apical height based on ultrasound), location within the uvea (choroid, iris, ciliary body, any or all sites), and cell type may represent subtypes of disease with differing etiology and prognosis; these subtypes may be distributed differently across populations or published studies. The advent of increasingly sophisticated diagnostic technology will permit more precise classification in future studies. Diagnostic accuracy and case definition may be less standard in older studies or those from the developing world; thus comparisons with other published studies must take these factors into account.

Comparison of incidence rates across populations and over time may be useful in generating etiologic hypotheses, but direct comparisons may be difficult due to variability in study design, including methods of adjusting for age. The incidence of uveal melanoma—i.e., the number of new cases occurring within a specified time period in a defined population—is generally derived from population-based registries. In countries with national systems of health care and central records, such as in northern Europe (e.g., Refs. 8,9), uveal melanoma registries are usually considered to be quite complete and the population base well defined. However, in all studies—and especially studies from societies with less structured or less universal health care systems—underascertainment is a concern. Methods of validating registry completeness exist [10] but have seldom been applied in uveal melanoma. Incidence estimates based on hospital-based case series are likely to be invalid due to lack of an appropriate population base.

In addition to documenting disease incidence, registries can be useful tools for conducting prospective or retrospective assessments of risk factors and prognosis [e.g., 11–14]. Retrospective, or case-control, studies are probably the most useful epidemiologic design for elucidating causative associations between risk factors and uveal melanoma because of the infrequent occurrence of this disease. This approach is subject to a number of inherent problems and biases that may complicate the interpretation of the results. Much has been written about selection of cases and controls, case definition, and potential difficulties with retrospective assessment of exposure (e.g., Refs. 15 and 16). Further complicating establishing etiologic associations in uveal melanoma is the presumed long latency period and the difficulty in quantifying exposures to hypothesized risks, such as to ultraviolet (UV) radiation [17]. For example, the literature contains many examples of case-control or cross-sectional investigations of the role of sunlight or UV exposure in causing uveal melanoma, with very mixed results. The inconsistencies in the findings may in part be due to variations in methods of defining and classifying exposure and the accuracy of retrospective assessment. Furthermore, it is generally very difficult in retrospective or cross-sectional studies to establish the temporal sequence of presumed exposures and initiation of disease.

II. MAGNITUDE AND DISTRIBUTION OF CASES OF UVEAL MELANOMA

In the United States, the estimated incidence of intraocular malignancies has remained relatively constant over the last 30 years. The annual age-adjusted incidence estimate was 6 per million population based on the Third National Cancer Survey conducted from 1969 to 1971 [13]. Since that time, the Surveillance, Epidemiology, and End Results (SEER) Program of the National Cancer Institute has compiled the largest public-use database for cancer incidence in the United States. Nine regional SEER registries have reported all new cancer cases since 1973–1975; two registries were added in 1992. The annual age-adjusted incidence of noncutaneous melanoma was reported as 7 per million population during the period from 1973 to 1977 [18]. More recently, SEER data indicate that the age-adjusted incidence of eye and orbit cancer has remained relatively constant from 1992 through 1999 (7.6 cases per million population to 7.3 cases per million population [19]. Across the years 1992–1999, the overall age-adjusted incidence rate is 7.98 cases per million population; it should be noted that the U.S. population from the year 2000 is used as the standard population for these adjustments and represents a change from previous estimates. However, estimates based on population-based surveys conducted in the United States yield similar findings. In an incidence survey carried out from 1984 to 1989 in the six New England states, the annual incidence was 7.4 cases per million population [2].

Similar incidence rates have been reported from surveys conducted in Canada [20], Sweden [21], Finland [9], and Denmark [8]. In most populations, these rates have remained constant over the past several decades [22]. The incidence of uveal melanoma has appeared stable at 6 cases per million population over a 35-year period from 1961 to 1996 in Israel [23]. A higher incidence rate was observed in a population-based study in the United Kingdom using the General Practice Research Database; the estimated incidence rate was 11.6 cases per million person-years [24]. Age-adjusted incidence rates of up to 10 per million person-years have been reported in Europe [25]. An excellent source of worldwide cancer registry information is an electronic database compiled by the International Agency for Research on Cancer (IARC), which contains data from 149 population-based cancer registries covering 183 populations in 50 countries [26].

Based on the incidence rates from the NCI SEER program 1979–1998, the American Cancer Society estimated that about 2200 new cases of all primary intraocular cancers (eye and orbit) will be diagnosed in the United States in the year 2002; approximately 200 deaths will be due to these malignancies [27]. Assuming that at least 70% of all primary eye malignancies are uveal melanoma [28], this translates into at least 1600 new cases of uveal melanoma and approximately 150 deaths each year.

In contrast, the age-adjusted incidence between 1995 and 1999 for skin melanoma in the United States was 163 cases per million population [19], roughly 20 times higher than that of eye and orbit cancers. A recent report reviewed 84,836 cases of cutaneous and noncutaneous melanoma in the United States [29] from the National Cancer Data Base from 1985 through 1994. This national cancer registry solicits all acute care hospitals to submit annually their cancer registry data. During this time period, 91.2% of cases were skin melanomas and 5.2% ($n = 4522$) were ocular melanomas. Of these 85% were uveal melanoma, 4.8% were conjunctival melanoma, and 10.2% occurred at other ocular sites.

III. PATIENT CHARACTERISTICS

Uveal melanoma occurs predominantly in individuals of Caucasian race, is associated with older age, and has been reported to occur more frequently in males than females. SEER data indicate increasing incidence with age in both males and females, with higher rates for males at all ages above 35 years [19]. The age-adjusted incidence rates by ethnicity are 8.9, 2.4, 3.9, 2.4, and 5.2 cases per million population for whites, blacks, American Indians/Alaskan Natives, Asian/Pacific Islanders, and Hispanics, respectively [19]. Recent statistics suggest that the age distribution of cases with new eye and orbit cancers is 32%, 24%, 22%, and 22% for individuals aged <50, 50–64, 65–74, and 75+ years, respectively [30]. Most studies suggest that the median age at diagnosis for the Caucasian population is approximately 60 years. In the review of ocular melanoma cases from the National Cancer Data Base, over 92% were white non-Hispanic, 52% were male, and the mean age at diagnosis was 60.4 years, with 75% aged 50 years or older [29]. This agrees with the mean age at diagnosis of 61 years obtained from the New England survey [2]. Similarly, a review of 184 Finnish patients with uveal melanoma diagnosed between 1994 and 1999 indicated that 47% were male and that the mean age at time of diagnosis was 60 years [31].

Race and ancestral origin appear to be associated with the development of uveal melanoma. Surveys among African and Asian populations indicate low risk of the disease [e.g., 32,33]. Similarly, in the United States, incidence in African Americans or other racial or ethnic groups is much lower than in Caucasians [2,34]. In a population-based study in Israel, there was considerable variation among ethnic groups; the highest incidence was observed in individuals with American- or eastern European-born parents [35]. Results from a previous case-control study suggest higher risk of uveal melanoma in individuals of northern European ancestry as compared to those of southern European or Mediterranean descent [36]. There appears to be ethnic variability in both incidence and age at diagnosis. The mean age at diagnosis of uveal melanoma in a series of Asian Indians was estimated as 46.1 years [37].

IV. RISK FACTORS FOR UVEAL MELANOMA AND PREDISPOSING ELEMENTS

A. Personal Characteristics

A number of personal characteristics have been associated with increased risk of uveal melanoma, including light irides [38–40], fair complexion [36] and melanocytic conditions such as ocular nevi [41], dysplastic nevus syndrome [42,43], and ocular and oculodermal melanocytosis [44]. In a recent population-based case-control study in Australia, there was increased risk of choroidal and ciliary body melanoma associated with non-brown eye color, four or more cutaneous nevi on the back, inability to tan, and squinting while outside in the sun as a child [45]. Previous history of nonocular malignancy also has been examined as a risk factor, with equivocal results [46–49].

B. Hormones and Reproductive Factors

The role of hormones and reproductive factors has been investigated, with equivocal results. Reports of increased incidence in women of childbearing age [13,50] or disease occurrence associated with pregnancy [40,51,52] suggest an effect of hormones, but results from case-control studies examining specific hormonal factors have been inconsistent [53,54]. A recent evaluation of enucleated eyes did not support the presence of type I estrogen receptors in human uveal melanoma [55], which concurred with a previous analysis using similar modern estrogen receptor testing methods [56].

C. Genetic Susceptibility

Physiological changes or genetic modifications may be associated with the occurrence of uveal melanoma, although there have not been consistent findings among studies. There are equivocal findings regarding the role of genetics in the development of uveal melanoma. Several studies have documented family clustering of uveal melanoma [57,58], bilateral occurrence of uveal melanoma [59,60], or associations with cutaneous melanoma [43,60], suggesting a genetic or heritable component. The occurrence of uveal melanoma within members of a family and across generations suggests inheritance may play a role [61–63]. Recently, the clinical cases of three siblings afflicted with uveal melanoma were reported; all three patients were diagnosed before the age of 40 years and developed aggressive disease [64].

The role of genes has been implicated in the pathogenesis of both cutaneous melanoma and breast cancer and also has been investigated in uveal melanoma. In a study of 49 samples, there was no association between uveal melanoma and c-Ha-*ras* proto-oncogene point mutations nor genetic alterations in the c-Ki-*ras*-2 gene at codons 12, 13, and 61 [65]. Similarly, allelic variations for the melancortin-1 receptor (MC1R) gene do not appear to play a role in the development of uveal melanoma [66]. There are inconclusive findings regarding the role of *CDKN2* (p16) gene as a tumor suppressor gene in uveal melanoma [67,68]. Specific genetic mutations, such as chromosomal deletions [69] or mutations in the p53 tumor-suppressor gene [70] have also been reported. In addition, germline *brca2* mutations may occur in a small proportion of uveal melanoma cases [71].

Although no common germline mutations have been identified in families with members having both ocular and cutaneous melanoma, animal models have suggested a common hereditary factor [72]. The identification of genetic loci that contribute to the family aggregation of ocular and cutaneous melanoma or other cancer requires further investigation. However, the majority of reported uveal melanoma cases are not associated with factors typical of diseases with strong genetic etiology; thus, even if there is a genetic component, it is likely that environmental or other factors are more important in triggering development of disease.

D. Environmental or Occupational Exposures

A key to the prevention of uveal melanoma is the identification of environmental or occupational exposures that place individuals at higher risk of developing the disease. Sunlight exposure and UV radiation have been implicated in the pathogenesis of cutaneous melanoma [73]. They also may play a role in the etiology of uveal melanoma but the association of environmental UV exposure and uveal melanoma is less clear than for cutaneous melanoma [17,74,75]. Studies evaluating tumor location in relation to presumed distribution of ultraviolet radiation exposure to the uvea have been contradictory [76,77], and the vulnerability of the uvea to UV radiation is not clear [78,79].

Occupational exposures to UV light or chemicals may also be involved in the etiology of uveal melanoma. Previous studies have suggested an association between uveal melanoma and use of sunlamps [36], intense sun exposure [80], and tendency to sunburn [36,39,81] . Occupational exposure to UV light among welders [82,83] or exposure to asbestos and chemicals in the workplace has been associated with increased risk of uveal melanoma [82,84–86]. However, differences in study designs and occupational coding schemes as well as selection biases influence both study findings and interpretation [87].

Exposure to radiofrequency radiation (in the form of radio sets and mobile phones) was recently shown to be associated with uveal melanoma in a case-control study from Germany [88]. Potential confounding variables that were not investigated in this study, such as occupational or recreational exposure to ultraviolet radiation, may account for the observed associations [89]. Conversely, an analysis of the incidence rate of uveal melanoma showed no correlation with the increase in mobile phone usage over time in Denmark [90]; further research is needed before recommendations can be made [91]. If radiofrequency radiation is in fact causative, future studies may demonstrate increasing incidence of uveal melanoma as these technologies become increasingly ubiquitous.

V. DETECTION OF UVEAL MELANOMA

Knowledge of the potential risk factors or predisposing elements for uveal melanoma would aid in early screening and detection of uveal melanoma. In Finland, 87% of patients had symptoms, mainly blurred vision and a visual field defect, before seeking an appointment with the health care system [31]. In the United Kingdom, most ocular melanomas are detected by optometrists [92]. An analysis of 223 patients presenting to optometrists between 1997 and 2000 revealed that as many as 45% of all detected tumors occurred in asymptomatic patients and would have been missed without appropriate screening. Also, tumors in patients with symptoms were less likely to be detected when there was reduced visual acuity, the anterior tumor margin was located anterior to the ora serrata, or the posterior margin was located in the pre-equatorial choroid [92]. The diagnosis of uveal melanoma by retinal specialists and other ophthalmologists has reached a high degree of accuracy due to improved indirect ophthalmoscopy, fluorescein angiography, and echography [3].

VI. FUTURE RESEARCH DIRECTIONS

In spite of the large amount of epidemiologic research that has been conducted to date, our understanding of the magnitude, distribution, and risk factors for uveal melanoma is incomplete. The future of research in the epidemiology of uveal melanoma will depend to a great extent on advances in molecular biology and genetics to facilitate more precise case definition and to form a more solid ground for evaluation of the interaction between host characteristics, genetic factors, and environment and in the pathogenesis of disease. Histopathology and tissue repositories such as that developed from the Collaborative Ocular Melanoma Study [93] provide a rich source for future exploration of genetic characteristics and susceptibility. Future epidemiologic investigations will also be important to better define subgroups of individuals at increased risk of disease so that screening and programs of primary and secondary prevention can be appropriately focused. Finally, research is needed to elucidate the potential biological mechanisms through which implicated exposures may cause melanoma.

REFERENCES

1. Seddon JM, Moy CS. Epidemiology of uveal melanoma. In: Ryan SJ, ed. Retina. Vol 1: Basic Sciences and Inherited Retinal Disease/Tumors, 3rd ed. St. Louis: Mosby, 2001, pp 664–672.
2. Seddon JM, Egan K. Application of epidemiologic methods to the study of eye disease: uveal melanoma. In: Albert DM, Jacobiec FA, eds. The Principles and Practice of Ophthalmology. Philadelphia: Saunders, 1993, pp 1245–1249.
3. Sahel JA, Polans AS, Mehta MP, Auchter RM, Albert DM. Intraocular melanomas. In: DeVita VT Jr, Hellman S, Rosenberg SA, eds. Cancer: Principles and Practice of Oncology, 6th ed. Philadelphia: Lippincott, 2001, pp 2070–2090.
4. Egan KM, Seddon JM, Glynn RJ, Gragoudas ES, Albert DM. Epidemiologic aspects of uveal melanoma. Surv Ophthalmol 32:239–251, 1988.
5. Collaborative Ocular Melanoma Study Group. Accuracy of diagnosis of choroidal melanoma in the Collaborative Ocular Melanoma Study. COMS Report No. 1. Arch Ophthalmol 108:1268–1273, 1990.
6. Margo CE. The accuracy of diagnosis of posterior uveal melanoma. Arch Ophthalmol 115:434–444, 1997.
7. Mahoney MC, Burnett WS, Majerovics A, Tanenbaum H. The epidemiology of ophthalmic malignancies in New York State. Ophthalmology 97:1143–1147, 1990.
8. Jensen OA, Prause JU. Malignant melanomas of the human uvea in Denmark: Incidence and a 25 year follow-up of cases diagnosed between 1943 and 1952. In: Lommatzsch PK, Blodi FC, eds: Intraocular Tumors. Berlin: Springer-Verlag, 1983, pp 85–92.
9. Teikari JM, Raivio I. Incidence of choroidal malignant melanomas in Finland in the years 1973–1980. Acta Ophthalmol 63:661–665, 1985.
10. Hook EB, Regal RR. The value of capture-recapture methods even for apparent exhaustive surveys. The need for adjustment for source of ascertainment intersection in attempted complete prevalence studies. Am J Epidemiol 135:1060–1067, 1992.

11. Jensen OA. Malignant melanomas of the uvea in Denmark 1943–1952: A clinical, histopathological and prognostic study. Acta Ophthalmol Suppl (Copenh) 75:17–78, 1963.

12. Osterlind A. Trends in incidence of ocular malignant melanoma in Denmark 1943–1982. Int J Cancer 40:161–164, 1987.

13. Scotto JS, Fraumeni JF, Jr, Lee JAH: Melanomas of the eye and other non-cutaneous site: Epidemiologic aspects. J Natl Cancer Inst 56:489–491, 1976.

14. Swerdlow AJ. Epidemiology of melanoma of the eye in the Oxford region, 1952–1978. Br J Cancer 47:311–313, 1983.

15. Moy CS. Case-control designs for clinical research in ophthalmology. Arch Ophthalmol 116:661–664, 1998.

16. Stang A, Ahrens W, Anastassiou G, Bornfeld N, Jockel KH. Methodological aspects and problems of a hospital-based case-control study on uveal melanoma. A case study. Stud Health Technol Inform 77:111–113, 2000.

17. Moy CS. Evidence for the role of sunlight exposure in the etiology of choroidal melanoma. Arch Ophthalmol 119:430–431, 2001.

18. Young JL, Percy CL, Asire AJ, Berg JW, Cusano MM, Gloeckler LA, Horn JW, Lourie WI, Jr, Pollack ES, Shambaugh EM. Cancer incidence and mortality in the United States, 1973–1977. Nat Cancer Inst Monogr 57:1–187, 1981.

19. Ries LAG, Eisner MP, Kosary CL, Hankey BF, Miller BA, Clegg L, Edwards BK, eds. SEER Cancer Statistics Review. 1973–1999. Bethesda, MD: National Cancer Institute, http://seer.cancer.gov/csr/1973_1999/

20. Birdsell JM, Gunther BK, Boyd TA, Grace M, Jerry LM. Ocular melanoma: A population-based study. Can J Ophthalmol 15:9–12, 1980.

21. Abrahamsson M. Malignant melanoma of the choroid and the ciliary body 1956–1975 in Halland and Gothenburg: Incidence, histopathology and prognosis. Acta Ophthalmol (Copenh) 61:600–610, 1983.

22. Hakulinen T, Teppo L, Saxen E. Cancer of the eye, a review of trends and differentials. World Health Stat Q 31:143–158, 1978.

23. Iscovich J, Abdulrazik M, Pe'er J. Posterior uveal malignant melanoma: Temporal stability and ethnic variation in rates in Israel. Anticancer Res 21(2B):1449–1454, 2001.

24. Huerta C, Garcia Rodriquez LA. Incidence of ocular melanoma in the general population and in glaucoma patients. J Epidemiol Community Health 55:338–339, 2001.

25. Parkin DM, Whelan SL, Ferlay J, Raymond L, Young J, eds. Cancer in Five Continents, vol. VIII. IARC Scientific Pub. No. 143. Lyon, France: International Agency for Research on Cancer, 1997.

26. Parkin DM, Bray F, Ferlay J, Pisani P. Estimating the world cancer burden. GLOBOCAN 2000. Int J Cancer 94:153–156, 2001.

27. American Cancer Society. Cancer Facts and Figures. American Cancer Society, Atlanta, GA. 2002.

28. Cutler SJ, Young JL, eds. Third National Cancer Survey: Incidence data. NCI Monogr 41:1–454, 1975.

29. Chang AE, Karnell LH, Menck HR. The National Cancer Data Base report on cutaneous and noncutaneous melanoma. Cancer 83:1664–1678, 1998.

30. Edwards BK, Howe HL, Ries LAG, Thun MJ, Rosenberg HM, Yancik R, Wingo PA, Jemal A, Feigal EG. Annual report to the nation on the status of cancer, 1973–1999, featuring implications of age and aging on US cancer burden. Cancer 94:2766–2792, 2002.

31. Eskelin S, Kivela T. Mode of presentation and time to treatment of uveal melanoma in Finland. Br J Ophthalmol 86:333–338, 2002.

32. Miller B, Abrahams C, Cole GC, Proctor NS. Ocular malignant melanoma in South African blacks. Br J Ophthalmol 65:720–722, 1981.

33. Kuo PK, Puliafito CA, Wang KM, Liu HS, Wu BF. Uveal melanoma in China. Int Ophthalmol Clin 22:57–71, 1982.

34. Neugut AI, Kizelnik-Freilich S, Ackerman C. Black-white differences in risk for cutaneous, ocular and visceral melanomas. Am J Public Health 84:1828–1829, 1994.

35. Iscovich J, Ackerman C, Andreev H, Pe'er J, Steinitz R. An epidemiological study of posterior uveal melanoma in Israel. 1961–1989. Int J Cancer 61:291–295, 1995.

36. Seddon JM, Gragoudas ES, Glynn RJ, Egan KM, Albert DM, Blitzer PH. Host factors, UV radiation, and risk of uveal melanoma. A case-control study. Arch Ophthalmol 108:1274–1280, 1990.

37. Biswas J, Krishnakumar S, Shanmugan MP. Uveal melanoma in Asian Indians: A clinicopathological study. Arch Ophthalmol 120:522–523, 2002.

38. Gallagher RP, Elwood JM, Rootman J, Spinelli JJ, Hill GB, Threlfall WJ, Birdsell JM. Risk factors for ocular melanoma: Western Canada Melanoma Study. J Natl Cancer Inst 74:775–778, 1985.

39. Holly EA, Aston DA, Char DH, Kristiansen JJ, Ahn DK. Uveal melanoma in relation to ultraviolet light exposure and host factors. Cancer Res 50:5773–5777, 1990.

40. Tucker MA, Shields JA, Hartge P, Augsburger J, Hoover RN, Fraumeni JF Jr. Sunlight exposure as risk factor for intraocular malignant melanoma. N Engl J Med 313:789–792, 1985.

41. Ganley JP, Comstock GW. Benign nevi and malignant melanomas of the choroid. Am J Ophthalmol 76:19–25, 1973.

42. Hammer H, Olah J, Toth-Molnar E. Dysplastic nevi are a risk factor for uveal melanoma. Eur J Ophthalmol 6:742–747, 1996.

43. Albert DM, Chang MA, Lamping K, Weiter J, Sober A. The dysplastic nevus syndrome: A pedigree with primary malignant melanomas of the choroid and skin. Ophthalmology 92:1728–1734, 1985.

44. Singh AD, De Potter P, Fijal BA, Shields CL, Shields JA, Elston RC. Lifetime prevalence of uveal melanoma in white patients with oculo(dermal) melanocytosis. Ophthalmology 105:195–198, 1998.

45. Vajdic CM, Kricker A, Giblin M, McKenzie J, Aitken J, Giles GG, Armstrong BK. Eye color and cutaneous nevi predict risk of ocular melanoma in Australia. Int J Cancer 92:906–912, 2001.

46. Holly EA, Aston DA, Ahn DK, Kristiansen JJ, Char DH. No excess prior cancer in patients with uveal melanoma. Ophthalmology 98:608–611, 1991.

47. Lischko AM, Seddon JM, Gragoudas ES, Egan KM, Glynn RJ. Evaluation of prior primary malignancy as a determinant of uveal melanoma: A case-control study. Ophthalmology 96:1716–1721, 1989.

48. Travis LB, Curtis RE, Boice JD, Platz CE, Hankey BF, Fraumeni JF. Second malignant neoplasms among long-term survivors of ovarian cancer. Cancer Res 56:1564–1570, 1996.

49. Turner BJ, Siatkowski RM, Augsburger JJ, Shields JA, Lustbader E, Mastrangelo MJ. Other cancers in uveal melanoma patients and their families. Am J Opthalmol 107:601–608, 1989.

50. Lee JA, Storer BE. Excess of malignant melanomas in women in the British Isles. Lancet 2:1337–1339, 1980.

51. Seddon JM, MacLaughlin DT, Albert DM, Gragoudas ES, Ferrence M. Uveal melanomas presenting during pregnancy and the investigation of estrogen receptors in melanomas. Br J Ophthlamol 66:695–704, 1982.

52. Shields CL, Shields JA, Eagle RC, DePotter P, Merduke H. Uveal melanoma and pregnancy: A report of 16 cases. Ophthalmology 98:1667–1673, 1991.

53. Hartge P, Tucker MA, Shields JA, Augsburger J, Hoover RN, Fraumeni JF. Case-control study of female hormones and eye melanoma. Cancer Res 49:4622–4625, 1989.

54. Holly EA, Aston DA, Ahn DK, Kristiansen JJ, Char DH. Uveal melanoma, hormonal and reproductive factors in women. Cancer Res 51:1370–1372, 1991.

55. Grostern RJ, Slusker-Shternfeld I, Bacus SS, Gilchrist K, Zimbric ML, Albert DM. Absence of type I estrogen receptors in choroidal melanoma: Analysis of Collaborative Ocular Melanoma Study (COMS) eyes. Am J Ophthalmol 131:788–791, 2001.

56. Foss AJ, Alexander RA, Guille MJ, Unngerford JI, McCartney ACE, Lightman S. Estrogren and progesterone receptor analysis in ocular melanoma. Ophthalmology 102:431–456, 1995.

57. Singh AD, Shields CL, Shields JA, Eagle RC, De Potter P. Uveal melanoma and familial atypical mole and melanoma (FAM-M) syndrome. Ophthalm Genet 16:53–61, 1995.

58. Young LH, Egan KM, Walsh SM, Gragoudas ES. Familial uveal melanoma. Am J Ophthalmol 117:516–520, 1994.

59. Singh AD, Shields CL, Shields JA, DePotter PL: Bilateral primary uveal melanomas. Bad luck or bad genes? Ophthalmology 103:256–262, 1996.

60. Oosterhuis JA, Went LN, Lynch HT. Primary choroidal and cutaneous melanomas, bilateral choroidal melanomas, and familial occurrence of melanomas. Br J Ophthalmol 66:230–233, 1982.

61. Walker JP, Weiter JJ, Albert DM, Osborn El, Weichselbaum RR. Uveal malignant melanoma in three generations of the same family. Am J Ophthalmol 88:723–726, 1979.

62. Canning CR, Hungerford J. Familial uveal melanoma. Br J Ophthalmol 72:241–243, 1988.

63. Singh AD, Wang MX, Donoso LA, Shields CL, DePotter PD, Shields JA, Elston RC, Fijal B. Familial uveal melanoma. III. Is the occurrence of family uveal melanoma conincidental? Arch Ophthalmol 114:1101–1104, 1996.

64. Krygier G, Lombardo K, Vargas C, Alvbez I, Costa R, Ros M, Echenique M, Navarro V, Delgado L, Viola A, Muse I. Familial uveal melanoma: Report on three sibling cases. Br J Ophthalmol 85:1007–1008, 2001.

65. Soparker CN, O'Brien JM, Albert DM. Investigation of the role of the *ras* proto-oncogene point mutation in human uveal melanomas. Invest Ophthalmol Vis Sci 34:2203–2209, 1993.

66. Metzelaar-Blok JAW, ter Huurne JAC, Hurks MHM, Keunen JEE, Jager MJ, Gruis NA. Characterization of melanocortin-1 receptor gene variants in uveal melanoma patients. Invest Ophthalmol Vis Sci 42:1951–1954, 2001.

67. Singh AD, Croce CM, Wary KK, Shields JA, Donoso LA, Shields CL, Huebner K, Ohta M. Familial uveal melanoma: Absence of germline mutations involving the cyclin dependent kinase-4 inhibitor gene (p16). Ophthalmic Genet 17:39–40, 1996.

68. Merbs SL, Sidransky D. Analysis of p16 (CDKN2/MTS-1/1NK4A) alterations in primary sporadic uveal melanoma. Invest Ophthalmol Vis Sci 40:779–783, 1999.

69. Mukai S, Dryja TP. Loss of alleles at polymorphic loci on chromosome 2 in uveal melanoma. Cancer Genet Cytogenet 22:45–53, 1986.

70. Jay M, McCartney AC. Familial malignant melanoma of the uvea and p53: A Victorian detective story. Surv Ophthalmol 37:457–462, 1993.

71. Sinilnikova OM, Egan KM, QuinnJL, Boutrand L, Lenoir GM, Stoppa-Lyonnet D, Desjardins L, Levy C, Goldgar D, Gragoudas ES. Germ-line *brca2* sequence variants in patients with ocular melanoma. Int J Cancer 82:325–328, 1999.

72. Bradl, Klein-Szanto A, Porter S, Mintz B. Malignant melanoma in transgenic mice. Proc Natl Acad Sci USA 88:164–168, 1991.

73. Whiteman DC, Green AC. Melanoma and sun exposure: Where are we now? Int J Dermatol 38:481–489, 1999.

74. Dolin PJ, Foss AJ, Hungerford JL. Uveal melanoma: Is solar ultraviolet radiation a risk factor? Ophthalmic Epidemiol 1:27–30, 1994.

75. Dolin PJ, Johnson GJ. Solar ultraviolet radiation and ocular disease: A review of the epidemiological and experimental evidence. Ophthalmic Epidemiol 1:155–164, 1994.

76. Schwartz LH, Ferrand R, Boelle PY, Maylin C, D'Hermies F, Virmont J. Lack of correlation between the location of choroidal melanoma and ultraviolet-radiation dose distribution. Radiat Res 147:451–456, 1997.

77. Li W, Judge H, Gragoudas ES, Seddon JM, Egan KM. Patterns of tumor initiaition in choroidal melanoma. Cancer Res 60:3757–3760, 2000.

78. Rosen ES. Filtration of non-ionizing radiation by the ocular media. In: Cronly-Dixon J, Rosen ES, Marshall J, eds. Hazards of light: Myths and realities on the eye and skin. Oxford: Pergamon Press, 1986, p 145.

79. Lerman S. Sunlight and intraocular melanoma. N Engl J Med 314:712–713, 1986.

80. Horn EP, Hartge P, Shields JA, Tucker MA. Sunlight and risk of uveal melanoma. J Natl Cancer Inst 86:1476–1478, 1994.

81. Pane AR, Hirst W. Ultraviolet light exposure as a risk factor for ocular melanoma in Queensland, Australia. Ophthalm Epidemiol 7:159–167, 2000.

82. Holly EA, Aston DA, Ahn DK, Smith AH. Intraocular melanoma linked to occupations and chemical exposures. Epidemiology 7:55–61, 1996.

83. Guenel P, Laforest L, Cyr D, et al. Occupational risk factors, ultraviolet radiation, and ocular melanoma: a case-control study in France. Cancer Cause Control 12:451–459, 2001.

84. Albert DM, Puliafito CA, Fulton AB, Robinson NL, Zakov ZN, Dryja TP, Smith AB, Egan E, Leffingwell SS. Increased incidence of choroidal malignant melanoma occurring in a single population of chemical workers. Am J Ophthalmol 89:323–337, 1980.

85. Ajani UA, Seddon JM, Hsieh CC, Egan KM, Albert DM, Gragoudas ES. Occupation and risk of uveal melanoma. Cancer 70:2891–2900, 1992.

86. Ganley JP, Fontenot K. Epidemiologic study of time and space clustering of 4 cases of choroidal malignant melanoma. Arch Ophthalmol 115:537–541, 1997.

87. Lutz J-M, Cree IA, Foss AJ. Risk factors for intraocular melanoma and occupational exposure. Br J Ophthlamol 83:1190–1193, 1999.

88. Stang N, Anastassiou G, Ahrens W, et al. The possible role of radiofrequency radiation in the development of uveal melanoma. Epidemiology 12:7–12, 2001.

89. Inskip PD. Frequent radiation exposures and frequency-dependent effects: The eyes have it. Epidemiology 12:1–4, 2001.

90. Johansen C, Boice JD Jr., McLaughlin JK, Christensen HC, Olsen JH. Mobile phones and malignant melanoma of the eye. Br J Cancer 86:348–349, 2002.

91. Bullimore MA. Are cell phones bad for your health? Optom Vis Sci 78:129, 2001.

92. Damato B. Detection of uveal melanoma by optometrists in the United Kingdom. Ophthalm Physiol Optom 21:268–271, 2001.

93. Collaborative Ocular Melanoma Study Group. Design and methods of a clinical trial for a rare condition: The Collaborative Ocular Melanoma Study. COMS Report No. 3. Control Clin Trials 14:326–391, 1993.

4

Epidemiology of Retinoblastoma

JAMES J. AUGSBURGER

University of Cincinnati College of Medicine, The University Hospital, Cincinnati Children's Hospital Medical Center, and Veteran's Affairs Medical Center, Cincinnati, Ohio, U.S.A.

I. OVERVIEW

This chapter contains information concerning (1) the frequency of retinoblastoma in the general population, (2) the demographics of retinoblastoma, (3) currently recognized risk factors for the disease, and (4) important extraophthalmic lesions and disorders associated with retinoblastoma.

II. FREQUENCY OF RETINOBLASTOMA

A. Incidence of Retinoblastoma

Incidence is an expression of the number of persons in a defined population who develop a disease or condition over a specified time interval. By definition, none of the persons in the population has the disease or condition of interest at the start of the interval. All of these unaffected persons are considered to be at risk for development of the disease or condition. The width of the evaluation interval may be quite short (e.g., hours, days or weeks, depending on the disease or condition) or quite long (e.g., months to years).

Incidence of a disease or condition is based on the number of new cases diagnosed within the specified interval. Diagnosis of a disease or condition does not occur at its onset but at some time after it has reached a detectable extent and become symptomatic. The age of a patient at initial diagnosis of a disease or condition is a function of the relative promptness versus lateness of patient presentation to his or her health care system and the quality and intensity of the health care services that are available in that system. In countries with a well-developed health care system and reasonably good patient access to that system, patients with a particular disease or condition are likely to be diagnosed on average at a less advanced stage of their disease. In contrast, in countries that have a poorly developed health care system and limited patient access to that system, patients tend to seek health care services later on average following recognition of symptoms and are likely to have more advanced disease on average at the time of diagnosis [1].

Multiple estimates of the incidence of retinoblastoma in various populations and countries have been published [2–19]. These reports differ greatly in the quality of the data on which the estimates are based and the width of the age intervals studied. Relatively few publications include both high-quality data and year-by-year estimates of retinoblastoma incidence from birth to age 15 years or older. The curves shown in Figure 1 are estimates of the year-by-year incidence of retinoblastoma from birth to 15 years in two very different populations. The solid curve is based on data from the United States of America [15]. It is a progressively decreasing function with a relatively steep slope during the first 2 years, a steadily lessening slope over the next 4 years, and an almost flat slope that approaches zero thereafter. In contrast, the dashed curve in Figure 1 is a hypothetical annual incidence curve for a country with a poorly developed health care system, limited patient access to that system, or both. In such a country, a higher percentage of detectable cases will remain undiagnosed during any given year than would be undiagnosed in the United States. This relative delay in diagnosis will lead to a lower estimated incidence for year 1 compared with that for the United States, an increasing incidence during year 2 compared with the decreasing incidence in the United States, and a displacement of the descending limb of the dashed curve to the right of the annual incidence curve of the United States.

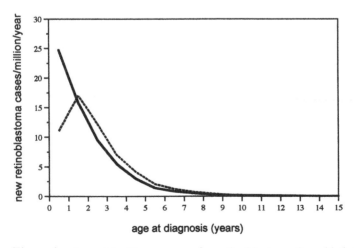

Figure 1   Annual incidence curves for retinoblastoma from birth to age 15 years. Solid line curve is based on data from the United States, while dashed line curve is hypothetical but approximates annual incidence values one would encounter in a third-world country. Relative shapes of these curves are discussed in text.

If one plots the sums of the yearly incidence figures shown in Figure 1 as a function of age at diagnosis, one obtains the curves shown in Figure 2. Both curves exhibit a rapid rise during the first 3 years, progressive flattening of slope over the next 5 years, and an almost flat slope thereafter for the remainder of life. The curves approach asymptotes of approximately 62.5 and 56.5 cases per million persons respectively. These asymptotic values are known as *cumulative lifetime incidence rates of retinoblastoma*. By dividing both the numerator and denominator of these cumulative incidence rates by the value of the numerator, one can express these rates as fractions with the value 1 in the numerator. By this transformation, the data presented in Figures 1 and 2 can be shown to correspond with cumulative lifetime incidence rates of approximately 1 in 15,000 to 1 in 18,000 individuals. For reasons unclear to this author, these cumulative lifetime incidence figures are commonly expressed as cases per million *live births*. Inspection of Figure 2 shows quite clearly that almost all cases of retinoblastoma are diagnosed prior to the age of 10 years, with the majority of cases being diagnosed prior to 3 years.

B. Prevalence of Retinoblastoma

In contrast with incidence, prevalence is an expression of the frequency of a disease or condition in a defined population at a specified point in time. The denominator is the number of individuals evaluated, and the numerator is the number found to have the disease or condition of interest at that evaluation. The specified point or window in time is the period during which all of the evaluations were carried out. This can be the same day relative to the date of birth or death of all subjects, the amount of time

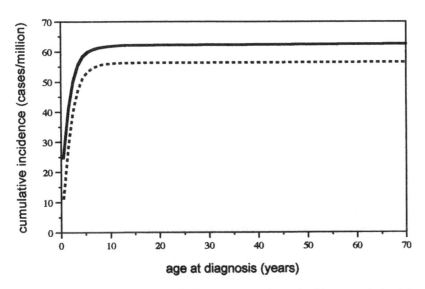

Figure 2   Cumulative lifetime incidence curves for retinoblastoma derived from the annual incidence curves shown in Figure 1. Solid line curve is based on data from the United States, while dashed line curve is hypothetical but approximates cumulative incidence values one would encounter in a third-world country. Asymptote for upper curve is approximately 62.5 cases per million and that for lower curve is approximately 57.5 cases per million.

required to perform a cross-sectional evaluation of a large population, or some other specified but limited time interval.

When one evaluates the prevalence of retinoblastoma, one must recognize that retinoblastoma is a disease that is almost always either completely cured or fatal within 2 to 3 years following initial diagnosis. Long remissions followed by local or metastatic recurrence of this malignancy are extremely uncommon. Unlike incidence, which relates to occurrence, prevalence falls as individuals who previously had the disease or condition are removed from the ranks of affected persons because of cure or death. An individual who is dead cannot be evaluated in a cross-sectional study of living patients. Similarly, an individual who previously had retinoblastoma but is now cured (e.g., following enucleation of the affected eye in a patient with unilateral intraocular disease) no longer has the disease and cannot be identified as having viable retinoblastoma in a cross-sectional survey. Consequently, the prevalence of retinoblastoma in any randomly selected segment of the population at any point in time will be exceptionally low. To this author's knowledge, no figures on prevalence of retinoblastoma have ever been published.

III. DEMOGRAPHICS OF RETINOBLASTOMA

A. Age at Diagnosis

As pointed our in the preceding section, retinoblastoma is almost exclusively a disease of childhood. If one plots the cumulative percentage of cases of retinoblastoma already diagnosed in a series of children with retinoblastoma as a function of age of the affected individual at initial diagnosis, one obtains a curve similar to the one shown in Figure 3. This particular curve is bases on data collected in the Retinoblastoma International Collaborative Study [20]. Inspection of Figure 3 reveals that over 90% of all cases of viable retinoblastoma are detected and diagnosed in children under the age of 6 years and approximately 99% of all cases are diagnosed prior to the age of 10 years. The point where the curve crosses the 50% line on the Y axis is referred to as the *median age at diagnosis* in the evaluated group of retinoblastoma patients. For the data plotted in Figure 3, the median age at diagnosis for the group is approximately 1.5 years (18 months). Retinoblastoma is occasionally detected as a congenital or even intrauterine disorder [21] (i.e., detected by a pelvic imaging study during pregnancy), especially in familial cases. At the other extreme, retinoblastoma is initially diagnosed after the age of 10 years in occasional cases and even after the age of 20 years in exceptional cases [22]. Many of newly diagnosed cases of retinoblastoma in juveniles and adults are currently believed to arise from a pre-existent *retinoma* (spontaneously arrested retinoblastoma, *retinocytoma*) that reverted to viable retinoblastoma.

Several factors influence the exact position of the curve on a graph of the cumulative percentage of cases of retinoblastoma already diagnosed versus age of the affected individual at diagnosis. The curve tends to be further to the left in countries with a high-quality health care delivery system and relatively prompt presentation of symptomatic persons to that system and further to the right in countries with a less well developed health care delivery system and relatively delayed presentation of symptomatic persons to eye care professionals. The impact of promptness versus

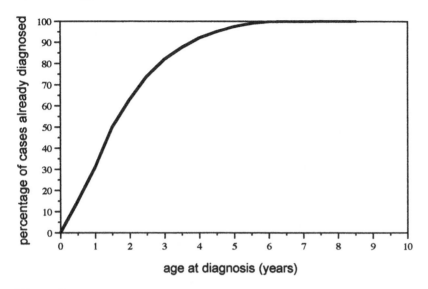

Figure 3 Graph showing percentage of cases already diagnosed as a function of age at diagnosis for newly diagnosed patients with retinoblastoma. Median age at diagnosis in group is approximately 18 months.

lateness of presentation of symptomatic patients to eye care professionals is reflected by the finding of a substantially higher proportion of patients with more advanced retinoblastoma at initial diagnosis in countries with a poorly developed health care delivery system for a substantial portion of their citizens [1].

B. Sex

Retinoblastoma affects males and females almost equally. Curves of cumulative percentage of cases already diagnosed versus age of the affected individual at initial diagnosis for males and females are virtually identical.

C. Race

Retinoblastoma occurs in all ethnic and racial groups. The cumulative lifetime incidence of the disease appears to be similar in all of these groups [16]. For reasons mentioned above, however, annual incidence curves and the exact positions of curves of the cumulative percentage of cases already diagnosed versus age of the affected individual at diagnosis for various racial groups may differ to some extent in different geographic locations.

D. Socioeconomic Group

Retinoblastoma appears to affect individuals in various socioeconomic groups equally. However, because patients of lower socioeconomic groups do not present as early on average for health care evaluations following onset of symptoms as do those from higher socioeconomic groups, the percentage of patients with more advanced forms of the disease at initial diagnosis and the median age at diagnosis both tend to be substantially higher among those of lower socioeconomic status [1].

E. Number of Eyes Affected

Retinoblastoma occurs in both unilateral and bilateral forms. In most large series, approximately 70% of cases are unilateral and 30% are bilateral. Most bilateral cases already exhibit bilateral ocular involvement when the disease is first detected, but occasional cases that are unilateral at initial diagnosis eventually become bilateral during follow-up [20]. Among individuals with unilateral retinoblastoma at initial diagnosis, the younger the child at the time of diagnosis, the higher the probability of subsequent conversion to bilaterality [23].

If one divides a group of patients with retinoblastoma into subgroups according to unilaterality or bilaterality of disease and then plots the cumulative percentage of cases already diagnosed as a function of age of the affected individual at initial diagnosis for each subgroup, one obtains curves similar to those shown in Figure 4. The data on which these curves are based again comes from the Retinoblastoma International Collaborative Study (RICS) [20]. Inspection of Figure 4 reveals a shift of the ascending limb of the curve of the bilateral cases to the left compared with the curve for unilateral cases. The median age at diagnosis of retinoblastoma in the RICS patients with bilateral ocular involvement was approximately 12 months, while that in the RICS patients with monocular ocular disease was approximately 24 months.

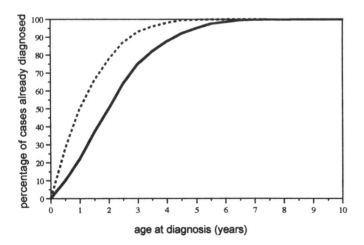

Figure 4 Graph showing percentage of cases already diagnosed as a function of age at diagnosis for patients with monocular retinoblastoma (solid line curve) and binocular retinoblastoma (dashed line curve). Median age at diagnosis is approximately 12 months for binocular cases and 24 months for monocular cases.

F. Number of Discrete Tumors

Retinoblastoma occurs in unifocal and multifocal forms in affected eyes. Individuals with bilateral disease have a much higher frequency of multifocal involvement in one or both eyes than do individuals with unilateral disease. Most persons with unilateral disease also have unifocal disease in the affected eye. In contrast, most persons with bilateral disease develop multifocal tumors in both eyes.

IV. RISK FACTORS FOR RETINOBLASTOMA

A risk factor is a feature or characteristic of persons in the general population that is strongly associated with a disease or condition of interest. Risk factors are generally identified by case-control studies in which the frequency of a feature or characteristic in individuals with the disease or condition of interest is compared with the frequency of the feature or characteristic in similar individuals without the disease or condition. Although risk factors are by definition strongly associated with the disease or condition of interest, they are not necessarily causative of the disease or condition.

Several risk factors for retinoblastoma have been identified over the years. These factors include a positive family history of retinoblastoma, deletion or inactivation of one allele of the retinoblastoma gene in somatic retinoblasts, advanced parental age at the time of an affected child's conception, and early-onset primitive neuroectodermal tumors in the pineal, suprasellar, or parasellar regions of the brain. Environmental factors such as intense sunlight exposure and ultraviolet light exposure have been linked by some investigators [24,25] but have not been confirmed by most researchers.

A. FAMILY HISTORY OF RETINOBLASTOMA

The risk of retinoblastoma is substantially increased if either of a child's parents had prior retinoblastoma [26]. The risk is most pronounced if the family member had bilateral disease, multifocal intraocular disease, or both. If one plots the cumulative percentage of cases already diagnosed versus age of the affected patient at the time of initial diagnosis for subjects with a positive versus negative family history of retinoblastoma, one obtains curves similar to those shown in Figure 5. Once again, these particular curves are based on data from the Retinoblastoma International Collaborative Study (RICS) [20]. Inspection of Figure 5 reveals that the median age at diagnosis in the patients with a positive family history of retinoblastoma was about 9 months, while that in the patients with a negative family history was approximately 1.7 years.

B. Loss or Inactivation of Retinoblastoma Gene in Somatic Cells

Whenever one allele of the retinoblastoma gene on the long arm of chromosome 13 is lost or inactivated in all somatic cells, the retinoblasts in the developing retina have a substantially increased risk of developing retinoblastoma by undergoing a deletion, translocation or other mutation of the remaining retinoblastoma gene allele.

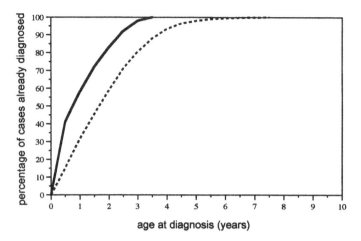

Figure 5 Graph showing percentage of cases already diagnosed as a function of age at diagnosis for patients with a positive family history of retinoblastoma (solid line curve) and a negative family history of retinoblastoma (dashed line curve). Median age at diagnosis is approximately 9 months for familial cases and 1.7 years for nonfamilial cases.

Estimates suggest that the average number of retinoblasts likely to undergo a spontaneous mutation of the intact retinoblastoma gene allele leading to retinoblastoma in the presence of loss or inactivation of one allele of the retinoblastoma gene in all somatic cells is approximately five to six per eye [27]. Methods of detection of such gene defects are described in Chapter 7.

    If a relatively major portion of the long arm of chromosome 13 is deleted from the either the sperm or the egg or does so in the early stages of development following fertilization, a child may be born with both a dysmorphic syndrome, the *chromosome 13q deletion syndrome* [28–30], and a predisposition to develop retinoblastoma. A spectrum of dysmorphic features can occur, the nature and severity of which appear related to the extent and location of the deletion. The most commonly reported dysmorphic features are prominent eyebrows, broad nasal bridge, bulbous tipped nose, large mouth, and a thin upper lip and long philtrum [30]. The recognized association between deletions of the long arm of chromosome 13 and retinoblastoma should remind ophthalmologists to recommend karyotype analysis whenever a dysmorphic syndrome is noted in a child with retinoblastoma and alert neonatalogists and pediatricians to request ophthalmic evaluation of any child with a dysmorphic syndrome associated with a deletion of the long arm of chromosome 13.

C.   Advanced Parental Age

The parents of children who develop sporadic hereditary retinoblastoma tend to be slightly but significantly older on average than parents of age and sex-matched children who do not develop this disease [31,32]. Some investigators have suggested that increased chromosomal fragility exists in older parents and such parents are therefore more likely to generate spermatocytes or oocytes having various chromosomal defects, including deletions or other defects that inactivate the retinoblastoma gene [32].

D. Early-Onset Primitive Neuroectodermal Intracranial Tumors

Development of a primitive neuroectodermal neoplasm in the pineal gland or in parasellar or suprasellar regions of the brain occasionally precedes development of intraocular retinoblastoma in children with hereditary disease. Because of this association, every child with an early onset primitive neuroectodermal tumor of the types mentioned above should probably be examined for retinoblastoma and followed as a retinoblastoma suspect. More information about such tumors is contained in the following section.

V. IMPORTANT EXTRAOPHTHALMIC LESIONS AND DISORDERS ASSOCIATED WITH RETINOBLASTOMA

A. Ectopic Intracranial Retinoblastoma

Ectopic intracranial retinoblastoma is a malignant central nervous system neoplasm that resembles intraocular retinoblastoma both histomorphologically and immuno-histochemically [33–35]. It arises either from the immature pineal gland, in which case it is termed *pineoblastoma*, or from ectopic suprasellar or parasellar rests of immature neuroectodermal tissue. This type of tumor is almost exclusively associated with germinal retinoblastoma. Because individuals with germinal retinoblastoma usually have bilateral ocular disease, the association of ectopic intracranial retinoblastoma with germinal retinoblastoma is commonly referred to as *trilateral retinoblastoma*. Approximately 6–10% of individuals with germinal retinoblastoma eventually develop trilateral retinoblastoma. If one evaluates a series of patients with trilateral retinoblastoma and plots the cumulative percentage of intraocular and ectopic intracranial retinoblastomas already diagnosed as a function of age at diagnosis of each form of this malignancy, one obtains a curve similar to that shown in Figure 6. Inspection of Figure 6 reveals that the median age at diagnosis of ectopic intracranial retinoblastoma in patients with germinal retinoblastoma is approximately 1.8 years. Note also that the median age at diagnosis of the intraocular retinoblastoma in these patients was only about 4.0 months.

In the majority of cases, ectopic intracranial retinoblastoma is diagnosed subsequent to detection and diagnosis of the intraocular tumors. In a metanalysis of reported cases of trilateral retinoblastoma, Kivela and coworkers [35] found a median interval between diagnosis of the retinal and central nervous system tumors of 21 months. However, the range was from 6 months prior to diagnosis of the retinal tumors to 141 months after diagnosis of the intraocular lesions.

The usual presenting symptoms of ectopic intracranial retinoblastoma (when the lesion is not detected at an asymptomatic stage by neuroimaging at the time of diagnosis of intraocular retinoblastoma) are somnolence, lethargy, vomiting, and failure to thrive. Older children may complain of headaches. In children with clinically apparent intraocular retinoblastoma, the finding of a pineal, suprasellar, or

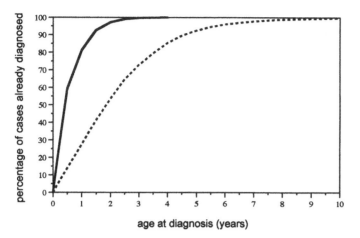

Figure 6   Graph showing percentage of cases of retinoblastoma (solid line curve) and ectopic intracranial retinoblastoma (dashed line curve) already diagnosed as a function of age at diagnosis for patients with trilateral retinoblastoma. Median age at diagnosis of retino-blastoma is about 4 months while that at diagnosis of ectopic intracranial retinoblastoma is about 1.8 years.

parasellar mass on central nervous system neuroimaging is usually considered sufficient for diagnosis of ectopic intracranial retinoblastoma. Lumbar puncture for cerebrospinal analysis and detection of malignant small round cells is indicated in such children to determine whether the ectopic intracranial retinoblastoma has been disseminated up and down the spinal cord within the cerebrospinal fluid. In contrast, in children without familial, bilateral, or multifocal intraocular retinoblastoma in whom the cerebrospinal fluid is negative for malignant cells, establishing the diagnosis of ectopic intracranial retinoblastoma generally entails neurosurgical biopsy of the mass. The survival prognosis for children with disseminated ectopic intracranial retinoblastoma via the cerebrospinal fluid is currently poor [35].

B. Second Primary Malignant Neoplasms

Survivors of germinal retinoblastoma have long been recognized to have a substantially increased risk of one or more extraophthalmic primary malignant neoplasms other than ectopic intracranial retinoblastoma [36–42]. These neoplasms are commonly referred to as *second primary tumors*. The most frequent of these neoplasms (in descending order, as identified by Moll and coworkers [37] in a large series of cases) are osteogenic sarcoma, various soft tissue sarcomas, and malignant melanomas of the skin. The cumulative incidence of a second primary malignant neoplasm of any type (excluding ectopic intracranial retinoblastoma) in survivors of germinal retinoblastoma, as estimated by Wong and coworkers [39], is shown in Figure 7. Inspection of this figure shows that the vast majority of second primary tumors develop in survivors of germinal retinoblastoma.

External-beam radiation therapy for retinoblastoma, especially if performed prior to the age of 6 months, appears to substantially increase the risk for a second

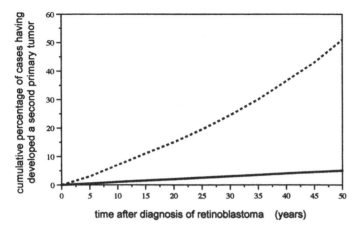

Figure 7   Cumulative incidence curves for second primary malignant neoplasms in patients with somatic retinoblastoma (solid line curve) and germinal retinoblastoma (dashed line curve). Cumulative incidence of second primary tumors is over 10 times as high in the germinal cases as in the somatic cases. The germinal case subgroup includes patients treated by external-beam radiation therapy for retinoblastoma early in life (see Fig. 8).

primary malignant neoplasm within the field of radiation. This effect is illustrated graphically in Figure 8. Inspection of this figure and comparison of the curve for unirradiated germinal retinoblastoma cases with that for somatic cases in Figure 7 reveals that the risk of second primary tumors is increased in germinal retinoblastoma by a factor of about 5. This added risk is attributable to the loss

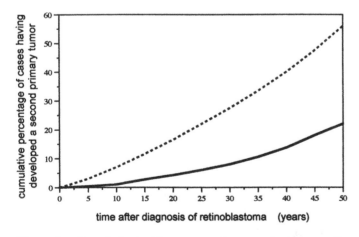

Figure 8   Cumulative incidence curves for second primary malignant neoplasms in survivors of germinal retinoblastoma if external-beam radiation therapy was employed as retinoblastoma treatment (dashed line curve) and if it was not (solid line curve). Cumulative incidence of second primary tumors in unirradiated germinal subgroup is about four times as high as the rate in the somatic cases (Fig. 7) but less than half the cumulative incidence in the irradiated germinal subgroup.

or inactivation of one allele of the retinoblastoma gene in virtually all somatic cells of such patients. Further inspection of Figure 8 shows that treatment by external-beam radiation therapy more than doubles the inherent added risk of second primary tumors in survivors of germinal retinoblastoma. This adverse effect of irradiation is less pronounced in children with germinal retinoblastoma treated after 6 months of age and appears to be extremely small in individuals with germinal retinoblastoma who underwent external-beam radiation therapy after the age of 1 year [41,42].

If one plots the percentage of retinoblastomas and second primary tumors already diagnosed as a function of age at diagnosis of the respective neoplasms in a group of retinoblastoma survivors who developed at least one second primary tumor, one obtains curves similar to those shown in Figure 9. These curves are based in part on data reported by Draper and coworkers [36]. Inspection of Figure 9 reveals that the curve for second primary tumors is displaced considerably to the right of that for retinoblastoma. The median age at diagnosis of retinoblastoma in this group of patients who developed a second primary tumor is approximately 1 year while that for initial diagnosis of a second primary tumor is about 15 years. Recent evidence suggests that retinoblastoma survivors who develop a second primary tumor and survive that tumor also have an extremely high risk of developing one or more subsequent second primary tumors.

The long-term impact of currently employed chemotherapy regimens for retinoblastoma on the cumulative incidence of second primary malignant neoplasms is unknown. This uncertainty is attributable to the fact that chemotherapy as primary treatment for germinal retinoblastoma only began to be used widely after the mid-1990s.

Although second primary tumors usually follow diagnosis, treatment, and eradication of retinoblastoma by months to years in survivors of germinal

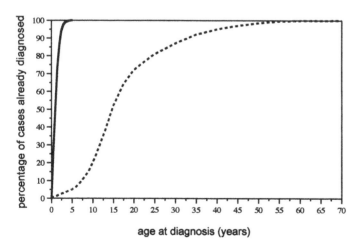

Figure 9   Graph showing percentage of cases of retinoblastoma (solid line curve) and second primary malignant neoplasm (dashed line curve) already diagnosed as a function of age at diagnosis in retinoblastoma survivors who developed at least one second primary tumor. Median age at diagnosis of retinoblastoma in this subgroup is about 1 year while that at diagnosis of the second primary tumor is about 15 years.

retinoblastoma, an occasional patient will present with an osteogenic or soft tissue sarcoma prior to detection of retinoblastoma. Because of its recognized association with germinal retinoblastoma, any person diagnosed with osteogenic or soft tissue sarcoma during the retinoblastoma-at-risk age period (birth to age 10 years) should probably be evaluated ophthalmologically to detect or rule out retinoblastoma.

REFERENCES

1. Erwenne CM, Franco EL. Age and lateness of referral as determinants of extraocular retinoblastoma. Ophthalm Paediatr Genet 10:179–184, 1989.
2. Tarkkanen A, Tuovinen E. Retinoblastoma in Finland 1912–1964. Acta Ophthalmol 49:293–300, 1971.
3. Horven I. Retinoblastoma in Norway. Acta Ophthalmol 123:103–109, 1973.
4. Devesa SS. The incidence of retinoblastoma. Am J Ophthalmol 80:263–265, 1975.
5. Freedman J, Goldberg L. Incidence of retinoblastoma in the Bantu of South Africa. Br J Ophthalmol 60:655–656, 1976.
6. Ben Ezra D, Chirambo MC. Incidence of retinoblastoma in Malawi. J Pediatr Ophthalmol 13:340–343, 1976.
7. O'Day J, Billson FA, Hoyt GS. Retinoblastoma in Victoria. Med J Aust 2:428–432, 1977.
8. Kock E, Naeser P. Retinoblastoma in Sweden 1958–1971. Acta Ophthalmol 57:344–350, 1979.
9. Pendergrass TW, Davis S. Incidence of retinoblastoma in the United States. Arch Ophthalmol 98:1204–1210, 1980.
10. Suckling RD. Fitzgerald PH, Stewart J, Wells E. The incidence and epidemiology of retinoblastoma in New Zealand: A 30-year survey. Br J Cancer 46:729–736, 1982.
11. Sanders BM, Draper GJ, Kingston JE. Retinoblastoma in Great Britain 1969–80: Incidence, treatment, and survival. Br J Ophthalmol 72:576–583, 1988.
12. Tamboli A, Podger MJ, Horm JW. The incidence of retinoblastoma in the United States: 1974 through 1985. Arch Ophthalmol 108:128–132, 1990.
13. Takano J, Akiyama K, Imamura N, Sakuma M, Amemiya T. Incidence of retinoblastoma in Nagasaki Prefecture, Japan. Ophthalmic Paediatr Genet 12:139–144, 1991.
14. Al-Idrissi I, Al-Kaff AS, Senft SH. Cumulative incidence of retinoblastoma in Riyadh, Saudi Arabia. Ophthalmic Paediatr Genet 13:9–12, 1992.
15. Gurney JG, Severson RK, Davis S, Robison LL. Incidence of cancer in children in the United States. Sex-, race- and 1-year age-specific rates by histologic type. Cancer 75:2186–2195, 1995.
16. Moll AC, Kuik DJ, Bouter LM, Den Otter W, Bezemer PD, Koten JW, Imhof SM, Kuyt BP, Tan KEWP. Incidence and survival of retinoblastoma in the Netherlands: A register based study 1862–1995. Br J Ophthalmol 81:559–562, 1997.
17. Wessels G, Hesseling PB. Incidence and frequency rates of childhood cancer in Namibia. S Afr Med J 87:885–889, 1997.
18. Kenney LB, Miller BA, Gloeckler Ries LA, Nicholson HS, Byrne J, Reaman GH. Increased incidence of cancer in infants in the US: 1980–1990. Cancer 82:1396–1400, 1998.
19. Saw SM, Tan N, Lee SB, Au Eong KG, Chia KS. Incidence and survival characteristics of retinoblastoma in Singapore from 1968–1995. J Paediatr Ophthalmol Strabismus 37:87–93, 2000.

20. Augsburger JJ, Oehlschlager U, Manzitti JE, RICS Group. Multinational clinical and pathologic registry of retinoblastoma. Retinoblastoma International Collaborative Study report 2. Graefes Arch Clin Exp Ophthalmol 233:469–475, 1995.

21. Salim A, Wiknjosastro GH, Danukusumo D, Barnas B, Zalud I. Fetal retinoblastoma. J Ultrasound Med 17:717–720, 1998.

22. Mietz H, Hutton WL, Font RL. Unilateral retinoblastoma in an adult. Report of a case and review of the literature. Ophthalmology 104:43–47, 1997.

23. Fontanesi J, Pratt C, Meyer D, Elverbig J, Parham D, Kaste S. Asynchronous bilateral retinoblastoma: The St. Jude Children's Research Hospital experience. Ophthalm Genet 16:109–112, 1995.

24. Hooper ML. Is sunlight an aetiological agent in the genesis of retinoblastoma? Br J Cancer 79:1273–1276, 1999.

25. Jemal A, Devesa SS, Fears TR, Fraumeni JF. Retinoblastoma incidence and sunlight exposure. Br J Cancer 82:1875–1878, 2000.

26. Memminki K, Mutanen P. Parental cancer as a risk factor for nine common childhood malignancies. Br J Cancer 84:990–993, 2001.

27. Lloyd RA, Papworth DG. Retinoblastoma: a model for deriving the mutation rate without using any estimate of the size of the population at risk. Mutat Res 326:117–124, 1995.

28. Seidman DJ, Shields JA, Augsburger JJ, Nelson LB, Lee ML, Sciorra LJ. Early diagnosis of retinoblastoma based on dysmorphic features and karyotype analysis. Ophthalmology 94:663–666, 1987.

29. Kennerknecht I, Barbi G, Greher J. Diagnosis of retinoblastoma in a presymptomatic stage after detection of interstitial chromosomal deletion 13q. Ophthalm Genet 15:19–24, 1994.

30. Baud O, Cormier-Daire V, Lyonnet S, Desjardins L, Turleau C, Doz F. Dysmorphic phenotype and neurological impairment in 22 retinoblastoma patients with constitutional cytogenetic 13q deletion. Clin Genet 55:478–482, 1999.

31. DerKinderen DJ, Koten JW, Pan KEWP, Beemer FA, Van Romunde LKJ, Den Otter W. Parental age in sporadic hereditary retinoblastoma. Am J Ophthalmol 110:605–609, 1990.

32. Moll AC, Imhof SM, Kuik DJ, Bouter LM, Den Otter W, Bezemer PD, Koten JW, Tan KEWP. High parental age is associated with sporadic hereditary retinoblastoma: The Dutch retinoblastoma register 1862–1994. Hum Genet 98:109–112, 1996.

33. Amoaku WMK, Willshaw HE, Parkes SE, Shah KJ, Mann JR. Trilateral retinoblastoma. A report of five patients. Cancer 78:858–863, 1996.

34. Paulino AC. Trilateral retinoblastoma. Is the location of the intracranial tumor important? Cancer 86:135–141, 1999.

35. Kivela T. Trilateral retinoblastoma: a meta-analysis of hereditary retinoblastoma associated with primary ectopic intracranial retinoblastoma. J Clin Oncol 17:1829–1837, 1999.

36. Draper GJ, Sanders BM, Kingston JE. Second primary neoplasms in patients with retinoblastoma. Br J Cancer 53:661–671, 1986.

37. Moll AC, Imhof SM, Bouter LM, Kuik DJ, Den Otter W, Bezemer PD, Koten JW, Tan KEWP. Second primary tumors in patients with hereditary retinoblastoma: A register-based follow-up study, 1945–1994. Int J Cancer 67:515–519, 1996.

38. Moll AC, Imhof SM, Bouter LM, Tan KEWP. Second primary tumors in patients with retinoblastoma. A review of the literature. Ophthalm Genet 18:27–34, 1997.

39. Wong FL, Boice JD, Abrahamson DH, Tarone RE, Kleinerman RA, Stovall M, Goldman MB, Seddon JM, Tarbell N, Fraumeni JF, Li FP. Cancer incidence after retinoblastoma. Radiation dose and sarcoma risk. JAMA 278:1262–1267, 1997.

40. Mohney BG, Robertson DM, Schomberg PJ, Hodge DO. Second nonocular tumors in survivors of heritable retinoblastoma and prior radiation therapy. Am J Ophthalmol 126:269–277, 1998.
41. Abramson DH, Frank CM. Second nonocular tumors in survivors of bilateral retinoblastoma: A possible age effect on radiation-related risk. Ophthalmology 105:573–580, 1998.
42. Moll AC, Imhof SM, Schouten-Van Meeteren AYN, Kuik DJ, Hofman P, Boers M. Second primary tumors in hereditary retinoblastoma: a register-based study, 1945–1997. Is there an age effect on radiation-related risk? Ophthalmology 108:1109–1114, 2001.

5

Genetics of Uveal Melanoma: Chromosomal Rearrangements and the Identification of Genes Involved in Tumorigenesis

KAREN SISLEY and IAN G. RENNIE

University of Sheffield, Sheffield, England

I. BACKGROUND

The study of chromosome abnormalities in tumors, otherwise known as cytogenetics, has played an effective and valuable role in improving our understanding of how cancers develop and progress. Chromosome analysis allows assessment of genetic alterations on a genomewide basis and—besides indicating losses and gains—provides information on structural rearrangements, including translocations and other aberrations, which, although resulting in no net loss or gain of genetic material, produce an unnatural juxtaposition of genes. Following the identification of the first chromosome abnormality associated with cancer, the Philadelphia chromosome in chronic myeloid leukaemia [1], many other changes have been also detailed in hematological malignancies, and found to be clinically relevant, to both diagnosis and prognosis [2]. Analysis of solid tumors for the most part tended to be a rather unfruitful exercise, as technically these tumors were difficult to work with and chromosomal abnormalities could be extensive and complex. Only in the last decade has our knowledge of the chromosome changes in solid tumors improved, in part because of an increase in the number of studies performed but also because of the introduction of new and powerful techniques [3]. Posterior uveal melanomas are a notable exception to the problems associated with the cytogenetic analysis of the majority of solid tumors. These ocular melanomas readily establish as short-term cultures and have consistent chromosomal alterations without the complexity and heterogeneity often experienced with most solid tumors. Such advantages have allowed an exponential growth in our knowledge of the relevant and specific changes associated with these primary eye tumors.

II. CYTOGENETIC STUDIES OF UVEAL MELANOMA

At the beginning of the last decade, five studies totaling 22 cases had reported observations on the chromosomal changes found in posterior uveal melanomas [4–8]. Even at this early stage a consistent pattern of chromosomal involvement began to emerge, with changes of chromosomes 1, 3, 6, 8, and the Y chromosome repeatedly found [6–8]. The simplest alterations in uveal melanoma are losses or gains of entire chromosomes. In the majority of tumors from male patients the Y chromosome is lost; but for both sexes, the commonest change, found in approximately 50% of posterior uveal melanomas, is the loss of one copy of chromosome 3 (monosomy 3). In most instances tumors with monosomy 3 were also found to have changes of chromosome 8, which effectively produced gain of material from the long arm of chromosome 8 (8q). There is now strong evidence to indicate that these alterations are associated and define a subsection of uveal melanomas [8–15]. Changes of chromosomes 1 and 6, although less frequent, seem equally important. For the most part they are present as structural alterations, which produce deletions of the short arm of chromosome 1 (1p), deletions of the long arm of chromosome 6 (6q), and gain of the short arm of chromosome 6 (6p). The aforementioned chromosomal alterations are not necessarily important to all uveal melanomas, and evidence suggests that melanomas of the anterior uvea, affecting the iris, may possess entirely different chromosomal alterations [16,17]. Iris melanomas are relatively benign in comparison to posterior uveal melanomas; it is possible that the distribution of chromosomal changes found in uveal melanoma contribute to these phenotypic differences.

Currently chromosomal studies in over 200 cases of posterior uveal melanomas have been detailed. Simple cytogenetic analysis of chromosomal changes has been increasingly supported by fluorescence in situ hybridization (FISH), comparative genomic hybridization (CGH), spectral karyotyping (SKY), and microsatellite analysis (MSA) [15,18–21]. In combination, these studies have confirmed the nonrandom involvement of these chromosomes with primary uveal melanoma and have began to delineate other less common alterations that may also have a direct bearing on the pathogenesis of these melanomas.

A. Monosomy 3 and Isochromosome 8q

The high frequency with which monosomy 3 is found in posterior uveal melanomas would seemingly implicate this change in the malignant transformation of the uveal melanocyte. It is also of interest that, at least at the level of cytogenetics, an entire copy of chromosome 3 appears to be deleted, and there is a virtual absence of chromosome 3 rearrangements. There is also little heterogeneity for monosomy 3; when present, for the majority of cases, it is so within all abnormal cells of the tumor population analyzed. Occasionally monosomy 3 also appears to be the only visible chromosomal alteration in some tumors; the evidence therefore suggests that this alteration is one of the earlier predisposing changes associated with uveal melanoma initiation and that other chromosome alterations subsequently follow [22–24]. Clearly related to the alterations of chromosome 3 are the gains of 8q, specifically in the form of an isochromosome in which both arms of the chromosome are derived for the most part, from the q arm of chromosome 8. The presence of these abnormalities together is much more frequent in melanomas involving the ciliary body (Fig. 1). However, the changes themselves are not exclusive to this location and are also found in choroidal melanomas, although usually not occurring together [8–15]. Just as the involvement of chromosome 3 is quite specific in uveal melanoma, occurring as it does in the form of monosomy, the abnormalities of chromosome 8 are equally reproducible, resulting in gain of almost the entire q arm. In some uveal melanomas, the amplification occurs in its simplest form as a straightforward gain of an entire chromosome 8 [14,24], but there is a progressive trend toward increasing amplification of 8q. The sequence of events appears to be as follows: chromosome 8 gain, followed by the development of an isochromosome 8q (or other form of amplification), finally culminating in the accumulation of multiple copies of i(8)(q10). In some individual tumors, sublines coexist demonstrating all phases, while other chromosomal abnormalities are maintained stably within all sublines

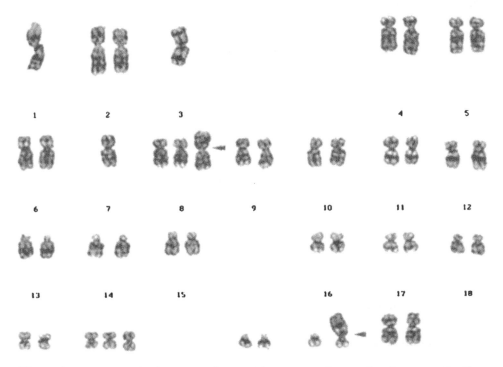

Figure 1 Representative karyotype from a primary posterior uveal melanoma with ciliary body involvement. Characteristic presence of monosomy 3 and i(8)(q10), also present, is an unbalanced translocation of chromosome 1, producing a deletion of the short arm. Structural abnormalities are indicated by arrows. 45,XX,-1,-3,-7,+i(8)(q10),+20,der(22)t(1;22) (p12;p11)

[13,22,24]. Loss of chromosome 3 arises prior to 8q amplification, and abnormalities of 8 are thought to be secondary chromosome changes associated with clonal evolution [6,18,19,22]. Indeed, in a total of eight metastatic lesions of uveal melanoma so far reported, all demonstrated abnormalities of chromosome 8 but not always monosomy 3 [4,25,26], suggesting that changes in chromosome 8 may be more important in the generation of a metastatic phenotype.

The association of certain chromosomal changes with clinical features established as prognostic parameters raised the possibility that chromosomal abnormalities themselves may correlate directly with the prognosis of uveal melanomas—a situation that is perhaps unparalleled in other adult solid tumors. In particular, monosomy 3 and 8q were found to be mainly correlated with ciliary body melanomas [8,10–12], and recent evidence suggests that these changes are also related to an epithelioid cell type [27]. Both of these factors are considered to be indicators of a poor prognosis [28]. The first chromosomal abnormality to be directly correlated to prognosis was also the most frequent—namely, monosomy 3. In this first report, by Prescher and coworkers, all patients with normal copies of chromosome 3 ($n = 24$) survived 3 years after diagnosis, whereas only 57% of those patients with monosomy 3 ($n = 30$) survived the same interval [15]. Loss of chromosome 3 was therefore suggested to correlate strongly with a poor prognosis of the patient. Following this initial report, the importance of monosomy 3 was again confirmed by a later study [18]. In addition, this later investigation also correlated extra copies of 8q with poor survival, suggesting a possible dosage effect, whereby increased amplification of 8q correlated with a reduced survival and a reduced disease-free interval [18]. White and associates again linked changes of both chromosomes 3 and 8 with poor prognosis, but they were predictive only when found together [29]. Besides cytogenetics, other techniques have also been employed to establish chromosomal abnormalities as prognostic indicators in uveal melanoma. CGH analysis contributed to the results of the first study associating chromosome alterations with prognosis [15]; of late, FISH in particular has been increasingly used. Initially, McNamara and associates used FISH to assess chromosome 3 copy number, but prognosis was not assessed [30]. More recently, Patel and associates applied FISH to determine the relative imbalance in copy numbers of chromosomes 3 and 8 and correlated these to patient survival [31]. An imbalance in chromosome 3 and 8 copy number was shown to significantly correlate with patient survival over a minimum follow-up of 9 years [31]. Only those patients with a genetic imbalance for chromosomes 3 and 8 died from metastatic disease, with the median survival being 37 months; while for the group with no abnormalities, median survival was 114 months [31]. In combination, the evidence from these studies suggests that monosomy 3 alone or when considered with amplification of 8q is a highly reliable indicator of prognosis.

B. Chromosome 6

Chromosome 6 abnormalities are perhaps some of the earliest changes to be associated with posterior uveal melanoma, and appear to be among the most consistent cytogenetic alterations in these tumors. Although both arms of the chromosome are affected, producing deletions of 6q and gains of 6p (Fig. 2), these changes can occur independently and, unlike monosomy 3, they appear to arise as a

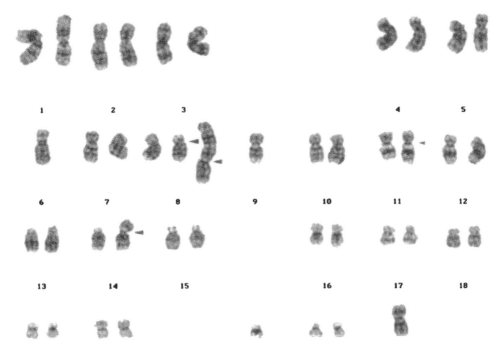

Figure 2 Representative karyotype from a primary posterior uveal melanoma. No obvious deletions of chromosome 3 are present, but an 8p deletion is present, and an additional large derivative chromosome 8. Also seen is involvement of band 11q23 and loss of 6q, resulting from an unbalanced translocation. Chromosomal painting confirmed that the large derivative chromosome 8 was almost entirely composed of additional chromosome 8 material. Small rearrangements of chromosome 3 appeared to be absent. 43,X-Y,-6,add(8)(p21), +add(8)(p23),-9,add(11)(q23),der(14)t(6;14)(p21;p11),-21

result of more complex mechanistic structural alterations. Needless to say, they are often present in the form of an isochromosome of the short arm, i(6)(p10); therefore, assuming that change is not additional, they encompass both the deletion of the long arm and the gain of the short arm in a single alteration [7,12,24]. Using CGH, isochromosome formation, whether of chromosome 1, 6, or 8, has been suggested to be more often associated with the presence of monosomy 3 [26], and certainly cytogenetic studies confirm that chromosome 3 loss and i(6)(p10) do occur together [7,12,24]. Paradoxically, an alternative pathway has also been suggested, one in which loss of chromosome 3 and the gain of 6p are mutually exclusive [19]. This apparent contradiction may be explained through the work of Tschentscher and associates, who used MSA to investigate chromosomal changes [32]. The study was able in part to confirm the mutual exclusivity of monosomy 3 and 6p gain [32], finding that their occurrence together was much less frequent, occurring in only 1 of 13 tumors [32]. It would appear that 6p alterations are infrequent in tumors with monosomy 3, and it is possible that two distinct pathways exist [19].

Equally confusing is the potential association between chromosome 6 and prognosis, unlike those changes of chromosomes 3 and 8, which are indicators of poor outcome. One study has shown that rearrangements of chromosome 6 predict better survival [29]. This effect appears to be maintained even in the presence of monosomy 3 and additional copies of 8q [29], but the relationship is complex, and it is unclear whether it is the overrepresentation of 6p or a loss of 6q that actually produces the association. The involvement of chromosome 6 changes in uveal melanoma seems at best to be contradictory. It is possible that by attempting to make comparisons between studies in which essentially different techniques are used—cytogenetics, FISH and MSA—a distortion of results may arise, providing contrary observations which, with continued study, may be resolved [32]. If two distinct pathways of genetic change do exist in uveal melanomas, one defined by monosomy 3 and i(8q) and indicting poor survival and the other by 6p gain, it would seem entirely plausible that 6p may under these circumstances give rise to an indication of favorable prognosis, thus leaving only those tumors in which visible changes of both chromosomes 3 and 6 occur together to be explained.

C. Chromosome 1

Changes in chromosome 1 are less frequent than those of 3, 6, and 8 but nevertheless are found in approximately 30% of all uveal melanomas [7,12,19,24,33]. Abnormalities mainly involve rearrangements or deletions of 1p, and the changes are comparable to those found in cutaneous melanomas, where distal alterations of 1p are one of the commonest changes, found in about 80% of cases [3,34]. Ciliary body melanomas tend to have more cytogenetic abnormalities of chromosome 1 than tumors arising from other parts of the uveal tract [7,12,24,33]. In cutaneous melanoma, rearrangements or deletions of 1p are thought to relate to tumor progression [7,35]. It is possible that a comparable situation exists in uveal melanoma, since deletions of 1p are less frequent than those of chromosomes 3 and 8 and may therefore be subsequent to these changes. In addition, a higher incidence of 1p rearrangements are reported in larger melanomas [24], and recent data have indicated that loss of chromosome 1p is present only in primary uveal melanoma that had metastasized and in metastases themselves [26]. It would seem likely that rearrangements of chromosome 1 are indicative of more advanced melanomas, suggesting that chromosome 1 is the location of a uveal melanoma metastatic suppressor gene or genes [26]. As changes in chromosome 1 have been directly correlated with aggressive uveal melanomas, it would be reasonable to anticipate that they may prove to be reliable indicators of poor prognosis, but confirmation is required by further study.

D. Other Chromosome Changes

As tumors progress, they appear to acquire more chromosomal abnormalities, and although uveal melanomas typically have relatively few chromosomal changes, they too show a correlation between additional chromosomal losses and gains and increasing tumor size, suggesting that such numerical alterations are random [24]. Some of these other changes, however, may be more specifically related, in particular those abnormalities producing structural rearrangements; evidence suggests that chromosomes 9, 10, 11, 21, and Y may be of more direct importance to uveal melanomas [7,11–14,24,33,36,37]. Most of these other alterations tend to occur in a limited number of cases, but the loss of the Y chromosome affects the majority of male patients. The involvement of the Y chromosome is a little ambiguous, and could be artifactual, related to patient age or cultural conditions. Conversely, as loss of the Y chromosome is not a frequent event in corresponding blood from patients, and given that its occurrence is mainly associated with the presence of other abnormalities [13,29,38], (unpublished data, Sheffield 2001), an as yet undetermined role, possibly related to tumor progression, has been postulated [7,12]. The gain of chromosome 21 appears to be secondary to those of other chromosomes including 3, 6 and 8, and as such is also speculated to be associated with tumour progression [24]. Melanomas with involvement of chromosomes 3 and 8 seemingly have higher incidences of trisomy 21, and as a consequence, the change is more frequent in melanomas with ciliary body involvement [7,11–14,24,33].

Chromosomal abnormalities of 9, 10, and 11 may indicate a degree of commonality between uveal and cutaneous melanoma, as nonrandom alterations of these chromosomes are found in cutaneous melanoma, but at a much higher frequency than that observed in uveal melanoma [39]. Comparable regions appear to be targeted in both forms of melanoma [7,11–14,24,33], but less is known about the role such changes may have in uveal melanoma and few associations have been drawn. Chromosomal analysis suggests that changes of chromosome 9 are present in only approximately 10% of cases, but this frequency includes abnormalities of both 9p and 9q, indicating that the incidence for rearrangements of each arm is actually much less [12–14,24,33,37]. In cutaneous melanoma, 9p appears the preferential target; in uveal melanoma, using techniques other than cytogenetics, slightly higher incidences have been recorded of approximately 20% for imbalances of 9p with MSA [19]. CGH studies have also indicated more involvement for 9p alteration, but they are contradictory, identifying both increased loss and gain for the region [40,41]. The role, and the true incidence of chromosome 9 abnormalities in uveal melanoma, has yet to be clarified, but the change may identify a shared inheritance with cutaneous melanoma, at least in some uveal melanomas.

Cytogenetic studies have also reported incidences of around 10% for deletions and rearrangements of 10q in uveal melanoma [12,14,24,41]. A much higher frequency is reported for cutaneous melanoma, and specific regions of 10q have been implicated [42]. In uveal melanoma however, the association is more tenuous, and because of the limited number of cases with such abnormalities, the specific region of 10q affected, and the implication, has yet to be defined. Stronger evidence exists for the changes affecting chromosome 11 in ocular melanoma, which are found in approximately 20% of reported cases [7,11–14,24,33]. In the majority of cases, these rearrangements are highly specific, targeting the regions 11p15 or 11q23-q25 [7,24] (Figs. 2 and 3). A comparable region of 11q is seemingly implicated in the cutaneous counterpart, where it is speculated to be associated with poor prognosis [43]. Insufficient evidence exists to draw similar conclusions in uveal melanoma. It is, however, possible that an opposite relationship may occur than that seen in the cutaneous form, since these changes are slightly more common among melanomas with choroidal involvement and or tumors of a spindle morphology; as such, they may correlate with a better prognosis [12,14,24,41].

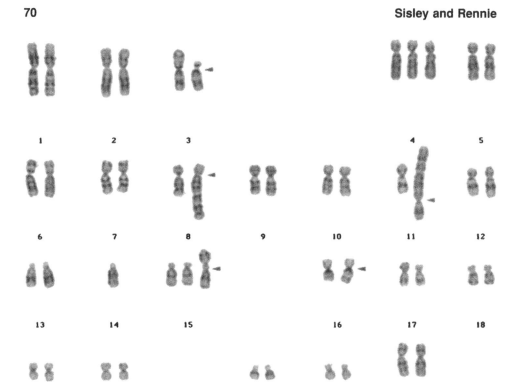

Figure 3 Representative karyotype from a primary posterior uveal melanoma. Structural rearrangements of chromosomes 3, 8, 11, 15, and 16 are present, as indicated by arrows, producing loss of 3p and gain of 8. Chromosome painting using FISH was used to confirm the partial involvement of chromosome 8 in both the derivative chromosomes 8 and 11.   47,XX,add(3)(p12–13),+4,add(8)(q24),add(11)(p15),-14,+add(15)(p11),der(16)t(6;16)(p21;q13)

E. The Future of Uveal Melanoma Cytogenetics

Abnormalities of all chromosomes have been reported in uveal melanoma. In some instances, associations have been made, but subsequent study has so far failed to substantiate such relationships. Until additional information is gained, it will not be possible to establish if these other abnormalities are of relevance or occur as a result of increasing instability associated with tumor progression. Cytogenetic analysis has played a valuable role in increasing our understanding of the genetic changes in uveal melanoma, allowing clear relationships between certain chromosome changes and prognosis to be determined. As more information accumulates, it is likely the involvement of other less common alterations will be further defined; in this respect cytogenetics still has much to offer. In addition, the correlation of certain chromosomal changes with prognosis, in particular chromosome 3, would suggest that cytogenetic analysis is a reliable and practicable method for determining prognosis in many uveal melanomas. The use of procedures such as FISH and MSA could, however, provide a valuable alternative, as they require smaller amounts of tumor material, and viability is not essential. With these techniques the procedure could be adapted to the assessment of small in situ lesions using fine-needle aspiration biopsies (FNAB). Despite sampling only a small portion of the lesion, chromosome analysis is feasible on these biopsies and results are apparently comparable to the bulk of the lesion [44]. Both FISH and MSA are suitable techniques to determine the prognostic significance of certain chromosomal abnormalities in uveal melanoma and could theoretically provide results in 100% of cases, as the need for culturing is abrogated [31]. Assessment of chromosomal changes may in the future become part of the standard practices applied to every uveal melanoma. As our knowledge of the relevant genetic alterations increases, additional potentially moderating chromosomal changes may also be identified. Ultimately the future lies in the detection of the underlying genetic alterations that form the basis of the visible chromosomal rearrangements. Only by identifying the genes responsible for uveal melanoma development can we develop new strategies designed to combat their influence.

III. THE IDENTIFICATION OF GENES INVOLVED IN UVEAL MELANOMA TUMORIGENESIS

To date, most reports of the genetic abnormalities associated with uveal melanoma have detailed the chromosomal alterations, mainly by cytogenetics but also by CGH. Fewer studies have attempted to establish the genes responsible for uveal melanoma initiation and progression. For the most part, the chromosomal regions implicated are large, representing as they do either entire chromosomes or chromosome arms; at best, the rearrangements still involve large chromosomal regions, which could encompass many biologically relevant genes. Equally important is the type of abnormality produced. In broad terms changes which result in a loss of genetic material, can be considered to target genes with a suppressive function, or so called *tumor suppressor genes*. Conversely, areas where amplification of regions has occurred may suggest the input of positive regulators of the process, otherwise termed *oncogenes*, which in some manner enhance uveal melanoma development and progression. Determining which are the candidate genes is a daunting task when such large regions are implicated. Cytogenetic analysis can most readily assist in the identification of relevant genes by implementing a more targeted research through the discovery of structural rearrangements and thus minimizing the chromosomal region where relevant genes may reside.

A. Chromosome 3

The most consistent genetic alteration of uveal melanoma is a case in point. It is rather perplexing that uveal melanomas can, broadly speaking, be divided into those tumors where monosomy of chromosome 3 is found and those where ostensibly two normal copies of chromosome 3 are present. This chromosome is only infrequently involved in structural abnormalities in uveal melanoma; in a series of over 100 tumors, only 4 cases actually had visible rearrangements of chromosome 3 (unpublished data, Sheffield 2001). Both arms were affected, and miscellaneous breakpoints were found, 3p24–25, 3p12–13, 3q13, and 3q21 (Fig. 2). Reports in the literature also indicate an equally diverse range, with the smallest regions of involvement shown to be at 3p25, 3p13, 3q13–21, and 3q24–26 [20,21,45]. Numerous cancer-related genes are located on chromosome 3 [46]. The virtual absence in uveal melanoma of structural rearrangements of this chromosome implies that its entire loss represents the most efficacious way to target multiple genes resident on a single chromosome [21]. The frequency with which this change occurs would suggest that it plays a pivotal role in the tumorigenesis of at least some uveal melanomas. Whether all uveal melanomas actually have small nonvisible deletions of chromosome 3 is unclear, but it is known that even apparently normal copies of chromosome 3 can harbor small deletions [21]. In extreme cases, isodisomy has been reported, where one copy of chromosome 3 is lost and the remaining homologue, presumably with all its deficiencies, is duplicated [47]. It is even possible that in uveal melanomas two pathways exist to target genes on chromosome 3. In the first, most of the relevant genes would effectively receive one "hit" by the loss of one entire copy, as seen with monosomy. In the second pathway, a more considered approach is taken, in which relevant genes are specifically targeted by nonvisible alterations or are the subject of structural rearrangements. From this point onwards it would seem that both pathways equally require the input of genes on chromosome 8; but, again, this may be effected by amplification of 8q in its entirety or through partial amplification. Seemingly a more conservative approach targeting genes on chromosome 3 gives rise to a similar approach to amplification of genes on 8q (Figs. 2 and 3), and several reports exist in the literature to support this theory [3].

In uveal melanoma, however, the relevant genes on chromosome 3 await identification, although recent evidence implicates one potential candidate gene, the *TGF-βR2* gene. Breakpoints and loss of heterozygosity (LOH) of the region containing the gene, at 3p21–22, have been reported in uveal melanoma [48], while TGF-β itself has been shown to regulate uveal melanoma proliferation negatively [48]. Many other potentially relevant genes await exploration, including genes related to cellular divisional control and longevity, such as hereditary nonpolyposis type 2 (*MLH1*) at 3p23-p21.3, and the telomerase RNA component (*TERC*) (hTR), located at 3q21-q28 [46]. Indeed, *TERC* may be of particular interest as it has the potential to regulate negatively telomerase activity, which is known to be upregulated in uveal melanomas, potentially contributing to avoidance of both cell senescence and death [46,49–51]. Other potential candidate genes, including Von Hippel Lindau (*VHL*) and thyroid hormone receptor β (*THRB*) genes, have recently been eliminated by more detailed molecular investigations, in which losses of markers on both arms of chromosomes 3 were assessed [21,47].

B. Chromosome 8

A comparable situation exists for the identification of relevant genes on chromosome 8, since in the majority of cases the entire long arm is affected. In this instance, however, amplification of genes, rather than loss, is the net result. These amplifications are predominantly in the form of an isochromosome in which both arms of the chromosome are derived from the long arm of chromosome 8, effecting a deletion of the short arm; thus gene loss on 8p may also be important. A comparable situation is found in some of the more common solid malignancies—such as breast and prostate, where potential candidate genes have been investigated—and may also be a feature in uveal melanoma development [52]. For 8q, cytogenetic studies in combination with CGH have defined the smallest region of amplification as 8q21-

qter [7,33,41]. More recently, studies using a combination of SKY and CGH, have found that in actuality two distinct regions of 8q may be specifically amplified, at 8q21.1–21.2 and again at 8q23–24 [20]. At present we can only speculate as to which genes in uveal melanoma may be the targets of such amplifications, as many genes of potential importance in biological processes associated with cancer are located on this chromosome. Included are some genes related to its potential role in the development of more advanced uveal melanoma, such as degradative enzymes and cell adhesion molecules [46], but as yet no evidence exists for their involvement in uveal melanoma. A clear candidate does, however, exist, the *myc* oncogene, which has diverse effects on cellular proliferation, and is located at 8q24, therefore falling within the second region identified by Naus and associates (20). Whether *myc* is the preferred target, or is coamplified because of its proximity to an otherwise unknown gene, remains to be established. Evidence does suggest that *myc* has some role to play in uveal melanoma tumorigenesis, as at least 30% of tumors appear to have specific amplification of *myc*, with the gain itself occurring later in the genetic progression [53]. If *myc* is the potential target, its ultimate effect appears to be contradictory, since expression is consistently associated with a good outcome [54–56]. Ultimately refining regional involvement on 8q will greatly assist in the hunt for the relevant amplified genes.

C. Chromosome 6

Essentially, cytogenetic changes of chromosome 6 would imply the contribution of two sets of genes; deletions of 6q would seemingly target negative regulators of the process, while the amplification of 6p would suggest the input of genes that enhance tumorigenesis. The situation may ultimately become more complex if the role of chromosome 6 as a moderating change is established. Breakpoints of 6p are consistently located toward the centromeric region, with the smallest regional gain established as 6pter-p21 [41], but on 6q they can be quite diverse, and often the whole arm is deleted through the formation of an isochromosome [7,12,24]. All uveal melanomas, including iris tumors, and more importantly cutaneous melanoma, appear to have comparable alterations of chromosome 6, suggesting the involvement of a common series of genes integral to melanocytic transformation [3,16,17,24]. Because of the nature of chromosome 6 rearrangements in uveal melanoma, again affecting both arms, it seems likely that numerous genes are important. In uveal melanoma there are several potential targets genes located in the region 6pter-p21; these include genes such as *CDKN1A* and *VEGF*, among whose functions are cell cycle control and angiogenesis [41,57,58]. The immunology of these melanomas could also be severely altered; as the genes encoding MHC class I molecules and TNF-α are also localized to this region [46]. Altered HLA expression in uveal melanoma is known; however, no clear relationship has been established with 6p abnormalities [59].

Potentially, at least two regions may be selectively deleted on 6q, but identifying the smallest regional involvement is hampered by the manner of rearrangements, which tend to produce loss from the breakpoint onward, rather than small interstitial deletions [7,12,–14,24,33,40]. Nevertheless, there appears to be a reasonably clear-cut distal deletion affecting 6q24-q27, but other breakpoints imply a second region at 6q13-q15, with potentially a third region at 6q21-q22 [7,12–

14,24,33,40]. Similar regions have been implicated in cutaneous melanoma, and it is entirely possible that the same panel of genes also has a functional role in uveal melanoma development. Much work still remains to be done regarding chromosome 6 in uveal melanoma. It is highly likely that aberrations of 6q in particular are far more complex than initially thought, but with the use of additional techniques such as SKY, the regions typically involved on 6q will be refined [20].

D. Chromosome 1

Although gain of 1q is occasionally found in uveal melanoma, in most instances deletions of 1p are the relevant alteration, either as loss of defined regions or as the result of unbalanced translocations in which the entire short arm is absent [7,12,24] (Fig. 1). These translocation events follow a specific pattern, and the recipient partner for 1q is often a member of the D group of chromosomes. Heterochromatic regions are heavily implicated in these transactions, and the presence of breakpoints in these regions may highlight the inherent weakness of highly repetitive DNA [7,12,24]. Other breakpoints, spanning a region of 1p12-p36, are reported, but a smallest regional involvement at 1p32-p36 has been established [7,12,24,33]. This more distal region appears different to a region identified by Aalto and associates [26], and it is likely that, as with other chromosomal changes in uveal melanoma, more than one gene is implicated by these rearrangements. Again, genes postulated to be involved in the cutaneous form could also be heavily implicated in uveal melanoma. In the cutaneous form, for example, deletions of a gene encoding a protein kinase isoform (*CDC2L*) located to 1p36, are found [60] and could potentially represent the target of the smallest regional involvement so far identified by cytogenetics [7,12,24,33].

E. Other Chromosomes Implicated in Uveal Melanoma

The gene targets of other chromosomal changes in uveal melanoma could again imply the input of genes involved in the pathogenesis of its cutaneous counterpart. Clear comparisons are provided by the comparable changes of chromosomes 9, 10, and 11 found in the two melanocytic malignancies. Deletions of chromosome 9 are considered to be an early event in the pathogenesis of cutaneous melanoma and target a familial melanoma susceptibility gene, p16, or *CDKN2/MTS-1/INK4A*, which is located at 9p21 [61,62]. In uveal melanoma, deletion of the p16 gene is rare [63]; inactivation is mainly thought to arise by other mechanisms, including altered methylation status and mutations, which have been identified in about 30% of uveal melanomas [64,65]. Inactivation of p16 appears to be a more important event in uveal melanoma tumorigenesis than might initially be thought on the basis of cytogenetic studies alone; it is possible that, as in cutaneous melanoma, it is a relatively early event. Similar importance may ultimately be attributed to the role of other chromosomal changes shared by both forms of melanoma. Currently, however, the targets on chromosome 10 appear to be different in the two forms of this malignancy, as the *PTEN* gene at 10q23 is implicated in cutaneous melanoma [66], but no mutations or deletions have been identified in uveal melanoma cell lines [67]. Finally, little is known about the target genes on chromosome 11 relevant for melanomas, but it is possible that genes implicated in other solid malignancies, at 11q23, could be the targets [68].

Increasingly more detailed investigation of the relevant chromosomal changes in uveal melanoma is being undertaken, and it is to be anticipated that the culprit genes cannot remain hidden for much longer.

IV. SUMMARY

In the last decade our knowledge of the genetic changes related to uveal melanoma tumorigenesis has increased exponentially, but it is apparent that we have much more to learn. Clearly, in uveal melanoma sequential chromosome changes are present, with alterations of chromosome 3 and 6 occurring earlier to those of 1, 8, and 21. As yet, it is not known if any of these changes are responsible for initiating uveal melanoma pathogenesis or whether otherwise undetected abnormalities instigate the transformation. Certainly the few MSA studies so far undertaken suggest that much higher levels of genetic changes exist than originally suggested by cytogenetic studies. It is therefore possible that an undisclosed succession of discreet submicroscopic events is responsible for uveal melanoma tumorigenesis. The search for the underlying genetic defects has begun in earnest, and with the increasing application of techniques such as FISH, CGH, SKY, and MSA and the continued input of cytogenetics, we have the potential to more fully refine and characterize regional chromosomal involvement. The clinical relevance of the established chromosomes changes, specifically monosomy 3, is now apparent; for uveal melanoma genetics, such studies have come of age. The potential exists to make real improvements in our understanding of the development of these melanomas, with the associated benefits that this may provide.

ACKNOWLEDGMENTS

We would like to express our gratitude to Yorkshire Cancer Research, Trent Regional Health Authority, and the Medical Research Council for support. Our thanks to the contributions made to studies by Mr. Kirtikbhai A. Patel, Mr. Neil Cross, Ms. Nicola Tattersall, and to Mr. Robin Farr for graphics.

REFERENCES

1. Nowell PC, Hungerford DA. A minute chromosome in human chronic granulocytic leukaemia. Science 132:1497, 1960.
2. Sandberg AA, Chen Z. Cancer cytogenetics and molecular genetics—Clinical implications (review). Int J Oncol 7:1241–1251, 1995.
3. Mitelman F, Johansson B, Merten F, eds. Mitelman Database of Chromosome Abberrations in Cancer. The Cancer Genome Anatomy Project. http://cgap.nci.nih.gov/Chromosomes/Mitelman 2001.
4. Rey JA, Bello MJ, DeCompos JM, Ramos MC, Benitez J. Cytogenetic findings in a human malignant melanoma metastatic to the brain. Cancer Genet Cytogenet 16:179–183, 1985.

5. Griffin CA, Long PP, Schachat AP. Trisomy 6p in an ocular melanoma. Cancer Genet Cytogenet 32:129–132, 1998.

6. Horsman DE, Sroka H, Rootman J, White VA. Monosomy 3 and isochromosome 8q in a uveal melanoma. Cancer Genet Cytogenet 45:249–253, 1990.

7. Prescher G, Bornfeld N, Becher R. Non-random chromosomal abnormalities in primary uveal melanoma. J Natl Cancer Inst 82:1765–1769, 1990.

8. Sisley K, Rennie IG, Cottam DW, Potter AM, Potter CW, Rees RC. Cytogenetic findings in six posterior uveal melanomas: involvement of chromosomes 3, 6 and 8. Genes Chromosomes Cancer 2:205–209, 1990.

9. Prescher G, Bornfeld N, Horsthemke B, Becher R. Chromosomal aberrations defining uveal melanoma of poor prognosis. Lancet 339:691–692, 1992.

10. Sisley K, Cottam DW, Rennie IG, Parsons MA, Potter AM, Potter CW, Rees RC. Non-random abnormalities of chromosomes 3, 6, and 8 associated with posterior uveal melanoma. Genes Chromosomes Cancer 5:197–200, 1992.

11. Dahlenfors R, Tornqvist G, Wettrell K, Mark J. Cytogenetical observations in nine malignant melanomas. Anticancer Res 13:1415–1420, 1993.

12. Horsman DE, White VA. Cytogenetic analysis of uveal melanoma. Consistent occurrence of monosomy 3 and trisomy 8q. Cancer 71, 811–819, 1993.

13. Wiltshire RN, Elner VM, Dennis T, Vine AK, Trent JM. Cytogenetic analysis of posterior uveal melanoma. Cancer Genet Cytogenet **66**: 47–53, 1993.

14. Singh AR, Boghosian-Sell L. Wary KK, Shields CL, De Potter P, Donoso LA, Shields JA, Cannizzaro LA. Cytogenetic findings in primary uveal melanoma. Cancer Genet Cytogenet 72, 109–115, 1994.

15. Prescher G, Bornfeld N, Hirche H, Horsthemke B, Karl-Heinz Jokel, Becher R. Prognostic implications of monosomy 3 in uveal melanoma. Lancet 347:1222–1225, 1996.

16. White VA, Horsman DE, Rootman J. Cytogenetic characterization of an iris melanoma. Cancer Genet Cytogenet 82:85–87, 1995.

17. Sisley K, Brand C, Parsons MA, Maltby E, Rees RC, Rennie IG. Cytogenetics of iris melanomas disparity with other uveal melanomas. Cancer Genet Cytogenet 101:128–133, 1998.

18. Sisley K, Rennie IG, Parsons MA, Jacques R, Hammond DW, Bell SM, Potter AM, Rees RC. Abnormalities of chromosomes 3 and 8, in posterior uveal melanoma, correlate with prognosis. Genes Chromosom Cancer 19:22–28, 1997.

19. Parrella P, Sidransky D, Merbs SL. Allelotype of posterior uveal melanoma: Implications for a bifurcated tumour progression pathway. Cancer Res 59:3032–3037, 1999.

20. Naus NC, van Drunen E, De Klein A, Luyten GPM, Paridaens DA, Alers JC, Ksander B, Beverloo HB, Slater RM. Characterization of complex chromosomal abnormalities in uveal melanoma by fluorescent in situ hybridization, spectral karyotyping and comparative genomic hybridization. Genes Chromosomes Cancer 30:267–273, 2001.

21. Tschentscher F, Prescher G, Horsman DE, White VA, Rieder H, Anastassiou G, Schilling H, Bornfeld N, Bartz-Schmidt KU, Horsthemke B, Lohmann DR, Zeschnigk M. Partial deletions of the long and short arm of chromosome 3 point to two tumour suppressor genes in uveal melanoma. Cancer Res 61:3439–3442, 2001.

22. Prescher G, Bornfeld N, Becher R. Two subclones in a case of uveal melanoma: Relevance of monosomy 3 and multiplication of chromosome 8q. Cancer Genet Cytogenet 77:144–2146, 1994.

23. White VA, McNeil K, Thiberville L, Horsman DE. Acquired homozygosity (isodisomy) of chromosome 3 during clonal evolution of a uveal melanoma: Association with morphologic heterogeneity. Genes Chromosomes Cancer 15:138–143, 1996.

24. Sisley K, Parsons MA, Garnham J, Potter AM, Curtis DI, Rees RC, Rennie IG. Association of specific chromosome alterations with tumour phenotype in posterior uveal melanoma. Br J Cancer 82:330–338, 2000.

25. Parada LA, Maranon A, Hallen M, Tranberg KG, Stenram U, Bardi G, Johansson B. Cytogenetic analysis of secondary liver tumours reveal significant differences in genomic imbalances between primary and metastatic colon carcinomas. Clin Exp Metastasis 17:471–479, 1999.

26. Aalto Y, Eriksson L, Seregard S, Larsson O, Knuutila S. Concomitant loss of chromosome 3 and whole arm losses and gains of chromosomes 1,6, or 8 in metastasizing primary uveal melanoma. Invest Ophthalmol Vis Sci 42:313–317, 2001.

27. Scholes AG, Liloglou T, Maloney P, Hagan S, Nunnj, Hiscott P, Damato BE, Grierson I, Field JK. Loss of heterozygosity on chromosomes 3, 9, 13, and 17 including the retinoblastoma locus, in uveal melanoma. Invest Ophthalmol Vis Sci 11:2472–2477, 2001.

28. Mooy CM, De Jong PT. Prognostic parameters in uveal melanoma: A review. Surv Ophthalmol 41:215–228, 1996.

29. White VA, Chambers JD, Courtright PD, Chang WY, Horsman DE. Correlation of cytogenetic abnormalities with the outcome of patients with uveal melanoma. Cancer 83:354–359, 1998.

30. McNamara M, Felix C, Davison EV, Fenton M, Kennedy SM. Assessment of chromosome 3 copy number in ocular melanoma using fluorescence in situ hybridization. Cancer Genet Cytogenet 98:4–8, 1997.

31. Patel KA, Edmondson ND, Talbot F, Parsons MA, Rennie IG, Sisley K. Prediction of prognosis in patients with uveal melanoma using fluorescence in situ hybridization. Br J Ophthalmol 85:1440–1444, 2001.

32. Tschentscher F, Prescher G, Zeschnigk M, Horsthemke B, Lohmann DR. Identification of chromosomes 3, 6, and 8 aberrations in uveal melanoma by microsatellite analysis in comparison to comparative genomic hybridization. Cancer Genet Cytogenet 122:13–17, 2000.

33. Prescher G, Bornfeld N, Friedrichs W, Seeber S, Becher R. Cytogenetics of twelve cases of uveal melanoma and patterns of nonrandom anomalies and isochromosome formation. Cancer Genet Cytogenet 80:40–46, 1995.

34. Zhang J, Glatfelter AA, Taetle R, Trent JM. Frequent alterations of evolutionary conserved regions of chromosome 1 in human malignant melanoma. Cancer Genet Cytogenet 111:119–123, 1999.

35. Dracopoli NC, Harnett P, Bale SJ, Stanger BZ, Tucker MA, Housman DE, Kefford RF. Loss of alleles from the distal short arm of chromosome 1 occurs late in melanoma progression. Proc Natl Acad Sci USA 86:4614–4618, 1989.

36. Mukai S, Dryja TP. Loss of alleles at polymorphic loci on chromosome 2 in uveal melanoma. Cancer Genet Cytogenet 22:45–53, 1986.

37. Magauran RG, Gray B, Small KW. Chromosome 9 abnormality in choroidal melanoma. Am J Ophthalmol 117:109–11, 1994.

38. Singh AD, Donoso LA, Jackson L, Shields CL, De Potter P, Shields JA. Familial uveal melanoma absence of constitutional cytogenetic abnormalities in 14 cases. Arch Ophthamol 114:502–503, 1996.

39. Nelson MA, Radmacher MD, Simon R, Aickin M, Yang JM, Panda L, Emerson J, Roe D, Adair L, Thompson F, Bangert J, Leong SPL, Taetle R, Salmon S, Trent J. Chromosome abnormalities in malignant melanoma: Clinical significance of non-random chromosome abnormalities in 206 cases. Cancer Genet Cytogenet 122:101–109, 2000.

40. Gordon KB, Thompson CT, Char DH, O'Brien JM, Kroll S, Ghazvini S, Gray JW. Comparative genomic hybridization in the detection of DNA copy number abnormalities in uveal melanoma. Cancer Res 54:4764–4768, 1994.

41. Speicher MR, Prescher G, du Manoir S, Jauch A, Horsthemke B, Bornfeld N, Becher R, Cremer T. Chromosomal gains and losses in uveal melanoma detected by comparative genomic hybridization. Cancer Res 54:3817–3823, 1994.

42. Robertson GP, Herbst RA, Nagane M, Huang HJ, Cavenee WK. The chromosome 10 monosomy common in human melanoma results from loss of two separate tumour suppressor loci. Cancer Res 59:3596–3601, 1999.

43. Herbst RA, Mommert S, Casper U, Podewski EK, Kiehl P, Kapp A, Weiss J. 11q23 allelic loss is associated with regional lymph node metastasis in melanoma. Clin Cancer Res 6:3222–2227, 2000.

44. Sisley K, Nichols C, Parsons MA, Farr R, Rees RC Rennie IG. Clinical applications of chromosome analysis, from fine needle aspiration biopsies, of posterior uveal melanoma. Eye 12:203–207, 1998.

45. Blasi MA, Roccella E, Balestrazzi E, Del Porto G, De Felice N, Roccella M, Rota R, Grammatico P. 3p13 region: A possible location of a tumour suppressor gene involved in uveal melanoma. Cancer Genet Cytogenet 108:81–83, 1999.

46. Online Mendelian Inheritance in Man (OMIM), Johns Hopkins University, 1966–2001, http://www.ncbi.nlm.nih.gov/Omim/

47. White VA, McNeil BK, Horsman DE. Acquired homozygosity (isodisomy) of chromosome 3 in uveal melanoma. Cancer Genet Cytogenet 102:40–45, 1998.

48. Myatt N, Aristodemou P, Neale MH, Foss AJE, Hungerford JL, Bhattacharya S, Cree IA. Abnormalities of the transforming growth factor-beta pathway in ocular melanoma. J Pathol 192:511–518, 2000.

49. De Lange T, Jacks T. For better or worse? Telomerase inhibition and cancer. Cell 98:273–275, 1999.

50. Mitchell JR, Collins K. Human telomerase activation requires two independent interactions between telomerase RNA and telomerase reverse transcriptase. Mol Cell 6:361–371, 2000.

51. Heine B, Coupland SE, Kneiff S, Demel G, Bornfeld N, Hummel M, Stein H. Telomerase expression in uveal melanoma. Br J Ophthalmol 84:217–223, 2000.

52. Ugolini F, Adelaide J, Charafe-Jauffret E, Nguyen C, Jacquemier J, Jordan B, Birnbaum D, Pebusque MJ. Differential expression assay of chromosome arm 8p genes identifies Frizzled-related (FRP1/FRZB) and fibroblast growth factor receptor 1 (FGFR1) as candidate breast cancer genes. Oncogene 18:1903–1910, 1999.

53. Parrella P, Caballero OT, Sidransky D, Merbs SL. Detection of c-myc amplification in uveal melanoma by fluorescent in situ hybridization. Invest Ophthalmol Vis Sci 42:1679–1684, 2001.

54. Mooy CM, Luyten GPM, de Jong PTVM, Luider TM, Stijnen T, van de Ham F, van Vroonhoven CC, Bosmam FT. Immunohistochemical and prognostic analysis of apoptosis and proliferation in uveal melanoma. Am J Pathol 147:1097–1104, 1995.

55. Chana JS, Cree IA, Foss AJE, Hungerford JL, Wilson GD. The prognostic significance of c-myc oncogene expression in uveal melanoma. Melanoma Res 8:139–144, 1998.

56. Chana JS, Wilson GD Cree IA, Alexander RA, Myatt N, Neale M, Foss AJE, Hungerford JL. c-myc, p53, and Bcl-2 expression and clinical outcome in uveal melanoma. Br J Ophthalmol 83:110–114, 1999.

57. Demetrick DJ, Matsumoto S, Hannon GJ, Okamoto K, Xiong Y, Zhang H, Beach DH. Chromosomal mapping of the genes for the human cell cycle proteins cyclin C (CCNC), cyclin E (CCNE), p21 (CDKN1) and KAP (CDKN3). Cytogenet Cell Genet 69:190–192, 1995.

58. Vincenti V, Cassano C, Rocchi M, Persico G. Assignment of the vascular enothelial growth factor gene to human chromosome 6p21.3. Circulation 93:1493–1495, 1996.

59. Metzelaar-Blok JA, Jager MJ, Moghaddam PH, van der Slik AR, Giphart MJ. Frequent loss of heterozygosity on chromosome 6p in uveal melanoma. Hum Immunol 60:962–962, 1999.

60. Nelson MA, Ariza ME, Yang JM, Thompson FH, Taetle R, Trent JM, Wymer J, Massey-Brown K, Broome-Powell M, Easton J, Lahti JM, Kidd VJ. Abnormalities in the p34cdc2-related PITSLRE protein kinase gene complex (CDC2L) on chromosome band 1p36 in melanoma. Cancer Genet Cytogenet 108:91–99, 1999.

61. Gruis NA, van der Velden PA, Sandkuijl LA, Prins DE, Weaver-Feldhaus J, Kamb A, Bergman W, Frants RR. Homozygotes for CDKN2 (p16) germline mutation in Dutch familial melanoma kindreds. Nat Genet 10:351–353, 1995.

62. Healy E, Rehman I, Angus B, Rees JL. Loss of heterozygosity in sporadic primary cutaneous melanoma. Genes Chromosomes Cancer 12:152–156, 1995.

63. Ohta M, Berd D, Shimizu M, Nagai H, Cotticelli MG, Mastrangelo M, Shields JA, Shields CL, Croce CM, Huebner K. Deletion mapping of chromosome region 9p21-p22 surrounding the CDKN2 locus inmelanoma. Int J Cancer 65:762–767, 1996.

64. Merbs SL, Sidransky D. Analysis of p16 (CDKN2/MTS-1/INK4A) alterations in primary sporadic uveal melanoma. Invest Ophthamol Vis Sci 40:779–783, 1999.

65. van der Velden PA, Metzelaar-Blok JA, Bergman W, Monique H, Hurks H, Frants RR, Gruis NA, Jager MJ. Promoter hypermethylation: A common cause of reduced p16 (INK4a) expression in uveal melanoma. Cancer Res 13:5303–5306, 2001.

66. Guldberg P, thor Straten P, Birck A, Ahrenkiel V, Kirkin AF, Zeuthen J. Disruption of the MMAC!/ PTEN gene by deletion or mutation is a frequent event in malignant melanoma. Cancer Res; 57:3660–3663, 1997.

67. Naus NC, Zuidervaart W, Rayman N, Slater RM, van Drunen E, Ksander B, Luyten GPM, De Klein A. Mutation analysis of the PTEN gene in uveal melanoma cell lines. Int J Cancer 87:151–153, 2000.

68. Gentile M, Ahnstrom M, Schon F, Wingren S. Candidate tumour suppressor genes at 11q23-q24 in breast cancer: Evidence of alterations in PIG8, a gene involved in p53-induced apoptosis. Oncogene 20:7753–7760, 2001.

6

Structural Alterations and Gene Expression in the Pathogenesis of Uveal Melanoma

PAUL R. VAN GINKEL

University of Wisconsin, Madison, Wisconsin, U.S.A.

I. INTRODUCTION

To develop into a uveal melanoma, melanocytes have to undergo genetic changes that enable these cells to re-enter the cell cycle and possibly at the same time repress apoptosis. As the size of the tumor increases, additional mutations can give tumor cells the potential to invade local barriers and to regulate their blood supply. Other mutations allow cells to enter the bloodstream, to extravasate elsewhere in the body, and to colonize these sites. All these changes are a result of random mutations, which will be selected for if they are beneficial to a tumor cell at some specific growth stage of the tumor. Chromosome-scale loss of genome integrity is usually a later event in many tumors, often related to the loss of *p53*. This may accelerate the rate of genetic changes acquired by tumor cells and thereby the progression to a malignant phenotype. A model for uveal melanoma oncogenesis predicts that three rate-limiting steps are required to develop a primary melanoma and a fourth to develop metastatic disease [1].

The initial change(s) necessary to set off these events in uveal melanocytes are currently unknown. A number of different studies have suggested that ultraviolet (UV) radiation (UVR) from sunlight exposure induces uveal melanoma. However, even though UV rays are a powerful mutagen and there is a strong link between skin cancer and sunlight exposure, many other studies have questioned any role of UVR in uveal melanomas [reviewed in Ref. 2]. A number of chemicals such as methylcholanthrene, N-2-fluorenylacetamide, nickel subsulfide, radium, and ethiorene have been linked to the pathogenesis in some cases of uveal melanoma [3]. In rare cases, uveal melanomas can occur in families (see below). However, no locus for hereditary uveal melanoma has been identified. A number of congenital conditions that can predispose to uveal melanoma have been described, including ocular melanocytosis, neurofibromatosis I, and possibly familial multiple mole syndrome. The molecular and genetic changes leading to the development of uveal melanoma in these conditions are not understood [2].

The histologic origin of uveal melanoma is not understood. One school of thought, based on clinical and histopathological studies, holds that the majority of uveal melanomas appear to develop from benign nevi. Yanoff and Zimmerman [4] found spindle-shaped nevus cells at the periphery of approximately three-quarters of these tumors. Furthermore, additional separate nevi were found to be common in eyes with uveal melanomas. However, given the relative abundance of ocular nevi in the population (3–7%) and the rarity of the disease (1400–2000 new cases in the United States each year), only a small minority of nevi (1:5000–15,000) are thought to transform to malignant melanoma per year [5]. This process is well recognized in the development of skin melanomas, where certain nevi may become dysplastic, leading to hyperplasia, in situ carcinoma, and subsequent invasion and metastasis [6]. Others dispute these ideas, however, and suggest that the nevus-like cells found at the base of many uveal melanomas may represent a local mechanical compressive effect on the cells of the choroid [7,8]. Furthermore, de novo formation of a uveal melanoma in the absence of pre-existing nevi has been documented [9]. An alternative hypothesis is that an oncogenic agent might produce both uveal melanoma as well as excessive number of benign melanocytic tumors [10]. A third, lesser-known hypothesis that uveal melanomas derive from Schwann cells from the sheaths of ciliary nerves that transverse the tumor was postulated by Dvorak-Theobald in 1937 [11] and later supported by data from Vogel [12] (1970). Currently, it is not known what the genetic basis is for the changes from uveal melanocyte (to benign nevus?) to malignant melanoma.

One of the prognostic factors for outcome of uveal melanoma is the type of cells that make up the tumor. Most iris melanomas consist of spindle A cells and these almost never show mitotic figures. Uveal melanomas can consist of spindle (A or B), mixed spindle (mostly B), and epithelioid or epithelioid cell types. The most common type of uveal melanoma is the mixed cell tumor. Spindle B cells rarely show mitotic figures, whereas epithelioid cells frequently do [13]. A larger component of epithelioid cells is linked to poorer outcome. At this time the genetic basis underlying these different uveal melanoma cell types is not known. It is also unclear whether spindle-type cells are in the same pathway as epithelioid cells in the progression of uveal melanoma or whether these cell types represent divergent pathways of uveal melanoma cells. Furthermore, iris melanomas seem to behave differently from other uveal melanomas. It has been shown that there are cytogenetic differences between iris melanomas and choroidal and ciliary body melanomas [14,15].

A great deal of research is currently being conducted in the cancer field to identify the molecular changes between nontransformed cells and primary tumors and between primary tumors and their metastases. Techniques such as microarray analysis, differential display, suppression subtractive hybridization (SSH), and serial analysis of gene expression (SAGE) are being used for these analyses. A number of these techniques are currently being applied to uveal melanomas to answer some of the questions raised above.

II. FAMILIAL UVEAL MELANOMA

Cases of familial uveal melanoma (FUM) are rare and comprise only 0.6% of all uveal melanoma cases; they have been postulated to follow an autosomal dominant mode of inheritance [16]. At least 53 families have been described with uveal melanoma. FUM most often affects first-degree relatives and rarely affects more than two people in a family [17]. However, in the largest family group, 7 family members over four generations had eyes enucleated, 5 with histologically proven choroidal or ciliary body melanomas [18–20]. In addition, these authors found that patients with FUM were four times as likely to have a second primary malignant neoplasm, suggesting that FUM may confer a generalized inherited predisposition to cancer. No linkage analysis has been reported for any of the reported families with uveal melanoma.

III. PREDISPOSING CONGENITAL CONDITIONS

Ocular melanocytosis is a mostly unilateral congenital condition characterized by hypermethylation of the uveal tract and the episclera. In cases where the eyelid or scalp is affected as well, the condition is called oculodermal melanocytosis (nevus of Ota). It is estimated that 2% or less of all uveal melanomas are associated with oculo (dermal) melanocytosis [21]. The lifetime risk for developing uveal melanoma is 1:400 for a patient with ocular melanocytosis. Remarkable in this regard is that, unlike normal eyes, eyes in this condition, with increased pigmentation, show an increased incidence of uveal melanoma [22].

Neurofibromatosis type I is primarily a disorder of neural crest–derived cells, characterized by congenital hyperchromia and an excessive number of melanocytic nevi in the uveal tract. In rare cases, these patients develop uveal melanoma [23]. This disease is inherited in an autosomal dominant fashion.

Familial atypical mole and melanoma syndrome may be associated with an increased risk of uveal melanoma. However, this link is controversial, since contradictory results have been obtained in different studies [24].

IV. SOMATIC MUTATIONS

A. Cytogenetics

In recent years a host of new techniques have become available to do karyotype analysis on tumor cells. Conventional banding techniques usually require cells in culture to obtain metaphase spreads. More recent techniques, such as fluorescence in situ hybridization (FISH), employ fluorescent probes to look for structural changes in tissue specimens, allowing detection of deletions, translocations, and amplifications. Comparative genomic hybridization (CGH) is a whole-genome screen for DNA copy number alterations. Furthermore, spectral karyotyping (SKY) analysis employing whole-chromosome specific fluorescent labeling can be used to refine analysis of complex genomic alterations involving marker chromosomes and various translocations. With the advent of these techniques, it is possible to study the karyotypes of uveal melanomas and to relate structural changes in the genome with certain aspects of the disease.

A number of chromosomal abnormalities have been identified that occur nonrandomly in uveal melanomas such as monosomy of 3, gain of 6p, loss of 6q, gain of 8q, and deletion of 1p. The specific oncogenes or tumor suppressor genes within these structural changes that are crucial for certain stages of tumor development are mostly unknown at this time.

1. Monosomy of 3

Several groups have identified monosomy of 3 as a nonrandom cytogenetic aberration that is specific to uveal melanomas [25–31]. CGH studies of copy number abnormalities in these tumors have confirmed these findings [32–34]. These studies showed that monosomy of 3 occurred in about 50% of the cases. Furthermore, cases have been reported with isodisomy of 3, whereby loss of heterozygosity is found even in the presence of two chromosomes 3, resulting in a functional monosomy [35]. The majority of tumors showed a complete loss of chromosome 3. However, in a more recent study, a few patients with uveal melanoma had a partial deletion of chromosome 3 [36]. Among these patients, the smallest region of overlap (SRO) spans 3q24–q26, with a second SRO of about 2.5Mb on 3p25. This suggests the presence of two tumor suppressor genes on chromosome 3. Mutation or deletion of the other allele at each of these locations may have led to gene inactivation, although this has not been detected by CGH or karyotyping. The well-known tumor suppressor gene *VHL* in this region on 3p is not located in the SRO at 3p25. Since the SROs are on different arms of chromosome 3, these findings may help explain the loss of the entire chromosome 3 in uveal melanomas. Other regions of 3p may also be important in uveal melanomas: a case was reported with the only structural rearrangement being a translocation involving chromosomes 3 and 22, with a breakpoint at 3p13 [37].

Loss of chromosome 3 correlates strongly with metastatic disease [38]. Long-term studies have shown that 4 years after diagnosis, about 70% of the patients with monosomy of 3 in their primary tumor had died of metastasis. Tumors with two copies of chromosome 3 rarely develop metastases [39]. Furthermore, monosomy of 3 has also been associated by some with ciliary body involvement of the tumor [40–42]. Therefore the basis of poor prognosis in patients with ciliary body tumors may be genetic. In fact, a patient was reported with a ciliary body uveal melanoma that had monosomy of 3 as the only visible cytogenetic abnormality [30]. The development of vascular networks is also associated with ciliary body involvement. This might suggest that monosomy of 3 has a role in vascular network formation, although local environment in the ciliary body could also explain this vascular behavior [43]. Local environment could also have a role in selecting for genetic changes required for tumor progression [44]. An important caveat in many of the correlations between cytogenetic abnormalities and clinical characteristics is the nature of the tumor population that is used. Results may vary depending on the size of the tumors used in the analyses. The advent of alternative therapies to enucleations might also change the type of tumors available for cytogenetic analysis, especially with regard to tumor size.

2. Gain of 8q

Uveal melanomas show a gain of chromosome 8q in about 50–60% of the tumors [45]. In about 45% of the cases, this gain coincides with monosomy of 3 [42]. Abnormalities of 8q in the form of translocations occur in 24% of the cases with disomy of 3. On the other hand, 82% of the cases with monosomy of 3 showed multiplication of 8q and the majority of these presented isochromosomes of 8q [26]. Since isochromosomes, not only of 8q but also of 6p, are almost exclusively found in the presence of monosomy of 3, it has been suggested that the loss of chromosome 3 may be associated with isochromosome formation itself. Several tumor suppressor genes residing on chromosome 3 may be involved in regulating the centromere or mitotic division, and loss of these genes may result in isochromosome formation [26,38].

There is also a correlation between gain of 8q and ciliary body location and poor prognosis, as is the case with monosomy of 3. The disease-free interval decreases with increased copy number of 8q [42]. This suggests that overexpression of a gene or genes on chromosome 8q is linked to development of the metastatic phenotype. This trend was also found when 8q gains were compared between nonmetastasizing primary tumors, metastasizing primary tumors, and metastases [38]. Gains of 8q were present in 14, 53, and 100% of these tumors, respectively.

Comparisons among tumors have narrowed the amplified region down to 8q23–24-qter [26,32–34]. This region contains the c-*myc* gene, which is frequently amplified as a later event during tumor progression in many different cancers. Detailed studies in uveal melanomas revealed that c-*myc* was amplified in 70% of the tumors. In about 43% of these tumors, c-*myc* amplification could not be explained by simple 8q abnormalities such as trisomy of 8 and isochromosome of 8q. In these tumors, c-*myc* amplification may be a result of intrachromosomal rearrangement or translocation of a small region of 8q [46]. Alternatively, c-*myc* amplification may occur as extrachromosomal amplification of c-*myc* on double minutes, as frequently occurs in other tumors like myeloid leukemias. Both the size, ranging into submicroscopic, and instability in culture might contribute to the apparent absence of double minutes in these tumors.

Since all tumors with c-*myc* amplification had monosomy of 3 but only 50% of the tumors with monosomy of 3 had c-*myc* amplification, this latter event may follow loss of a gene or genes on chromosome 3.

3. Chromosome 6 Abnormalities

Chromosome 6 anomalies are found in about 40% of uveal melanomas [33,41,44,47]. These anomalies occur as gains of 6p and/or losses of 6q. In fact, SKY analysis of uveal melanomas and melanoma cell lines suggests that abnormalities involving chromosome 6 may be more frequent than reported by cytogenetic analysis [48]. The majority of anomalies of chromosome 6 are associated with choroidal melanomas only and not with those of the ciliary body [26,28,29,31,44,49,50]. They occur mostly in the absence of abnormalities of 3 and 8, which are associated with ciliary body uveal melanomas [49] although tumors of mixed location show aberrations from both locations [41,44]. Prognosis is generally better even in the presence of abnormalities of 3 and 8 [41]. Alterations of chromosome 6 in uveal melanoma are similar to those in cutaneous melanoma [51–53], although this still has to be proven at the gene level. Parrella et al. [45] have suggested a model with a bifurcated progression of the tumor with monosomy of 3 and gain of 6p as separate pathways, both followed by the loss of 8q. Losses of 6q are significantly higher in metastasizing primary uveal tumors and metastases than in nonmetastasizing primary tumors [38]. The smallest region for deletion of 6q is 6q22-qter [33].

Gains of 6p on the other hand, were found to occur in only slightly higher numbers in the nonmetastasizing primary uveal melanomas than metastasizing primary tumors and metastases [38]. The SOR on 6p is 6p21-pter [33]. A gene(s) that is the crucial target for this abnormality has not been identified. However, p21 has been mapped to 6p and is thought to be involved in cutaneous melanoma as well as the HLA class I genes, whose expression has been found to be altered in uveal melanomas [54]. Interestingly, it has also been reported that uveal melanomas show frequent loss of heterozygosity at 6p [55].

4. Loss of 1p

It has been reported that loss of chromosome 1p occurs in about 25% of uveal melanomas [34,42,45]. Losses on chromosome 1p were found in primary uveal melanomas that have metastasized and metastases but not in nonmetastasizing primary tumors. This suggested that this region could harbor a tumor suppressor gene important for tumor progression [38]. The SRO was at 1p21-23 and was detected only in metastasizing tumors. Loss of 1p36 is a recurrent event in about 35% these tumors [48], a region that is also frequently deleted in metastatic skin melanomas [56–58]. In many other tumors, loss of 1p is also a late event in tumor progression [59]. Structural abnormalities of 1 are most frequently observed for ciliary body melanomas and those of mixed location (ciliary body and choroid) and correlate with poor prognosis [44]. Translocations involving 1p consistently yielded deletion of 1p. Furthermore, translocation partners for chromosome 1 seem to be nonrandom, with preference for chromosome 8, 13, and 15 involving similar breakpoints. We have karyotyped an epithelioid melanoma cell line (Mel290) and found the only visible cytogenetic abnormality to be duplication of the short arm of chromosome 1 from 1p13-32 and its translocation to chromosome 8q. In addition there is an internal deletion of 1p32-36. This karyotype has remained relatively stable for over 60 passages in culture [60].

5. Other Chromosomal Abnormalities

Uveal melanomas often have minimal cytogenetic changes as compared to many other solid tumors, although the numerical changes (but not the structural changes) increase as tumor size increases. In addition to the frequent karyotypic changes described above, a number of other recurrent changes like trisomy of 21 (often associated with ciliary body tumors), rearrangements of 11 (often associated with choroidal tumors), and loss of the Y chromosome (more frequent as the tumor progresses) have been reported. Loss of heterozygosity of chromosome 9p21, which is the locus of the p16 gene, has been reported in about 28% of uveal melanomas, although mutation of the p16 gene is rarely observed [50,61,62].

B. Alterations in Gene Expression

In addition to nonrandom structural changes in uveal melanoma, a large number of genes have been studied that may have a role in some stage of the development of these tumors. In the next section these genes are roughly divided into categories representing essential alterations for cells to manifest malignant growth. For most of these genes, the basis for their overexpression is not known and changes in expression may be a result of a direct mutation in the gene or a mutational event in a pathway upstream of the gene. This may lead to altered patterns of gene expression in different signal transduction pathways.

1. Cell Cycle Regulation/Proliferation

A critical stage for cells to monitor their environment and to sense signals—which determine whether the cell will proliferate or become quiescent or postmitotic—is the G1 phase of the growth cycle. The retinoblastoma protein (pRb) and other proteins in the pRb pathway have a central role in this decision point [reviewed in Ref. 63]. When hypophosphorylated, pRb blocks cell cycle progression by preventing the transcription factor E2F from transactivating genes important for G1-S phase progression. Cell cycle progression proceeds when pRb is phosphorylated by the cyclin dependent kinases cdk2 and cdk4/6. These kinases are bound to regulatory cyclin units to form active kinase complexes. Upstream of these kinases are inhibitory factors such as p16, p21, and p27. Another factor upstream of pRb is transforming growth factor beta (TGFβ), which can prevent phosphorylation of pRb by upregulation of p15 and p21 and suppression of c-*myc* expression [64,65]. The Ras protein is a positive regulator upstream of cyclin D. Many of the positive and negative effectors of this pathway have been shown to be altered in different cancers.

The retinoblastoma protein itself is infrequently mutated in uveal melanomas. However, pRb was frequently phosphorylated on residues 807 and 811, which leads to inactivation of its tumor suppressor activity [66]. These residues are targets for cyclin D-cdk4/6 kinase activity. Since cyclin D1 was expressed in most tumors in this study and not in normal uveal melanocytes, it suggested a role for this cyclin-cdk complex in the inactivation of pRb. The reason for cyclin D overexpression is not clear in uveal melanomas although in other cancers this has been a result of gene amplification, translocation or disruption of upstream regulatory pathways. The c-*myc* proto-oncogene has been shown to induce expression of cyclin D, and since c-*myc* is frequently overexpressed in uveal melanomas, it may alter cyclin D levels [46]. Cyclin D1 expression has been positively associated with epithelioid cell type, anterior location, and extraocular extension and growth fraction and generally with unfavorable outcome in uveal melanomas [67,68]. Overexpression of c-*myc* demonstrated by immunohistochemistry and flow cytometry has been correlated both to worse prognosis [69] and better prognosis [70–72]. Studies of *ras*, a proto-oncogene upstream of cyclin D, revealed no activating mutations at codons 12, 13, and 61 in uveal melanomas [73,74].

Abnormalities of p16 are often associated with skin melanoma [75]. Although a significant amount of the uveal melanomas showed loss of heterozygosity (LOH) at 9p21, where the p16 gene resides, deletion mapping and mutation screening have not shown p16 inactivation in uveal melanoma [62]. Promoter hypermethylation of the p16 promoter, however, occurs in 32% of primary uveal melanomas and 50% of uveal melanoma cell lines [76]. Expression of p16 could be restored in these cell lines by adding a demethylating agent, suggesting that hypermethylation caused the inactivation of the gene. Significantly, one cell line (Mel270) underwent growth arrest for a considerable time. Colonies that resumed growth were shown to have undergone hypermethylation of the promoter again. In addition to its important role in regulating the cell cycle, p16 may also prevent invasion and angiogenesis [77,78]. Others have described the lack of p16-cdk4 complexes in transformed cells in a small study comparing cultured uveal melanomas to uveal melanocytes [79]. Deficiency in p16 binding to cdk4 has also been found in some familial cutaneous melanomas [80]. TGF-β, like p16, is a negative factor upstream of cyclin D. TGF-β binding to the TGF-β receptor (TGF-βR2) can activate signal transduction pathways involving SMAD proteins, leading to upregulation of cdk inhibitors [81]. Normally TGF-β suppresses growth of human melanocytes but this response is lost in melanoma cells [82–84]. Abnormalities of the TGF-β pathway have been found in 61% of uveal melanomas, potentially occurring at the level of TGF-βR2 or the SMAD 2, 3, and 4 proteins. However, in another study, all uveal melanomas were found to stain positive for TGF-β [85]. Recently, reduced expression of myristoylated alanine-rich C kinase substrate (MARCKS) was found in the choroidal melanoma cell line OCM-1 as compared to primary cultures of choroidal melanocytes [86]. MARCKS levels sharply increase when 3T3 cells exit the cell cycle into G0 during serum starvation, suggesting a role in cell proliferation. Since MARCKS is a calmodulin binding protein, it may modulate calmodulin's function in G1 progression and mitogenesis. Increasing levels of this protein in OCM-1 by transfection reduces cell proliferation.

Another control on unlimited cell proliferation is telomere erosion. This process leads to cell senescence and acts via p16. Telomerase activity, which maintains telomere length, is upregulated in all uveal melanomas [87].

2. Apoptosis

In addition to alterations in the proliferation, differentiation, and senescence pathways, tumor cells often also manifest alterations in the apoptotic pathway. A very common target for inactivation in cancers is the proapoptotic regulator p53 [88]. It senses DNA damage and other abnormalities, such as oncogene over-expression and hypoxia, and activates the apoptotic cascade via Bax. At the same time, p53 activates p21, which blocks the cell cycle. p53 forms an autoregulatory loop with MDM2, in which p53 positively regulates MDM2, which functionally inactivates p53 by binding to it and targeting it for degradation. MDM2 also has oncogenic potential independent of p53 [89].

Mutation of p53 is an uncommon event in uveal melanoma [72,90]. Tumor positivity of p53 in uveal melanomas varies among different studies from 0 to 100%, which may be the result of different fixation techniques, antibodies, and antigen retrieval techniques [68,72,90–92]. Results may also depend on the source of the melanoma cells, since p53 is rapidly upregulated when tumor cells are brought into culture. Mdm2 is upregulated in most uveal melanomas and is also correlated with poor clinical outcome [66,68]. The mechanism by which this occurs is as yet unclear. Bcl-2 is a survival factor; it can counteract Bax activity and can also block p53 independent apoptosis. Bcl-2 is upregulated in more than 70% of uveal melanomas [70,72,93]. Bcl-2 expression does not have an effect on prognosis, although an inverse relation was found between Bcl-2 expression and *myc* expression in uveal melanomas.

We have recently identified the apoptosis linked protein ALG-2 in uveal melanomas cells. ALG-2 is a calcium-binding protein that is involved in apoptosis in T-cell hybridomas [94]. Its expression is necessary for response to a number of apoptotic signals. Levels of this protein are decreased in certain more malignant uveal melanoma cell lines as compared to normal uveal melanocytes.

3. Angiogenesis

Another important acquired property of tumor cells is their ability to induce angiogenesis when the size of the primary tumor exceeds 1–2 mm. This allows the primary tumor to continue growing while simultaneously allowing tumor cells to intravasate and metastasis to occur. The leakiness of the new vessels is thought to aid in this process. Tumor angiogenesis is especially important for uveal melanomas, since the eye lacks lymphatics and metastasis occurs almost exclusively via the hematogenous route. Vascular endothelial growth factor (VEGF) is a well-described angiogenic factor; it is induced by hypoxia and is upregulated in many tumors. Reports of VEGF expression in uveal melanomas have been inconsistent. While some studies have found no expression [95,96], others have found diffuse or inconsistent expression of VEGF within the tumor [60,97,98]. More recently, VEGF expression was reported in the majority of uveal melanomas analyzed, although levels were variable [99]. VEGF levels correlated with the presence of necrosis but not with angiogenesis or metastasis. In a study of uveal melanoma cell lines, high levels of VEGF expression were found in all lines [100]. In the same study, expression of angiopoietin 2 was found in all cell lines, and of interleukin 8 in some cell lines. These factors may increase the angiogenic properties of these melanomas.

We have recently identified two additional angiogenic factors, tissue factor and Cyr61, which are upregulated in uveal melanomas and certain uveal melanoma cell lines [60]. Tissue factor correlated with blood vessel density in paraffin sections from uveal melanomas.

Recently, a process called vasculogenic mimicry has been described for certain aggressive uveal melanomas in which tumor cells form patterned tubular networks that mimic endothelial-formed vasculogenic networks [101]. It is not clear whether these networks have a role in perfusion of the tumor, though they are associated with aggressive growth. Comparison by chip array analysis of aggressive tubular network–forming uveal melanoma cells to poorly aggressive ones that lack this ability identified various protein kinases such as epithelial cell kinase (Eck/EphA2). This kinase was exclusively expressed and phosphorylated in the aggressive cells [102]. When this protein was transiently knocked out, these tumor cells lost the ability to form tubular networks. Eck/Eph2A has been previously implicated in angiogenesis, growth and proliferation as well as induction of vascularization of melanoma cells [103,104]. Several other genes associated with the endothelial/vascular phenotype, such TIE-1, an endothelial receptor kinase, urokinase-type plasminogen activator (uPA), and keratin 8 intermediate filament were also identified by this same technique [101]. Other genes that were upregulated and could be involved in the microvascular channel formation include connective tissue growth factor (CTGF), fibrillin, collagens VI and I, and fibronectin.

4.   Invasion and Metastasis

An important property of many tumors, and of uveal melanomas in particular, is the ability to escape the primary tumor mass and then to invade neighboring tissues and metastasize to more distant sites. One of the natural barriers against tumor spread is the extracellular matrix (ECM). Many tumor cells excrete proteolytic enzymes, such as matrix metalloproteinases (MMPs) and plasminogen activators, to degrade basal membranes and ECM components. At least half of the uveal melanomas express MMP2 and or MMP9 [105–108]. In a different study, all epithelioid tumors and only 30% of the spindle cell tumors were found to be positive for MMP2 [107]. MMP9 is mainly expressed in the more malignant epithelioid uveal melanomas [109]. Tumors positive for MMP2 and/or 9 are associated with a significantly higher metastatic incidence and lower survival rate. In addition, 65% of uveal melanomas express MMP3, which can activate pro-MMP9. Microarray gene chip analysis revealed increased expression of MMP1, 2, 9, and 14 in aggressive, compared to poorly aggressive, uveal melanoma cells [110]. It has been suggested that another function of MMPs is in vasculogenic mimicry, a process whereby tumor cells form ECM-rich patterned tubular networks [101]. Both MMPs and laminin 5, which is also overexpressed, may be involved in this remodeling of the ECM [110].

Tissue inhibitors of MMPs (TIMP) are natural inhibitors of MMPs. Levels of TIMP1 and 2 tend to be lower in patients with uveal melanomas that had developed metastatic disease [109]. TIMP1 may also have growth factor-like effects, as has been described in colon cancer cells [111]. This might explain why upregulation of this protein may lead to increased tumorigenicity in some tumors. In addition, TIMP2 also induces activation of proMMP2 [112], thus leading to increased tumorigenicity at intermediate levels. MMPs work synergistically with plasminogen activators. Urokinase-type activator (uPA) and tissue plasminogen activator (tPA) have been implicated in metastasis. The presence of uPA on primary uveal tumors correlates with metastatic disease and poor prognosis [113]. uPA and inhibitors of plasminogen activity (PAI-1, PAI-2) were detected on all of a series of 10 uveal melanomas [106]. tPA activity from primary cultures of uveal melanoma correlates with scleral invasion in the tumor lesion. Furthermore, tPA activity is present in the invasive front of uveal melanoma [113]. The importance of the plasminogen activator system in metastasis was also apparent from gene transfer experiments of PAI-1 into uveal melanoma cells, which inhibits metastasis of uveal melanoma [114].

For tumor cells to colonize new sites, adaptations in their cell surface receptors occur in order to adhere to their new microenvironment. These interactions are mediated by integrins, which consist of an alpha and a beta subunits. Sixteen alpha and eight beta subunits can form 20 different integrins. The combination of these subunits displayed on the cell surface determines the adhesive properties of the cell to the matrix in a certain environment. Some integrins induce expression of MMP's and are thus involved in the invasive process.

Integrin expression is heterogeneous in both cutaneous and uveal melanoma cell lines [115]. Although no link between invasiveness or cell type and integrin expression has been observed in one study [116]; others have reported a correlation between spindle cell morphology and the lack of $\alpha6\beta1$ integrin expression in a group of 10 uveal melanomas [108]. In addition, all uveal melanomas were positive for $\alpha1\beta1$, whereas ocular melanocytes were negative. Both $\alpha1$ and $\alpha6$ integrins bind laminin, which is a constituent of basement membranes and may thus be important for invasive potential. $\alpha v\beta3$, an important integrin for the invasive potential of cutaneous melanoma, does not appear to be important to uveal melanoma: some studies do not find it on these tumors whereas others find it on melanoma cells and melanocytes [108,115,116]. A potential caveat in some of these studies is that integrin expression can be altered as a result of culturing cells [106].

Expression of the $\alpha4$ subunit gene was found to be downregulated in a uveal melanoma cell line and its metastatic derivatives as compared to uveal melanocytes [117]. Study of the promoter of this gene showed that transcriptional activity and transcription factor binding was inversely correlated with metastatic potential of the lines.

Another class of proteins involved in cell adhesion and implicated in invasion and metastasis are the cell adhesion molecules (CAM), which mediate calcium-dependent adhesion. The role of the intercellular adhesion molecule 1 (ICAM-1) in uveal melanoma seems unclear [118–120]. Neural cell adhesion molecule (NCAM) expression was correlated to metastatic potential of uveal melanomas [121]. NCAM isoforms that lack the HNK-1 epitope may play a role in organ specific metastatic behavior of uveal melanomas. This epitope may serve as a ligand for cell adhesion.

Organ-specific metastasis is not only a result of organ-specific homing mediated by cell surface receptors on the tumor cells but also paracrine stimulation of tumor cells by organ-derived growth factors. It has been shown that expression of the epidermal growth factor receptor (EGFR) in uveal melanoma cell lines correlates with the capacity of tumor cells to localize in the liver [122]. These tumor cells may be stimulated to proliferate by transforming growth factor alpha (TGF-α) and hepatocyte growth factor (HGF), similar to colon carcinoma cells, which also preferentially metastasize to the liver [123]. EGFR receptor also protects uveal melanoma cells against lysis mediated by TNF-α. There is some controversy regarding a correlation of EGFR expression and metastatic disease. Hurks et al. [124] have shown that such a correlate exists in patients with uveal melanoma. However, Scholes et al. [125] find no such correlation and, in addition, find EGFR immunoreactivity restricted to macrophages.

Another receptor involved in dissemination of uveal melanoma cells to the liver is the proto-oncogene c-*met*, the receptor for HGF/scatter factor (SF) [126]. Expression of c-*met* correlates with the appearance of cells coexpressing vimentin and keratin intermediate filaments (interconverted phenotype) [127] and invasive ability. HGF/SF is expressed both in the primary uveal tumor and in metastatic foci in the liver. An important source of HGF in the primary tumor may be the tumor-infiltrating lymphocytes. Two-thirds of surgically removed uveal melanomas contain moderate to high numbers of these cells [128]. A downstream target of c-*met* is ezrin, which acts as a linker between the plasma membrane and the actin cytoskeleton [129,130]. Ezrin is involved in cell motility, cell adhesion, and intracellular signaling [131,132]. It is expressed in a number of different tumors and tumor cell lines. More than 60% of uveal melanomas express ezrin [133]. The presence of ezrin in these melanomas is associated with higher mortality, increased microvascular density, and the presence of infiltrating macrophages.

Another growth factor that is mainly produced in the liver is insulin-like growth factor 1 (IGF-1), which binds to the IGF-1 receptor (IGF-1R). Activation of the IGF-1R leads to activation of the mitogenic cascade. IGF-1R is upregulated in many different tumor types and is important in tumorigenesis and cell transformation. It also protects cells from apoptosis [134]. In uveal melanomas, high IGF-1R expression is associated with death due to metastatic disease [135]. In addition, decreasing the IGF-1R levels of uveal melanoma cell lines in vitro decreased cell viability.

We have recently found that the tyrosine kinase receptor Axl is upregulated in uveal melanoma [136]. We show that Axl can mediate mitogenesis and survival of cultured uveal melanoma cells through its ligand Gas6. Therefore this receptor may enable uveal melanoma cells to remain dormant in the liver as micrometastases till outgrowth occurs years later.

The gene *nm23* is a metastasis suppressor that is downregulated in many human cancers. The mechanism by which this suppression occurs is unclear. In a mouse model of uveal melanoma, the level of *nm23* expression and the development of liver metastases were inversely correlated, demonstrating the importance of *nm23* in limiting metastasis in uveal melanoma [137].

Table 1   Suppression Subtractive Hybridization of Mel290 vs. Uveal Melanocytes

Clone	Identity
2-290UM	Na/H exchange regulatory cofactor
4-290UM	Nonmuscle myosin heavy chain
5-290UM	Cyclin-dependent kinase inhibitor p21
6-290UM	Ubiquitin-like protein 1
7-290UM	F-Box only protein 32
8-290UM	Plasminogen activator inhibitor 1
9-290UM	TI-227H
13-290UM	5′ nucleotidase
1.4	Tyrosine kinase receptor AXL
1.5	Inosine 5′-monophosphate dehydrogenase
1.7	Promyelocytic leukemia cell RNA
1.8	CYR61 protein
2.1	Tissue factor
2.3	Leman coiled-coil protein
2.4	CDC42 GTPase-activating protein
2.9	Amphiglycan
3.2	Tumor antigen (L6)
3.3	Elongation factor 1 alpha
3.4	Smooth muscle myosin light-chain kinase
4.1	PED phosphoprotein
4.3	Similar to ovarian carcinoma immunoreactive antigen
5.2	S3 ribosomal protein
5.3	Oxytocin receptor
5.6	Glycoprotein
5.7	Ferritin H

V. CONCLUSION

It has become apparent over the years that no single gene mutation underlies uveal melanoma. As this review shows, many genes have been implicated in different stages of tumor growth and development in this tumor type. In addition, a large number of chromosomal abnormalities have been described. New screening

Table 2 Suppression Subtractive Hybridization of OCM-3 vs. OCM-1[a]

Clone	Identity
SSH1.4	c-*myc*
SSH1.5	Yeast Sps1/Ste20-related kinase 1 (YSK1)
SSH1.7	mRNA export protein RAE1
SSH1.8	GCN1-like 1 protein (GCN1L1)
SSH1.11	Skeletal muscle-specific calpain
SSH223	Splicing factor 3B
SSH23.1	B-tubulin
SSH23.2	Sortilin
SSH23.3	Melanoma-associated ME20 antigen
SSH23.4	Actin-binding protein
SSH23.5	p100 gene
SSH2.13	Gamma actin
SSH2.15	Pituitary tumor transforming1-interacting protein 1 (PTT1-IP1)
SSH2.18	E16
SSH2.19	Procollagen lysine, 2-oxoglutarate 5-dioxygenase 3 (PLOD3)
SSH2.20	TI-227H
SSH2.21	Beta-site app-cleaving enzyme 2 (BACE2)
SSH3.1	Adenylate kinase 2B
SSH3.2	Cathepsin D
SSH3.3	CAPG
SSH3.11	S100C
SSH4.1	Unknown, similar to mouse calsyntenin
SSH4.2	Ribosomal protein L18
SSH4.7	HLA-DR-associated invariant chain P33
SSH4.8	Ribosomal protein L28
SSH4.9	TH1
SSH4.10	VATI
SSH4.11	Protein kinase C and casein kinase substrate 2 (PACSIN2)
SSH4.13	Aminopeptidase B
SSH4.15	G2 and S-phase expressed 1 (GTSE1)
SSH5.9	Tumor DNAJ-like protein
SSH5.10	CKII beta binding protein 2 (CKBB2)
SG3	Acidic ribosomal phosphoprotein
SG4	ALG-2
SG8	TIMP-3
SG12	Apoptosis-related gene 3 (APR3)
SG13	eIF-4AI
SGO4	Unknown (similar to rat CAS-associated zinc-finger protein (CIZ)

[a]A number of metabolic and mitochondrial genes were not included in this table.

technologies to scan for genomewide changes in gene expression will identify many more gene products that are relevant for the growth of these uveal tumors. Many of these genes will be part of different signal transduction pathways. Identification of these key pathways holds prospects for treatment even in the absence of one distinct disease causing gene mutation. We have used SSH [138] to compare the epithelioid uveal melanoma cell line Me1290 to cultured normal uveal melanocytes. This cell line is especially interesting because of the relatively few genomic changes it has undergone and the stability of the changes in tissue culture [60]. We obtained a list of genes that were upregulated in the tumor cell line and may be relevant to the disease (Table 1). Many of these genes play a role in other types of cancers. The described functions of these genes span the different categories of alterations in cell physiology necessary for malignant growth—namely, cell cycle regulation/proliferation, apoptosis, angiogenesis and invasion, and metastasis [139]. We have similarly compared an epithelioid (OCM-3) to a spindle-type (OCM-1) uveal melanoma cell line using SSH to begin to study the molecular basis for the difference between these two types of uveal melanoma cells (Table 2). Although these are one-way comparisons screening only for genes upregulated in Me1290 and OCM-3 cells respectively, it does show the wealth of data that can be obtained by these sorts of studies. The use of increasingly sophisticated gene expression analysis software will allow the further sorting of these data for example by signal transduction pathways [140]. Similarly, chip arrays have been used to do cluster analysis to compare tumor cell lines that differ in their ability to form tubular networks (vasculogenic mimicry) [141]. The growing complement of human expressed sequences represented on the chips and their relative ease of use make them a powerful tool for further identification of genes that are important for the growth and development of uveal melanoma. However, ultimately, these descriptive data will have to lead to biological experiments that identify the roles of these gene products and their pathways in this specific cancer. Development of suitable animal models will then allow for the design of therapeutic interventions.

REFERENCES

1. Foss AJE, Cree IA, Dolin PJ, Hugerford JL. Modelling uveal melanoma. Br J Ophthalmol 83:588–594, 1999.
2. Egan KM, Seddon JM, Glynn RJ, Gragoudas ES, Albert DM. Epidemiologic aspects of uveal melanoma. Surv Ophthalmology 32:239–251, 1988.
3. Albert DM, Puliafito CA, Fulton AB, Robinson NL, Zakov ZN, Dryja TP, Smith AB, Egan E. Increased incidence of choroidal malignant melanoma occurring in a single population of chemical workers. Am J Ophthalmol 89:323–337, 1980.
4. Yanoff M, Zimmerman LE. Histogenesis of malignant melanomas of the uvea. Cancer 20:493–507, 1967.
5. Ganley JP, Comstock GW. Benign nevi and malignant melanomas of the choroid. Am J Ophthalmol 76:19–25, 1973.
6. Clark BH, Elder DE, Guerry D, Epstein IV MN, Greene MH. The development of and subsequent cellular evolution of the primary human cutaneous melanomas. Hum Pathol 15:1147–1165, 1984.

7. Albert DM, Gaasterland DE, Caldwell JB, Howard RD, Zimmerman LE. Bilateral metastatic choroidal melanoma, nevi, and cavernous degeneration. Arch Ophthalmol 87:39–47, 1972.
8. Albert DM, Lahav M, Packer S, Yimoyines D. Histogenesis of malignant melanomas of the uvea: Occurrence of nevus-like structures in experimental choroidal tumors. Arch Ophthalmol 92:318–323, 1974.
9. Sahel JA, Pesavento R, Frederick AR, Albert DM. Melanoma arising de novo over a 16 month period. Arch Ophthalmol 106:381–386, 1988.
10. Zimmerman LE. Malignant melanoma of the uveal tract. In: Spencer WH, ed. Ophthalmic Pathology. Philadelphia: Saunders, pp 2072–2139, 1986.
11. Dvorak-Theobald G. Neurogenic origin of choroidal sarcoma. Arch Ophthalmol 18:971–997, 1937.
12. Vogel MH. Malignes Aderhautmelanom und Ziliarnerv. Klin Monatsbl Augenheilkd 157:215–224, 1970.
13. Grossniklaus HE, Green WR. Uveal tumors. In: Garner A, Klintworth GK, eds. Pathobiology of Ocular Disease. New York: Marcel Dekker, pp 1423–1477, 1994.
14. White VA, Horsman DE, Rootman J. Cytogenetic characterization of an iris melanoma. Cancer Genet Cytogenet 82:85–87, 1995.
15. Sisley K, Brand C, Parsons A, Maltby E, Rees RC, Rennie IG. Cytogenetics of iris melanomas: Disparity with other uveal tract melanomas. Cancer Genet Cytogenet 101:128–133, 1998.
16. Lynch HT, Anderson DE, Krush AJ. Hereditary and intraocular melanomas. Cancer 21:119–125, 1968.
17. Singh AD, Shields CL, De Potter P, Shields JA, Troch B, Cater J, Pastore D. Familial uveal melanoma—Clinical observations on 56 patients. Arch Ophthalmol 114:392–399, 1996.
18. Silcock AQ. Hereditary sarcoma of the eyeball. Trans Pathol Soc London 43:140–141, 1892.
19. Parsons JH. Some anomalous sarcomata of the choroid. Trans Ophthalmol Soc U K 25:205–211, 1905.
20. Davenport RC. Family history of choroidal melanoma. Br J Ophthalmol 11:443–445, 1927.
21. Gonder JR, Shields JA, Albert DM, Augsburger JJ, Lavin PT. Uveal malignant melanoma associated with ocular and oculodermal melanocytosis. Ophthalmology 89:953–960, 1982.
22. Nik ND, Glew WB, Zimmerman LE. Malignant melanoma of the choroids in the nevus of Ota of a black patient. Arch Ophthalmol 100:1641–1643, 1982.
23. Specht CS, Smith TW. Uveal malignant melanoma and vonRecklinghausen's neurofibromatosis. Cancer 62:812–817, 1988.
24. Singh AD, Wang MX, Donoso LA, Shields CL, De Potter P, Shields JA. Genetic aspects of uveal melanoma: A brief review. Semin Oncol 23:768–772, 1996.
25. Prescher G, Bornfeld N, Becher R. Nonrandom chromosomal abnormalities in primary uveal melanoma. J Natl Cancer Inst 82:1765–1769, 1990.
26. Prescher G, Bornfeld N, Friedrichs W, Seeber S, Becher R. Cytogenetics of twelve cases of uveal melanoma and patterns of nonrandom anomalies and isochromosome formation. Cancer Genet Cytogenet 80:40–46, 1995.
27. Horsthemke B, Prescher G, Bornfeld N, Becher R. Loss of chromosome 3 alleles and multiplication of chromosome 8 alleles in uveal melanoma. Genes Chromosomes Cancer 4:217–222, 1992.
28. Sisley K, Rennie IG, Cottam DW, Potter AM, Potter CW, Rees RC. Cytogenetic findings in six posterior melanomas. Genes Chromosomes Cancer 2:205–209, 1990.

29. Horsman DE, White VA. Cytogenetic analysis of uveal melanoma. Cancer 71:811–819, 1992.

30. Wiltshire RN, Elner VM, Dennis T, Vine AK, Trent JM. Cytogenetic analysis of posterior uveal melanoma. Cancer Genet Cytogenet 66:47–53 1993.

31. Dahlenfors R, Törnqvist G, Wettrell K, Mark J. Cytogenetical observations in nine ocular melanomas. Anticancer Res 13:1415–1420, 1993.

32. Gordon KB, Thompson CT, Char DH, O'Brien JM, Kroll S, Ghazvini S, Gray JW. Comparative genomic hybridization in the detection of DNA copy number abnormalities in uveal melanoma. Cancer Res 54:4764–4768, 1994.

33. Speicher MR, Prescher G, Du Manoir S, Jauch A, Horsthemke B, Bornfeld N, Becher R, Cremer T. Chromosomal gains and losses in uveal melanomas detected by comparative genomic hybridization. Cancer Res 54:3817–3823, 1994.

34. Ghazvini S, Devron H, Kroll S, Waldman FM, Pinkel D. Comparative genomic hybridization analysis of archival formalin-fixed paraffin-embedded uveal melanomas. Cancer Genet Cytogenet 90:95–101, 1996.

35. White VA, McNeil BK, Horsman DE. Acquired homozygosity (isodisomy) of chromosome 3 in uveal melanoma. Cancer Genet Cytogenet 102:40–45, 1998.

36. Tschentscher F, Prescher G, Horsman DE, White VA, Rieder H, Anastassiou G, Schilling H, Bornfeld N, Bartz-Schmidt KU, Horsthemke B, Lohmann DR, Zeschnigk M. Partial deletions of the long and short arm of chromosome 3 point to two tumor suppressor genes in uveal melanoma. Cancer Res 61:3439–3442, 2001.

37. Blasi MA, Roccella F, Balestrazzi E, Del Porto G, De Felice N, Roccella M, Rota R, Grammatico P. 3p13 region: A possible location of a tumor suppressor gene involved in uveal melanoma. Cancer Genet Cytogenet 108:81–83, 1999.

38. Aalto Y, Eriksson L, Seregard S, Larsson O, Knuutila S. Concomitant loss of chromosome 3 and whole arm losses and gains of chromosome 1, 6, and 8 in metastasizing primary uveal melanoma. Invest Ophthalmol Vis Sci 42:313–317, 2001.

39. Prescher G, Bornfeld N, Hirche H, Horsthemke B, Jöckel K-H, Becker RL. Prognostic implications of monosomy 3 in uveal melanomas. Lancet 347:1222–1225, 1996.

40. Prescher G, Bornfeld N, Horsthemke B, Becher R. Chromosomal aberrations defining uveal melanoma of poor prognosis. Lancet 339:691–692, 1992.

41. White VA, Chambers JD, Courtright PD, Chang WY, Horsman DE. Correlation of cytogenetic abnormalities with the outcome of patients with uveal melanoma. Cancer 83:354–359, 1998.

42. Sisley K, Rennie IG, Parsons MA, Jacques R, Hammond DW, Bell SM, Potter AM, Rees RC. Abnormalities of chromosomes 3 and 8 in posterior uveal melanoma correlate with prognosis. Genes Chromosomes Cancer 19:22–28, 1997.

43. Rummelt V, Folberg R, Woolson RF, Hwang T, Pe'er J. Relationship between the microcirculation architecture and the aggressive behaviour of ciliary body melanomas. Ophthalmology 102:844–851, 1994.

44. Sisley K, Parsons MA, Garnham J, Potter AM, Curtis D, Rees RC. Association of specific chromosome alterations with tumor phenotype in posterior uveal melanoma. Br J Cancer 82:330–338, 2000.

45. Parrella P, Sidransky D, Merbs SL. Allelotype of posterior uveal melanoma: Implications for a bifurcated tumor progression pathway. Cancer Res 59:3032–3037, 1999.

46. Parrella P, Caballero OL, Sidransky D, Merbs SL. Detection of c-myc amplification in uveal melanoma by fluorescent in situ hybridization. Invest Ophthalmol Vis Sci 42:1679–1684, 2001.

47. Tschentscher F, Prescher G, Zeschnigk M, Horsthemke B, Lohmann DR. Identification of chromosomes 3, 6, and 8 aberrations in uveal melanoma by microsatellite analysis in

comparison to comparative genomic hybridization. Cancer Genet Cytogenet 122:13–17, 2000.

48. Naus NC, Van Drunen E, de Klein A, Luyten GP, Paridaens DA, Alers JC, Ksander BR, Beverloo HB, Slater RM. Characterization of complex chromosomal abnormalities in uveal melanoma by fluorescence in situ hybridization, spectral karyotyping, and comparative genomic hybridization. Genes Chromosomes Cancer 30:267–273, 2001.

49. Sisley K, Cottam DW, Rennie IG, Parsons MA, Potter AM, Potter CW, Rees RC. Non-random abnormalities of chromosome 3, 6, and 8 associated with posterior melanoma. Genes Chromosomes Cancer 5:197–200, 1992.

50. Singh AD, Boghosian-Sell L, Wary KK, Shields CL, De Potter P, Donoso LA, Shields JA, Cannizzaro LA. Cytogenetic findings in primary uveal melanoma. Cancer Genet Cytogenet 72:109–115, 1994.

51. Trent JM, Rosenfeld SB, Meyskens FL. Chromosome 6q involvement in human malignant melanoma. Cancer Genet Cytogenet 9:177–180, 1983.

52. Cowan JM, Halaban R, Lane AT, Francke U. The involvement of 6p in melanoma. Cancer Genet Cytogenet 20:255–261, 1986.

53. Bastian BC, LeBoit PE, Hamm H, Brocker E-V, Pinkel D. Chromosomal gains and losses in primary cutaneous melanomas detected by comparative genomic hybridization. Cancer Res 58:2170–2175, 1998.

54. Blom DJR, Schurmans LRHM, De Waard-Siebinga I, De Wolff-Rouendaal D, Keunen JEE, Jager MJ. HLA expression in a primary uveal melanoma, its cell line, and four of its metastases. Br J Ophthalmol 81:989–993, 1997.

55. Metzelaar-Blok JAW, Jager MJ, Hanifi Moghaddam P, van der Slik AR, Giphart MJ. Frequent loss of heterozygosity on chromosome 6p in uveal melanoma. Hum Immunol 60:962–969, 1999.

56. Poetsch M, Woenckhaus C, Dittberner T, Pambor M, Lorenz G, Herrmann FH. Significance of the small subtelomeric area of chromosome 1 (1p36.3) in the progression of malignant melanoma: FISH deletion screening with YACDNA probes. Virchows Arch Int J Pathol 435:105–111, 1999.

57. Poetsch M, Dittberner T, Cowell JK, Woenckhaus C. *TTC4*, a novel candidate tumor suppressor gene at 1p31 is often mutated in malignant melanoma of the skin. Oncogene 19:5817–5820, 2000.

58. Böni R, Matt D, Voetmeyer A, Burg G, Zhuang Z. Chromosomal allele loss in primary cutaneous melanoma is heterogeneous and correlates with proliferation. J Invest Dermatol 110:215–217, 1998.

59. Dracopoli NC, Harnett P, Bale SJ, Stanger BZ, Tucker MA, Housman DE, Kefford RF. Loss of alleles from the distal short arm of chromosome 1 occurs late in melanoma progression. Proc Natl Acad Sci USA 86:4614–4618, 1989.

60. Walker TM, van Ginkel PR, Gee RL, Ahmadi H, Subramanian L, Ksander BR, Meisner LF, Albert DM, Polans AS. Expression of angiogenic factors Cyr61 and tissue factor in uveal melanoma. Arch Ophthalmol 120:1719–1725, 2002.

61. Ohta M, Berd D, Shimizu M, Nagai H, Cotticelli M-G, Mastrangelo MJ, Shields JA, Shields CL, Croce CM, Huebner K. Deletion mapping of chromosome region 9p21-p22 surrounding the CDKN2 locus in melanoma. Int J Cancer 65:762–767, 1996.

62. Merbs SL, Sidransky D. Analysis of p16 (cdkn2/mts-1/ink4A) alterations in primary sporadic uveal melanoma. Invest Ophthalmol Vis Sci 40:779–783, 1999.

63. Weinberg RA. The retinoblastoma protein and cell cycle control. Cell 81:323–330, 1995.

64. Hannon GJ, Beach D. p15ink4B is a potential effector of TGF-beta–induced cell cycle arrest. Nature 371:257–261, 1994.

65. Moses HL, Yang EY, Pietenpol JA. TGF-β stimulation and inhibition of cell proliferation: new mechanistic insights. Cell 63:245–256, 1990.

66. Brantley MA, Jr., Harbour JW. Deregulation of the Rb and p53 pathways in uveal melanoma. Am J Pathol 157:1795–1801, 2000.

67. Coupland SE, Bechrakis N, Schüler A, Anagnostopoulos I, Hummel M, Bornfeld N, Stein H. Expression patterns of cyclin D1 and related proteins regulating G1-S phase transition in uveal melanoma and retinoblastoma. Br J Ophthalmol 82:961–970, 1998.

68. Coupland SE, Anastassiou G, Stang A, Schilling H, Anagnostopoulos I, Bornfeld N, Stein H. The prognostic value of cyclin D1, p53, and MDM2 protein expression in uveal melanoma. J Pathol 191:120–126, 2000.

69. Royds JA, Sharrard RM, Parsons MA, Lawry J, Rees RC, Cottam DW, Wagner B, Rennie IG. c-myc oncogene expression in ocular melanomas. Graefes Arch Clin Exp Ophthalmol 230:366–371, 1992.

70. Mooy CM, Luyten GPM, De Jong PTVM, Luider TM, Stijnen T, van de Ham F, et al. Immunohistochemical and prognostic analysis of apoptosis and proliferation in uveal melanoma. Am J Pathol 147:1097–1104, 1995.

71. Chana JS, Cree IA, Foss AJE, Hungerford JL, Wilson GD. The prognostic significance of c-myc oncogene expression in uveal melanoma. Melanoma Res 8:139–144, 1998.

72. Chana JS, Wilson GD, Cree IA, Alexander RA, Myatt N, Neale M, Foss AJE, Hungerford JL. *c-myc, p53*, and *Bcl-2* expression and clinical outcome in uveal melanoma. Br J Ophthalmol 83:110–114, 1998.

73. Mooy CM, van der Helm MJ, van der Kwast ThH, De Jong PTVM, Ruiter DJ, Zwarthoff EC. No N-*ras* mutations in human uveal melanoma: The role of ultraviolet light revisited. Br J Cancer 64:411–413, 1991.

74. Soparker CN, O'Brien JM, Albert DM. Investigation of the role of the *ras* protooncogene point mutation in human uveal melanomas. Invest Ophthalmol Vis Sci 34:2203–2209, 1993.

75. Hussussian CJ, Struewing JP, Goldstein AM, Higgins PA, Ally DS, Sheahan MD, Clark WH, Jr, Tucker MA, Dracopoli NC. Germline p16 mutations in familial melanoma. Nat Genet 8:15–21, 1994.

76. Van der Velden PA, Metzelaar-Blok JAW, Bergman W, Hurks HMH, Frants RR, Gruis NA, Jager MJ. Promoter hypermethylation: A common cause of reduced *p16^{INK4a}* expression in uveal melanoma. Cancer Res 61:5303–5306, 2001.

77. Chintala SK, Fueyo J, Gomez-Manzano C, Venkaiah B, Bjerkvig R, Yung WK, Sawaya R, Kyritsis AP, Rao JS. Adenovirus-mediated *p16/CDKN2* gene transfer suppresses glioma invasion *in vitro*. Oncogene 15:2049–2057, 1997.

78. Harada H, Nakagawa K, Iwata S, Saito M, Kumon Y, Sakaki S, Sato K. Restoration of wild-type p16 down-regulates vascular endothelial growth factor expression and inhibits angiogenesis in human gliomas. Cancer Res 59:3783–3789, 1999.

79. Mouriaux F, Casagrande F, Pillaire M-J, Manenti S, Malecaze F, Darbon JM. Differential expression of G1 cyclins and cyclin-dependent kinase inhibitors in normal and transformed melanocytes. Invest Ophthalmol Vis Sci 39:876–884, 1998.

80. Reymond A, Brent R. p16 proteins from melanoma-prone families are deficient in binding to Cdk4. Oncogene 11:1173–1178, 1995.

81. Heldin CH, Miyazono K, ten Dijke P. TGF-β signalling from cell membrane to nucleus via SMAD proteins. Nature 390:465–471, 1997.

82. Hu D-N, McCormick SA, Ritch R, Pelton-Henrion K. Studies of human uveal melanocytes in vitro: Isolation, purification and cultivation of human uveal melanocytes. Invest Ophthalmol Vis Sci 34:2210–2219, 1993.

83. Rodeck U, Bossler A, Graeven U, Fox FE, Nowell PC, Knabbe C, Kari C. Transforming growth factor β production and responsiveness in normal human melanocytes and melanoma cells. Cancer Res 54:575–581, 1994.

84. Myatt N, Aristodemou P, Neale MH, Foss AJE, Hungerford JL, Bhattacharya S, Cree IA. Abnormalities of the transforming growth factor-beta pathway in ocular melanoma. J Pathol 192:511–518, 2000.

85. Esser P, Grisanti S, Bartz-Schmidt KU. TGF-β in uveal melanoma. Microsc Res Tech 52:396–400, 2001.

86. Manenti S, Malecaze F, Chap H, Darbon JM. Overexpression of the myristoylated alanine-rich C kinase substrate in human choroidal melanoma cells affects cell proliferation. Cancer Res 58:1429–1434, 1998.

87. Heine B, Coupland SE, Kneiff S, Demel G, Bornfeld N, Hummel M, Stein H. Telomerase expression in uveal melanoma. Br J Ophthalmol 84:217–223, 2000.

88. Harris CC. p53 tumor suppressor gene: From the basic research laboratory to the clinic—an abridged historical perspective. Carcinogenesis 17:1187–1198, 1996.

89. Freedman DA, Wu L, Levine AJ. Functions of the MDM2 oncoprotein. Cell Mol Life Sci 55:96–107, 1999.

90. Kishore K, Ghazvini S, Char DH, Kroll S, Selle J. p53 gene and cell cycling in uveal melanoma. Am J Ophthalmol 121:561–567, 1996.

91. Janßen K, Kuntze J, Busse H, Schmid KW. *p53* oncoprotein overexpression in choroidal melanoma. Mod Pathol 9:267–272, 1996.

92. Tobal K, Warren W, Cooper AS, McCartney A, Hungerford J, Lightman S. Increased expression and mutation of p53 in choroidal melanoma. Br J Cancer 66:900–904, 1992.

93. Jay V, Yi Q, Hunter WS, Zielenska M. Expression of *bcl-2* in uveal malignant melanoma. Arch Pathol Lab Med 120:497–498, 1996.

94. Vito P, Lacana E, D'Adamio L. Interfering with apoptosis: Calcium-binding protein ALG-2 and Alzheimer's disease gene ALG-3. Science 271:521–525, 1996.

95. Kvanta A, Steen B, Seregard S. Expression of vascular endothelial growth factor (VEGF) in retinoblastoma but not in posterior uveal melanoma. Exp Eye Res 63:511–518, 1996.

96. Pe'er J, Folberg R, Itin A. Vascular endothelial growth factor upregulation in human central vein occlusion. Ophthalmology 105:412–416, 1998.

97. Stitt AW, Simpson DAC, Boocock C, Gardiner TA, Murphy GM, Archer DB. Expression of vascular endothelial growth factor (VEGF) and its receptors is regulated in eyes with intra-ocular tumours. J Pathol 186:306–312, 1998.

98. Vinores SA, Küchle M, Mahlow J, Chiu C, Green WR, Campochiaro PA. Blood-ocular barrier breakdown in eyes with ocular melanoma—A potential role for vascular endothelial growth factor vascular permeability factor. Am J Pathol 147:1289–1297, 1995.

99. Sheidow TG, Hooper PL, Crukley C, Young J, Heathcote JG. Expression of vascular endothelial growth factor in uveal melanoma and its correlation with metastasis. Br J Ophthalmol 84:750–756, 2000.

100. IJland SA, Jager MJ, Heijdra BM, Westphal JR, Peek R. Expression of angiogenic and immunosuppressive factors by uveal melanoma cell lines. Melanoma Res 9:445–450, 1999.

101. Maniotis AJ, Folberg R, Hess A, Seftor EA, Gardner LMG, Pe'er J, Trent JM, Meltzer PS, Hendrix MJC. Vascular channel formation by human melanoma cells *in vivo* and *in vitro*: Vasculogenic mimicry. Am J Pathol 155:739–752, 1999.

102. Hess AR, Seftor EA, Gardner LMG, Carles-Kinch K, Schneider GB, Seftor REB, Kinch MS, Hendrix MJC. Molecular regulation of tumor cell vasculogenic mimicry by tyrosine phosphorylation: Role of epithelial cell kinase (Eck/EphA2). Cancer Res 61:3250–3255, 2001.

103. Pasquale EB. The Eph family of receptors. Curr Opin Cell Biol 9:608–615, 1997.

104. Easty DJ, Hill SP, Hsu M, Fallowfield ME, Florenes VA, Herlyn M, Bennet DC. Up-regulation of Ephrin-A1 during melanoma progression. Int J Cancer 84:494–501, 1999.

105. El-Shabrawi Y, Langmann G, Hutter H, Kenner L, Hoefler G. Comparison of current methods and PCR for the diagnosis of metastatic disease in uveal malignant melanoma. Ophthalmologica 212:80, 1998.

106. Baker JKL, Elshaw SR, Mathewman GEL, Nichols CE, Murray AK, Parsons MA, Rennie IG, Sisley K. Expression of integrins, degradative enzymes and their inhibitors in uveal melanoma: Differences between *in vitro* and *in vivo* expression. Melanoma Res 11:265–273, 2002.

107. Väisänen A, Kallioinen M, von Dickhoff K, Laatikainen L, Höyhtyä M, Turpeenniemi-Hujanen T. Matrix metalloproteinase-2 (MMP-2) immunoreactive protein—A new prognostic marker in uveal melanoma? J Pathol 188:56–62, 1999.

108. Elshaw SR, Sisley K, Cross N, Murray AK, MacNeil SM, Wagner M, Nichols CE, Rennie IG. A comparison of ocular melanocyte and uveal melanoma cell invasion and the implications of [alpha]1[beta]1, [alpha]4[beta]1 and [alpha]6[beta]1 integrins. Br J Ophthalmol 85:732, 2001.

109. El-Shabrawi Y, Ardjomand N, Radner H, Ardjomand N. MMP-9 is predominantly expressed in epithelioid and not spindle cell uveal melanoma. J Pathol 194:201–206, 2001.

110. Seftor REB, Seftor EA, Koshikawa N, Meltzer PS, Gardner LMG, Bilban M, Stetler-Stevenson WG, Quaranta V, Hendrix MJC. Cooperative interactions of laminin 5 γ2 chain, matrix metalloproteinase-2, and membrane type-1-matrix/metalloproteinase are required for mimicry of embryonic vasculogenesis by aggressive melanoma. Cancer Res 61:6322–6327, 2001.

111. Hewitt RE, Brown KE, Corcoran M, Stetler-Stevenson WG. Increased expression of tissue inhibitor of metalloproteinase type 1 (TIMP-1) in more tumourigenic colon cancer cell line. J Pathol 192:455–459, 2000.

112. Hernandez-Barrantes S, Toth M, Bernardo MM, Yurkova M, Gervasi DC, Raz Y, Sang QA, Fridman R. Binding of active (57kDa) membrane type 1-matrix metalloproteinase (MT1-MMP) to tissue inhibitor of metalloproteinase (TIMP)-2 regulates MT1-MMP processing and pro-MMP-2 activation. J Biol Chem 275:12080–12089, 2002.

113. de Vries TJ, Mooy CM, van Balken MR, Luyten GPM, Quax PHA, Verspaget HW, Weidle UH, Ruiter DJ, Van Muijen GNP. Components of the plasminogen activation system in uveal melanoma—A clinico-pathological study. J Pathol 175:59–67, 1995.

114. Ma D, Gerard RD, Li XY, Alizadeh H, Niederkorn JY. Inhibition of metastasis of intraocular melanomas by adenovirus-mediated gene transfer of plasminogen activator inhibitor type I (PAI-1) in an athymic mouse model. Blood 90:2738–2746, 1997.

115. Marshall JF, Rutherford DC, Happerfield L, Hanby A, McCartney ACE, Newton-Bishop J, Hart IR. Comparative analysis of integrins in vitro and in vivo in uveal and cutaneous melanomas. Br J Cancer 77:522–529, 1998.

116. Ten Berge PJM, Danen EHJ, Van Muijen GNP, Jager MJ, Ruiter DJ. Integrin expression in uveal melanoma differs from cutaneous melanoma. Invest Ophthalmol Vis Sci 34:3635–3640, 1993.

117. Larouche N, Larouche K, Béliveau A, Leclerc S, Salesse C, Pelletier G, Guérin SL. Transcriptional regulation of the α4 integrin subunit gene in the metastatic spread of uveal melanoma. Anticancer Res 18:3539–3548, 1998.

118. Natali PG, Bigotti A, Nicotra MR, Nardi RM, Delovu A, Segatto O, Ferrone S. Analysis of the antigenic profile of uveal melanoma lesions with anti-cutaneous melanoma-associated antigen and anti-HLA monoclonal antibodies. Cancer Res 49:1269–1274, 1989.

119. van der Pol JP, Jager MJ, De Wolff-Rouendaal D, Ringens PJ, Vennegoor C, Ruiter DJ. Heterogeneous expression of melanoma-associated antigens in uveal melanomas. Curr Eye Res 6:757–765, 1987.

120. Carrel S, Schreyer M, Gross N, Zografos L. Surface antigenic profile of uveal melanoma lesions analyzed with a panel of monoclonal antibodies directed against cutaneous melanoma. Anticancer Res 10:81–90, 1990.

121. Mooy CM, Luyten GPM, De Jong PTVM, Jensen OA, Luider TM, Van der Ham F, Bosman FT. Neural cell adhesion molecule distribution in primary and metastatic uveal melanoma. Hum Pathol 26:1185–1190, 1995.

122. Ma D, Niederkorn JY. Role of epidermal growth factor receptor in the metastasis of intraocular melanomas. Invest Ophthalmol Vis Sci 39:1067–1075, 1998.

123. Radinsky R. Molecular mechanisms for organ-specific colon carcinoma metastasis. Eur J Cancer 31:1091–1095, 1995.

124. Hurks HMH, Metzelaar-Blok JAW, Barthen ER, Zwinderman AH, De Wolff-Rouendaal D, Keunen JEE, Jager MJ. Expression of epidermal growth factor receptor: risk factor in uveal melanoma. Invest Ophthalmol Vis Sci 41:2023–2027, 2000.

125. Scholes AGM, Hagan S, Hiscott P, Damato BE, Grierson I. Overexpression of epidermal growth factor receptor restricted to macrophages in uveal melanoma. Arch Ophthalmol 119:373–377, 2001.

126. Hendrix MJC, Seftor EA, Seftor REB, Gardner LM, Boldt HC, Meyer M, Pe'er J, Folberg R. Biologic determinants of uveal melanoma metastatic phenotype: Role of intermediate filaments as predictive markers. Lab Invest 78:153–163, 1998.

127. Hendrix MJC, Seftor EA, Seftor REB, Kirschmann DA, Gardner LM, Boldt HC, Meyer M, Pe'er J, Folberg R. Regulation of uveal melanoma interconverted phenotype by hepatocyte growth factor scatter factor (HGF/SF). Am J Pathol 152:855–863, 1998.

128. Mäkitie T, Summanen P, Tarkkanen A, Kivelä T. Tumor-infiltrating macrophages (CD68^{+} cells) and prognosis in malignant uveal melanoma. Invest Ophthalmol Vis Sci 42:1414–1421, 2001.

129. Vaherie A, Carpen O, Heiska L. The ezrin protein family: Membrane-cytoskeleton interactions and disease associations. Curr Opin Cell Biol 9:659–666, 2002.

130. Crepaldi T, Gautreau A, Comoglio PM, Louvard D, Arpin M. Ezrin is an effector of hepatocyte growth factor-mediated migration and morphogenesis in epithelial cells. J Cell Biol 138:423–434, 1997.

131. Lamb RF, Ozanne BW, Roy C. Essential functions of ezrin in maintenance of cell shape and lamellipodial extensions in normal and transformed fibroblasts. Curr Biol 7:682–688, 1997.

132. Hiscox S, Jiang WG. Ezrin regulates cell-cell and cell-matrix adhesion, a possible role with E-cadherin/β-catenin. J Cell Sci 112:3081–3090, 1999.

133. Mäkitie T, Carpén O, Vaherie A, Kivelä T. Ezrin as a prognostic indicator and its relationship to tumor characteristics in uveal malignant melanoma. Invest Ophthalmol Vis Sci 42:2442–2449, 2001.

134. Yu H, Rohan T. Role of the insulin-like growth factor family in cancer development and progression. J Natl Cancer Inst 92:1472–1489, 2000.

135. All-Ericsson C, Girnita L, Seregard S, Bartolazzi A, Jager MJ, Larsson O. Insulin like growth factor-1 receptor in uveal melanoma: a predictor for metastatic disease and a potential therapeutic target. Invest Ophthalmol Vis Sci 43:1–8, 2002.

136. van Ginkel PR, Gee RL, Subramanian L, Walker TM, Albert DM, Meisner LF, Varnum BC, Polans AS. Over-expression of the receptor tyrosine kinase axl promotes ocular melanoma cell survival. submitted 2002.

137. Ma D, Luyten GP, Luider TM, Jager MJ, Niederkorn JY. Association between nm23-H1 gene expression and metastasis of human uveal melanoma in an animal model. Invest Ophthalmol Vis Sci 37:2293–2301, 1996.

138. Diatchenko L, Lau Y-FC, Campbell AP, Chenckik A, Mooadam F, Huang B, et al. Suppression subtractive hybridization: a method for generating differentially regulated

or tissue-specific cDNA probes and libraries. Proc Natl Acad Sci USA 93:6025–6030, 1996.

139. Hanahan D, Weinberg RA. The hallmarks of cancer. Cell 100:57–70, 2000.

140. Novatchkova M, Eisenhaber F. Can molecular mechanisms of biological processes be extracted from expression profiles? Case study: Endothelial contribution to tumor-induced angiogenesis. Bioessays 23:1159–1175, 2002.

141. Bittner M, Meltzer P, Chen Y, Jiang Y, Seftor E, Hendrix M, Radmacher M, Simon R, Yakhini Z, Ben-Dor A, Sampas N, Dougherty E, Wang E, Marincola F, Gooden C, Lueders J, Glatfelter A, Pollock P, Carpten J, Gillanders E, Leja D, Dietrich K, Beaudry C, Berens M, Alberts D, Sondak V, Hayward N, Trent J. Molecular classification of cutaneous melanoma by gene expression profiling. Nature 406:536–540, 2000.

7

A Cascade of Genomic Changes Leads to Retinoblastoma

VIVETTE D. BROWN

University Health Network, Toronto, Ontario, Canada

HELEN S. L. CHAN and BRENDA L. GALLIE

University of Toronto, Toronto, Ontario, Canada

Retinoblastoma is a malignant tumor of the eye in children that arises in a uniquely susceptible human developing retinal cell when both alleles of the retinoblastoma gene (*RB1*) are mutated (M1, M2) [1–3]. However, all retinoblastoma tumors have additional mutational events (M3, M4, ..., Mn) and other unknown stochastic events that may be required for full malignant transformation [4,5]. In most tissues except retina, the loss of both *RB1* alleles results in cell death. Therefore, in predisposed human infants, a unique characteristic of the undefined retinal cell that is dependent on *RB1* to prevent cancer might be a dependence on a specific mechanism for physiological cell death. Other cells in tissues at risk of cancer in $RB1^{+/-}$ patients (e.g., differentiating bone) might share such cell death attributes.

In this chapter, we describe the known initiating mutations in the *RB1* gene (M1, M2) and outline the evidence for a cascade of mutational events in other candidate genes (M3 to Mn) that result in cancer of the developing retina (Fig. 1). Mutational instability continues in cancer cells, with selection of the tumor cells that have acquired mutations which enhance survival of that tumor cell over others and contribute selective advantage. Two genes that lead to multidrug resistance are commonly overexpressed in retinoblastoma, and other undefined genes are anticipated to play additional roles in the malignant progression that leads to failure to cure. When the oncogenic events beyond the *RB1* gene are clearly

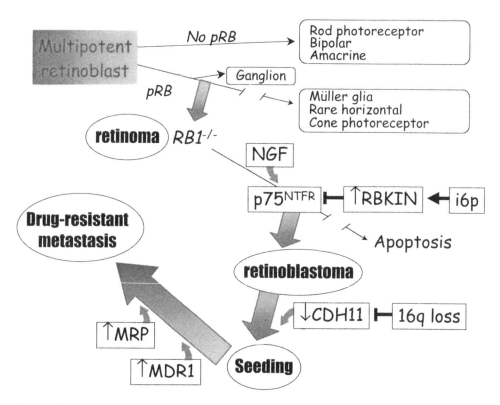

Figure 1 Theoretical events driving progression from normal multipotent retinoblasts to retinoma, retinoblastoma, dissemination by vitreous and subretinal seeding, and ultimately multidrug-resistant metastasis. The initiating loss of pRB by mutation of both alleles of RB1 and the promotion of drug resistance by MDR1 are well established. The hypothetical roles of p75NTFR, RBKIN, CDH11, and MRP are not yet established.

understood, they may constitute good targets for retinoblastoma treatment and prevention strategies to cure tumors, decreasing the risk of blindness and loss of life in predisposed children.

I. FEATURES OF THE RETINAL CELL UNIQUELY SENSITIVE TO LOSS OF *RB1* ALLELES

A. Developmental Window

1. The Retina: Between Precursor and Mature Cells

Only cells that normally require the intact *RB1* gene for the critical role played by its protein product, pRB, can give rise to retinoblastoma. All retinal cells arise from a common precursor of neural origin. In the fully mature retina, cells are organized into three nuclear layers: the ganglion cell layer (GCL); the inner nuclear layer (INL), containing horizontal, bipolar, amacrine, and Müller glia cells; and the outer nuclear layer (ONL), containing rod and cone photoreceptor cells. There is a well-defined temporal pattern of progression in which proliferating pluripotent precursor cells undergo terminal mitosis ("birth"), followed by terminal differentiation. In rodents, the ganglion, amacrine, horizontal, and cone photoreceptor cells are "born prenatally," whereas the bipolar and Müller glia cells are mainly "born postnatally." Rod photoreceptor cells, by far the predominant retinal cell type, are "born both pre- and postnatally," with the peak terminal mitosis occurring around birth [reviewed in Ref. 6]. Ganglion cells are unique in that their birth and terminal differentiation occur over a very short, early period of time. In contrast, acquisition of features of terminal differentiation in other retinal cell types is delayed for several days after terminal mitosis [7]. Although postmitotic, multipotent progenitors give rise to mature retinal cells in a predictable fashion, their specific fates may be altered by growth factors [e.g., rod photoreceptors may be respecified by the ciliary neurotrophic factor (CNTF)] [8,9].

Our preliminary data suggests that only a few retinal cell types express detectable *RB1*: the postmitotic cone photoreceptor, Müller glia, ganglion, and a rare horizontal cell type. Both murine models of retinoblastoma and human retinoblastoma frequently arise from the inner nuclear layer (Fig. 2), making the developing Müller glia or horizontal cells prime candidates to be the retinoblastoma precursor (Fig. 1). In humans, the loss of both alleles of the *RB1* gene in the precursor cells predisposes to development of retinoblastoma. In mice, loss of *RB1* from the earliest stages of retinal development does not cause retinoblastoma, but loss of both *RB1* and p107 does [10]. Jacks et al. now suggest that acute loss of *RB1* alone within the window of ongoing retinal development, rather than before retinal differentiation starts, results in retinoblastoma [11].

B.   Learning from Differences and Similarities in Mice and Humans

1.   Impact of Loss of *RB1* in the Mouse Embryo

Homozygous deletion of the *RB1* gene in mice results in embryonic lethality at day E13.5–15.5 gestation [12–14], with death from abnormal hematopoiesis and neurogenesis. The embryos show a significant increase in immature erythrocytes, and massive apoptosis and ectopic mitoses in the central and peripheral nervous system. There are also significant defects in lens development and myogenesis, showing the important role of pRB in proliferation and differentiation in many tissues [15,16].

2.   Different Impact of Loss of *RB1* in Mouse Embryos and in Humans

Surprisingly, the neural retina of $RB1^{-/-}$ mice is normal up to day E15.5 gestation, compared to wild type $RB1^{+/+}$ mice [12–14]. Beyond day E16, however, loss of pRB in individual cells of $RB1^{-/-};RB1^{+/-}$ chimeric mice in which embryonic lethality has been prevented by the presence of $RB1^{+/-}$ still resulted in abnormal development of the lens, with ectopic mitoses and cellular degeneration of the retina [17,18]. $RB1^{+/-}$ mice and chimeric $RB1^{-/-};RB1^{+/-}$ mice tend to develop pituitary adenoma in which the second *RB1* allele has been lost, as in human retinoblastoma [14,17,19]. However, $RB1^{+/-}$ humans do not develop pituitary adenoma, whereas $RB1^{+/-}$ and

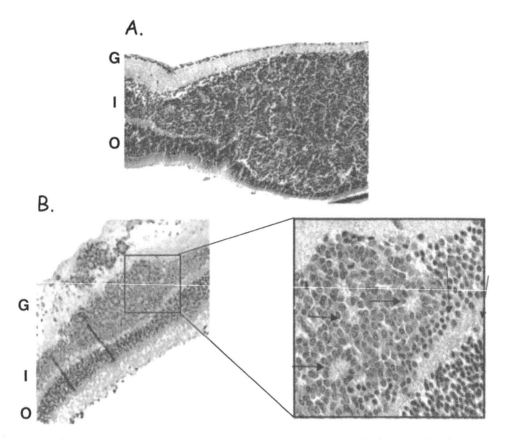

Figure 2 Murine and human retinoblastomas commonly arise in the inner nuclear layer. A. SV40 TAg–induced murine retinoblastoma arises from the inner nuclear layer of developing retina. B. Human retinoblastoma arises from the inner nuclear layer of the retina. G, ganglion cell layer; I, inner nuclear layer; O, outer nuclear layer; arrows point to Flexner–Wintersteiner rosettes.

chimeric $RB1^{-/-};RB1^{+/-}$ mice do not develop retinoblastoma. This suggests that loss of pRB prior to the development of mouse retina results in cell death rather than increased retinal cell proliferation, in contrast to loss of pRB in developing human retina, which results in cell cycle progression.

3. Other pRB Family Members Compensate for Loss of *RB1* in the Murine Embryo

In mice, the other pRB family members may partially compensate for loss of pRB by suppressing the development of retinoblastoma. For instance, both p107$^{-/-}$ and p130$^{-/-}$ mice are viable without retinal dysplasia [20,21], whereas loss of p107 as well as one copy of the *RB1* gene in $RB1^{+/-}$;p107$^{-/-}$ mice causes retinal dysplasia [20]. Loss of p107 as well as both copies of the RB1 gene in $RB1^{-/-}$;p107$^{-/-}$ mice causes death at E11.5 so the impact on the developing retina cannot be determined [20], whereas only simultaneous loss of both p107 and pRB proteins in the retinoblasts can cause retinoblastoma in $RBI^{-/-}$;p107$^{-/-}$ chimeric mice [22]. This retinoblastoma tumor originates in cells in the inner nuclear layer (Fig. 2) and expresses amacrine cell markers.

4. A Murine Model Comparable to Human Retinoblastoma

In an attempt to make a mouse model for pituitary adenoma, the simian virus-40 large T antigen (SV40 TAg) was linked to the promoter of the human luteinizing hormone beta subunit, LHβ, so as to restrict expression to gonadotrophic cells [23]. Surprisingly, one founder lineage developed focal bilateral retinal tumors as a result of the high expression of TAg also in the retina, the first transgenic mouse model of retinoblastoma. These focal tumors are histologically, ultrastructurally, and immunohistochemically identical to human retinoblastoma. The pRB interacts with the high expression of TAg in the murine retinoblastoma cells. The retina-specific promoter, interphotoreceptor retinoid-binding protein (IRBP), which differentiates the photoreceptors and is expressed early in retinal cell differentiation, is used to produce TAg transgenic mice [24–26]. However, the opsin promoter resulted in no retinal tumors, presumably because opsins are expressed later in photoreceptor differentiation when the retinal cells no longer have the potential for mitosis. In the murine retinoblastoma model, the entire photoreceptor layer was malignant, probably reflecting the early timing of inactivation of all the pRB family proteins by TAg rather than specific binding to pRB.

5. Loss of pRB and Default Pathway of Retinal Differentiation

Our preliminary data indicate that pRB is not expressed in adult rod photoreceptors or bipolar cells of human or mouse, and only in a very narrow window of differentiation, if at all, in murine development. However, loss of pRB may result in the transformed cells assuming a default pathway of differentiation that does not require pRB. Indeed, retinal progenitor cells go through a series of changes in intrinsic properties that control their competence to make different cell types [27]. If a pRB-dependent lineage is disrupted, a cell may follow another lineage pathway, depending on extrinsic cues from the neighboring cells. Therefore, identification of retinal specific pathways that are regulated by pRB will provide clues to the identity of the cell of origin in retinoblastoma. This will not only provide a system to test experimental therapies for prevention of human retinoblastoma but also help define the fundamental properties of the stem cells that are capable of forming cancer. This has relevance beyond the rare disease of retinoblastoma.

C. The Retinoma Way Station

1. Attributes of the Benign Human Retinoma

Nonprogressing retinal lesions were originally considered to represent "spontaneous regression" of retinoblastoma. Then Gallie et al. proposed designating nonmalig-nant-looking retinal lesions associated with retinoblastoma as retinoma since there was no clear evidence that they were "regressed retinoblastomas" [28,29]. A retinoma is typically a translucent-gray retinal mass frequently associated with calcification and hyperplasia of the retinal pigment epithelium [28,30–32], unlike the actively proliferating retinoblastoma, which shows calcification but appears opaque-white [30]. Electron microscopy of six retinomas showed a haphazard arrangement of neuronal cells with photoreceptor differentiation, a few axons, Müller glia, and astrocytes [29]. Alió and coworkers found, in intraocular fine-needle aspiration biopsy of a retinoma, mainly degenerated cells with lipid cytoplasmic vacuoles and disintegrating mitochrondria, but no Flexner-Wintersteiner rosettes characteristic of retinoblastoma [33].

2. Retinoma Predisposed by *RB1* Mutations

Although retinomas are "benign," they may rarely undergo malignant progression to retinoblastoma. *RB1* germline mutations predispose to both retinoma and retinoblastoma. Therefore individuals with retinoma should be followed regularly [30]. Of 32 individuals with retinoma studied, two-thirds had a family history of retinoblastoma or had retinoblastoma in their other eye, and 23 of 37 (62%) of their offspring developed retinoblastoma [30]. Another study showed 11 individuals with retinoma in 103 retinoblastoma families, 7 of which had a family history of retinoblastoma, and 12 of their 16 offspring developed retinoblastoma [34,35]. Keith and Webb reported a chromosome 13q-deleted patient with active retinoblastoma in one eye and a retinoma in the other eye, suggesting that retinoma and retinoblastoma were induced by similar genetic changes [36]. Although no molecular analysis of retinoma has been reported, we have identified the germline *RB1* mutations in several patients with bilateral or unilateral multifocal retinomas as their only clinical manifestation.

3. Malignant Transformation of Retinoma to Retinoblastoma

Retinoma has been reported to undergo malignant transformation to retinoblastoma [32,37–39]. Histopathology of a rapidly growing, newly elevated area of a retinoma that had remained stable for 3 years showed undifferentiated retinoblastoma, while the retinoma base was characteristic of benign retinoma [32]. This suggests that additional mutations, presumably in genes involved in cell cycle regulation or apoptosis, are necessary to convert a benign retinoma cell into a malignant retinoblastoma cell [40].

II. INITIATION OF RETINOBLASTOMA: M1 AND M2 EVENTS

Since the discovery of the retinoblastoma gene, *RB1*, in 1986 [41], molecular identification of *RB1* mutations has been used to determine the risk of retinoblastoma in other family members [42–44]. Bilaterally affected patients all have one germline *RB1* mutant allele, which results in autosomal dominant transmission of the predisposition to retinoblastoma. Clinical testing requires study of blood DNA to identify the precise mutant allele in each affected family. Unilaterally affected patients have only a 15% chance that they carry a germline *RB1* mutant allele. Since 85% of unilateral sporadic patients have no germline mutations, testing of blood would be prohibitively expensive and inconclusive if no mutation is found. Therefore the standard approach for unilateral patients is testing the retinoblastoma tumor DNA to identify the two mutant *RB1* alleles, followed by testing the blood DNA for each of those mutations. In this way, a negative result generally rules out a heritable retinoblastoma in the proband, which is useful for risk prediction for the relatives. However, a small possibility of mosaicism remains, as discussed below.

A. Spectrum of *RB1* Mutant Alleles

1. Expeditious Strategies for Screening for *RB1* Mutations

RB1 mutations occur throughout the gene and the majority are "null," resulting in no detectable pRB. More than 50% of *RB1* mutations have been found once only, and the majority of germline mutations have originated with the proband. Therefore the job of identifying the *RB1* mutation in each family is onerous. To detect the mutation in each family, a series of assays and different technologies are required. Various scanning techniques help identify suspect exons, and follow-up sequencing detects approximately 60% of the mutations. Somatic mutations in tumors that involve methylation of the promoter occur in about 10% of tumors [45]. To achieve 90% sensitivity of identifying the *RB1* mutation in each family, we have added quantitative multiplex polymerase chain reaction (QM-PCR) to detect copy number changes of single and multiple exons. The types of mutations include single base substitutions, resulting in amino acid substitutions or altered splice sites, small deletions and large ones up to deletion of the whole gene, exonic deletions, intraexon deletions, and insertions and methylation of promoter regions. *RB1* mutations are spread throughout the gene including the promoter, occurring in most exons and some introns, with no significant hot spots for null mutations.

2. Our Results for *RB1* Mutation Screening

We have identified more than 450 mutant *RB1* alleles [45a]. In bilateral probands, 93% of the mutations have been null, 6% are in-frame, and 1% are promoter. The *RB1* germline mutations in unilateral probands (both familial and sporadic) are 57% null only, while 40% are in-frame and 3% are promoter. The reduced expressivity manifests as fewer than expected tumors, therefore more often occurring as unilateral rather than bilateral disease. This correlates with the presence of "weak" *RB1* mutant alleles that retain enough activity to prevent some but not all retinoblastoma tumors. The mutant alleles that have been identified in retinoblastoma tumors but not in blood, therefore presumably somatic, are 88% null, 3% in-frame, and 8% promoter methylation. In summary, the overall rate to successfully complete the clinical analysis (persons diagnosed/persons analyzed) was 86% for families with unilateral germline mutations, 89% for families with bilateral probands, and 82% for unilateral retinoblastoma probands with no family history for which both mutant alleles must be found in each of the tumors.

For sporadic retinoblastoma tumors, the second allele was mutated by loss of heterozygosity (LOH) in 52%. The likelihood that the M2 event would be LOH varied with the type of M1 event. Only 22 (27%) of the tumors with M1 whole gene and exonic deletions, respectively, showed LOH, while 89% of tumors with methylation of the promoter showed LOH.

Some "recurrent" mutations, including large deletions and methylation of the promoter, have not been defined at a nucleotide level. Thirteen true recurrent point mutations occurred four or more times in our dataset, all resulting from CT transitions at CpG dinucleotides because of deamination of 5-methylcytosine [46,47]. Twelve affect arginine codons, and one creates a splice mutation. There is a true "hot spot" for missense mutations, involving the A/B "pocket" domain of pRB, which is critical in the interaction of pRB with the transcription factor E2F [48]. Presumably, missense mutations in the remainder of *RB1* are insufficient to initiate retinoblastoma.

B. Practical Clinical Detection

1. Clinical Importance of *RB1* Mutation Identification

Precise identification of the *RB1* mutations that account for retinoblastoma in each family enhances the quality of clinical management of the affected patient and relatives at risk. Individuals with *RB1* mutations have a higher-than-normal lifetime risk to develop additional cancers [49]. Exposure to external beam radiation further increases that risk. In the absence of knowledge of the precise *RB1* mutation in the family, children at risk to have retinoblastoma undergo a series of clinical examinations, including examination under anesthetic (EUA), in order to diagnose and treat tumors as early as possible. If the *RB1* gene status of the proband has been determined by molecular testing, only those relatives with the mutation require clinical surveillance, while those proven not to be carriers require no further testing. The direct costs of molecular testing are significantly less than conventional clinical examinations for each family [50]. If a family's mutation is known, prenatal molecular testing allows careful planning of perinatal management for infants with *RB1* mutations. We have delivered five infants prematurely to facilitate early treatment of macular tumors. Two of the babies had macular tumors at 35 weeks gestation, and all of the children had bilateral retinoblastoma within the first 3 months of age.

2. "Best Practice" Guidelines for *RB1* Mutation Identification

Despite clear clinical benefits of molecular testing for retinoblastoma, mutation detection in the *RB1* gene has not been widely implemented. The wide variety of inactivating mutations, and their distribution along the entire length of the gene without any significant hot spots, have made *RB1* mutation identification difficult and expensive. In addition, the heterogeneity of the *RB1* mutation spectrum suggests that no one single mutation identification technology could be totally sensitive and fully efficient. Several testing laboratories have focused on clinical *RB1* mutation testing and refined their technologies and interpretation to enable implementation in practice. These laboratories include the Institut für Humangenetik, Essen, Germany (D. Lohmann), and Retinoblastoma Solutions (http://www.solutionsbysequence.com). The European Molecular Quality Network has already formalized the validation of *RB1* testing and published this on the EMQN website (http://www.emqn.org/guidelines/rb.php).

C.   Origin of *RB1* Mutations and Mosaicism

1.   Frequent Mutation of the Paternal *RB1* Allele

The majority of children with heritable retinoblastoma have newly acquired *RB1* mutations. Most frequently, it is the paternal *RB1* allele that is mutated [51], presumably due to the increased exposure risks of sperms relative to ova. This observation is consistent with the epidemiologic data suggesting an increased risk for fathers in metal works and the military to have children with retinoblastoma [52,53].

2.   Mosaicism of *RB1* Mutations

About 10% of new *RB1* germline mutations may be present in only a fraction of the cells of the proband. These individuals, therefore, are considered to be mosaic for the mutant allele. Mosaicism becomes obvious only when a parent with more than one child with retinoblastoma does not show the same mutant *RB1* allele present in the children [54,55]. Of the 10% bilaterally affected probands in whom we cannot identify the *RB1* mutant allele, perhaps 1% may be mosaic, such that the fraction of mutant cells in their blood leukocytes is insufficient for detection of the mutation. Therefore, when the two *RB1* mutant alleles are characterized in the retinoblastoma tumor tissue but cannot be found in the blood DNA of a unilaterally affected proband, we report that there remains a 2–3% chance that the child is mosaic. Since mosaicism could not be inherited, ancestors and siblings are not considered at risk for retinoblastoma. However, each future offspring of such a proband should be checked for the two mutant alleles found in the retinoblastoma tumor.

D.   Phenotype-Genotype Correlations

1.   *RB1* "Null" Mutations and Penetrance

The vast majority of *RB1* mutant alleles are "null," resulting in premature truncation of translation, unstable mRNA [42] and no detectable pRB protein, and predispose to bilateral retinoblastoma tumors in close to 100% of children. Of the probands with null germline mutations, 92% had bilateral tumors, while only 50% of probands with in-frame mutations developed bilateral tumors. The disease/eye ratio (DER), or ratio of clinically affected eyes to mutation carriers [56], for persons with null *RB1* alleles is approximately 2.0 [57]. *RB1* mutations that result in a stable but less active protein are associated with reduced penetrance and a reduced number of tumors (30% of eyes affected) versus 100% of eyes in persons with null alleles. The recurrent missense mutation R661W has been associated with reduced penetrance with an average DER of 0.73 [58,59]. The R661W protein has been shown to have partial activity, including retention of nuclear localization and hyperphosphorylation, but reduced or absent pRB-binding protein interactions [57,60,61]. Sporadic unilateral patients with R661W germline mutations are founders of reduced penetrance families. Other low penetrance missense mutations affect the promoter, the A/B domain of pRB, or splicing functions, resulting in a reduction of the amount of pRB [62–64].

2.   Examples of Low-Penetrance Families

We reported a low penetrance family with an in-frame deletion of *RB1* exon 24 and 25, resulting in a protein with altered nuclear localization, reduced ability to repress E2F-mediated transcription, inability to bind the MDM2 pRB-binding protein, and the inability to suppress growth [65]. Of 18 members of this large family known to carry the Δ24–25 mutation, only 11 of 18 individuals developed retinoblastoma, 1 had retinoma, and only 3 had bilateral tumors (low expressivity). The DER for this family was 0.78, consistent with reduced penetrance. Other small deletions that resulted in low penetrance retinoblastoma include ΔN480 that deletes asparagine 480, and Δ4 that contains an in-frame deletion of exon 4. Each of these mutants retained the ability to suppress growth but differed in their ability to bind pRB-binding proteins [57].

3.   Other Primary Tumors from pRB Inactivation

Inactivation of pRB and other proteins in the pRB cell cycle regulatory pathway contribute to a wide array of cancers including osteosarcoma, small cell lung carcinoma, breast carcinoma, and other malignancies [66]. Inactivation of the pathway can occur by mutation of *RB1*, mutation of p16 which inhibits pRB phosphorylation by inhibiting cyclin D1, or amplification of cyclin D1, which phosphorylates pRB to its inactive form.

4.   Exogenous Inactivation of pRB

Some of the missing *RB1* mutations in retinoblastoma tumors theoretically may involve other parts of the RB pathway [67]. It has also been suggested that exogenous factors may induce retinoblastoma, since the DNA of the human papillomavirus has been detected in 36% of retinoblastoma tumors [68]. This virus is well known to produce proteins that can inactivate pRB. However, more work is needed to clarify these observations, since the *RB1* mutations have not been studied in this particular set of tumors.

III.   CANDIDATE M3-TO-MN EVENTS

A.   Genomic Gains and Losses

1.   Gains at 1q and 2p and Loss at 16q as M3-to-Mn Events

All retinoblastoma tumors are initiated by mutation of both copies of the *RB1* gene. There is no evidence that any other gene besides *RB1* initiates the predisposition to human retinoblastoma. Knudson's two-hit hypothesis states that these two mutational events (M1 and M2) are rate-limiting for development of retinoblastoma [69]. However, additional mutations (M3-Mn) are almost certainly required before full malignant transformation results, since there are genetic alterations in addition to *RB1* in all retinoblastoma tumors [4,5]. Karyotypic analysis and comparative genomic hybridization (CGH) have been used to characterize genomic gains and losses within retinoblastoma tumors [70–72]. The minimal regions most frequently gained were 1q31 (52%), 6p22 (44%), 2p24–25 (30%), and 13q32–34 (12%) [72]. The minimal region most frequently lost was 16q22 (14%). In one study, gains at 1q and 2p and loss of 16q were restricted to more advanced tumors in older children, suggesting that these changes might correlate with tumor progression. However, 6p gains might be associated more with tumor initiation [71]. Chromosome 1q gain is common in many cancers besides retinoblastoma [73–77]. However, almost unique to retinoblastoma is a specific pattern of 6p gain, i(6p), identified in 60% of retinoblastoma tumors [78]. This marker chromosome results in four copies of genes on chromosome 6p, or low-level amplification [79].

2. Maintenance of Genetic Stability by pRB

Interestingly, recent data from the mouse suggests that pRB is involved in maintaining genetic stability within the cell. Using a retrovirus carrying negative and positive selectable markers which integrated randomly into individual chromosomes, the authors were able to determine the frequency of loss of the chromosomal marker in mammalian cells [80]. In normal mouse embryonic stem (ES) cells, the frequency for loss of the marker was less than 10^{-8} per cell per generation. In $RB1^{-/-}$ ES cells, the frequency was increased to 10^{-5} per cell per generation, while in $RB1^{+/-}$ ES cells, the frequency was 10^{-7} per cell per generation. Such a process may account for the emergence of M3 events after the loss of $RB1$. However, in contrast to adult-onset tumors, retinoblastoma tumors have abnormal karyotypes with a finite number of genomic changes that remain stable over years.

B. Isochromosome 6p Contains a Candidate Oncogene, *RBKIN*

We hypothesized that the region of chromosome 6p gain may contain an oncogene necessary for progression of retinoblastoma. To identify candidate oncogenes, we narrowed the region of gain on 6p to a minimal 0.6-Mb region of 6p22 using quantitative multiplex polymerase chain reaction (QM-PCR) for sequence-tagged sites (STS) [81], and cloned a novel human kinesin-like gene, *RBKIN*. *RBKIN* expression is increased in retinoblastoma compared to normal human retina, and inhibition of *RBKIN* in retinoblastoma cell lines using an antisense oligonucleotide results in a block in cell growth, consistent with *RBKIN* acting as an oncogene [81]. However, further experimentation is necessary to confirm the role of *RBKIN* as an oncogene in retinoblastoma development. Chromosome 6p gain is also common in bladder cancer and is associated with an elevated risk of progression of bladder cancer [82,83], suggesting that *RBKIN* may have a much broader role in cancer.

C. Chromosome 16q Loss Narrowed to a Member of the Cadherin Family

Using loss of heterozygosity and QM-PCR, we narrowed the loss of chromosome 16q22 in retinoblastoma to a region that contains the cadherin 11 (*CDH11*) and *CDH13* genes. Allelic loss on 16q22 has been frequently shown in liver [84], breast [85], prostate [86], and Wilms' [87] tumors, suggesting the presence of a gene or genes in this region that may be important in carcinogenesis. Three members of the cadherin family have previously been implicated in carcinogenesis. Downregulation of *CDH1* gene expression correlates with invasive potential and poor prognosis in human carcinoma, sometimes combined with functional loss of *CDH11* [88]. *CDH11* is also downregulated in 23 cases of osteosarcoma but not in normal osteoblasts, and in astrocytoma but not in normal brain tissues [89,90]. The *CDH13* gene has been deleted or inactivated by promoter methylation in more than 50% of advanced-stage ovarian cancers [91] and in breast, lung, and osteosarcoma tumors [92,93]. We have shown the expression of *CDH11* in normal retina, but not in 2 of 3 primary retinoblastoma tumors and 3 of 4 retinoblastoma cell lines. One primary retinoblastoma and one cell line showed a faster migrating form of *CDH11*. The role of cadherins in progression of retinoblastoma requires further investigation.

IV. SLIPPING PAST CELL DEATH

A. Importance of Programmed Cell Death in Retinal Development

The retina is one of the tissues whose final architecture is achieved by the precise balance between proliferation, differentiation, and apoptosis. During retinal development, the number of cells produced exceeds the number of cells ultimately required, so that many cells are removed by apoptosis to achieve the final retinal structure.

1. Role of p75^{NTR} in the Retina and in Retinoblastoma

Nerve growth factor (NGF) signals for survival through TrkA, and for apoptosis through p75^{NTR} in retina [94–96]. Induction of cell death through p75^{NTR} may be preceded by the unscheduled re-entry of postmitotic neurons into the cell cycle [95]. We have evidence that downregulation of the p75^{NTR} protein might be important for M3-Mn events in retinoblastoma by promoting proliferation of $RB1^{-/-}$ retinal cells and disrupting apoptosis induced by NGF produced by Müller glia.

The p75^{NTR} protein is highly expressed in Müller glia of wild-type retina and in the benign retinoma but is undetectable in retinoblastoma (unpublished data). Although we found significant cell division in retinoma, indicated by expression of proliferating cell nuclear antigen (PCNA), there is probably also significant apoptotic activity in retinoma compared to retinoblastoma. Therefore there may be a homeostatic balance between cell growth and cell death within a retinoma, explaining why retinomas are generally stable. One or more additional mutations that prevent apoptosis may tip over this balance and convert a retinoma into a retinoblastoma.

B. Telomerase and Immortality

1. Telomerase Activity in Cancers

The role of telomerase in the development of cancer has been suggested based on the presence of telomerase activity in many human cancers, whereas normal cells are devoid of telomerase activity [97]. Telomeres are specialized protein-DNA structures at the ends of chromosomes that protect the chromosome from end-to-end fusion and eventual cell death [98]. Telomerase is the reverse transcriptase that maintains the ends of chromosomes. During normal cellular replication, the lagging strand is replicated by short RNA primers, which are made by RNA primase. These primers are extended by DNA polymerase to form Okazaki fragments [99]. However, when these primers are removed, there is no way to replicate the small fragment of DNA at the ends of the chromosomes. Therefore, with each cell division, the chromosomes are shortened a bit more and eventually become inadequate, causing the cell to enter crisis. In order for a cell to become immortal, it must overcome the end replication problem and maintain intact telomeres. Cancer cells are thought to do this by reactivating telomerase, which has been found to be highly expressed in a number of cancers, including metastatic ovarian carcinoma, colorectal adenocarcinoma, and aggressively proliferating myeloid leukemia [100–103].

However, few retinoblastoma tumors activate telomerase en route to malignancy. Of 34 retinoblastoma tumors studied, 17 (50%) did not express telomerase [104]. Telomerase activity even in the 17 telomerase-positive retinoblastoma tumors was low relative to the telomerase-positive adenovirus-transformed 293 cells. As expected, normal human embryonic retina was negative for telomerase activity. Unilateral and bilateral tumors were almost equally represented in the telomerase-positive and telomerase-negative groups. Additionally, those telomerase-negative tumors contained significantly longer telomeres than the telomerase-positive tumors. Telomerase-negative retinoblastoma tumors containing longer telomeres may have acquired mutations that utilize different mechanisms, such as activation of an oncogene or loss of a tumor suppressor gene, thereby bypassing the need for reactivation of telomerase.

V. RETINOBLASTOMA RESISTANCE TO THERAPY

Chemotherapy followed by focal therapy with laser and cryotherapy has become the primary treatment for large intraocular retinoblastomas and visually threatening small tumors. Extraocular retinoblastoma can also respond to chemotherapy, and in combination with orbital radiation and bone marrow or stem cell transplantation, there is the possibility of long-term remissions and even cures of extraocular retinoblastoma [105,106]. A large series treated with a unified protocol has yet to be reported.

A. Multidrug-Resistance Genes

1.   Overview of Multidrug Resistance in Cancer

Retinoblastoma tumors are rarely cured by chemotherapy alone, since they frequently contain cells that are resistant and survive chemotherapy to regrow. Multidrug resistance (MDR) in the human host could be caused by a number of genes and factors acting cooperatively (Fig. 3). Upstream factors include genetic factors intrinsic to the host, tumor factors, drug metabolism, drug clearance, and drug distribution, all potentially affecting the response to chemotherapy. Tumor factors include a variety of genes that confer multidrug resistance, such as MDR1 (P-glycoprotein), MRP (multidrug-resistance protein), LRP (lung resistance protein), Topo II (topoisomerase II enzymes), and GSH (glutathione enzymes), all potentially affecting the response to chemotherapy. Downstream factors include yet other genes

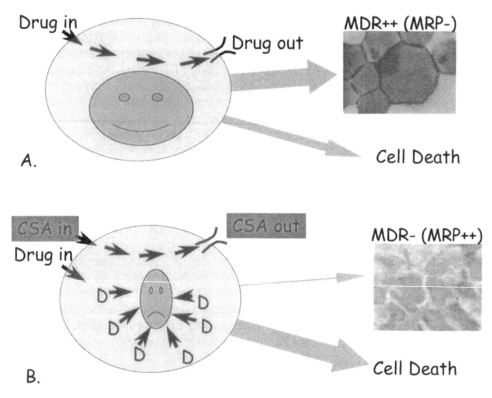

Figure 3 Model of multidrug resistance and mechanism of cyclosporine (CSA) action. A. Chemotherapy drugs diffuse into the tumor cell but are rapidly removed by the MDR membrane pump, allowing tumor cell survival. Some cells die, but many are resistant. Multidrug resistance correlates with the level of expression of the MDR protein (shown using immunohistochemistry), so residual and recurrent retinoblastomas stain positive for MDR and negative for MRP (not shown). B. CSA given at the same time as the chemotherapy drugs is removed from the tumor cell by the MDR membrane pump, competing with extrusion of chemotherapy drugs. The chemotherapy drugs remain in the tumor cell, achieving a high rate of cell death. Retinoblastoma multidrug resistance is less likely; but when it arises, the recurrent cells are MDR-negative and MRP-positive (not shown).

that regulate cell cycle progression, cell death, and differentiation, including the *bcl*-2 family of apoptosis genes, oncogenes (e.g., *myc* family genes), and tumor suppressor genes (e.g., p53 family genes) [107,108].

2. Classic Multidrug-Resistance P-Glycoprotein in Cancer

Ling and coworkers first described the classic MDR phenotype in human cancer, which they have shown to be due to upregulation of the MDR1 gene, with increased expression of P-glycoprotein [109]. This MDR protein broadly reduces intracellular levels of vinca alkaloids (vincristine, vinblastine), epipodophyllotoxins (etoposide, teniposide) and other natural-product antineoplastic agents, by functioning as an ATP-dependent plasma membrane pump that expels drugs from human cancer cells

[110] (Fig. 3). Platinum compounds are not substrates of the P-glycoprotein drug efflux mechanism.

Relatively high expression of P-glycoprotein is found in normal epithelial tissues and in cancers derived from epithelial tissues arising from the adrenal cortex, breast, kidney, liver, ovary and colon [111–114]. Increased expression of P-glycoprotein has been reported in leukemia, lymphoma and myeloma, neuroblastoma, osteosarcoma, rhabdomyosarcoma, and retinoblastoma [115–128]. Increased P-glycoprotein at diagnosis in these cancers generally correlates with failure of therapy, whereas undetectable P-glycoprotein at diagnosis correlates with lasting remission [115–131].

The increased P-glycoprotein that we found in many retinoblastoma tumors when the eye was removed for relapse may have accounted for the frequent chemotherapy failures observed in the past 30 years [122,126,128]. Likewise, the good response of retinoblastoma to carboplatin, teniposide, and vincristine that we have reported might be due to concurrent use of cyclosporin A (CSA) [132,133], a known inhibitor of P-glycoprotein in vitro, that inhibits the efflux of drugs by the MDR pump, allowing the drugs to be effective [128].

For intraocular retinoblastoma, it is not possible to correlate P-glycoprotein levels before therapy with the outcome of chemotherapy since biopsies are known to incur an increased risk of systemic spread [134]. In metastatic retinoblastoma, however, P-glycoprotein expression before therapy correlates precisely with failure of therapy (Fig. 3), and initially undetectable P-glycoprotein correlates with long-term remission [122,126,128]. We have found that P-glycoprotein is increased in one-third of eyes with large retinoblastoma enucleated primarily at diagnosis and is present in all eyes with large retinoblastoma enucleated at failure of different primary therapies. This suggests that the intrinsic presence of P-glycoprotein before therapy and/or its subsequent induction by therapy may both be responsible for the resistance of large retinoblastoma to chemotherapy [122,126,128]. Eyes with medium and small retinoblastoma often respond well to chemotherapy, but they almost always require focal therapy for residual or recurrent disease [135–139].

In retinoblastoma cell lines, the MDR phenotype correlated with increased P-glycoprotein in the original retinoblastoma tumors that were resistant to chemotherapy in vitro [122,126,128,140] (Fig. 3). Conversely, P-glycoprotein was undetectable in retinoblastoma cell lines and the original retinoblastoma tumors that appeared sensitive to chemotherapy in vitro [122,126,128,140]. Poor penetration of chemotherapy into the eye might also contribute to drug resistance in retinoblastoma. The use of CSA doubled the intravitreal carboplatin levels in animals [141], possibly by circumventing the effect of the highly expressed P-glycoprotein at the "blood-eye barrier" [142–144]. The mechanism has not been determined for this observation.

3. Other Multidrug-Resistance Genes Expressed in Retinoblastoma

Intraocular retinoblastoma that failed chemotherapy despite CSA use expressed another multidrug-resistance protein (MRP) rather than P-glycoprotein, whereas retinoblastoma that failed chemotherapy prior to the use of CSA showed increased P-glycoprotein [128]. MRP belongs to the same ATP-dependent membrane transporter superfamily as P-glycoprotein [145], and transfection of the MRP gene confers a similar broad-spectrum pattern of drug resistance to antineoplastic agents [122,146]. Whereas CSA inhibits P-glycoprotein in vitro, CSA does not block MRP, for which there is presently no effective inhibitor. We have shown that the presence of MRP in retinoblastoma may be associated with failure despite using CSA concurrently with chemotherapy [128]. However, MRP is less frequently found at diagnosis in retinoblastoma (1 of 18) than P-glycoprotein (8 of 38).

B. Modification of Therapy to Avoid Multidrug Resistance

Eye irradiation of bilateral patients with *RB1* germline mutations and large intraocular tumors results in an at least 30% risk of secondary bone or soft tissue sarcoma, brain tumor, lung tumor, or malignant melanoma by 30 years [67,148–151] and a 90% risk of orbital deformities and lacrimal dysfunction [152,153]. To avoid radiation-induced secondary tumors, chemotherapy has become the primary treatment in most centers. To circumvent multidrug resistance, we have added CSA to block the P-glycoprotein-induced drug efflux (Fig. 3). CSA and chemotherapy (vincristine and etoposide or teniposide with or without carboplatin) controls intraocular retinoblastoma without requiring radiation: 91% of newly untreated tumors remained relapse-free, and 70% of tumors that had relapsed from a previous therapy were cured [132,133]. In addition, tumors with the worst prognosis (vitreous seeds) were 88% relapse-free, better than previously reported [132,133].

The Toronto retinoblastoma protocol with short 3-hr infusions of high-dose CSA showed increased efficacy but no concurrent increase in chemotherapy toxicity, as is observed with prolonged infusions of CSA [154–158]. Besides reversing MDR, preclinical data suggest that CSA might increase the efficacy of carboplatin by modulating non-P-glycoprotein mechanisms of drug resistance. CSA given in short high doses may also prevent P-glycoprotein upregulation by chemotherapy agents [159,160]. A recent in vitro study also suggests that CSA might induce cancer progression by a cell-autonomous mechanism [161]. Therefore we will continue to cautiously use CSA for modulation of chemotherapy, because our own clinical data strongly suggest that CSA improves the long-term response of retinoblastoma to chemotherapy [162].

VI. THERAPY-INDUCED MUTATIONS LEAD TO SECOND PRIMARY TUMORS IN RETINOBLASTOMA PATIENTS

A. Radiation Therapy

The radiation-induced tumors are aneuploid, with many chromosomal markers and genetic rearrangements. Presumably, the susceptibility of $RB1^{+/-}$ persons to second primary tumors is due to the mutation of the second *RB1* allele induced by radiation.

B. Chemotherapy

1. Epipodophyllotoxin-Induced Secondary Leukemia

The epipodophyllotoxins, etoposide and teniposide, are included in most of the protocols for retinoblastoma. By inhibiting the normal religation activity of the nuclear enzyme topoisomerase II, these drugs can induce secondary leukemia characterized by site-specific DNA rearrangements. Secondary leukemia often has a short latency period, appearing within 2 years of epipodophyllotoxin therapy. Both high cumulative doses [164–167] and intensive schedules of administration [168] may contribute to the clinical risk.

Smith et al. recently reported the cumulative 6-year risk of leukemia for patients treated on 12 prospectively tracked protocols with different epipodophyllotoxin schedules combined with other chemotherapy and radiation, suggesting that factors other than epipodophyllotoxin cumulative doses may determine the risk of secondary leukemia [169]. There are also no data addressing the possibility that a greater systemic exposure to etoposide in the presence of CSA [170,171] increases the risk of secondary leukemia. Recently, high cumulative carboplatin doses have also been implicated as a risk factor for induction of secondary leukemia in ovarian cancer patients [172].

2. The Leukemic Risk of Patients with Retinoblastoma

Fortunately, children with *RB1* germline mutations do not have an increased predisposition for leukemia [173,174], despite their increased risk for other types of solid tumors [174]. M5 acute myelogenous leukemia developed after a latent period of only 2 months in a retinoblastoma patient treated with vincristine, doxorubicin, and cyclophosphamide [175]. There are five unpublished cases of myeloid leukemia in retinoblastoma patients who reportedly had received both etoposide and carboplatin. It is important to remain vigilant regarding this rare but catastrophic complication of treatment of retinoblastoma with chemotherapy [137].

VII. CONCLUSIONS

When it is fully understood why *RB1* mutations (M1, M2) initiate cancer development specifically in developing retina, the genes and processes that are unbalanced after loss of *RB1* (M3 to Mn) will become targets for interventions to prevent the emergence of retinoblastoma in children known to be predisposed. Similarly, knowledge of the genes and growth factors that act independently and cooperatively on retinoblastoma—promoting tumorigenesis, cell cycle progression, differentiation, and programmed cell death (Fig. 1) and their interaction with multidrug-resistance genes (Fig. 3)—will form the basis of novel strategies to cure retinoblastoma.

REFERENCES

1. Godbout R, Dryja TP, Squire J, Gallie BL, Phillips RA. Somatic inactivation of genes on, chromsome 13 is a common event in retinoblastoma. Nature 1983; 304:451–453.
2. Cavenee WK, Hansen MF, Nordenskjold M, et al. Genetic origin of mutations predisposing to retinoblastoma. Science 1985; 228:501–503.
3. Friend SH, Bernards R, Rogelj S, et al. A human DNA segment with properties of the gene that predisposes to retinoblastoma and osteosarcoma. Nature 1986; 323:643–646.
4. Squire JA, Gallie BL, Phillips RA. A detailed analysis of chromosomal changes in heritable and non-heritable retinoblastoma. Hum Genet 1985; 70:291–301.
5. Potluri VR, Helson L, Ellsworth RM, Reid T, Gilbert F. Chromosomal abnormalities in human retinoblastoma. A review. Cancer 1986; 58:663–671.
6. Cepko CL, Austin CP, Yang X, Alexiades M, Ezzeddine D. Cell fate determination in the vertebrate retina. Proc Natl Acad Sci USA 1996; 93:589–595.
7. Belecky-Adams T, Cook B, Adler R. Correlations between terminal mitosis and differentiated fate of retinal precursor cells in vivo and in vitro: Analysis with the "window-labeling" technique. Dev Biol 1996; 178:304–315.
8. Lin LF, Mismer D, Lile JD, et al. Purification, cloning, and expression of ciliary neurotrophic factor (CNTF). Science 1989; 246:1023–1025.
9. Ezzeddine ZD, Yang X, DeChiara T, Yancopoulos G, Cepko CL. Postmitotic cells fated to become rod photoreceptors can be respecified by CNTF treatment of the retina. Development 1997; 124:1055–1067.
10. Robanus-Maandag E, Dekker M, van der Valk M, et al. p107 is a suppressor of retinoblastoma development in pRb-deficient mice. Genes Dev 1998; 12:1599–1609.
11. Wells W. The Rb pretenders: Report from the American Association for Cancer Research, San Francisco, 2002. J Cell Biol 2002; 157:549.
12. Clarke AR, Maandag ER, vanRoon M, et al. Requirement for a functional Rb-1 gene in murine development. Science 1992; 359:328–330.
13. Jacks T, Fazeli A, Schmitt EM, Bronson RT, Goodell MA, Weinberg RA. Effects of an Rb mutation in the mouse. Science 1992; 359:295–300.
14. Lee EY-HP, Chang C-Y, Hu N, et al. Mice deficient for Rb are nonviable and show defects in neurogenesis and haematopoiesis. Science 1992; 359:288–294.
15. Morgenbesser SD, Williams BO, Jacks T, DePinho RA. p53-dependent apoptosis produced by Rb-deficiency in the developing mouse lens. Nature 1994; 371:72–74.
16. Zacksenhaus E, Jiang Z, Chung D, Marth JD, Phillips RA, Gallie BL. pRb controls proliferation, differentiation, and death of skeletal muscle cells and other lineages during embryogenesis. Genes Dev 1996; 10:3051–3064.
17. Maandag EC, van der Valk M, Vlaar M, et al. Developmental rescue of an embryonic-lethal mutation in the retinoblastoma gene in chimeric mice. EMBO J 1994; 13:4260–4268.
18. Williams BO, Schmitt EM, Remington L, et al. Extensive contribution of Rb-deficient cells to adult chimeric mice with limited histopathological consequences. EMBO J 1994; 13:4251–4259.
19. Hu N, Gutsmann A, Herbert DC, Bradley A, Lee W-H, Lee EY-HP. Heterozygous Rb-$1^{\Delta 20}/^+$ mice are predisposed to tumors of the pituitary gland with a nearly complete penetrance. Oncogene 1994; 9:1021–1027.
20. Lee M-H, Williams BO, Mulligan G, et al. Targeted disruption of $p107$: Functional overlap between $p107$ and Rb. Genes Dev 1996; 10:1621–1632.
21. Cobrinik D, Lee M-H, Hannon G, et al. Shared role of the pRB-related p130 and p107 proteins in limb development. Genes Dev 1996; 10:1633–1644.
22. Robanus-Maandag E, Dekker M, Van der Valk M, et al. p107 is a suppressor of retinoblastoma development in pRb-deficient mice. Genes Dev 1998; 12:1599–1609.

23. Windle JJ, Albert DM, O'Brien JM, et al. Retinoblastoma in transgenic mice. Nature 1990; 343:665–669.
24. al-Ubaidi MR, Font RL, Quiambao AB, et al. Bilateral retinal and brain tumors in transgenic mice expressing simian virus 40 large T antigen under control of the human interphotoreceptor retinoid-binding protein promoter. J Cell Biol 1992; 119:1681–1687.
25. Howes KA, Lasudry JG, Albert DM, Windle JJ. Photoreceptor cell tumors in transgenic mice. Invest Ophthalmol Vis Sci 1994; 35:342–351.
26. Marcus DM, Lasudry JG, Carpenter JL, et al. Trilateral tumors in four different lines of transgenic mice expressing SV40 T-antigen. Invest Ophthalmol Vis Sci 1996; 37:392–396.
27. Cepko CL. The roles of intrinsic and extrinsic cues and bHLH genes in the determination of retinal cell fates. Curr Opin Neurobiol 1999; 9:37–46.
28. Gallie BL, Ellsworth RM, Abramson DH, Phillips RA. Retinoma: Spontaneous regression of retinoblastoma or benign manisfestation of the mutation? Br J Cancer 1982; 45:513–521.
29. Margo C, Hidayat LCA, Kopelman J, Zimmerman LE. Retinocytoma. A benign variant of retinoblastoma. Arch Ophthalmol 1983; 101:1519–1531.
30. Gallie BL, Phillips RA, Ellsworth RM, Abramson DH. Significance of retinoma and phthisis bulbi for retinoblastoma. Ophthalmology 1982; 89:1393–1399.
31. Aaby AA, Price RL, Zakov ZN. Spontaneously regressing retinoblastomas, retinoma or retinoblastoma group 0. Am J Ophthalmol 1983; 96:315–320.
32. Eagle RCJ, Shields JA, Donoso L, Milner RS. Malignant transformation of spontaneously regressed retinoblastoma, retinoma/retinocytoma variant. Ophthalmology 1989; 96:1389–1395.
33. Alió J, Ludeña M, Millan A, Caballero V, Guinaldo V. Ultrastructural study of a retinoma by intraocular fine-needle aspiration biopsy. Ophthalmologica 1988; 196:192–199.
34. Balmer A, Munier F, Gailloud C. Retinoma and phtisis bulbi: Benign expression of retinoblastoma. Klin Monatsbl Augenheilkd 1992; 200:436–439.
35. Balmer A, Munier F, Gailloud C. Retinoma. Case studies. Ophthalm Paediatr Genet 1991; 12:131–137.
36. Keith CG, Webb GC. Retinoblastoma and retinoma occurring in a child with a translocation and deletion of the long arm of chromosome 13. Arch Ophthalmol 1985; 103:941–944.
37. Rychener RO. Retinoblastoma in the adult. Trans Am Ophthalmol Soc 1948; 46:318–326.
38. Balmer A, Munier F, Gailloud C. Retinoma. Case Studies. Ophthalm Paediatr Genet 1991; 12:131–137.
39. Lueder GT, Heon E, Gallie BL. Retinoma associated with vitreous seeding. Am J Ophthalmol 1995; 119:522–523.
40. Gallie BL, Campbell C, Devlin H, Duckett A, Squire JA. Developmental basis of retinal-specific induction of cancer by RB mutation. Cancer Res 1999; 59:1731s–1735s.
41. Friend SH, Bernards R, Rogelj S, et al. A human DNA segment with properties of the gene that predisposes to retinoblastoma and osteosarcoma. Nature 1986; 323:643–646.
42. Dunn JM, Phillips RA, Zhu X, Becker AJ, Gallie BL. Mutations in the RB1 gene and their effects on transcription. Mol Cell Biol 1989; 9:4594–4602.
43. Harbour JW. Overview of RB gene mutations in patients with retinoblastoma. Implications for clinical genetic screening. Ophthalmology 1998; 105:1442–1447.
44. Lohmann DR. RB1 gene mutations in retinoblastoma. Hum Mutat 1999; 14:283–288.
45. Zeschnigk M, Lohmann D, Horsthemke B. A PCR test for the detection of hypermethylated alleles at the retinoblastoma locus (letter). J Med Genet 1999; 36:793–794.

45a. Richter S, Vandezande K, Chen N, Zhang K, Sutherland J, Anderson J, Han L, Panton R, Branco P, Gallie B. Sensitive and efficient detection of *RB1* gene mutations enhances care for families with retinoblastoma. Am J Hum Genet 2003; 72:253–269.

46. Rideout WM, 3rd, Coetzee GA, Olumi AF, Jones PA. 5-Methylcytosine as an endogenous mutagen in the human LDL receptor and p53 genes. Science 1990; 249:1288–1290.

47. Schmutte C, Jones PA. Involvement of DNA methylation in human carcinogenesis. Biol Chem 1998; 379:377–388.

48. Dyson N. The regulation of E2F by pRB-family proteins. Genes Dev 1998; 12:2245–2262.

49. Eng C, Li FP, Abramson DH, et al. Mortality from second tumors among long-term survivors of retinoblastoma. J Natl Cancer Inst 1993; 85:1121–1128.

50. Noorani HZ, Khan HN, Gallie BL, Detsky AS. Cost comparison of molecular versus conventional screening of relatives at risk for retinoblastoma. Am J Hum Genet 1996; 59:301–307.

51. Zhu X, Dunn JM, Goddard AD, et al. Preferential germline mutation of the paternal allele in retinoblastoma. Nature 1989; 340:312–313.

52. Bunin GR, Petrakova A, Meadows AT, et al. Occupations of parents of children with retinoblastoma: A report from the Children's Cancer Study Group. Cancer Res 1990; 50:7129–7133.

53. Bunin GR, Meadows AT, Emanuel BS, Buckley JD, Woods WG, Hammond GD. Pre- and postconception factors associated with sporadic heritable and nonheritable retinoblastoma. Cancer Res 1989; 49:5730–5735.

54. Munier FL. Evidence of somatic and germinal mosaicism in pseudo-low penetrance hereditary retinoblastoma by constitutional and single-sperm mutation analysis. Am J Hum Genet 1998; 63:1903–1908.

55. Sippel KC, Fraioli RE, Smith GD, et al. Frequency of somatic and germ-line mosaicism in retinoblastoma: implications for genetic counseling. Am J Hum Genet 1998; 62:610–619.

56. Lohmann DR, Brandt B, Höpping W, Passarge E, Horsthemke B. Distinct RB1 gene mutations with low penetrance in hereditary retinoblastoma. Hum Genet 1994; 94:349–354.

57. Otterson GA, Chen W, Coxon AB, Khleif SN, Kaye FJ. Incomplete penetrance of familial retinoblastoma linked to germ-line mutations that result in partial loss of RB function. Proc Natl Acad Sci USA 1997; 94:12036–12040.

58. Lohmann D, Horsthemke B, Gillessen KG, Stefani FH, Hofler H. Detection of small RB1 gene deletions in retinoblastoma by multiplex PCR and high-resolution gel electrophoresis. Hum Genet 1992; 89:49–53.

59. Onadim A, Hogg A, Baird PN, Cowell JK. Oncogenic point mutation in exon 20 of the RB1 gene in families showing incomplete penetrance and mild expression of the retinoblastoma phenotype. Proc Natl Acad Sci USA 1992; 89:6177–6181.

60. Kratzke RA, Otterson GA, Hogg A, et al. Partial inactivation of the RB product in a family with incomplete penetrance of familial retinoblastoma and benign retinal tumors. Oncogene 1994; 9:1321–1326.

61. Whitaker LL, Su H, Baskaran R, Knudsen ES, Wang JY. Growth suppression by an E2F-binding-defective retinoblastoma protein (RB): Contribution from the RB C pocket. Mol Cell Biol 1998; 18:4032–4042.

62. Schubert EL, Strong LC, Hansen MF. A splicing mutation in RB1 in low penetrance retinoblastoma. Hum Genet 1997; 100:557–563.

63. Otterson GA, Modi S, Nguen K, Coxon AB, Kaye FJ. Temperature-sensitive *RB* mutations linked to incomplete penetrance of familial retinoblastoma in 12 families. Am J Hum Genet 1999; 65:1040–1046.

64. Cowell JK, Bia B. A novel missense mutation in patients from a retinoblastoma pedigree showing only mild expression of the tumor phenotype. Oncogene 1998; 16:3211–3213.

65. Bremner R, Du DC, Connolly-Wilson MJ, et al. Deletion of *RB* exons 24 and 25 causes low penetrance retinoblastoma. Am J Hum Genet 1997; 61:556–570.

66. Nevins JR. The Rb/E2F pathway and cancer. Hum Mol Genet 2001; 10:699–703.

67. Orjuela M, Orlow I, Dudas M, et al. Alterations of cell cycle regulators affecting the RB pathway in nonfamilial retinoblastoma. Hum Pathol 2001; 32:537–544.

68. Orjuela M, Castaneda VP, Ridaura C, et al. Presence of human papilloma virus in tumor tissue from children with retinoblastoma: An alternative mechanism for tumor development. Clin Cancer Res 2000; 6:4010–4016.

69. Knudson JAG. Mutation and cancer: Statistical study of retinoblastoma. Proc Natl Acad Sci USA 1971; 68:820–823.

70. Mairal A, Pinglier E, Gilbert E, et al. Detection of chromosome imbalances in retinoblastoma by parallel karyotype and CGH analyses. Genes Chromosomes Cancer 2000; 28:370–379.

71. Herzog S, Lohmann DR, Buiting K, et al. Marked differences in unilateral isolated retinoblastomas from young and older children studied by comparative genomic hybridization. Hum Genet 2001; 108:98–104.

72. Chen D, Gallie BL, Squire JA. Minimal regions of chromosomal imbalance in retinoblastoma detected by comparative genomic hybridization. Cancer Genet Cytogenet 2001; 129:57–63.

73. Guan XY, Fang Y, Sham JS, et al. Recurrent chromosome alterations in hepatocellular carcinoma detected by comparative genomic hybridization. Genes Chromosomes Cancer 2000; 29:110–116.

74. Kytola S, Farnebo F, Obara T, et al. Patterns of chromosomal imbalances in parathyroid carcinomas. Am J Pathol 2000; 157:579–586.

75. Zettl A, Strobel P, Wagner K, et al. Recurrent genetic aberrations in thymoma and thymic carcinoma. Am J Pathol 2000; 157:257–266.

76. Alers JC, Rochat J, Krijtenburg PJ, et al. Identification of genetic markers for prostatic cancer progression. Lab Invest 2000; 80:931–942.

77. Bergamo NA, Rogatto SR, Poli-Frederico RC, et al. Comparative genomic hybridization analysis detects frequent over-representation of DNA sequences at 3q, 7p, and 8q in head and neck carcinomas. Cancer Genet Cytogenet 2000; 119:48–55.

78. Squire J, Phillips RA, Boyce S, Godbout R, Rogers B, Gallie BL. Isochromosome 6p, a unique chromosomal abnormality in retinoblastoma: Verification by standard staining techniques, new densitometric methods, and somatic cell hybridization. Hum Genet 1984; 66:46–53.

79. Horsthemke B, Greger V, Becher R, Passarge E. Mechanism of i(6p) formation in retinoblastoma tumor cells. Cancer Genet Cytogenet 1989; 37:95–102.

80. Zheng L, Flesken-Nikitin A, Chen P-L, Lee W-H. Deficiency of *retinoblastoma* gene in mouse embryonic stem cells leads to genetic instability. Cancer Res 2002; 62:2498–2502.

81. Chen D, Pajovic S, Duckett A, Brown VD, Squire JA, Gallie BL. Genomic amplification in retinoblastoma narrowed to 0.6Mb on chromosome 6p containing a kinesin-like gene, RBKIN. Cancer Res 2002; 63:967–971.

82. Bruch J, Schulz WA, Haussler J, et al. Delineation of the 6p22 amplification unit in urinary bladder carcinoma cell lines. Cancer Res 2000; 60:4526–4530.

83. Richter J, Wagner U, Schraml P, et al. Chromosomal imbalances are associated with a high risk of progression in early invasive (pT1) urinary bladder cancer. Cancer Res 1999; 59:5687–5691.

84. Bando K, Nagai H, Matsumoto S, et al. Identification of a 1-Mb common region at 16q24.1–24.2 deleted in hepatocellular carcinoma. Genes Chromosomes Cancer 2000; 28:38–44.

85. Skirnisdottir S, Eiriksdottir G, Baldursson T, Barkardottir RB, Egilsson V, Ingvarrson S. High frequency of allelic imbalance at chromosome region 16q22–23 in human breast cancer: Correlation with high PgR and low S phase. Int J Cancer 1995; 64:112–116.

86. Suzuki H, Komiya A, Emi M, et al. Three distinct commonly deleted regions of chromosome arm 16q in human primary and metastatic prostate cancers. Genes Chromosomes Cancer 1996; 17:225–233.

87. Mason JE, Goodfellow PJ, Grundy PE, Skinner MA. 16q loss of heterozygosity and microsatellite instability in Wilms' tumor. J Pediatr Surg 2000; 35:891–896; discussion 896–897.

88. Braungart E, Schumacher C, Hartmann E, et al. Functional loss of E-cadherin and cadherin-11 alleles on chromosome 16q22 in colonic cancer. J Pathol 1999; 187:530–534.

89. Kashima T, Kawaguchi J, Takeshita S, et al. Anamolous cadherin expression in osteosarcoma. Possible relationships to metastasis and morphogenesis. Am J Pathol 1999; 155:1549–1555.

90. Zhou R, Skalli O. Identification of cadhere-11 down-regulation as a common response of astrocytoma cells to transforming growth factor-alpha. Differentiation 2000; 66:165–172.

91. Kawakami M, Staub J, Cliby W, Hartmann L, Smith DI, Shridhar V. Involvement of H-cadherin (CDH13) on 16q in the region of frequent deletion in ovarian cancer. Int J Oncol 1999; 15:715–720.

92. Sato M, Mori Y, Sakurada A, Fujimura S, Horii A. The H-cadherin (CDH13) gene is inactivated in human lung cancer. Hum Genet 1998; 103:96–101.

93. Toyooka KO, Toyooka S, Virmani AK, et al. Loss of expression and aberrant methylation of the CDH13 (H-cadherin) gene in breast and lung carcinomas. Cancer Res 2001; 61:4556–4560.

94. Frade JM, Bovolenta P, Rodriguez-Tebar A. Neurotrophins and other growth factors in the generation of retinal neurons. Microsc Res Tech 1999; 45:243–251.

95. Frade JM. Unscheduled re-entry into the cell cycle induced by NGF precedes cell death in nascent retinal neurones. J Cell Sci 2000; 113:1139–1148.

96. Frade JM, Rodriguez-Tebar A, Barde YA. Induction of cell death by endogenous nerve growth factor through its p75 receptor. Nature 1996; 383:166–168.

97. Chadeneau C, Siegel P, Harley CB, Muller WJ, Bacchetti S. Telomerase activity in normal and malignant murine tissues. Oncogene 1995; 11:893–898.

98. Stewart SA, Weinberg RA. Telomerase and human tumorigenesis. Semin Cancer Biol 2000; 10:399–406.

99. Wynford-Thomas D, Kipling D. Telomerase. Cancer and the knockout mouse. Nature 1997; 389:551–552.

100. Kim NW, Piatyszek MA, Prowse KR, et al. Specific association of human telomerase activity with immortal cells and cancer. Science 1994; 266:2011–2015.

101. Chadeneau C, Hay K, Hirte HW, Gallinger S, Bacchetti S. Telomerase activity associated with acquisition of malignancy in human colorectal cancer. Cancer Res 1995; 55:2533–2536.

102. Counter CM, Hirte HW, Bacchetti S, Harley CB. Telomerase activity in human ovarian carcinoma. Proc Natl Acad Sci USA 1994; 91:2900–2904.

103. Counter CM, Gupta J, Harley CB, Leber B, Bacchetti S. Telomerase activity in normal leukocytes and in hematologic malignancies. Blood 1995; 85:2315–2320.

104. Gupta J, Han L-P, Wang P, Gallie BL, Bacchetti S. Development of retinoblastoma in the absence of telomerase activity. J Natl Cancer Inst 1996; 88:1152–1157.

105. Doz F, Neuenschwander S, Plantaz D, et al. Etoposide and carboplatin in extraocular retinoblastoma: A study by the Société Française d'Oncologie Pédiatrique. J Clin Oncol 1995; 13:902–909.

106. Namouni F, Doz F, Tanguy ML, et al. High-dose chemotherapy with carboplatin, etoposide and cyclophosphamide followed by a haematopoietic stem cell rescue in patients with high-risk retinoblastoma: A SFOP and SFGM study. Eur J Cancer 1997; 33:2368–2375.

107. Lehnert M. Clinical multidrug resistance in cancer: a multifactorial problem. Eur J Cancer 1996; 32A:912–920.

108. Chan HSL, Grogan TM, DeBoer G, Haddad G, Gallie BL, Ling V. Diagnosis and reversal of multidrug resistance in paediatric cancers. Eur J Cancer 1996; 32A:1051–1061.

109. Gerlach JH, Kartner N, Bell DR, Ling V. Multidrug resistance. Cancer Surveys 1986; 5:25–46.

110. Gerlach JH, Endicott JA, Juranka PF, et al. Homology between P-glycoprotein and a bacterial haemolysin transport protein suggests a model for multidrug resistance. Nature 1986; 324:485–489.

111. Fojo AT, Whang-Peng J, Gottesman MM, Pastan I. Amplification of DNA sequences in human multidrug-resistant KB carcinoma cells. Proc Natl Acad Sci USA 1985; 82:7661–7665.

112. Goldstein LJ, Galski H, Fojo AT, et al. Expression of a multidrug resistance gene in human cancers. J Natl Cancer Inst 1989; 81:116–124.

113. Weinstein RS, Kuszak JR, Kluskens LF, Coon JS. P-glycoproteins in pathology: The multidrug resistance gene family in humans. Hum Pathol 1990; 21:34–48.

114. Gamelin E, Mertins SD, Regis JT, et al. Intrinsic drug resistance in primary and metastatic renal cell carcinoma. J Urol 1999; 162:217–224.

115. Pirker R, Wallner J, Geissler K, et al. MDR1 gene expression and treatment outcome in acute myeloid leukemia. J Natl Cancer Inst 1991; 83:708–712.

116. Campos L, Guyotat D, Jaffar C, Solary E, Archimbaud E, Treille D. Correlation of MDR1/P-170 expression with daunorubicin uptake and sensitivity of leukemic progenitors in acute myeloid leukemia. Eur J Haematol 1992; 48:254–258.

117. Dalton WS, Grogan TM, Rybski JA, et al. Immunohistochemical detection and quantitation of P-glycoprotein in multiple drug-resistant human myeloma cells: Association with level of drug resistance and drug accumulation. Blood 1989; 73:747–752.

118. Miller TP, Grogan TM, Dalton WS, Spier CM, Scheper RJ, Salmon SE. P-glycoprotein expression in malignant lymphoma and reversal of clinical drug resistance with chemotherapy plus high-dose verapamil. J Clin Oncol 1991; 9:17–24.

119. Goasguen JE, Dossot JM, Fardel O, et al. Expression of the multidrug resistance-associated P-glycoprotein (P-170) in 59 cases of de novo acute lymphoblastic leukemia: Prognostic implications. Blood 1993; 81:2394–2398.

120. Bourhis J, Goldstein LJ, Riou G, Pastan I, Gottesman MM, Benard J. Expression of a human multidrug resistance gene in ovarian carcinomas. Cancer Res 1989; 49:5062–5065.

121. Chan HSL, Thorner PS, Haddad G, Ling V. Immunohistochemical detection of P-glycoprotein: Prognostic correlation in soft tissue sarcoma of childhood. J Clin Oncol 1990; 8:689–704.

122. Chan HSL, Thorner PS, Haddad G, Gallie BL. Multidrug-resistant phenotype in retinoblastoma correlates with P-glycoprotein expression. Ophthalmology 1991; 98:1425–1431.

123. Chan HSL, Haddad G, Thorner PS, et al. P-glycoprotein expression as a predictor of the outcome of therapy for neuroblastoma. N Engl J Med 1991; 325:1608–1614.

124. Baldini N, Scotlandi K, Barbanti-Bròdano G, et al. Expression of P-glycoprotein in high-grade osteosarcomas in relation to clinical outcome. N Engl J Med 1995; 333:1380–1385.

125. Kang Y-K, Zhan Z, Regis J, et al. Expression of *mdr*-1 in refractory lymphoma: Quantitation by polymerase chain reaction and validation of the assay. Blood 1995; 86:1515–1524.

126. Chan HSL, Thorner PS, Haddad G, Gallie BL. Effect of chemotherapy on intraocular retinoblastoma. Int J Pediatr Hematol/Oncol 1995; 2:269–281.

127. Chan HSL, Grogan TM, Haddad G, DeBoer G, Ling V. P-Glycoprotein expression: Critical determinant in the response to osteosarcoma chemotherapy. J Natl Cancer Inst 1997; 89:1706–1715.

128. Chan HSL, Lu Y, Grogan TM, et al. Multidrug resistance protein (MRP) expression in retinoblastoma correlates with rare failure of chemotherapy despite cyclosporine for reversal of P-glycoprotein. Cancer Res 1997; 57:2325–2330.

129. Bates SE, Shieh CY, Tsokos M. Expression of mdr-1/P-glycoprotein in human neuroblastoma. Am J Pathol 1991; 139:305–315.

130. Nakagawara A, Kadomatsu K, Sato S, et al. Inverse correlation between expression of multidrug resistance gene and N-myc oncogene in human neuroblastomas. Cancer Res 1990; 50:3043–3047.

131. Niehans GA, Jaszcz W, Brunetto V, et al. Immunohistochemical identification of P-glycoprotein in previously untreated, diffuse large cell and immunoblastic lymphomas. Cancer Res 1992; 52:3768–3775.

132. Gallie BL, Budning A, DeBoer G, et al. Chemotherapy with focal therapy can cure intraocular retinoblastoma without radiation. Arch Ophthalmol 1996; 114:1321–1328.

133. Chan HSL, DeBoer G, Thiessen JJ, et al. Combining cyclosporin with chemotherapy controls intraocular retinoblastoma without requiring radiation. Clin Cancer Res 1996; 2:1499–1508.

134. White L. Chemotherapy in retinoblastoma: Current status and future directions. Am J Pediatr Hematol Oncol 1991; 13:189–201.

135. Murphree AL, Villablanca JG, Deegan WF, et al. Chemotherapy plus local treatment in the management of intraocular retinoblastoma. Arch Ophthalmol 1996; 114:1348–1356.

136. Shields CL, Shields JA, DePotter P, Himelstein BP, Meadows AT. The effect of chemoreduction on retinoblastoma-induced retinal detachment. J Pediatr Ophthalmol Strabismus 1997; 34:165–169.

137. Beck MN, Balmer A, Dessing C, Pica A, Munier F. First-line chemotherapy with local treatment can prevent external-beam irradiation and enucleation in low-stage intraocular retinoblastoma. J Clin Oncol 2000; 18:2881–2887.

138. Friedman DL, Himelstein B, Shields CL, et al. Chemoreduction and local ophthalmic therapy for intraocular retinoblastoma. J Clin Oncol 2000; 18:12–17.

139. Shields CL, Honavar SG, Meadows AT, et al. Chemoreduction plus focal therapy for retinoblastoma: Factors predictive of need for treatment with external beam radiotherapy or enucleation. Am J Ophthalmol 2002; 133:657–664.

140. Chan HSL, Canton MD, Gallie BL. Chemosensitivity and multidrug resistance to antineoplastic drugs in retinoblastoma cell lines. Anticancer Res 1989; 9:469–474.

141. Wilson TW, Chan HSL, Moselhy GM, Heydt DD Jr, Frey CM, Gallie BL. Penetration of chemotherapy into vitreous is increased by cryotherapy and cyclosporin in rabbits. Arch Ophthalmol 1996; 114:1390–1395.

142. Stewart PA, Tuor UI. Blood-eye barriers in the rat: Correlation of ultrastructure with function. J Comp Neurol 1994; 340:566–576.

143. Holash JA, Stewart PA. The relationship of astrocyte-like cells to the vessels that contribute to the blood-ocular barriers. Brain Res 1993; 629:218–224.

144. Schlingemann RO, Hofman P, Klooster J, Blaauwgeers HG, Van der Gaag R, Vrensen GF. Ciliary muscle capillaries have blood-tissue barrier characteristics. Exp Cell Res 1998; 66:747–754.

145. Cole SPC, Bhardwaj G, Gerlach JH, et al. Overexpression of a transporter gene in a multidrug-resistant human lung cancer cell line. Science 1992; 258:1650–1654.

146. Grant CE, Valdimarsson G, Hipfner DR, Almquist KC, Cole SP, Deeley RG. Overexpression of multidrug resistance-associated protein (MRP) increases resistance to natural product drugs. Cancer Res 1994; 54:357–361.

147. Cole SPC, Sparks KE, Fraser K, et al. Pharmacological characterization of multidrug resistant MRP-transfected human tumor cells. Cancer Res 1994; 54:5902–5910.

148. Eng C, Li FP, Abramson DH, et al. Mortality from second tumors among long-term survivors of retinoblastoma. J Natl Cancer Inst 1993; 85:1121–1128.

149. Wong FL, Boice JD, Jr., Abramson DH, et al. Cancer incidence after retinoblastoma. Radiation dose and sarcoma risk. JAMA 1997; 278:1262–1267.

150. Li FP, Abramson DH, Tarone RE, Kleinerman RA, Fraumeni JF Jr, Boice JD Jr. Hereditary retinoblastoma, lipoma, and second primary cancers. J Natl Cancer Inst 1997; 89:83–84.

151. Abramson DH, Frank CM. Second nonocular tumors in survivors of bilateral retinoblastoma: A possible age effect on radiation-related risk. Ophthalmology 1998; 105:573–579.

152. Imhof SM, Hofman P, Tan KE. Quantification of lacrimal function after D-shaped field irradiation for retinoblastoma. Br J Ophthalmol 1993; 77:482–484.

153. Imhof SM, Mourits MP, Hofman P, et al. Quantification of orbital and mid-facial growth retardation after megavoltage external beam irradiation in children with retinoblastoma. Ophthalmology 1996; 103:263–268.

154. Fojo AT, Ueda K, Slamon DJ, Poplack DG, Gottesman MM, Pastan I. Expression of a multidrug-resistance gene in human tumors and tissues. Proc Natl Acad Sci USA 1987; 84:265–269.

155. Cordon-Cardo C, O'Brien JP, Casals D, et al. Multidrug-resistance gene (P-glycoprotein) is expressed by endothelial cells at blood-brain barrier sites. Proc Natl Acad Sci USA 1989; 86:695–698.

156. Drach D, Zhao S, Drach J, et al. Subpopulations of normal peripheral blood and bone marrow cells express a functional multidrug resistant phenotype. Blood 1992; 80:2729–2734.

157. Smit JJM, Schinkel AH, Oude Elferink RPJ, et al. Homozygous disruption of the murine mdr2 P-glycoprotein gene leads to a complete absence of phospholipid from bile and to liver disease. Cell 1993; 75:451–462.

158. Schinkel AH, Mayer U, Wagenaar E, et al. Normal viability and altered pharmacokinetics in mice lacking mdr1-type (drug-transporting) P-glycoproteins. Proc Natl Acad Sci USA 1997; 94:4028–4033.

159. Beketic-Oreskovic L, Durán GE, Chen G, Dumontet C, Sikic BI. Decreased mutation rate for cellular resistance to doxorubicin and suppression of mdr1 gene activation by the cyclosporin PSC 833. J Natl Cancer Inst 1995; 87:1593–1602.

160. Jetté L, Beaulieu E, Leclerc JM, Béliveau R. Cyclosporin A treatment induces overexpression of P-glycoprotein in the kidney and other tissues. Am J Physiol 1996; 270:F756-F765.

161. Hojo M, Morimoto T, Maluccio M, et al. Cyclosporine induces cancer progression by a cell-autonomous mechanism. Nature 1999; 397:530–534.

162. Chan HSL, Heon E, Budning A, Gallie BL. Retinoblastoma shows dose-response to cyclosporine-modulated chemotherapy. Proc Am Assoc Cancer Res 2000; 41:abstr 3866.

163. Kleinerman RA, Tarone RE, Abramson DH, Seddon JM, Li FP, Tucker MA. Hereditary retinoblastoma and risk of lung cancer. J Natl Cancer Inst 2000; 92:2037–2039.

164. Pedersen-Bjergaard J, Daugaard G, Hansen SW, Philip P, Larsen SO, Rorth M. Increased risk of myelodysplasia and leukaemia after etoposide, cisplatin, and bleomycin for germ-cell tumours. Lancet 1991; 338:359–363.

165. Pui CH, Ribeiro RC, Hancock ML, et al. Acute myeloid leukemia in children treated with epipodophyllotoxins for acute lymphoblastic leukemia. N Engl J Med 1991; 325:1682–1687.

166. Winick NJ, McKenna RW, Shuster JJ, et al. Secondary acute myeloid leukemia in children with acute lymphoblastic leukemia treated with etoposide. J Clin Oncol 1993; 11:209–217.

167. Kollmannsberger C, Beyer J, Droz JP, et al. Secondary leukemia following high cumulative doses of etoposide in patients treated for advanced germ cell tumors. J Clin Oncol 1998; 16:3386–3391.

168. Chen CL, Fuscoe JC, Liu Q, Pui CH, Mahmoud HH, Relling MV. Relationship between cytotoxicity and site-specific DNA recombination after in vitro exposure of leukemia cells to etoposide. J Nat Cancer Inst 1996; 88:1840–1847.

169. Smith MA, Rubinstein L, Anderson JR, et al. Secondary leukemia or myelodysplastic syndrome after treatment with epipodophyllotoxins. J Clin Oncol 1999; 17:569–577.

170. Lum BL, Kaubisch S, Yahanda AM, et al. Alteration of etoposide pharmacokinetics and pharmacodynamics by cyclosporine in a phase I trial to modulate multidrug resistance. J Clin Oncol 1992; 10:1635–1642.

171. Yahanda AM, Alder KM, Fisher GA, et al. Phase I trial of etoposide with cyclosporine as a modulator of multidrug resistance. J Clin Oncol 1992; 10:1624–1634.

172. Travis LB, Holowaty EJ, Bergfeldt K, et al. Risk of leukemia after platinum-based chemotherapy for ovarian cancer. N Engl J Med 1999; 340:351–357.

173. Phillips RA, Gill RM, Zacksenhaus E, et al. Why don't germline mutations in RB1 predispose to leukemia? In: Potter M, Melchers F, eds. Current Topics in Microbiology & Immunology. Vol. 182. Berlin: Springer-Verlag, 1992, pp 485–491.

174. Draper GJ, Sanders BM, Kingston JE. Second primary neoplasms in patients with retinoblastoma. Br J Cancer 1986; 53:661–671.

175. Felice MS, Zubizarreta PA, Chantada GL, et al. Acute myeloid leukemia as a second malignancy: Report of 9 pediatric patients in a single institution in Argentina. Med Pediatr Oncol 1998; 30:160–164.

8

The Role of the Retinoblastoma Protein in Health, Malignancy, and the Pathogenesis of Retinoblastoma

KURTIS R. VAN QUILL and JOAN M. O'BRIEN

University of California–San Francisco, San Francisco, California, U.S.A.

I. INTRODUCTION

Retinoblastoma (RB) is the most common primary eye cancer of childhood, affecting approximately 1 in 20,000 live births [1] and accounting for 12% of infant cancer [2]. The disease results from loss or mutation of both alleles of the retinoblastoma gene (*RB1*). Between 60 and 70% of affected children have sporadic or nonheritable retinoblastoma [1]. In this form of the disease, both *RB1* alleles are inactivated somatically in a single developing retinal cell, resulting in unifocal, unilateral tumor development. The remaining 30–40% of affected children have familial or heritable retinoblastoma. These individuals carry an inactivated *RB1* allele in their germline, and loss or mutation of the second allele occurs somatically. In the great majority of kindreds, heritable RB is characterized by virtually complete penetrance (nearly all carriers develop the disease) and high expressivity (disease is characterized by multifocal, bilateral tumor development). In some kindreds, however, the disease demonstrates reduced penetrance and expressivity ("low-penetrance RB"). Penetrance may be as low as 20% in these kindreds, and affected carriers often have only unilateral RB or benign retinal lesions (called retinoma or retinocytoma) [3–7]. It is estimated that between 10 and 15% of children with unilateral RB harbor a mutant allele in their germline [1,8,9].

Children with heritable RB are predisposed to develop other malignancies throughout life. In their early years many of these children develop characteristic midline brain tumors called trilateral retinoblastoma (Trb) or primitive neuroectodermal tumor (PNET). The cumulative incidence of PNET is 9% by 5 years of age [10], and these children remain at risk for this tumor until early adolescence [11,12]. Individuals with heritable RB also have a high lifetime risk of developing osteogenic and soft-tissue sarcomas [10,13–15]. Radiation therapy increases this sarcoma risk up to 10-fold depending on the dose [14], and this risk may be higher if radiation is administered within the first year of life [16,17]. Heritable RB patients also face an elevated risk of developing cutaneous melanoma [13,14,18,19]. The cumulative incidence of a second tumor in this population is as high as 50% at 50 years post-diagnosis [14].

Knudson provided critical insight into the genetic basis of RB in 1971, when he proposed that two mutations were required to transform a susceptible retinal cell ("two-hit" hypothesis) [8]. Knudson derived this conclusion from his observation that patients with heritable RB tend to present earlier with multiple, bilateral tumors, whereas patients with nonheritable RB tend to present later with exclusively unilateral disease. Children with heritable RB develop tumors earlier and at a higher frequency, Knudsen argued, because they already harbor one of the causative mutations in their germline. This reduces the mutational requirement for new tumor formation in these children to a single somatic mutation. Comings later extended Knudsen's proposal by suggesting that retinoblastoma arises due to mutations in both alleles of the same gene, which he posited to exert a haplosufficient tumor suppressive function [20].

The proposed RB predisposition gene was localized to chromosome 13q14 through deletion studies [21] and linkage analysis [22,23]. The critical role of this locus in RB was verified by the finding of frequent loss of the normal allele (loss of heterozygosity, or LOH) in RB tumors [24–26]. A candidate gene, *RB1*, was later cloned from this locus [27,28], and its causal role in retinoblastoma was supported by the finding that both alleles of the gene were frequently lost or mutated in RB tumor specimens [29–31]. Other studies confirmed the presence of a germline *RB1* mutation in virtually all RB kindreds examined and demonstrated that inheritance of the mutant *RB1* allele predicted disease development within these kindreds [32]. The tumor suppressor function of the gene was also suggested by transfection studies showing that introduction of wild-type expression in *RB1*-defective cell lines partially reverses the malignant phenotype [33–38].

RB1 was the first tumor suppressor gene to be identified. Over the past 15 years, researchers have made remarkable advances in understanding the functions of its protein product, pRb, and the pathways that it regulates. This research has demonstrated that pRb's tumor suppressive function extends well beyond the prevention of this rare retinal tumor. pRb functions to suppress tumor development in most if not all cell types by negatively regulating cell cycle progression. In this role, pRb mediates antiproliferative signals by inhibiting E2F family transcription factors, which regulate the expression of a large set of genes required for cellular proliferation. Control of E2Fs by pRb may result in cell cycle arrest which is reversible, as in the case of quiescent cells, or permanent, as in the case of cells which have undergone replicative senescence or terminal differentiation. Evidence from many malignancies suggests that derangement of the *RB1* pathway is a fundamental requirement for tumorigenesis [39–41]

pRb also promotes terminal differentiation through mechanisms distinct from the induction of cell cycle arrest. These additional mechanisms include suppression of apoptosis and activation of tissue-specific gene expression [42]. Early evidence in bone suggests that activation of differentiation genes by pRb may also serve a tumor suppressive function [43,44]. To date, pRb has been implicated in the terminal differentiation of neurons, skeletal muscle, bone, adipose tissue, erythrocytes, monocytes, keratinoctyes, and fiber cells of the ocular lens [44–52]. In most cell types where pRb plays a critical role in terminal differentiation, including neurons of the brain and peripheral nervous system, skeletal muscle, erythrocytes, and lens fiber cells, developmental loss of pRb is associated with apoptosis or perturbed terminal differentiation [45–49,53–55]. In a limited number of other tissues, including retina and bone, loss of pRb can initiate tumorigenesis [10,13,14]. Of all tissues, the developing retina is most acutely sensitive to tumorigenesis upon pRb loss, and it has been estimated that carriers of a mutant *RB1* allele bear a 30,000-fold relative risk for the development of retinoblastoma [56].

This chapter reviews current understanding of the function of pRb and the role of pRb loss in retinoblastoma. Despite enormous recent advances, our understanding of the molecular pathogenesis of this disease remains incomplete. Observations in pRb-deficient knockout, chimeric, and transgenic mice suggest that events in addition to pRb loss are required for retinal tumorigenesis, at least in mice. Analyses of human RB tumors have identified consistent chromosomal alterations apart from *RB1* mutation, suggesting that other genes may also be important for retinoblastoma development in man. However, it remains unclear whether any of these additional genetic alterations plays a role in the initiation of human RB. Competing models of RB tumorigenesis have been proposed, but these models are necessarily rudimentary. Definitive understanding of the pathogenesis of retinoblastoma should enhance our ability to diagnose, treat, and prevent this disease. Such understanding also promises to provide further insight into general mechanisms of malignant transformation.

II. pRb REGULATION AND FUNCTION

The human *RB1* gene contains 180 kb and 27 exons, and it encodes a 4.8-kb mRNA [57–59]. Its protein product, pRb, is a nuclear transcription factor composed of 928 amino acids. pRb is the best described member of the pocket protein family, which also includes p107 and p130. All three family members share a highly conserved pocket domain and exert similar, often overlapping functions in cell cycle control and in the promotion of terminal differentiation [60,61].

Isolated loss of p107 or p130 is not rate-limiting for tumorigenesis [60,61], but some evidence suggests that inactivation of either protein may contribute to tumor development in the absence of pRb. Notably, combined loss of p107 and pRb appears to be required for the development of retinoblastoma in mice [62]. In humans, however, mutational inactivation of p107 has been described in only one tumor specimen to date, a lymphoma cell line [63]. In contrast, mutations in *p130* have been reported in a pRb-deficient lung carcinoma cell line and in several other human tumors [64–68]. On the basis of this and other evidence, p130 has been proposed to function as a *bona fide* tumor suppressor protein in humans [69].

A. pRb and Phosphorylation

The activity of the retinoblastoma protein is controlled by phosphorylation. pRb is active in its hypophosphorylated form, which complexes with a variety of cellular proteins. pRb has been reported to associate with over 100 cellular proteins, but the functional significance of many of these interactions remains unclear [70]. Many pRb binding partners are transcription factors with activities that are negatively or positively regulated by pRb binding. The best understood of these protein partners are the E2F family transcription factors. pRb inhibits cell cycle progression by binding and negatively regulating E2Fs, which are essential for cellular proliferation [71].

pRb is normally inactivated by phosphorylation events, the effects of which can be mimicked by *RB1* mutation or by viral oncoprotein binding. The addition of phosphate groups to pRb inhibits its ability to bind other proteins, through the induction of conformational changes [72] or by promoting competitive displacement of binding partners by phosphorylated peptide segments of pRb [73–75]. Sixteen potential phosphorylation sites have been identified on pRb, many of which are phosphorylated in vivo [76–78].

pRb is phosphorylated by cyclin—cyclin-dependent kinase (cyclin-cdk) complexes [79]. These include cyclin D-cdk4/6, which is produced early in the presynthetic (G1) phase of the cell cycle in response to mitogenic signaling, and cyclinE-cdk2, which is upregulated downstream of cyclin D-cdk4/6 in mid to late G1. According to a current model, cyclin D-cdk4/6 and cyclin E-cdk2 play complementary roles in the phosphorylation of pRb during G1 [72]. In this model, sequential addition of phosphate groups by cyclin D-cdk4/6 and, later in G1, cyclin E-cdk2 progressively inhibits pRb's ability to bind E2Fs and other protein partners, resulting in derepression of E2F target genes and progression into the DNA synthesis (S) phase of the cell cycle. Levels of cyclin E-cdk2 are quickly reduced upon the cell's entry into S phase, but pRb remains in a hyperphosphorylated state until late mitosis. Persistent hyperphosphorylation of pRb is thought to be maintained by cyclin A- and cyclin B-dependent kinases, which are important in later phases of the cell cycle [79].

Dephosphorylation and activation of pRb is controlled by cyclin-dependent kinase inhibitors (CDKIs) of the Ink4 (inhibitors of cdk4) and Cip/Kip (cdk interacting protein/cdk inhibitor protein) families [80]. While upstream regulation of CDKIs is little understood, activation of these proteins has been associated with diverse antiproliferative signals, including DNA damage, senescence, and differentiation signals; transforming growth factor β (TGFβ); and cell-to-cell contact (contact inhibition) [81–85]. Collectively, Ink4 and Cip/Kip CDKIs positively regulate pRb by inhibiting its negative regulators, the activated cyclin-cdk complexes. Ink4 CDKIs—which include p16Ink4a, p15Ink4b, p18Ink4c, and p19Ink4d—specifically inactivate cyclinD-cdk4/6 by binding and inhibiting the catalytic cdk4 or cdk6 subunit. Cip/Kip CDKIs, including p21Cip1, p27Kip1, and p57Kip2, inhibit cyclinE-cdk2 and cyclin A-cdk2 by binding to both the cyclin and cdk subunits of these complexes. However, it should be noted that Cip/Kip proteins also positively regulate cyclin D-cdk4/6 and are required for their assembly [86,87]. These findings suggest that the initial identification of Cip/Kip proteins as cdk "inhibitors" is an oversimplification and that these proteins actually function as negative regulators of pRb in early G1 and positive regulators of pRb at later stages of the cell cycle. Since the half-life of phosphate groups on pRb is approximately 30 minutes [90], inactivation of cyclin-cdks by CDKIs may be sufficient to induce rapid dephosphorylation and activation of pRb. This action results in cell cycle arrest. Regulation of pRb by cyclin-cdks and CDKIs will be described in more detail in our discussion of pRb's role in the cell cycle, below.

B. Inhibition of Cell Cycle Progression by pRb

Well before the identification of *RB1*, Knudsen suggested that the product of the proposed RB predisposition gene functioned as an inhibitor of DNA synthesis and of cellular proliferation [89]. The first experimental support for this proposal arose from the discovery that viral oncoproteins—including adenovirus E1A, simian virus 40 (SV40), large T-antigen (TAg), and human papillomavirus (HPV) E7—all bind pRb by means of conserved domains required for transformation [90–95]. These findings suggested that pRb inhibits cellular proliferation by means of a functional domain that can be inactivated by viral oncoprotein binding or by mutation, resulting in deregulated proliferation and risk for malignant transformation.

Further insight into the mechanism of pRb's antiproliferative action arose from the finding that hypophosphorylated pRb forms complexes with the transcription factor E2F [98–101], which had been implicated in the activation of proliferation genes [100–102]. Later studies confirmed that pRb binding of E2F occurs principally in the G1 phase of the cell cycle [103,104], that pRb binding blocks the transactivating function of E2F [105–107], and that pRb binding of E2F is abrogated by phosphorylation and in the presence of viral oncoproteins [108]. Taken together, these studies suggest that hypophosphorylated pRb inhibits cell cycle progression in G1 by binding and inhibiting E2F, and that this function of pRb is inactivated by phosphorylation or by viral oncoprotein binding of pRb.

To date, six E2F family members (E2F1-E2F6) have been identified [109–111]. pRb interacts preferentially with E2F1-4, while p107 and p130 interact almost exclusively with both E2F4 and E2F5 [61,111]. E2F proteins function in heterodimeric complexes with one of two DP (E2F dimerization partner) family proteins (DP1 and DP2). These E2F-DP dimers, which we will call simply E2Fs, regulate transcription by binding to a specific nucleotide recognition sequence in the promoter of E2F target genes. Cellular proliferation is associated principally with the activity of E2F1-E2F3 (the "activating" E2Fs) [111], which are required for cellular proliferation [71]. These E2Fs stimulate cell cycle progression by activating the expression of a large set of genes required for G1/S phase progression, including cell cycle regulatory genes (e.g., cyclin E, cyclin A, and cdk2) and DNA replication genes (e.g., thymidine kinase, dihydrofolate reductase, and DNA polymerases) [112]. Recent evidence indicates that E2F family members also regulate the expression of a large number of genes involved in development, differentiation, and apoptosis [113].

While early evidence suggested that pRb induces cell cycle arrest by blocking the transactivation domain of E2Fs, other evidence pointed to mechanisms of active transcriptional repression by pRb [114,115]. These repressor mechanisms were later shown to be the principle means whereby pRb induces cell cycle arrest [116]. pRb actively represses transcription by recruiting several classes of chromatin remodeling complexes to E2F sites [117]. The term chromatin refers to the densely packed form of DNA found in eukaryotes, composed of nucleosomes. The nucleosome consists of a histone core wrapped twice around by a continuous sequence of DNA, which serves to connect one core to the next in a structural arrangement that resembles beads on a string (Fig. 1). Each histone core is comprised of two copies of each of four distinct histone proteins, H2A, H2B, H3, and H4. Chromatin remodeling complexes influence transcription by altering chromatin structure, thereby modulating access of transcription factors to DNA [118–122].

In the best described mechanism of active repression, pRb recruits chromatin remodeling complexes containing the class I histone deacetylases HDAC1, HDAC2, and HDAC3 [123–126]. When recruited to E2F sites by pRb, HDACs inhibit transcription by deacetylating the exposed tails of histone cores and condensing chromatin structure [118]. HDAC activity is required for repression of a subset of E2F target genes in G1, notably cyclin E but not cyclin A [124,125,127]. While pRb was initially thought to bind HDACs directly, it now appears that pRb tethers HDAC complexes to E2F sites by means of a linking protein called retinoblastoma binding protein 1 (RBP1) (Fig. 1A) [126,128]. Interestingly, RBP1 induces growth arrest when overexpressed and demonstrates a repressor function which is independent of HDACs [126,129].

pRb also recruits to E2F sites a chromatin remodeling complex containing the histone methylase SUV39H1 and a methyl-lysine binding protein called HP1 (Fig. 1B) [130,131]. SUV39H1 methylates a lysine residue on the histone protein H3, creating a binding site for HP1 [132–134]. This cooperative mechanism results in transcriptional repression. Interestingly, SUV39H1 activity requires prior deacetylation of the lysine residue on H3 [132], a step which could be performed by the HDAC complexes [130]. This suggests a model in which repression of some E2F target genes by pRb requires consecutive recruitment of HDAC and SUV39HI-HP1 complexes to E2F sites [130]. Consistent with this model, the SUV39HI-HP1 complex specifically binds and represses the promoter of cyclin E, an E2F target gene that is also regulated by HDAC [130]. Targeted disruption of SUV39H1 results in elevated levels of cyclin E as well as cyclin A [130].

pRb also forms complexes with the ATPases BRG1 and hBRM [135–138], which function as the catalytic subunits of SWI/SNF chromatin remodeling complexes (Fig. 1C) [121,122]. pRb-hBRM represses E2F1-mediated transcription, and pRb-BRG1 is required for the repression of critical E2F target genes, including both cyclin E and cyclin A [127,138]. BRG1 induces cell cycle arrest when overexpressed and is required for pRb-mediated cell cycle arrest [135,139]. Consistent with its proposed tumor suppressive function, BRG1 is mutated in multiple human tumor cell lines [140]. Trimolecular HDAC1-pRb-BRG1 complexes have been detected in cells transfected with all three proteins, suggesting a model in which pRb simultaneously recruits HDAC and BRG1/hBRM complexes to E2F sites (Fig. 1D) [127]. The three components of this complex are proposed to cooperate in silencing E2F target genes in early G1 [127]. This action results in cell cycle arrest that may be reversible (quiescence) or permanent (replicative senescence or terminal differentiation). Quiescence is also associated with formation of p130-E2F4/5 complexes [61], suggesting that pRb and p130 play complimentary role in the maintenance of this state.

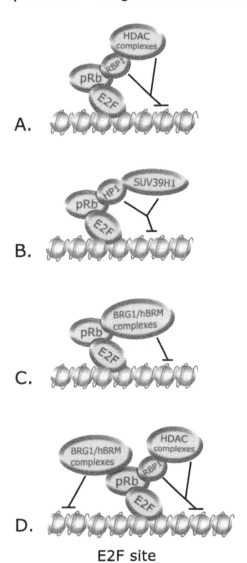

Figure 1 Chromatin remodeling complexes are recruited by pRb to promoter-bound E2F. These complexes function to repress transcription of E2F-responsive genes. (A) pRb-RBP1-HDAC complex. (B) pRb-HP1-SUV39H1 complex. (C) pRb-BRG1/hBRM complex. (D) Proposed pRb corepressor complex containing both HDAC and BRG1 complexes.

C. Promotion of Terminal Differentiation by pRb

pRb promotes terminal differentiation through diverse mechanisms, including induction of cycle arrest, inhibition of apoptosis, and activation of tissue-specific gene expression. The first insight into pRb's critical role in differentiation arose from findings in germline *RB1−/−* mice. These animals demonstrate a requirement for pRb in the terminal differentiation of neurons, erythrocytes, fiber cells of the ocular lens, and skeletal muscle [45–47,49]. Unexpectedly, embryonic cells appear to cycle normally in *RB1*-nullizygous mice throughout the first half of the gestational period [45–47], suggesting that pRb does not play an essential role in actively proliferating cells [141]. However, these mice die by embryonic day 15.5 (E15.5) with severe defects in neurogenesis, fetal liver erythropoiesis, and ocular lens development. Cells in these compartments demonstrate aberrant S phase entry and massive apoptosis in areas where terminal differentiation would normally be observed [45–48,142]. A recent study by Lee and coworkers describes a similar pattern of ectopic S phase entry and apoptosis in the retina of *RB1*-nullizygous mice between E11.5 and E15.5 [143]. Partial developmental rescue of *RB1*−/− mice has been achieved through introduction of an *RB1* minigene that expresses low levels of *RB1*. E14 neuronal and erythropoietic defects are suppressed in these mice, but subnormal pRb levels result in massive skeletal muscle defects at later stages of development and the mice die at birth [49]. Studies of *RB1* expression in mice have confirmed that tissue defects in *RB1*−/− mice correspond precisely to those tissues in which *RB1* is normally expressed during terminal differentiation [144]. Ex vivo studies have implicated pRb in the terminal differentiation of additional cell types, including adipose tissue, monocytes, keratinocytes, bone, and possibly also lung epithelial cells [44,50–52,145].

Terminal differentiation is a coordinated process that begins with the commitment of precursor cells to a particular cell fate. The process of commitment involves the tissue-specific expression of early differentiation genes. Immediately after this point, or in some cases after an intervening phase of clonal expansion, committed cells exit permanently from the cell cycle. At this time, susceptibility to apoptosis is reduced, and cell begins to express late differentiation markers. Changes in cellular morphology result, as the cell develops characteristics of the fully differentiated tissue. pRb has been observed to perform at least four distinct functions during this process, including induction of terminal cell cycle arrest, suppression of apoptosis, transcriptional activation of tissue-specific differentiation genes, and inhibition of cell cycle re-entry [42,146]. These functions and the pRb binding partners associated with these processes are depicted in Figure 2.

1. Induction of Terminal Cell Cycle Arrest

pRb is thought to induce terminal cell cycle arrest principally through repression of E2F target genes (Fig. 1). However, pRb has also been proposed to promote terminal cell cycle arrest through other repressor mechanisms that appear to operate only in differentiating cells. The best described of these mechanisms involves pRb binding to the HMG family transcription factor HBP1 (HMG-box containing protein 1) [42,146]. HBP1 is upregulated during terminal differentiation and represses genes involved in cell cycling, including the E2F-responsive genes, *N-myc* and cyclin D1 [147, 148]. HBP1 inhibits cell cycle progression when overexpressed in vitro and when expressed ectopically in transgenic mice [147,149]. HBP1-mediated repression of the *N-myc* promoter is alleviated by deletion of HBP1's high-affinity pRb binding motif [147]. These data suggest that pRb can negatively regulate cell cycle progression by augmenting the repressor function of HBP1.

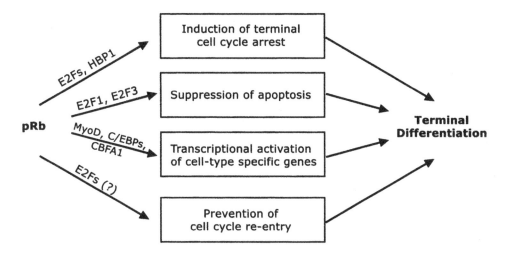

Figure 2 pRb is capable of performing at least four distinct functions during the process of terminal differentiation. Proteins partners associated with these functions are indicated. Mechanisms by which pRb promotes terminal differentiation vary by cell type and do not necessarily include all four mechanisms depicted here. See text for details.

2. Suppression of Apoptosis

Apoptosis or programmed cell death is a highly conserved regulatory mechanism employed during development for tissue modeling and for the elimination of inappropriately cycling cells. The role of apoptosis has been especially well described in neuronal and muscle development [150–154]. The importance of pRb in the suppression of apoptosis during development was first suggested by tissue defects in *RB1*−/− mice. These findings suggested that cells which require pRb for terminal differentiation, including neurons, erythrocytes, and lens fiber cells, undergo apoptosis in its absence [45–49,142]. However, it should be noted that the requirement for pRb in these cells may be cell-autonomous or noncell-autonomous, and that environmental factors can rescue certain *RB1*−/− cell types from apoptosis. For example, the presence of neighboring *RB1* wild-type cells in chimeric *RB1*−/− mice suppresses apoptosis and promotes differentiation of *RB1*−/− neurons and erythrocytes (see full discussion below) [53,54]. *RB1*−/− neuronal and muscle precursor cells can also be rescued from apoptosis and induced to differentiate in vitro [155, 156], although, in contrast to their normal counterparts, differentiated *RB1*−/− neuronal and muscle cells remain acutely vulnerable to apoptosis [42,157].

Apoptosis is often associated with the activity of the tumor suppressor protein p53, which triggers apoptosis or cell cycle arrest in response to stress signals [158–161]. In the case of *RB1*−/− mice, apoptosis occurs through both p53-dependent and p53-independent mechanisms. On embryonic day 13.5 (E13.5), for example, pRb loss results in the activation of p53-dependent apoptosis in the central nervous system and p53-independent apoptosis in the peripheral nervous system. Targeted disruption of the *p53* gene in *RB1*−/− mice suppresses apoptosis in the CNS at this stage of development, but does not prevent abnormal proliferation associated with pRb loss [162]. Apoptosis in the ocular lens of $RB1-/-$ mice is also p53 dependent at E13.5 [48].

pRb prevents apoptosis principally by controlling the activity of E2Fs, which can trigger apoptosis when inadequately regulated. Overexpression of E2F1 in cell culture systems reliably induces apoptosis [109,163–166], which occurs through both p53-dependent [163,164,166,167] and p53-independent mechanisms [168,169]. While some researchers have argued that apoptosis induction is a specialized function of E2F1 [170–173] at least two groups have reported that overexpression of E2F2 or E2F3 also produces apoptosis in vitro [111,174].

So far, only E2F1 and E2F3 have been shown to play a role in the induction of apoptosis in vivo in the absence of pRb. Targeted disruption of $E2F1$ in $RB1-/-$ mice suppresses apoptosis as well as ectopic S-phase entry in the developing CNS and lens, suggesting a critical role for E2F1 in the induction of apoptosis in these tissues. However, these mice die around E17 with anemia and defects in skeletal muscle and lung tissue, suggesting that pRb regulates apoptosis through other effectors in these tissues [172]. Targeted disruption of $E2F3$ in $RB1-/-$ mice also suppresses both apoptosis and ectopic S-phase entry in the developing CNS and lens [175] but mice die at E17 with defects in erythrocytes, muscle, and lung tissue. To our knowledge, similar studies of $E2F2$ disruption in $RB1-/-$ mice have not yet been performed.

E2F1 induces apoptosis by mechanisms distinct from its ability to induce cell cycle progression. E2F1 mutants have been created that are incapable of inducing S-phase entry but that retain the ability to induce apoptosis [169]. It has been widely suggested that E2F1 induces p53-dependent apoptosis through the activation of $p14ARF$ ($p19ARF$ in mice), an E2F target gene which is an important positive regulator of p53 [176,177]. However, recent studies in $RB1-/-;p19ARF-/-$ mice indicate that $p19ARF$ is not critical for p53-dependent apoptosis in the $RB1$-deficient CNS or lens [178].

Findings in $E2F3$-deficient $RB1-/-$ mice suggest that E2F3 also induces apoptosis and S-phase entry by separable mechanisms, with higher levels of free E2F3 required for the induction of apoptosis than are required for S phase entry [175]. Specifically, inactivation of a single $E2F3$ allele in $RB1-/-$ mice is sufficient to suppress p53-dependent apoptosis in the CNS and lens but has no discernible effect on ectopic S-phase entry. In contrast, disruption of both E2F3 alleles in $RB1-/-$ mice suppresses both apoptosis and ectopic S-phase entry in the CNS and lens. In light of these findings, Lees and coworkers have suggested a threshold model in which the combined dosage of E2F1 and E2F3 determines whether a cell proliferates or undergoes apoptosis [111,175]. Recently, E2Fs have been found to activate several critical regulators of apoptosis, including caspase 3 and caspase 7. These observations provide fresh insight into the mechanisms of apoptosis induction by E2F1 and E2F3 [113].

Remarkably, the targeted mutation of an unrelated transcription factor, $Id2$, in $RB1-/-$ mice completely suppresses both apoptosis and inappropriate cellular proliferation throughout the developing nervous system. Erythropoietic abnormalities are also virtually absent in $RB1-/-;Id2-/-$ mice, although these animals die at birth with defects in skeletal muscle tissue [179]. These observations suggest a role for Id2 in apoptosis regulation by pRb.

Id2 is a member of the Id (inhibitor of differentiation) family of helix-loop-helix (HLH) transcription factors. This family serves important functions in the induction of cell cycle progression and in the negative regulation of differentiation [180–184]. As in the case of E2Fs, overexpression of Id2 has been associated with both proliferation and apoptosis [184]. pRb binds Id2 [185], suggesting that survival of differentiating neurons and erythrocytes requires direct physiological control of Id2 by pRb [179,183]. The precise nature of pRb's interaction with Id2 remains to be defined.

3. Transcriptional Activation of Tissue-Specific Genes

While the retinoblastoma protein is best known for its repressor functions, pRb also serves to activate tissue-specific gene expression in terminally differentiating cells in several lineages. In the best studied example, pRb plays an indispensable role in the expression of late skeletal muscle genes through its interaction with MyoD [186], a basic helix-loop-helix (bHLH) family transcription factor which plays a central role in myogenesis [187]. It has been proposed that pRb stimulates the transactivating function of MyoD through direct binding and enhancement of MyoD's DNA binding ability [188], but data are inconsistent on this point [70]. Recent findings suggest a novel mechanism of transcriptional activation involving the chromatin remodeling enzyme HDAC1. In an early study, HDAC1 was shown to repress the transcriptional activity of MyoD by direct binding to its bHLH domain [189]. Subsequent experiments revealed that during myogenesis, hypophosphorylated pRb competes for HDAC1, displacing it from MyoD. This results in the derepression of MyoD and the activation of late muscle differentiation genes [190]. This model provides an attractive mechanism for precise coordination of terminal cell cycle arrest and induction of differentiation genes by pRb in skeletal muscle tissue.

Some researchers have suggested that pRb also activates bHLH family transcription factors in differentiating neurons [191,192], but evidence for this hypothesis is currently circumstantial. bHLH family proteins do play a critical role in the induction of differentiation genes in nervous tissue, including retina [193–196]. In addition, pRb loss is associated with decreased expression of neuronal differentiation genes in RB1−/− mice [142]. However, it remains unclear whether pRb loss plays a proximal role in this outcome [197]. There is also no evidence that pRb directly associates with bHLH proteins in nervous tissue. On the other hand, it is possible the pRb regulates bHLH transcription factors indirectly through interaction with Id2. Like other Id family proteins, Id2 negatively regulates bHLH family proteins by forming inactive Id-bHLH heterodimers. Hence, pRb could positively regulate bHLH-mediated induction of differentiation genes in nervous tissue by negatively regulating Id2 [192]. This proposed mechanism is consistent with recent findings in differentiating cortical progenitor cells [198]. Id2 overexpression in these cells results in the complete suppression of neuron-specific genes and ultimately in apoptosis; both of these effects are prevented by the added introduction of constitutively activated pRb. Conceivably, pRb could also activate bHLH transcription factors in differentiating neurons through an HDAC1-mediated mechanism, as observed in skeletal muscle differentiation (see above).

pRb induces differentiation gene expression in several cell types by enhancing the activity of CCAAT/enhancer-binding protein (C/EBP) family transcription factors, which are important in adipogenesis, hematopoiesis, and hepatogenesis [199–203]. pRb is required for the differentiation of cultured fibroblasts into adipose tissue, and it promotes this process by stimulating the transcriptional activity of C/EBPα [204] and C/EBPβ [50]. pRb binds C/EBPα, C/EBPβ, as well as C/EBPδ [50,145] suggesting that pRb regulates these C/EBPs through direct interaction [50]. However, abrogation of the pRb binding domain of C/EBPα has no detectable effect on adipogenesis, making this conclusion less certain [205]. pRb also promotes monocyte/macrophage differentiation in lymphoma cells by enhancing the transactivating function of C/EBPβ (also called NF-IL6 [199]) [51]. C/EBPs have been implicated in lung development, and pRb has recently been shown to stimulate the transcription of a differentiation-specific gene (surfactant protein D) in embryonic lung epithelial cells through the formation of cooperative, DNA-binding complexes containing C/EBPα, C/EBPβ, and C/EBPδ [145].

    pRb is also required to activate the osteoblast transcription factor CBFA1 [44], which is essential for the expression of late bone differentiation markers [206]. pRb binds CBFA1 and facilitates the ability of CBFA1 to bind osteoblast-specific promoters [44]. In another example, pRb has been proposed to play a role in tissue-specific gene expression in differentiating keratinocytes, where it binds and activates the AP-1 transcription factor c-jun [52]. A general role for pRb in the induction of differentiation-specific genes has been proposed by Khochbin and coworkers [207]. These investigators found that pRb cooperates with HBP1 to induce the expression of histone $H1^0$ and possibly other important chromatin remodeling genes which are expressed ubiquitously in terminally differentiated cells. The transactivating function of the pRb-HBP1 complex in this context contrasts with the proposed repressor function of the pRb-HBP1 complex in the induction of cell cycle arrest (see above), but both mechanisms could serve to promote terminal differentiation.

4. Inhibition of Cell Cycle Re-entry

In some cell types, constitutive cell cycle control by pRb is important for maintaining the postmitotic state. For example, pRb is required for the prevention of cell cycle re-entry in differentiated muscle cells [155,186]. Mechanisms whereby pRb prevents differentiated cells from re-entering the cell cycle remain unclear, although the involvement of E2Fs and HBP1 has been proposed [42]. *RB1* is highly expressed in terminally differentiated nervous tissue [208], including several cell types within the retina [209], suggesting a similar role for pRb in the prevention of cell-cycle re-entry in postmitotic neurons. However, ex vivo studies have demonstrated that pRb and other pocket family proteins are dispensable for the maintenance of terminal cell cycle arrest and dispensable for survival in fully differentiated neurons [156]. Consistent with these findings, pRB-E2F complexes are undetectable in the mature nervous system [210]. While the function of pRb in mature neurons remains to be defined, these observations suggest that its function in such tissues is unrelated to cell cycle control.

III. pRb STRUCTURE

pRb has several important functional domains, the chief of which is an A/B pocket domain, also called the small pocket. The C-terminal region of pRb is also important, containing sequences contiguous with the A/B pocket that are critical for growth suppression. While the role of the N-terminal region of pRb is least defined, it also affects pRb function. pRb contains 16 potential phosphorylation sites, at least 7 of which are phosphorylated in vivo [76–78]. The structural features of pRb are depicted in Figure 3.

A. The A/B Pocket

The A/B pocket is highly conserved among all three pocket family proteins. This region is formed by covalent bonding of the A box (amino acids 379 through 572) and the B box (amino acids 646 through 772). The spacer separating the A and B boxes is not well conserved and is dispensable for A/B pocket formation [74]. The small pocket is the minimum region required for viral oncoprotein binding and the majority of mutations cluster in this region of pRb [211–213]. This domain is both necessary and sufficient for transcriptional repression by pRb [115,214]. The binding requirements for most of pRb's binding partners fall within or overlap this region.

The small pocket includes a binding site for an LxCxE motif (L = leucine, C = cysteine, E = glutamic acid, and x = any amino acid), a peptide sequence that is conserved among viral oncoproteins and is shared by a number of cellular proteins that bind pRb. RBP1, which tethers HDAC complexes to pRb, binds to pRb by means of an LxCxE domain [126,128]. HP1, a subunit of the SUV39H1-HP1 chromatin remodeling complex, also contains an LxCxE domain, and this domain is required for the formation of pRb-HP1-histone complexes [130]. The presence of a LxCxE domain on both RBP1 and HP1 suggests that pRb does not simultaneously bind HDAC and SUV39H1-HP1 complexes, and this is consistent with the proposal

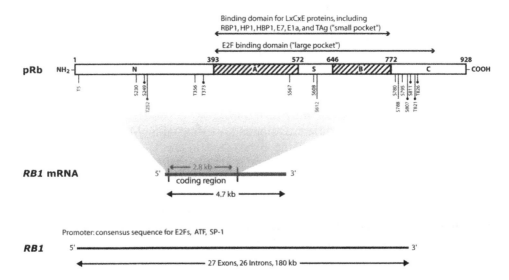

Figure 3 Features of *RB1*, *RB1* mRNA, and pRb. The coding sequence on *RB1* mRNA begins with the second methionine at nucleotide 139 and results in protein product containing 928 amino acids. Proposed phosphorylation sites on pRb are indicated; those that are known to be phosphorylated in vivo are indicated by closed circles. Sequences corresponding to small pocket, large pocket, N terminus, A box, spacer, B box, C terminus are indicated.

that pRb recruits these complexes consecutively to E2F sites [130]. The chromatin remodeling ATPase BRG1 also contains an LxCxE domain but does do not require this sequence to bind pRb [127,215]. This observation is consistent with the proposal that pRb can simultaneously recruit HDAC and BRG1 to E2F sites [127]. Finally, HBP1, which cooperates with pRb in the induction of terminal cell cycle arrest and differentiation-specific gene expression, also binds to pRb by means of an LxCxE domain [147,207]. The crystal structure of the pRb A/B pocket domain bound to a conserved E7 peptide containing the LxCxE motif has been described [74]. Crystallography demonstrates that the LxCxE motif binds to highly conserved residues in a shallow groove on the B box. While the A box does not bind directly to the LxCxE motif, it is required for LxCxE binding and probably facilitates stable folding of the B box.

The A/B interface, formed by the interaction of the A and B boxes, is also highly conserved. This high degree of conservation suggests that this interface serves as another pocket binding site, possibly for E2Fs, which lack an LxCxE motif [74]. pRb binding of E2F at the A/B interface could provide a means for pRb to simultaneously bind E2Fs and chromatin remodeling complexes. Several missense mutations affecting the A/B interface have been described, providing supporting evidence that this structure is important for tumor suppression by pRb [74]. The precise mechanism whereby viral oncoprotein binding to pRb disrupts E2F binding remains unclear, but it has been suggested that viral oncoproteins compete with E2F for a non-LxCxE binding site [74].

B. The C Terminus

The large pocket domain comprises the A/B pocket plus a portion of the C-terminal domain through residue 869. This domain is required for E2F binding and for pRb-mediated growth suppression [216]. The vast majority of naturally occurring *RB1* mutations (98% in one large study [217]) affect the large pocket, suggesting the critical significance of this domain for tumor suppression by pRb. The C terminal sequences of the large pocket contain a second binding site for E2Fs as well as a distinct binding site for the c-Abl tyrosine kinase [218,219]. This c-Abl binding site contributes to growth suppression by pRb [219].

pRb binding of several differentiation factors—including MyoD, CBFA1, and c-Jun—requires sequences in both the B box and in the C terminus [44,52,188]. Exon 25 encodes a region of the C terminus that contains a nuclear localization sequence required for full wild-type activity [220,221]. The C-terminal domain also contains a binding site for the oncoprotein mdm2, which negatively regulates p53 by promoting its degradation [222]. While the functional significance of the pRb-mdm2 interaction remains unclear [70,223], pRb has been shown to promote the apoptotic function of p53 by binding to mdm2 [224].

C. The N Terminus

The N-terminal region of pRb is the least studied region of this protein, and its functional significance is not well defined. This region does contain binding sites for several proteins [225–228], including p202, a protein that negatively regulates the cell cycle through the pRB/E2F pathway and is targeted by the adenovirus E1A oncoprotein [229–231]. In addition, in vitro analyses of N-terminally mutated pRb indicate that this domain is important for normal protein function [43,232].

Deletion analyses in mice suggest that this region does play a significant role in tumor suppression by pRb. Introduction of N-terminal-deleted *RB1* fails to rescue pituitary tumors which arise in *RB1+/−* mice (discussed below), suggesting that the N-terminal region contributes to tumor suppression by pRb [233]. N-terminal deletions have also been reported in low-penetrance retinoblastoma kindreds, providing further evidence for this region's importance in tumor suppression [43,234,235]. Surprisingly, however, N-terminally truncated pRb has also been associated with enhanced tumor suppressive function in cell culture systems [236,237], and it has been suggested that N-terminal truncation of pRb may represent a cellular mechanism for modulating pRb function [237].

D.   Insights from Low-Penetrance pRb Mutants

Although *RB1* has no known hot spots for mutation, truncating mutations are very common. Ninety percent of clinically significant mutations are characterized by frameshift, nonsense, or splice site mutations, which produce a premature stop codon and a truncated transcript [217]. These mutations are distributed fairly evenly throughout the N-terminal and large-pocket domains, invariably resulting in partial or complete loss of large pocket coding sequences. The high frequency of truncating mutations in retinoblastoma suggests that tumorigenesis is most favored by mutations that globally inactivate pRb. This provides further support for the view that multiple functional domains contribute to tumor suppression by pRb.

This view is also consistent with genetic findings in low-penetrance retinoblastoma kindreds, where truncating *RB1* mutations are notably absent and disease is less severe. *RB1* mutations reported in low-penetrance kindreds include point mutations in the promoter region [239,240], splice site mutations [241–243], amino acid substitutions (missense mutations) [242,244–249], and in-frame deletions [221,234,245]. These mutations have consistently been predicted to only mildly alter pRb expression or structure, permitting residual protein function [250]. Consistent with these predictions, retinoblastoma in these kindreds often skips generations [23,221,234,235,239,240,244,245,247,251,252], and is associated with unilateral involvement [23,221,235,239,245,247], benign retinoma [23,221,235,244,246], delayed onset [243], few intraocular recurrences [244], and early and complete response to therapy [244].

A model has been proposed to explain how minimally deranging germline *RB1* mutations results in low-penetrance, low-expressivity retinoblastoma (Fig. 4) [234,239,253]. This model relies on the observation that in approximately 70% of cases, the second hit leading to RB tumor formation occurs following loss of heterozygosity (LOH) for the normal *RB1* allele. In heritable RB, the usual consequence of LOH is two copies of the germline mutant allele. In cases where the germline mutant allele encodes a protein with residual activity, biallelic expression of the mutant protein as a consequence of LOH is proposed to result in pRb activity which is suboptimal yet sufficient to prevent tumorigenesis (Fig. 4).

Functional studies of low-penetrance pRb mutants have provided further insight into both the mechanisms of low-penetrance retinoblastoma and the tumor suppressive functions of the retinoblastoma protein. In vitro analysis of two low-penetrance pRb mutants by Kaelin and coworkers revealed that these proteins were incapable of E2F binding (and hence, unable to induce cell cycle arrest), yet they retained the ability to promote MyoD-mediated differentiation in a standard "flat cell" assay of *RB1*−/− SAOS-2 osteosarcoma cells [43]. These researchers suggest that tumor suppression by pRb involves separable functions: (1) induction of cell cycle arrest, and (2) activation of differentiation genes. Retention of the latter function by these low-penetrance pRb mutants, they argue, could account for the reduced risk for retinoblastoma in individuals who carry these mutations (for further discussion, see Ref. 79).

In light of the recently proposed mechanism of MyoD activation by pRb in myoblasts (see above), it seems likely that these low-penetrance pRb mutants are able to induce differentiation in this osteosarcoma cell line because they retain a functional LxCxE binding site [190]. This binding site is required for pRb to induce myogenic differentiation [260], presumably because this site is required for pRb binding of RBP1-HDAC complexes [130] and for alleviation of HDAC-mediated repression of MyoD [192]. It is also worth noting that cultured, *RB1*-deficient myoblasts remain capable of undergoing cell cycle arrest, which is required for the activation of muscle-specific gene expression [155,186]. Kaelin et al.'s results suggest that *RB1*−/− SAOS-2 osteosarcoma cells possess a similar capability, which could explain why these two low-penetrance pRb mutants do not require E2F binding ability to induce differentiation in this cell line [190]. To date, regulation of HDAC-mediated repression of differentiation by pRb has been described only in skeletal

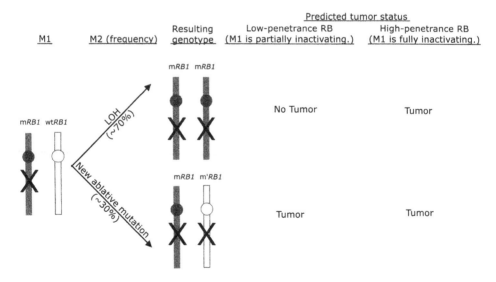

Figure 4 Model for low-penetrance retinoblastoma. Loss of heterozygosity (LOH) at the *RB1* locus with duplication of the mutant *RB1* allele occurs in about 70% of tumors. If the germline mutant allele is associated with residual function (low-penetrance mutant), biallelic expression due to LOH results in sufficient pRb function to prevent tumorigenesis. (M1 = first mutational event, M2 = second mutational event.)

muscle, so the precise role of the LxCxE binding site in retinogenesis and retinoblastoma tumorigenesis remains unclear.

IV. pRb AND THE CELL CYCLE

pRb functions at the nexus of a signaling network that controls the cell's replicative and developmental fate. The upstream effectors of this network include mitogenic and antiproliferative factors that act in an antagonistic fashion. On the one hand, mitogens produce their effects through activation of cyclin D-cdk4/6 complexes, which phosphorylate and inactivate pRb. This critical action derepresses E2F target genes, enabling the cell to begin its progression through the cell cycle. In contrast, antiproliferative signals induce the expression of CDKIs, which positively regulate pRb by inactivating its negative regulators, the cyclin-cdk complexes. When activated by CDKIs, hypophosphorylated pRb induces cell cycle arrest through the repression of E2F target genes. In this manner, pRb functions as a sensitive indicator and effector of the balance of proliferative and antiproliferative signals emanating both from within the cell and from its external environment [39,40].

The cell cycle consists of a presynthetic gap phase (G1), followed by a DNA synthesis phase (S), a second gap phase (G2), and finally mitosis (M). Expression of cdks is relatively invariant, but the kinase activity of these enzymes requires association with cyclins, whose expression is strictly regulated throughout the cell cycle [40,255,256] (Fig. 5). Tightly controlled fluctuations in cyclin expression result in assembly and activation of distinct cyclin-cdk complexes at sequential stages throughout the cell cycle, beginning in early G1 with the assembly of cyclinD-cdk4/6. Cyclin E-cdk2 complexes are assembled in mid to late G1, and cyclin A- and B-dependent kinases are activated later in the cell cycle.

As discussed previously, pRb induces reversible cell cycle arrest (quiescence) through formation of corepressor complexes at E2F-responsive promoters (Fig. 1). Continuous mitogenic signaling is required to induce the cell out of quiescence (also termed G0) and back into the cell cycle. The cell remains dependent on this stimulation until it passes through a critical checkpoint in late G1 called the *restriction point*, after which it becomes irreversibly committed to progressing through the cell cycle (mitogen-independent). A current model for the cell's progression out of quiescence is depicted in a simplified fashion in Figure 6 (for critical discussion, see Refs. 79 and 257).

The cell's emergence from quiescence requires the activity of Ras family proteins. These proteins relay exogenous growth signals from the inner cell membrane to the nucleus via a cascade that activates transcription of cyclin D [258–260]. Induced cyclin D binds to its partners cdk4 or cdk6 to form complexes whose assembly requires the cooperation of the CDKIs p21Cip1 and p27Kip1 [82]. Hence, these cdk "inhibitors" actually serve as positive regulators of cell cycle progression in early G1. Once assembled, cyclin D-cdk4/6 must also be activated by cdk activating kinase (CAK), which adds a phosphate group.

Activated cyclin D-cdk4/6 partially inactivates pRb by phosphorylating the protein at specific sites [72,79,257]. This phosphorylation results in disassociation of HDAC complexes from pRb and derepression of HDAC-regulated E2F target genes, notably cyclin E (Fig. 6). Upregulation of cyclin E expression results in the

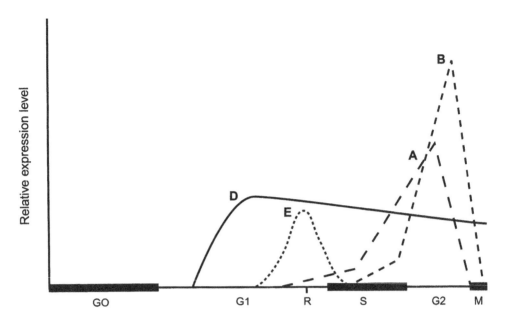

Figure 5 Cell cycle-dependent expression of cyclins. While cdk expression is relatively constant throughout the cell cycle, cyclin expression fluctuates in a cell cycle-dependent manner. D-type cyclins are induced in early G1 by mitogenic signaling, and their activity results in the expression of cyclin E later in G1. Cyclin E is required for S-phase entry and for expression of cyclin A, which is in turn required for the completion of S phase. Cyclin B is induced during S phase and regulates the cell's progression through mitosis.

formation of activated cyclin E-cdk2 complexes, which further inactivate pRb through additional phosphorylation events. This action disrupts pRb's binding to E2F and BRG1 and results in the derepression of BRG1-regulated E2F target genes. These genes include additional cell cycle genes (notably cyclin A) and DNA synthesis genes with activities that promote S phase progression.

While it is widely held that upregulation of cyclin E and functional inactivation of pRb is critical for the cell's passage through the restriction point (Fig. 6), recent evidence suggests that the converse may be true. Detailed analysis of individual cycling cells indicates that passage through the restriction point occurs prior to the accumulation of cyclin E [261]. These findings suggest that upregulation of cyclin E is more closely associated with the initiation of DNA synthesis than with the establishment of mitogen independence.

Levels of cyclin E-cdk2 decline precipitously upon the cell's entry into S phase. According to an early model, cyclin A- and B-dependent kinases maintain pRb in a hyperphosphorylated, functionally inactivated state as the cell progresses through S and G2/M [40]. However, more recent data suggests that pRb is only partially inactivated in G1 and that pRb performs significant functions during later phases of the cell cycle, including induction of cell cycle arrest in G2/M [262–269].

pRb is dephosphorylated in late M phase by a type 1 protein phosphatase (PP1α) [270–272]. According to the current consensus, dephosphorylation of pRb at

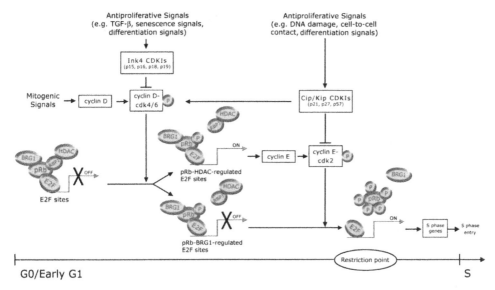

Figure 6 Model for the cell's emergence from quiescence. pRb blocks cell cycle progression by binding and inhibiting E2Fs and by recruiting repressor complexes to E2F sites. For simplicity, only one of the pRb corepressor complexes depicted in Figure 1 is depicted in this model. Chronic mitogenic signaling induces the expression of D-type cyclins, resulting in the assembly and activation of cyclin D-cdk4/6 complexes. Cyclin D–dependent kinase phosphorylates pRb at specific sites, abrogating the association between pRb and RBP1-HDAC complexes. This results in the derepression of HDAC-regulated E2F target genes, including cyclin E. Induced cyclin E complexes with cdk2, and activated cyclin E-cdk2 phosphorylates pRb at additional sites, disrupting its association with E2F and BRG1 complexes. This results in the derepression of BRG1-regulated E2F target genes, stimulating the cell's entry into S phase. The restriction point is depicted in its customary position subsequent to the induction of cyclin E. However, recent evidence suggests that cyclin E is actually induced only after the cell attains mitogen independence (see text for details). Ink4 family CDKIs positively regulate pRb by inhibiting the action of cyclin D–dependent kinase. Cip/Kip family proteins promote the assembly of cyclin D-cdk4/6 complexes in early G1 but also serve as potent inhibitors of cyclin E-cdk2 and cyclin A-cdk2.

the mitotic exit enables pRb to resume its function as a negative regulator of the G1/S phase transition during the cell's next passage through G1 [39,40]. However, exclusively hyperphosphorylated Rb has been detected in several exponentially growing cell lines, suggesting that cell-cycle dependent phosphorylation and dephosphorylation of pRb is not necessary for passage through the cell cycle in actively proliferating cells [273,274]. This view is consistent with the observation that embryonic cells in *RB1*−/− mice appear cycle normally until relatively late in development [45–47,141].

Cell cycle arrest is effected by antiproliferative signals that convey their effects through upregulation of Ink4 and Cip/Kip family CDKIs (Fig. 6). Ink4 family proteins (p15Ink4b, p16Ink4a, 18Ink4c, and p19Ink4d) specifically inactivate cyclin D-cdk4/6 complexes. Cip/Kip family proteins (p21Cip1, p27Kip1, and p57 Kip2) function as potent inhibitors of cyclin E-cdk2 and cyclin A-cdk2 complexes. Antiproliferative signals that regulate CDKIs include transforming growth factor β, which induces p15Ink4b [85], and cell-to-cell contact, which is associated with the induction of Cip/Kip family proteins [85]. Senescence signals, which are often associated with shortening of telomeres at the distal ends of chromosomes, induce both p16Ink4a [82] and p27Kip1 [275]. p53 induces pRb-mediated cell cycle arrest in response to DNA damage by upregulating p21Cip1 [286,287]. Finally, Cip/Kip family proteins also respond to differentiation signals. Interestingly, like pRb, Cip/Kip family proteins have been shown to activate the expression of differentiation genes by mechanisms distinct from their cell cycle regulatory functions [83,84,282].

V. pRb AND CANCER

Malignant transformation is generally regarded as a multistep, Darwinian process in which the cell sustains a series of mutations that endow it with growth and survival advantages [279]. The earliest traits required for malignant transformation include replicative self-sufficiency, insensitivity to antiproliferative signals, and resistance to apoptosis. Later requirements for tumor growth and spread include avoidance of replicative senescence, new blood vessel formation (angiogenesis), and the acquisition of tissue invasiveness (metastatic potential). Consistent with a proposed universal requirement for deregulated antiproliferative signaling in malignancy, functional inactivation of pRb is observed in most if not all tumors. It should be emphasized, however, that inactivation of pRb occurs most frequently through dysfunction of its upstream regulators. For example, mutational inactivation of p16Ink4a is commonly observed in many malignancies [280]. Amplification of cyclin D is another common mechanism of pRb inactivation in tumorigenesis [281]. These findings support the concept of a core "Rb pathway," p16Ink4a ⊣cyclin D-cdk4/6 ⊣pRb, which must be disabled for malignant transformation to occur [39–41].

The high frequency of Rb pathway defects upstream of pRb nevertheless suggests that this pathway is not linear, and that other proteins in the pocket family, i.e., p107 and p130, are also important downstream effectors of this pathway. This conclusion is supported by recent findings indicating that p16-mediated cell cycle arrest depends upon the activity of both pRb and either p107 or p130 [282]. Since p16 is a critical positive regulator of all three pocket proteins, mutational inactivation of *p16* may be functionally equivalent to loss of both alleles of all three pocket proteins, a set of events that is unlikely to occur in a single cell [60]. Similarly, the induction of cell cycle progression by cyclin D-dependent kinase activity appears to involve phosphorylation and inactivation of not only of pRb but also p107 and p130 [283–286]. Constitutive phosphorylation of all pocket family proteins by deregulated cyclin D–dependent kinase represents an oncogenic mechanism similar to that which has evolved in viral oncoproteins, which bind and inactivate all pocket family proteins [61]. Employing a mechanism that is even more akin to the action of viral oncoproteins, the helix-loop-helix (HLH) transcription factor Id2 also binds and inactivates all pocket family proteins when it is overexpressed in cell culture [185,287]. This mechanism has recently been described in human malignancy. Tumorigenesis initiated by *N-myc* amplification in neuroblastoma is dependent on upregulation of Id2 by oncogenic N-myc [179,288]. This finding suggests a novel mechanism for functional inactivation of pRb and other pocket family proteins in malignant transformation.

The limited spectrum of second tumors associated with heritable RB suggests that loss of pRb *per se* is an initiating event in only a small subset of malignancies, including retinoblastoma, osteosarcoma, and some soft tissue sarcomas. Biallelic loss of *RB1* appears to be required for retinoblastoma tumorigenesis. Biallelic loss of *RB1* is also frequently observed in osteosarcoma. *RB1* mutations are found consistently not only in osteosarcoma specimens from heritable RB patients, but also in sporadically occurring osteosarcomas [27,29,289–292]. There are fewer data available on the status of *RB1* in soft tissue sarcomas. Biallelic *RB1* inactivation has been demonstrated in subtypes of soft tissue sarcoma that have been reported in association with heritable RB, including malignant fibrous histiocytoma (MFH) and leiomyosarcoma [289,291,293–296]. Recent genetic and immunohistochemical analyses strongly suggests that pRb loss is a primary factor in the development of MFH [295], and immunohistochemical studies of pRb expression in leiomyosarcomas suggest that pRb loss is also critical in the pathogenesis of this tumor [297–300].

Biallelic *RB1* inactivation is frequently observed in a handful of other tumors, including bladder, lung, and breast carcinomas, and glioblastoma [41]. The absence of elevated risk for these tumors in familial RB patients suggests that loss of pRb does not play an initiating role in these tumors but rather contributes to tumor progression [238]. In the case of bladder carcinoma, this conclusion is supported by correlation between loss of pRb and malignant progression [301,302]. Alternatively, because both bladder and lung carcinomas tend to appear late in life, the absence of excessive risk for these tumors among individuals with heritable RB may be an artifact of limited follow-up time [14], or of mortality from other cancers.

The unusual vulnerability to tumorigenesis of *RB1*-deficient cells in the retina and connective tissues presumably arises from a critical requirement for pRb in terminal differentiation. However, the nature of pRb's tumor suppressive function in these tissues remains ill defined. Evidence on pRb's role in bone differentiation suggests that in this system at least, pRb's role in tumor suppression extends beyond its ability to induce terminal cell cycle arrest through control of E2Fs. Specifically, Hinds and coworkers propose that pRb's activation of CBFA1-mediated gene expression in differentiating osteoblasts serves a tumor suppressive function [44]. These investigators propose that loss of this activating function may result in the failure of differentiating osteoblasts to upregulate the cyclin-dependent kinase inhibitors, p21Cip1 and p27Kip1, which both exert important antiproliferative functions in this system. This model provides a preliminary rationale for the propensity of carriers of a mutant *RB1* allele to develop bony sarcomas.

Individuals with heritable RB are also at risk of developing cutaneous melanoma, which represents 7 to 25% of second tumors in this population [10,14,15,18]; (see also Ref. 303)]. While this observation suggests the pRb loss can initiate this tumor, this conclusion is at odds with current data on the pathogenesis of cutaneous melanoma. Normal pRb expression has been detected in 64 of 67 (96%) unrelated melanoma cell lines [238,304–306], and in 57 of 57 (100%) metastatic melanomas [305]. In contrast, Rb pathway defects upstream of pRb have been detected in 62 of 64 (97%) unrelated melanoma cell lines [304,306]. To our knowledge, the status of *RB1* in cutaneous melanomas specifically associated with heritable retinoblastoma remains undescribed. These findings suggest that isolated pRb loss in melanocytes does not initiate tumorigenesis and that transformation in this cell type requires functional inactivation of all three pocket proteins. This conclusion is supported by a recent study demonstrating high levels of constitutively phosphorylated pRb, p107, and p130 in melanoma cell lines [307,308].

VI. pRb IN RETINOGENESIS

Understanding the precise role of pRb loss in retinoblastoma will require a clearer understanding of pRb's normal role in retinogenesis. Unfortunately, we currently have little direct evidence concerning the role of pRb in retinal development. With respect to the CNS in general, suppression of both abnormal S-phase entry and apoptosis in the brains of *RB1−/−;E2F1−/−* and *RB1−/−;E2F3−/−* mice [172,175] suggests that the principle developmental functions of pRb in this compartment are induction of terminal cell cycle arrest and inhibition of apoptosis through control of E2Fs. However, given recent evidence that E2Fs repress genes involved in cell fate determination, it seems likely that pRb also promotes tissue-specific gene expression in the CNS and other tissues through control of E2Fs. For example, E2Fs repress transcription of inhibin β A, a gene which induces the differentiation of a variety of neuronal cell types, including rod photoreceptors. Inhibition of this E2F function by pRb would promote neuronal differentiation [113]. Early evidence suggests that pRb's interaction with Id2 in differentiating nervous tissue may also be similarly complex, involving the regulation of cell cycle progression, apoptosis, and the expression of differentiation genes [179,198].

A few studies have provided direct insight into pRb's role in retinogenesis. These include studies of *RB1* expression in the developing murine retina, as well as studies of *RB1*-deficient knockout and chimeric mice.

A. *RB1* Expression in the Developing Retina

The mature retina consists of three nuclear layers, the ganglion cell layer, inner nuclear layer, and outer nuclear layer (GCL, INL, and ONL). The GCL is comprised of ganglion cells and displaced amacrine cells. Amacrine, horizontal, and bipolar cells make up the INL, and the ONL consists of cone and rod photoreceptors. During development, the retina begins as a single layer of proliferating neuronal stem cells (neuroblastic layer). In the course of differentiation, neuroblasts enter terminal mitosis at the outer neuroblastic layer and subsequently migrate to the inner margin of the primordial retina, forming a distinct layer of postmitotic, differentiating cells. The first cells to populate this layer are the ganglion cells of the GCL. The INL emerges later in embryogenesis, whereas the ONL does not fully differentiate until after birth [309].

In situ hybridization studies of *RB1* expression during murine retinal development suggest that pRb plays an important yet cell-type restricted role in retinal differentiation. Gallie and coworkers have demonstrated that *RB1* is first expressed as early as E13.5 in ganglion cells, the first retinal cell type to differentiate [144]. Following a more detailed analysis, Gallie and colleagues reported strong *RB1* expression in every cell of the GCL by E15 [209], while at the same time *RB1* is expressed in only a small number of cells in the neuroblastic layer. These latter cells were presumed to be migrating post-mitotic cells. *RB1* is also strongly expressed in the incipient inner nuclear layer of the retina by around E17 [209]. Among the three neuronal cell types found in the INL, *RB1* is expressed in differentiating amacrine and horizontal cells only, and not in bipolar cells. *RB1* is only sparsely expressed in the outer nuclear layer, even in adult mice, and *RB1* is expressed in cone photoreceptors only, not rods. Lastly, these investigators describe a similar pattern of *RB1* expression in adult human retina; in adults *RB1* expression is absent in bipolar cells and rod photoreceptor cells. Taken together, these data indicate that endogenous *RB1* expression is not important for differentiation of bipolar or rod cells, and that retinoblastoma does not originate from these cells.

B.   Insights from *RB1*-Deficient Knockout and Chimeric Mice

Retinal findings in germline *RB1−/−* mice provide additional insight into the functions of pRb in developing retina. Unfortunately, data is limited to early retinal development due to embryonic lethality in these mice. Until recently, there was no evidence of retinal abnormalities in these mice; however, using more sensitive analyses, including BrdU incorporation and TUNEL assays, Lee and coworkers demonstrated the presence of ectopic S phase entry and enhanced apoptosis in the inner retinal progenitor layers of these mice at E13.5 [143]. These observations are consistent with findings elsewhere in the CNS of these animals, indicating that pRb is required for terminal cell cycle arrest and suppression of apoptosis in this compartment. These investigators also report that ectopic proliferation and apoptosis appear sequentially in the developing *RB1−/−* retina from E11.5 to the time of death at E15.5. This suggests that *RB1* is expressed in the retina as early as E11.5, rather than E13.5 as previously reported [144].

The role of pRb at later stages of retinal development has been examined in chimeric *RB1−/−* mice, created by injection of *RB1−/−* embryonic stem cells into *RB1+/+* embryos [53,54]. Unexpectedly, these mice develop almost normally, and *RB1−/−* cells contribute significantly to several tissues in which pRb plays a critical developmental role, including retina, brain, blood, and skeletal muscle. This suggests that pRb-dependent *RB1−/−* cells in these tissues can be developmentally rescued by neighboring wild-type cells, and that the requirement for pRb in terminal differentiation of these cells is therefore non-cell-autonomous. Some defects were nevertheless observed in these chimeras. Like germline *RB1+/−* mice (see below), *RB1−/−* chimeras develop pituitary tumors with nearly complete penetrance. The latency period of tumorigenesis is considerably shorter in the chimeras, strongly suggesting that pRb loss is a rate-limiting step in the development of these tumors. Massive apoptosis was also detected in lens fiber cells of these chimeras, indicating that the requirement for pRb in fiber cell differentiation is cell-autonomous. Less severe abnormalities were also observed in these mice, including hyperplasia of the adrenal medulla and enlargement of Purkinje cells in the cerebellum. Notably, these chimeras do not develop retinoblastoma (see full discussion below). Other retinal findings described in these mice differed between studies, probably due to different developmental timepoints chosen for histopathologic examination.

te Riele and coworkers examined both germline and chimeric $RB1-/-$ retina by standard light microscopy, reporting no abnormal findings through E14.5 [53] (for positive findings, see Ref. 143). However, these investigators did detect ectopic mitoses and significant pyknosis (indicating apoptosis) in the inner half of the developing chimeric retina at E16.5–18.5 [53], when $RB1$ expression becomes evident in the emerging inner nuclear layer [209]. The finding of retinal apoptosis in post-E16.5 chimeras is consistent with the results of recent experiments in which murine retinas from E11.5–12.5 germline $RB1-/-$ mice were transplanted intracranially into $RB1+/-$ mice (145). One week after transplantation, at the equivalent of E18.5–19.5, $RB1-/-$ retinal cells demonstrated elevated apoptosis in comparison to transplanted $RB1+/+$ retinal cells used as controls. Also, as in the case of $RB1-/-$ cells in chimeric retina, many intracranially transplanted $RB1-/-$ retinal cells were developmentally rescued and demonstrated evidence of differentiation, including rod-specific opsin expression, at one month post-transplantation. te Riele and coworkers also described retinal dysplasia in the inner and outer nuclear layers of adult chimeras. In addition, the contribution of $RB1-/-$ cells to the retina was lower than to other tissues and less than the retinal contribution of $RB1+/-$ cells in $RB1+/-$ chimeras used as controls.

te Riele and coworkers' findings in embryonic and adult chimeras suggest that while many cells in the retina are able to differentiate in the absence of autonomously produced pRb, a significant number of $RB1-/-$ retinal cells are deleted by apoptosis at the time of terminal differentiation. The most likely candidates for apoptosis are $RB1$-expressing ganglion, amacrine, horizontal, and cone cells. It may be that one or more of these cell types depend on pRb for survival in a cell-autonomous manner, as in the case of $RB1-/-$ lens fiber cells, which are eliminated by apoptosis in both germline and chimeric $RB1-/-$ mice [48,53,54]. Alternatively, mechanisms of non-cell-autonomous developmental rescue may simply be less efficient in the retina than in other tissues, such as brain, blood, and skeletal muscle, resulting in elevated levels of apoptosis observed in chimeric $RB1-/-$ retina.

In another study of chimeric $RB1-/-$ mice, Jacks and coworkers examined the eyes of chimeras after birth and reported no abnormal findings [54]. The absence of ectopic mitoses and apoptosis in the retina of newborn chimeras could be explained by the fact that virtually all retinal cell types which express $RB1$ during terminal differentiation, including ganglion, amacrine, horizontal, and cone cells, have entered final S phase by the time of birth [310]. While rod and bipolar cells continue to mature in large numbers postnatally, these cells do not express $RB1$ and therefore would not be affected by inactivation of this gene [209].

Follow-up studies of the individual fate of $RB1-/-$ cells in the CNS of these chimeras have provided preliminary insight into the mechanism of developmental rescue [55]. These studies demonstrate that while $RB1-/-$ cells in the brain are rescued, they do not differentiate normally. At the time of terminal differentiation, these cells undergo ectopic S-phase entry but do not proceed to mitosis; instead, they undergo G2 phase arrest and ultimately differentiate with 4N DNA content. These findings suggest that in the developing CNS, pRb is required in a cell-autonomous manner for the orderly induction of terminal cell cycle arrest. In contrast, the requirements for pRb in apoptosis protection and in induction of differentiation genes are non-cell-autonomous. Normal pRb activity in neighboring wild-type cells appears to be sufficient to achieve these latter effects.

The neuronal findings in *RB1*−/− chimeras are remarkably similar to findings in skeletal muscle in germline *RB1*−/− mice which were partially developmentally rescued by the introduction of an *RB1* minigene [49]. Restoration of low levels of pRb expression in these mice is sufficient for near-normal neurogenesis and erythropoiesis, but mice die at birth from severely impaired skeletal muscle development. While the majority of myoblasts in these undergo apoptosis mice, some myoblasts do manage to differentiate, albeit abnormally. As is the case in neuroblast differentiation in *RB1*−/− chimeras, myoblast differentiation in this model is characterized by ectopic S-phase entry and endoreduplication without mitosis.

The precise manner in which neighboring wild-type cells rescue *RB1*-deficient cells in the neuronal, erythroid, and skeletal muscle compartments of *RB1*−/− chimeras remains unclear. Jacks and coworkers suggest that wild-type cells may secrete factors required for the survival of differentiating neurons, such as neurotrophins [55]. Helin and coworkers speculate that activin A may be involved; this protein functions both as a nerve cell survival molecule and as an erythroid differentiation factor [113]. Activin A is a dimer composed of two inhibin β A molecules. Activated E2Fs strongly repress inhibin β A expression while strongly inducing expression of follistatin, an inhibitor of activin A [113]. Deregulation of E2Fs in the absence of pRb should negatively affect activin A levels within the cell and in its external microenvironment; however, secretion and local diffusion of activin A by neighboring wild-type cells in *RB1*−/− chimeras could promote neuronal and erythroid differentiation in *RB1*-deficient cells in these compartments [113]. Interestingly, apart from neurotrophin 3, activin A is the only protein known to induce cell cycle arrest and differentiation in retinal progenitor cells [311]. Specifically, activin A induces rod photoreceptor differentiation in E18 rat retinal cell cultures [311].

VII. pRb IN THE PATHOGENESIS OF MURINE RB

Retinoblastoma has been reported in several different lines of transgenic and chimeric mice [197,312–315]. Findings from these studies provide suggestive evidence regarding the role and sufficiency of pRb loss in the genesis of human RB. While RB in humans is thought to arise due to inactivation of only a single pocket family protein, pRb, studies in chimeric mice indicate that retinoblastoma in this species requires inactivation of at least two pocket family members, pRb and p107. However, incomplete disease penetrance in chimeric *RB1*−/−;p107−/− mice indicate that even these two events are insufficient for the development of murine RB. Studies in transgenic mice suggest that inactivation of the tumor suppressor p53 may also be required, but this view remains inadequately substantiated. Definitive identification of the additional genetic events required for murine RB promises to provide insight into the possible requirement for additional genetic alterations in human RB. Findings from all reported genetic mouse models of retinoblastoma are summarized in Table 1. In the sections that follow, transgenic models of retinoblastoma will be discussed first, followed by a discussion of pocket family gene-deficient knockout and chimeric mice, in which the genetic requirements for murine retinoblastoma have been most rigorously evaluated.

A. Insights from Transgenic Mice

Retinoblastoma has been described in several lines of transgenic mice that express SV40 TAg or HPV E6 and E7 within the developing retina. TAg induces cellular transformation by binding to and inactivating all pocket family proteins; p53; the transcriptional coactivators and putative tumor suppressors p300 and CBP; and possibly other cellular proteins [316]. HPV E6 mediates transformation by binding to and inducing the degradation of p53, as well as by interacting with other cellular proteins, including p300 and CBP [317]. HPV E7 complements the transforming activity of E6 by binding to and inactivating all pocket family proteins, as well as the CDKIs p21Cip and p27Kip1, and the transcription factor AP-1 [318,319]. Studies of viral oncoprotein-induced retinoblastoma represent the earliest evidence that pRb inactivation plays a role in retinoblastoma development in the mouse. However, the complex protein binding properties of TAg and E6/E7 also suggest the involvement of other proteins, particularly other pocket family proteins and p53, in the initiation of murine retinoblastoma.

1. LHβ-TAg Mice

Murine retinoblastoma was first described in a line of mice carrying a *TAg* transgene under the control of the luteinizing hormone β-subunit promoter (LHβ) [320]. This promoter is normally expressed in the pituitary, but it is expressed ectopically in the retina in this line of mice. Beginning at 8 weeks of age, all LHβ-*TAg* mice develop multifocal, bilateral tumors with microscopic features similar to human RB [320–323]. However, tumors consistently arise from the inner nuclear layer in these mice, and immunohistochemical analysis suggests an origin in the amacrine compartment [324,325]. In contrast, current evidence suggests a photoreceptor origin for human RB [209,326].

   These mice also develop primitive neuroectodermal midbrain tumors (PNETs) with a penetrance of 15–27%, although the cell of origin differs from that of PNETs found in patients with heritable RB [11,328,329]. Similar PNETs have been described in mice expressing *TAg* under the control of at least six different promoters, including the IRBP-*TAg* and PNMT-*TAg* mice discussed below [327–331]. Albert and coworkers suggest that the *TAg* gene contains a regulatory region which is specific to the subependymal midbrain, where these tumors originate [331].

2. Opsin-TAg Mice

TAg expression has been directed to the photoreceptor compartment in mice using the mouse opsin promoter, which is specifically expressed in postmitotic rods on postnatal day 1 (P1) [332,333]. While *TAg*-expressing photoreceptors in these mice do demonstrate ectopic S-phase entry, they do not proliferate to form tumors. Instead, these cells undergo apoptosis at the time of mitosis [332,333]. Severe degeneration of the outer nuclear layer results by P10, and photoreceptor cells are nearly eliminated by adulthood [332]. These findings suggest that *TAg* expression is insufficient to transform differentiated photoreceptors in vivo.

Table 1 Retinal Findings in pRb-Deficient Transgenic, Knockout, and Chimeric Mice

Transgenic mice	Cell-type specificity of promoter in retina	Principle retinal phenotype(s)	Penetrance	Retinal layer(s)	Cell type(s)	Refs.
LHβ-TAg	Unknown	Retinoblastoma	100%	INL	Amacrine cells (?)	320
Opsin-TAg	Postmitotic rod photoreceptors	Degeneration	100%	ONL	Rod photoreceptor cells	332, 333
IRBP-TAg	Photoreceptor cells	Retinoblastoma	100%	ONL	Photoreceptor cells	327, 328
PNMT-TAg	Amacrine, horizontal cells	Degeneration Retinoblastoma	100%	OPL GCL, INL	Horizontal cells Amacrine, horizontal cells	329, 337, 338
αAcry-E6+E7	Unknown	Retinoblastoma	~90%[1]	INL	Photoreceptor cells (?)	342
IRBP-E7	Photoreceptor cells	Degeneration	100%	ONL	Photoreceptor cells	343
IRBP-E7;p53-/-	Photoreceptor cells	Degeneration and retinoblastoma	100%	ONL	Photoreceptor cells	343, 344
IRBP-E7;p53+/-	Photoreceptor cells	Degeneration and retinoblastoma	nr	ONL	Photoreceptor cells	343, 344
Knockout mice						
RB1+/-	—	Normal	—	—	—	45, 46, 354
RB1-/-	—	Normal at time of death (~ E14)	—	—	—	45–47
RB1+/-;p53-/-	—	Dysplasia	~40%	nr	nr	358
RB1+/-;p107-/-	—	Dysplasia	100%	ONL (?)	Photoreceptor cells (?)	355
RB1+/-;p130-/-	—	Normal	—	—	—	355
Chimeric mice						
RB1-/-	—	Apoptosis at E16.5 Dysplasia in adults	nr nr	VL nr	nr nr	53, 54
RB1+/-;p107-/- [RB1-/-;p107-/-]	—	Dysplasia Apoptosis and dysplasia at E17.5 Retinoblastoma	~20% nr[2] 33%[3]	INL VL INL	nr nr Amacrine cells	62
RB1-/-;p107-/-; IRBP-p53DD	Photoreceptor cells	Apoptosis and dysplasia at E17.5 Retinoblastoma	nr[2] 38%[4]	VL INL	nr Amacrine cells	62

[1] When bred on a C57BL/6 genetic background.
[2] Phenotype observed in 11/23 (48%) eyes of RB1-/-;p107-/- mice.
[3] Unilateral RB detected in 2/6 chimeras.
[4] RB detected in 3/8 chimeras (one bilateral case).
Abbreviations: INL, inner nuclear layer; ONL, outer nuclear layer; OPL, outer plexiform layer; GCL, ganglion cell layer; VL, ventricular layer; nr, not reported.

Interestingly, explanted *TAg*-expressing retinal cells from 10-day-old opsin-*TAg* mice replicate efficiently in vitro and form tumors when injected into nude mice. Environmental factors such as apoptotic signals or inadequate trophic support may account the death of postmitotic photoreceptors which reenter the cell cycle in vivo [332,333].

3.   IRBP-*TAg* Mice

Two groups have directed *TAg* expression to mitotically active photoreceptor precursor cells using the human or mouse interstitial retinol binding protein (IRBP) promoter [327,328]. IRBP is expressed exclusively in rod and cone photoreceptors in human retina [334] and expressed as early as E17 in mice [335]. IRBP promoter expression is also photoreceptor-specific [336] and is detectable in the retina by day E13 [327]. In contrast to opsin-*TAg* mice, IRBP-*TAg* mice develop bilateral retinal tumors with complete penetrance at 1 week after birth [334]. In contrast to human RB, tumors in these mice arise nonfocally, with uniform transformation of the developing photoreceptor cell layer [327,328].

4.   PNMT-*TAg* Mice

Both retinal degeneration and retinoblastoma have been observed in mice expressing *TAg* under the control of the human phenylethanolamine *N*-methyltransferase (PNMT) promoter [329,337,338]. In the rat retina, PNMT is localized to amacrine and horizontal cells [338], and is detected as early as postnatal day 1 [339]. PNMT-*TAg* mice exhibit massive degeneration of horizontal cells in the central retina and tumors of mixed amacrine and horizontal cell origin in the ganglion cell and inner nuclear layers of the peripheral retinal [337,338]. As the authors of these studies suggest, the alternative fates of *TAg*-expressing cells in these mice may be attributable to the fact that retinal development proceeds outwardly from the central to the peripheral retina [340,341]. Since cells mature first in the central retina, *TAg* expression in this portion of the retina may be consistently postmitotic, producing cell death similar to that observed in *TAg*-expressing postmitotic photoreceptors in opsin-*TAg* mice. In contrast, *TAg* expression may occur prior to terminal S phase entry in target cells of the peripheral retina, resulting in tumorigenesis.

5.   α Acry-*E6*+*E7* Mice

Retinoblastoma has also been described in a line of mice expressing HPV *E6* and *E7* under the control of the αA crystallin promoter [342]. Expression of this promoter is normally restricted to the lens, but *TAg* expression is observed in both the lens and the retina in this line of mice, resulting in lens and retinal tumors [342]. The proportion of ocular tumors that originate in the retina in these mice varies from 1–90%, depending upon genetic background. This finding suggests the existence of genes which modify risk for retinoblastoma development in mice. When bred on a permissive genetic background (C57BL/6 inbred strain) multifocal retinal tumors arise in approximately 90% of mice by age 13 months. Microscopically, these tumors appear strikingly similar to human RB. Although these tumors originate in the inner nuclear layer, cells with histopathological and ultrastructural features of photoreceptors are observed within tumor foci. However, it remains uncertain whether these photoreceptor cells are neoplastic.

6. IRBP-*E7* and IRBP-*E7;p53*−/− Mice

In all the transgenic murine models of retinoblastoma reviewed so far, tumorigenesis is associated with inactivation of pocket family members and p53. In order to examine the effects of pocket protein family inactivation in the presence of normal p53 function, transgenic mice were created which carried HPV *E7* under control of the photoreceptor-specific IRBP promoter [343]. Unexpectedly, IRBP-*E7* mice do not develop retinoblastoma, suggesting that inactivation of pRb and other pocket family members is insufficient for transformation of photoreceptors in the mouse. Instead, *E7* expression in these cells produces apoptosis at the time of terminal differentiation, resulting in degeneration of the entire photoreceptor layer. IRBP-*E7* mice do develop retinoblastoma when bred on a *p53*−/− background. These animals develop nonfocal bilateral photoreceptor cell tumors similar to those described in IRBP-*TAg* mice, and tumors arise with complete penetrance by one month of age [343]. IRBP-*E7;p53*+/− mice also develop retinal tumors which demonstrate loss of the remaining *p53* allele. These tumors develop with lower frequency and after a latency period of several months [344]. At first appraisal, these findings suggest that the apoptosis observed in IRBP-*E7* mice is p53-dependent and can be suppressed by inactivation of p53, resulting in tumorigenesis [343].

However, closer histopathologic examination of IRBP-*E7;p53*−/− mice at earlier and later stages of development revealed that photoreceptors undergo apoptosis at nearly the nearly the same rate observed in IRBP-*E7* mice, although with slightly delayed onset [344]. Tumors which develop in IRBP-*E7;p53*−/− mice arise from surviving precursor cells within the degenerating outer nuclear layer. In light of these later findings, Windle and colleagues have concluded that E7-mediated apoptosis in IRBP-*E7* mice is largely p53-independent, and that p53 inactivation in IRBP-*E7;p53*−/− mice contributes to tumorigenesis through mechanisms other than suppression of apoptosis [315].

Both of these conclusions merit further comment. In the first place, in light of the finding that apoptosis is exclusively p53-dependent in the CNS of *RB1*−/− mice [164], it is initially surprising that retinal apoptosis is largely p53-independent in IRBP-*E7* mice. It could be that mechanisms of apoptosis in the retina differ from those operating elsewhere in the CNS. Alternatively, given that p53-dependent apoptosis has been demonstrated in the *RB1*−/− CNS only as late as E13.5 [164] and retinal apoptosis in IRBP-*E7* mice occurs postnatally, it may be that role of p53-dependent apoptosis in the CNS varies as a function of developmental stage. Findings in the *RB1*-deficient murine lens support this possibility. Apoptosis in the lens is also p53-dependent in E13.5 *RB1*−/− mice [162]; however, separate studies of *E7* expression in the lens indicate that the role p53-dependent apoptosis in this tissue diminishes as a function of developmental stage [345].

Secondly, in regard to alternative mechanisms whereby germline p53 inactivation might promote tumorigenesis in IRBP-*E7;p53*−/− mice, it should be noted that p53-deficiency is associated with genomic instability and the accumulation of secondary mutations [346–352]. This mechanism could also account for photoreceptor tumors that arise IRBP-*E7;p53*−/− mice. Germline *p53* inactivation contributes to tumorigenesis without affecting apoptosis in a mouse mammary tumor model, and genomic instability due to loss of p53 has also been proposed to account for these results [353].

7. IRBP-*E2F1* and IRBP-*E2F1;p53*-/- Mice

Transgenic IRBP-*E2F*1 mice were created to test the sufficiency of deregulated E2F1 to induce photoreceptor tumors, either in the presence or absence of p53 [143]. Overexpression of *E2F1* in these mice results in ectopic proliferation, apoptosis, and delayed differentiation of developing photoreceptor cells. These findings suggest a role for deregulated E2F1 protein in the photoreceptor degeneration which is observed in IRBP-*E7* and IRBP-*E7;p53*-/- mice. Dysplastic lesions are also observed in IRBP-*E2F1* mice between post-natal days 9 and 28, but these lesions are eliminated by 3 months of age along with the majority of the photoreceptor cell layer. When IRBP-*E2F1* mice were bred on a *p53*-/- background, absence of p53 partially suppresses E2F1-mediated apoptosis during the first two weeks after birth, resulting in earlier appearing dysplasia as well as hyperplasia of multiple cell types. However, these lesions are also transient in these mice and no tumors develop. By 3 weeks of age, the degree of retinal degeneration in IRBP-*E2F1;p53*-/- and IRBP-*E2F1* mice is comparable, suggesting that apoptosis of photoreceptors in the mature retina is p53-independent. These results suggest that deregulated E2F1 may be involved in the retinal dysplasia observed in adult *RB1*-/- chimeras [53].

B. Insights from Pocket Family Gene-Deficient Knockout and Chimeric Mice

In order to better understand the genetic requirements for retinoblastoma development in the mouse, several groups have examined the effects of targeted disruption of pocket family members and the *p53* gene in knockout and chimeric mice.

1. Germline RB1+/- Mice

To reflect the genotype of individuals with heritable RB, mice with a mutant *RB1* allele were generated. *RB1*+/- mice do not develop retinoblastoma, but do develop pituitary tumors with nearly complete penetrance. These tumors arise in the pars intermedia and consistently demonstrate loss of the remaining normal *RB1* allele [45,46,354]. The pars intermedia is vestigial in humans, which could explain the absence of such tumors in individuals who carry a germline mutation in *RB1*.

2. Chimeric *RB1*-/- Mice

The absence of retinoblastoma in *RB1*+/- mice was initially attributed to factors that reduced the opportunity for mutation of the remaining *RB1* allele; these factors include a smaller pool of retinal target cells and a shorter period of retinal development. Alternatively, it was proposed that mutations in addition to biallelic *RB1* inactivation were required for the development of retinoblastoma in this species [141]. Embryonic lethality in germline *RB1*-/- mice precluded evaluation of retinoblastoma development in these animals. This difficulty was circumvented by the production of chimeric *RB1−/−* mice [53,54]. These mice also failed to develop retinoblastoma, confirming that biallelic *RB1* inactivation is insufficient for the development of retinoblastoma in mice.

3. Introduction of Additional Mutations in *RB1+/−* Mice

The effects of pRb loss in combination with p107, p130, or p53 loss were examined by breeding *RB1+/−* mice on *p107−/−* , *p130−/−* , and *p53−/−* backgrounds. Mice that are nullizygous for *p107* or *p130* are viable and do not develop retinal abnormalities [355,356]. While *RB1+/−;p107−/−* mice likewise do not develop retinoblastoma, these animals invariably develop bilateral, multifocal dysplastic retinal lesions [355]. These lesions may represent focal deformities of the retina which result from ectopic cellular proliferation and apoptosis following somatic inactivation of the remaining *RB1* allele [60,313]. The description of similar dysplastic lesions in IRBP-*E2F1* mice suggests that these lesions may be attributable to deregulated E2F1 [145]. In contrast, dysplastic retinal lesions are not observed in *RB1+/−;p130−/−*, *p107+/−;p130−/−* , or *p130+/−;p107−/−* mice [355]. Findings in *RB1+/−;p107−/−* mice suggest that pRb and p107 have overlapping functions in murine retinal development and that compensatory cell cycle control by p107 may suppress ectopic proliferation in *RB1−/−* retinoblasts. *p53*-null mice are also viable [357], and retinal dysplasia has been observed in 1 of 14 (7%) *p53−/−* mice [358]. Retinal dysplasia develops at higher frequency in *RB1+/−;p53−/−* mice, with penetrance of 41% (7 of 17 mice) [358]. The increased frequency of retinal lesions in these mice is presumably due to somatic inactivation of the remaining *RB1* allele. The absence of retinoblastoma in these mice suggests that loss of dual loss of pRb and p53 is insufficient for tumorigenesis.

4. *RB1−/−;p107−/−* Chimeras

The role of combined pRb and p107 loss in the development of murine retinoblastoma has been examined through the creation of chimeric *RB1−/−;p107−/−* mice [62]. The combined loss of pRb, p107, and p53 in developing photoreceptors was also examined in this study through the creation of an additional line of chimeric mice containing *RB1−/−;p107−/−* cells that also carried a dominant negative p53 mutant minigene (*p53DD*) under the control of the human IRBP promoter (*RB1−/−;p107−/−;*IRBP-*p53DD* chimeras). p53DD expression functionally inactivates p53 and mimics the effect of genetic p53 loss in transgenic mice [359].

Retinoblastoma was detected in 2 of 6 eyes in *RB1−/−;p107−/−* chimeras and in 4/8 eyes of *RB1−/−;p107−/−;*IRBP-*p53DD* chimeras, suggesting that pRb and p107 cooperate to suppress tumorigenesis in the murine retina. In addition, retinal dysplasia was detected at low incidence in *RB1+/−;p107−/−* chimeras (controls). Interestingly, retinoblastoma in both lines of mice originated exclusively from the non-IRBP expressing amacrine compartment of the inner nuclear layer, and tumorigenesis in *RB1−/−;p107−/−;*IRBP-*p53DD* chimeras was not associated with IRBP-*p53DD* activity. Instead, IRBP-*p53DD*-expressing cells destined for the outer nuclear layer were eliminated from the retina.

The individual fate of *RB1−/−;p107−/−* cells lacking the *p53DD* transgene could not be assessed, and the retinal contribution of *RB1−/−;p107−/−* cells was not described. It therefore remains unclear why retinoblastoma did not develop in some chimeras. It seems likely that in retinoblastoma-free chimeras, $RB1-/$ $-;p107-/-$ retinal cells were either developmentally rescued or eliminated by apoptosis. The authors do report that the contribution of $RB1-/-;p107-/-$ cells to adult tissues was approximately half the contribution of $RB1$-null cells in $RB1-/-$ chimeras; this suggests mechanisms of developmental rescue are significantly less effective in the case of cells lacking both pRb and p107.

The absence of retinoblastoma in a number of chimeric $RB1-/-;p107-/-$ eyes, despite confirmation of chimerism in the retinal pigment epithelium, strongly suggests that dual inactivation of these genes is insufficient to induce retinoblastoma in the mouse [62]. However, while transgenic TAg, $E6+E7$, and $E6;p53-/-$ models of retinoblastoma all suggest that additional loss of p53 is required for murine retinoblastoma development, no evidence for p53 mutation could be obtained by p53 sequence analysis or by immunohistochemistry in retinoblastoma tumors which developed in these chimeras. Therefore, it remains unclear whether p53 loss plays a direct role in the development of retinoblastoma in target cells of the murine inner nuclear layer. With respect to the outer nuclear layer, the finding that IRBP-$p53DD$-expressing, $RB1-/-;p107-/-$ cells undergo apoptosis rather than tumorigenesis, suggests that combined functional inactivation of pRb, p107, and p53 is insufficient to induce tumorigenesis in photoreceptor precursor cells. Other unidentified genetic events must be required for these cells to escape apoptosis and to develop into retinoblastoma.

VIII. pRb IN THE PATHOGENESIS OF HUMAN RB

Despite continuing uncertainties regarding the precise mutational requirements for retinoblastoma in mice, it is evident that the murine retina is better protected from tumorigenesis upon pRb inactivation than is the human retina. Studies in chimeric mice suggest that nullizygosity for $RB1$ and even nullizygosity for both $RB1$ and $p107$ are insufficient for retinoblastoma development and that in the absence of additional mutations, $RB1-/-$ and $RB1-/-;p107-/-$ cells in the developing chimeric retina undergo either apoptosis or differentiation. Epidemiological evidence suggests that the developing retina in other vertebrates is similarly well protected against tumorigenesis, and that humans are uniquely vulnerable to retinoblastoma upon loss of pRb. Spontaneous retinoblastoma is virtually unreported in other species [360] and has been demonstrated persuasively in nonhumans only once, in a dog [361]. In contrast, retinoblastoma develops with nearly complete penetrance in humans who inherit a null $RB1$ allele.

While it is generally accepted that loss or mutation of both alleles of $RB1$ ("M1" and "M2") are necessary and rate-limiting events in the development of human retinoblastoma, the sufficiency of these two events for tumorigenesis remains a matter of controversy. Gallie and coworkers, for example, have proposed that malignant transformation in human retinoblastoma requires a third mutation ("M3"), which allows the developing, pRb-deficient retinoblast to escape apoptosis and to proliferate [209]. Findings of ectopic apoptosis in embryonic $RB1-/-$ knockout and chimeric retina, as well as dysplastic lesions in adult $RB1-/-$ chimeric retina, suggest the existence of apoptotic mechanisms which compensate for pRb loss during murine retinal development [53,143]. Similar yet less effective mechanisms of apoptosis induction could also exist in the human retina to safeguard against abnormal cellular proliferation in the event of pRb loss. This possibility is consistent with a proposal that the acquired ability to evade apoptosis is a universal requirement for human tumorigenesis [279].

The importance of additional mutations in the genesis of human retinoblastoma is also supported by findings of other consistent genetic alterations in human RB tumors. In addition to alterations in region 13q14 (the locus of *RB1*), frequently described genetic alterations include + 1q, + 6p, − 16/del(16q), and − 17/del(17p). All these alterations (summarized in Table 2) have been proposed as early events in the malignant progression of human retinoblastoma, most recently on the basis of reconstruction of chromosomal evolution in RB tumors [362].

Most consistent genetic alterations in retinoblastoma were originally identified through cytogenetic analysis. This technique detects gross chromosomal rearrangements and often requires propagation of tumor cells in vitro or in immunodeficient mice, increasing the risk for artifact. More recently, results of cytogenetic analysis in RB have been confirmed by more sophisticated genetic approaches, including comparative genomic hybridization (CGH) and quantitative-multiplex polymerase chain reaction (QM-PCR). These techniques do not involve cell propagation and allow more precise localization of regions of consistent gain or loss.

A. Consistent Chromosomal Gains

Regions of consistent chromosomal gain in a malignancy suggests the presence of one or more oncogenes which contribute to tumor development. Increased gene dosage represents an efficient means for a tumor cell to acquire selective advantage, since only a single genetic event is required. Frequently reported genetic gains in RB include + 1q and + 6p (Table 2). Gain of 1q [363] or 6p [362–364] has been correlated with increased chromosomal instability in tumor specimens, suggesting that these genetic alterations contribute to the accumulation of additional mutations. 6p gain has been associated with higher risk histopathological features in RB, including less differentiated histology and optic nerve invasion [362,364]. Others have failed to confirm these observations [365], and larger studies will be required to resolve these discrepancies.

1. + 1q

1q gain is a frequent finding in many malignancies, especially breast cancer [366–368]. This alteration is observed in half of RB tumors by cytogenetic or CGH analysis (Table 2). A common region of gain has been localized to 1q25-q32 by cytogenetic analysis [369] and further narrowed by CGH to 1q31 (26 of 50 [52%] tumors [369]), or 1q32 (10 of 26 [38%] tumors [370]), with the great majority of 1q amplifications by CGH encompassing both regions [363,365,370]. Gain of 1q32 is also observed in glioma, and a causal gene has been proposed at this locus, GAC1 (glioblastoma amplification on chromosome 1) [371]. The role of this gene in RB is presently unclear [370].

Table 2   Frequencies of Chromosomal Gain or Loss in RB

Study	Method of analysis	+1q	+6p	+i(6p)	+1q and/or +6p	−16 /del(16q)	−17/del(17p)	Refs.
					Frequency of chromosomal gain or loss			
Balaban et al. (1982)	Cytogenetic	2/6	2/6	1/6[1]	4/6	0/6	0/6	409
Kusnetsova et al. (1982)	Cytogenetic	2/9[2]	7/9	6/9	8/9	4/9	0/9	372
Benedict et al (1983)	Cytogenetic	5/20	7/20	6/20	12/20	4/20	3/20	410
Workman et al. (1984)	Cytogenetic	2/2	1/2	0/2	2/2	2/2	2/2	411
Chaum et al. (1984)	Cytogenetic	2/10	1/10	1/10	3/10	3/10	2/10	412
Squire et al. (1985)[3]	Cytogenetic	21/27	15/27	15/27	26/27	3/27	2/27	413
Potluri et al. (1986)[4]	Cytogenetic	2/5	3/5	2/5	4/5	0/5	0/5	374
Cano et al. (1994)	Cytogenetic	nr	14/34[5]	9/34	nr	nr	nr	364
Oliveros et al. (1995)	Cytogenetic	23/43	20/43[5]	nr	17/19[6]	26/43	10/43	362
Yan et al. (2000)	Cytogenetic	8/12	5/12	5/12	10/12	4/12	0/12	414
Mairal et al. (2000)	Cytogenetic	10/20	10/20	6/20	14/20	11/20	3/20	365
Mairal et al. (2000)	CGH	12/24	13/24	—	18/24	11/24	3/24	365
Herzog et al. (2001)	CGH	10/26	11/26	—	14/26	9/26	0/26	370
Chen et al. (2001)	CGH	28/50	23/50	—	45/50	9/50	1/50	363
Naumova et al. (1994)	SH and PCR	nr	29/66	—	nr	nr	nr	415
Chen et al. (2002)	QM-PCR	nr	50/70[7]	—	nr	nr	nr	382
Total frequency (%), cytogenetic studies		77/154 (50%)	71/154 (46%)	51/145 (35%)	100/130 (77%)	57/154 (37%)	22/154 (14%)	—
Total frequency (%), CGH studies		50/100 (50%)	47/100 (47%)		77/100 (77%)	29/100 (29%)	4/100 (4%)	—
Total frequency (%), SH and PCR study		—	29/66 (44%)					—
Total frequency (%), QM-PCR study		—	50/70 (71%)					—

[1] Initially reported as i17q [see Balaban et al. (1981) and Potluri et al. (1986), Refs. 374, 416].

[2] See also Potluri et al. (1986), Ref. 380.

[3] See also prior analyses in Gardner et al. (1982) and Squire et al. (1984), Refs. 369, 373.

[4] Figures cited reflect findings only in the 5 previously unpublished cases included in this review.

[5] Due to an overlap in tumor specimens examined for 6p gain in these two studies, results of the earlier study are not reflected in the total frequency of 6p gain for cytogenetic studies, below.

[6] Data available for only 19/43 specimens examined in this study.

[7] Figure reflects frequency of gain within 6p21.3p23; 41/70 (59%) specimens showed a 0.6 megabase minimal region of 6p22 gain (see text).

Abbreviations: CGH, comparative genomic hybridization; SH, Southern hybridization; QM-PCR, quantitative-multiplex PCR; nr, not reported.

2. +6p/i(6p)

6p gain is also observed in half of RB tumors by cytogenetic, CGH analysis, or Southern hybridization with PCR (Table 2). In the majority of cases, 6p gain occurs in the form of an isochromosome i(6p), containing two extra copies of the short arm of chromosome 6 and producing tetrasomy for 6p. While this marker is highly characteristic of RB [364,372,375], it is also found in other malignancies [376]. Less frequent mechanisms for 6p gain in RB include loss of entire chromosome 6 with translocations of 6p to other chromosomes [370].

Identification of partial gains of 6p by CGH has allowed localization of a minimal region of 6p gain to 6p22 in 22 of 50 (44%) tumors [363]. 6p22 gain has also been observed in bladder cancer [377], another malignancy in which RB1 loss is well documented [301,302,378,379]. Gain of 6p in bladder carcinoma has been correlated with elevated risk for disease progression [380,381]. Quantitative-multiplex PCR has recently been used to sublocalize frequent regions of genomic amplification on 6p22 [382]. In this analysis, 50 of 70 (71%) tumors demonstrated gain within 6p21.3p23, and 41 of 70 (59%) demonstrated a 0.6 megabase minimal region of 6p22 gain containing three predicted genes. One of these genes was cloned and identified as a novel kinesin superfamily motor protein gene, RBKIN (RB kinesin-like) [382]. Kinesin-related proteins function as molecular cargo vehicles which bind and navigate microtubules. These proteins function in vesicle transport and may also regulate spindle assembly and chromosomal segregation during meiosis and mitosis [383]. Overexpression of RBKIN (also known as KIF13A) results in misallocation of the transcription factor AP-1 and the cell-surface mannose-6-phosphate receptor (M6PR) [384]. M6PR is a putative tumor suppressor gene whose loss has been predicted to result in reduced apoptosis and in increased cellular proliferation [385]. RBKIN is expressed at high levels in RB, and an antisense oligonucleotide targeting the RBKIN gene inhibits proliferation of RB cell lines [382]. Oncogenic expression of RBKIN could account for the finding of 6p gain in RB, although two other genes identified in the minimal region of 6p22 gain remain promising candidates.

3. +1q and/or +6p

On average, gain of either 1q or 6p has been observed in 77% of tumors on cytogenetic or CGH analysis (Table 2). Gallie and coworkers report gain of either 1q or 6p in 100% of specimens by karyotyping or CGH [373]. In light of these findings, these authors suggest that gain of either 1q or 6p may be necessary for malignant transformation. Gallie also proposes that retinoblastoma cells lacking these alterations may represent premalignant growths, or retinomas [209,363].

B. Consistent Chromosomal Losses

Consistent loss of chromosomal material suggests the possible existence of one or more tumor suppressor genes. A single deletion resulting in monosomy could have tumorigenic consequences if the encompassed locus includes a haploinsufficient tumor suppressor, such as p27Kip1 [386]. In contrast, a second event resulting in loss of the remaining wild-type allele would be necessary for tumorigenic inactivation by a haplosufficient tumor suppressor, such as pRb. Consistent chromosomal losses in retinoblastoma include loss of entire chromosome 16 or 16q loss [-16/del(16q)] and, less frequently, loss of entire chromosome 17 or 17p loss [-17/del(17p)] (Table 2).

1. – 16/del(16q)

Loss of entire chromosome 16 or 16q loss has been reported in 40% of tumors by cytogenetic analysis and in 30% of tumors by CGH (Table 2). A common region of 16q22 loss has been identified in 7 of 50 (15%) retinoblastomas by CGH [363]. Cadherin-11 (located on 16q22.1) and cadherin-13 (located on 16q24.2q24.3) have been proposed as candidate tumor suppressor genes on 16q [382,387]. Cadherin family proteins are transmembrane cell adhesion molecules, and members of this family have been implicated both in tumor suppression and in tumor progression [387–389]. Other researchers have emphasized the potential significance of 16q12 [376], another region of frequent 16q loss by CGH [365,370]. This region is frequently deleted in other cancers, including Wilms' tumor and ovarian carcinoma [390–392]. 16q12 contains the *p130* gene, which could partially compensate for pRb loss within the developing retina [370]. As noted above, p130 mutations have been described in a number of malignancies, and *p130* inactivation may confer selective advantage in pRb-deficient cells [64]. The status of *p130* in human RB remains to be defined.

2. – 17/del(17p)

This genetic alteration is found in 14% of retinoblastomas by cytogenetic analysis and in 4% by CGH (Table 2). Oliveros and Yunis detected −17/del(17p) in 10 of 43 (23%) retinoblastomas, and on the basis of reconstructed chromosomal evolution proposed that this alteration could occur as an early or a late event in the progression of retinoblastoma [362]. These authors suggest that the causative gene may be *p53*, located on 17p13. Potential involvement of p53 in human RB has been a topic of intense controversy [393], particularly in light of a possible requirement for p53 inactivation in murine RB. However, sequencing studies have confirmed the presence of exclusively wild-type p53 in retinoblastoma specimens [56,209,394]. No *p53* mutation has ever been characterized in primary RB, despite the fact that *p53* is the most commonly altered gene in cancer [395,396]. A *p53* mutation has been described in a metastatic focus of retinoblastoma, but the gene was found to be wild-type in primary tumor tissue from the same individual [397]. Studies in RB tumor specimens also suggest the presence of normal p53 function [398]. Induction of apoptosis in RB tumor cells is correlated with increased distance from blood vessels and upregulation of p53 expression, suggesting that p53-mediated apoptosis may be secondary to ischemia or to loss of nutritional support [398]. Interestingly, abnormal cytoplasmic staining for p53, indicating dysfunction through nuclear exclusion, has been reported in more invasive portions of primary RB tumors and in immortalized RB cell lines [394]. Taken together, these findings suggest that p53 pathway inactivation may represent a late event in this disease, related to invasion and metastatic progression, and that *p53* mutation does not play a role in the initiation of human RB.

C. Other Events

1. LOH for 1p

LOH for 1p has been reported in 9 of 43 (21%) tumors, and has been statistically correlated with metastasis, suggesting that this could represent a late event contributing to tumor progression [399].

2. +2p

Localized regions of 2p gain are detected in 28% of RB tumors by CGH (Table 2). 2p23p25 gain has been described in 13 of 50 (26%) cases [365,370]. In 15 of 50 (30%) additional cases this region of gain has been narrowed to 2p24p25, the location of both *N-myc* (*MYCN*) and *Id2* [363]. 2p gain is rarely detected by cytogenetic studies [372]. However, cytogenetic analyses do report homogeneously staining regions (HSR) and double minute (dmin) chromosomes associated with gene amplification in 9% of RB tumors [362,374]. These markers have been associated with *N-myc* amplification [365,400,403] and have been demonstrated to contain the *N-myc* locus [371]. While one group detected *N-myc* amplification (defined as more than 10 copies) in only 1 of 45 RB tumors [399], the finding of increased copy number of *N-myc* in 4 of 8 tumors with 2p amplification by CGH suggests that this event may actually occur more frequently [365]. The functional link between *N-myc* amplification and Id2-mediated inactivation of pRb in the genesis neuroblastoma (see above) provides an attractive mechanism whereby alterations at this locus could contribute to the development of retinoblastoma.

3. Telomerase Activity

Telomerase is an enzyme that adds length to telomeres. Upregulation of telomerase is a common means for cells to avoid replicative senescence. Half of retinoblastomas demonstrate elevated telomerase activity. As in other tumors, this appears to be a late event associated with tumor progression and immortalization in cell culture [404].

4. *p107*

While *p107* mutation may be required for the development of murine RB, there is little indication that this gene plays a role in human RB. *p107* maps to 20q11.2 [405], but of 100 RB tumors demonstrated 20q loss by CGH [369,371,376]. In a single report, p107 was reported to be undetectable by adenovirus E1A binding in an RB cell line [406]. Studies on the mutational status of *p107* in RB remain to be performed.

D. Models of RB Pathogenesis

Despite recent advances, it is unclear whether other consistent chromosomal alterations in retinoblastoma represent initiating events or secondary events which contribute to tumor progression. At least two models for RB tumorigenesis have been proposed, which differ with respect to the requirement for an additional mutation ("M3") in tumor formation. Both models suggest that biallelic inactivation of pRb in susceptible retinoblasts results in abnormal proliferation. However, these models propose differing mechanisms to explain how these proliferating retinoblasts escape apoptosis to form tumors.

Brantley and Harbour propose that biallelic *RB1* loss may be sufficient for RB tumorigenesis [407]. Citing data from chimeric *RB1*−/− mice, these authors suggest that biallelic *RB1* inactivation in a developing human retinoblast results in abnormal proliferation because of a cell-autonomous requirement for pRb in induction of cell cycle arrest. In addition, they propose that ectopically proliferating retinoblasts are protected from apoptosis by neighboring *RB1* wild type cells through non-cell-autonomous mechanisms similar to those observed in chimeric *RB1*−/− mice. The combination of these factors results in unchecked cellular proliferation and frank tumor development.

However, other observations in chimeric *RB1*−/− mice raise doubts about this hypothesis. Close examination of mechanisms of developmental rescue in the brain of chimeric *RB1*−/− mice has demonstrated that protection from apoptosis of *RB1*−/− cells in this tissue is consistently associated with non-cell-autonomous mechanisms of differentiation induction, which prevent ectopic proliferation [55] (see above). Similar mechanisms of developmental rescue have been observed in pRb-deficient skeletal muscle [49]. If we presume that similar mechanisms also account for developmental rescue of pRb-null retinal cells in *RB1*−/− chimeras, it remains unclear why these noncell-autonomous mechanisms of apoptosis protection and differentiation induction would be uncoupled in the developing human retina. It also worth noting that *RB1*−/− cells in chimeric retina are not consistently rescued. As indicated by findings of retinal apoptosis and dysplasia in *RB1*−/− chimeras [53], certain ectopically cycling *RB1*−/− cells in the murine retina undergo apoptosis despite the presence of neighboring *RB1* wild-type cells, The identity of these apoptotic cells remains unclear, but these cells could well include those which are susceptible to retinoblastoma development upon combined loss of pRb and p107 [62]. If this were the case, it would be necessary to explain in mice as well as in humans why some ectopically cycling pocket family protein-deficient retinal cells (*RB1*−/−;*p107*−/− cells in mice and *RB1*−/− cells in humans) are able to escape apoptosis to form tumors.

Gallie and coworkers have proposed an alternative explanation for the unique vulnerability of human *RB1*−/− retinoblasts to tumorigenesis [209]. In their view, *RB1*-deficient retinoblasts are prone to tumor formation due to the retina's extreme dependence on programmed cell death for development. During retinal development, an overabundance of cells is produced and formation of retinal architecture requires massive elimination of developing cells by programmed cell death. The mechanisms of this specialized form of apoptotic signaling in the retina remain undefined but could involve interneuronal connections as well as diffusible intercellular signals [209].

According to this model of retinoblastoma pathogenesis, biallelic *RB1* inactivation results in a retinoblast's failure to undergo final mitosis, an event which normally occurs in the proliferating outer neuroblastic layer of the developing retina. This *RB1*−/− precursor cell migrates to its normal destination point in the inner retina, but continues to proliferate. This model proposes that retinal apoptotic signaling deletes these ectopically cycling cells just as other unnecessary cells are deleted in the course of normal development. However, inefficient elimination of these cells by programmed cell death could result in linear expansion of these cells.

Despite this expansion, it is proposed that in the absence of a required third mutation (M3) all *RB1−/−* cells eventually undergo apoptosis or differentiation. These authors suggest that this mechanism could explain the occurrence of retinoma/retinocytoma in patients with heritable RB. Consistent with this model, histopathological analysis of retinomas suggests that these lesions arise following ectopic proliferation and eventual, although markedly abnormal, differentiation [408].

Gallie proposes that the third mutation required for the development of frank malignancy is one which renders ectopically proliferating *RB1−/−* cells insensitive to apoptotic signaling. Such a mutation would enable cells to expand exponentially rather than in a linear fashion. These authors suggest one of at least two different genetic events could serve as M3, most likely involving genes on 1q or 6p [209].

IX. SUMMARY

The past 15 years have witnessed an explosion in knowledge about the function of the retinoblastoma protein and its role in tumorigenesis. Despite these advances, we still know relatively little about the function of pRb in retinal tissue. The precise role of pRb loss in the development of retinoblastoma remains similarly unclear. Because retinoblastoma is a tumor which presents shortly after birth without a background of other acquired mutations, it may be possible to precisely define the molecular requirements for tumorigenesis and tumor progression in this disease. Further characterization of the pathways involved in the pathogenesis of retinoblastoma promises to shed light on fundamental mechanisms of tumorigenesis. This understanding also promises to reveal novel targets for molecular intervention in the treatment and prevention of this disease.

REFERENCES

1. Vogel F. Genetics of retinoblastoma. Hum Genet 1979; 52:1–54.
2. Gurney JG, Smith MA, Ross JA. Cancer Among Infants. In: Ries LAG, Smith MA, Gurney JG, Linet M, Tamra T, Young JL, Bunin GR, eds. Cancer Incidence and Survival Among Children and Adolescents: United States SEER Program, 1975–1995 (SEER Pediatric Monograph). NIH Pub. No. 99-4649. Bethesda, Md.: National Cancer Institute, SEER Program. 1999:149–156.
3. Matsunaga E. Hereditary retinoblastoma: Delayed mutation or host resistance? Am J Hum Genet 1978; 30:406–424.
4. Bonaiti-Pellie C, Briard-Guillemot ML. Segregation analysis in hereditary retinoblastoma. Hum Genet 1981; 57:411–419.
5. Bonaiti-Pellie C, Clerget-Darpoux F, Babron MC. Hereditary retinoblastoma: Can balanced insertion entirely explain the differences of expressivity among families? Hum Genet 1990; 86:203–208.
6. Genuardi M, Klutz M, Devriendt K, Caruso D, Stirpe M, Lohmann DR. Multiple lipomas linked to an RB1 gene mutation in a large pedigree with low penetrance retinoblastoma. Eur J Hum Genet 2001; 9:690–694.

7. Gallie BL, Ellsworth RM, Abramson DH, Phillips RA. Retinoma: spontaneous regression of retinoblastoma or benign manifestation of the mutation? Br J Cancer 1982; 45:513–521.

8. Knudson AG, Jr. Mutation and cancer: Statistical study of retinoblastoma. Proc Natl Acad Sci USA 1971; 68:820–823.

9. Wiggs JL, Dryja TP. Predicting the risk of hereditary retinoblastoma. Am J Ophthalmol 1988; 106:346–351.

10. Moll AC, Imhof SM, Bouter LM, Kuik DJ, Den Otter W, Bezemer PD, Koten JW, Tan KE. Second primary tumors in patients with hereditary retinoblastoma: A register-based follow-up study, 1945–1994. Int J Cancer 1996; 67:515–519.

11. Marcus DM, Brooks SE, Leff G, McCormick R, Thompson T, Anfinson S, Lasudry J, Albert DM. Trilateral retinoblastoma: Insights into histogenesis and management. Surv Ophthalmol 1998; 43:59–70.

12. Kivelä T. Trilateral retinoblastoma: A meta-analysis of hereditary retinoblastoma associated with primary ectopic intracranial retinoblastoma. J Clin Oncol 1999; 17:1829–1837.

13. Eng C, Li FP, Abramson DH, Ellsworth RM, Wong FL, Goldman MB, Seddon J, Tarbell N, Boice JD, Jr. Mortality from second tumors among long-term survivors of retinoblastoma. J Natl Cancer Inst 1993; 85:1121–1128.

14. Wong FL, Boice JD, Jr., Abramson DH, Tarone RE, Kleinerman RA, Stovall M, Goldman MB, Seddon JM, Tarbell N, Fraumeni JF, Jr., Li FP. Cancer incidence after retinoblastoma. Radiation dose and sarcoma risk. Jama 1997; 278:1262–1267.

15. Mohney BG, Robertson DM, Schomberg PJ, Hodge DO. Second nonocular tumors in survivors of heritable retinoblastoma and prior radiation therapy. Am J Ophthalmol 1998; 126:269–277.

16. Abramson DH, Frank CM. Second nonocular tumors in survivors of bilateral retinoblastoma: A possible age effect on radiation-related risk. Ophthalmology 1998; 105:573–579.

17. Moll AC, Imhof SM, Schouten-Van Meeteren AY, Kuik DJ, Hofman P, Boers M. Second primary tumors in hereditary retinoblastoma: a register-based study, 1945–1997: Is there an age effect on radiation-related risk? Ophthalmology 2001; 108:1109–1114.

18. Traboulsi EI, Zimmerman LE, Manz HJ. Cutaneous malignant melanoma in survivors of heritable retinoblastoma. Arch Ophthalmol 1988; 106:1059–1061.

19. Abramson DH, Melson MR, Dunkel IJ, Frank CM. Third (fourth and fifth) nonocular tumors in survivors of retinoblastoma. Ophthalmology 2001; 108:1868–1876.

20. Comings DE. A general theory of carcinogenesis. Proc Natl Acad Sci USA 1973; 70:3324–3328.

21. Yunis JJ, Ramsay N. Retinoblastoma and subband deletion of chromosome 13. Am J Dis Child 1978; 132:161–163.

22. Sparkes RS, Sparkes MC, Wilson MG, Towner JW, Benedict W, Murphree AL, Yunis JJ. Regional assignment of genes for human esterase D and retinoblastoma to chromosome band 13q14. Science 1980; 208:1042–1044.

23. Connolly MJ, Payne RH, Johnson G, Gallie BL, Allderdice PW, Marshall WH, Lawton RD. Familial, EsD-linked, retinoblastoma with reduced penetrance and variable expressivity. Hum Genet 1983; 65:122–124.

24. Godbout R, Dryja TP, Squire J, Gallie BL, Phillips RA. Somatic inactivation of genes on chromosome 13 is a common event in retinoblastoma. Nature 1983; 304:451–453.

25. Cavenee WK, Dryja TP, Phillips RA, Benedict WF, Godbout R, Gallie BL, Murphree AL, Strong LC, White RL. Expression of recessive alleles by chromosomal mechanisms in retinoblastoma. Nature 1983; 305:779–784.

26. Dryja TP, Cavenee W, White R, Rapaport JM, Petersen R, Albert DM, Bruns GA. Homozygosity of chromosome 13 in retinoblastoma. N Engl J Med 1984; 310:550–553.

27. Friend SH, Bernards R, Rogelj S, Weinberg RA, Rapaport JM, Albert DM, Dryja TP. A human DNA segment with properties of the gene that predisposes to retinoblastoma and osteosarcoma. Nature 1986; 323:643–646.

28. Lee W-H, Bookstein R, Hong F, Young L-J, Shew J-Y, Lee EY-HP. Human retinoblastoma susceptibility gene: Cloning, identification, and sequence. Science 1987; 235:1394–1399.

29. Fung Y-KT, Murphree AL, T'Ang A, Qian J, Hinrichs SH, Benedict WF. Structural evidence for the authenticity of the human retinoblastoma gene. Science 1987; 236:1657–1661.

30. Dunn JM, Phillips RA, Becker AJ, Gallie BL. Identification of germline and somatic mutations affecting the retinoblastoma gene. Science 1988; 241:1797–1800.

31. Dunn JM, Phillips RA, Zhu X, Becker A, Gallie BL. Mutations in the RB1 gene and their effects on transcription. Mol Cell Biol 1989; 9:4596–4604.

32. Wiggs J, Nordenskjold M, Yandell D, Rapaport J, Grondin V, Janson M, Werelius B, Petersen R, Craft A, Riedel K, et al. Prediction of the risk of hereditary retinoblastoma, using DNA polymorphisms within the retinoblastoma gene. N Engl J Med 1988; 318:151–157.

33. Huang HJ, Yee JK, Shew JY, Chen PL, Bookstein R, Friedmann T, Lee EY, Lee WH. Suppression of the neoplastic phenotype by replacement of the RB gene in human cancer cells. Science 1988; 242:1563–1566.

34. Bookstein R, Shew JY, Chen PL, Scully P, Lee WH. Suppression of tumorigenicity of human prostate carcinoma cells by replacing a mutated RB gene. Science 1990; 247:712–715.

35. Sumegi J, Uzvolgyi E, Klein G. Expression of the RB gene under the control of MuLV-LTR suppresses tumorigenicity of WERI-Rb-27 retinoblastoma cells in immunodefective mice. Cell Growth Differ 1990; 1:247–250.

36. Takahashi R, Hashimoto T, Xu HJ, Hu SX, Matsui T, Miki T, Bigo-Marshall H, Aaronson SA, Benedict WF. The retinoblastoma gene functions as a growth and tumor suppressor in human bladder carcinoma cells. Proc Natl Acad Sci USA 1991; 88:5257–5261.

37. Chen PL, Chen Y, Shan B, Bookstein R, Lee WH. Stability of retinoblastoma gene expression determines the tumorigenicity of reconstituted retinoblastoma cells. Cell Growth Differ 1992; 3:119–125.

38. Muncaster MM, Cohen BL, Phillips RA, Gallie BL. Failure of RB1 to reverse the malignant phenotype of human tumor cell lines. Cancer Res 1992; 52:654–661.

39. Weinberg RA. The retinoblastoma protein and cell cycle control. Cell 1995; 81:323–330.

40. Sherr CJ. Cancer cell cycles. Science 1996; 274:1672–1677.

41. Sellers WR, Kaelin WG, Jr. Role of the retinoblastoma protein in the pathogenesis of human cancer. J Clin Oncol 1997; 15:3301–3312.

42. Lipinski MM, Jacks T. The retinoblastoma gene family in differentiation and development. Oncogene 1999; 18:7873–7882.

43. Sellers WR, Novitch BG, Miyake S, Heith A, Otterson GA, Kaye FJ, Lassar AB, Kaelin WG, Jr. Stable binding to E2F is not required for the retinoblastoma protein to activate transcription, promote differentiation, and suppress tumor cell growth. Genes Dev 1998; 12:95–106.

44. Thomas DM, Carty SA, Piscopo DM, Lee JS, Wang WF, Forrester WC, Hinds PW. The retinoblastoma protein acts as a transcriptional coactivator required for osteogenic differentiation. Mol Cell 2001; 8:303–316.

45. Lee EY, Chang CY, Hu N, Wang YC, Lai CC, Herrup K, Lee WH, Bradley A. Mice deficient for Rb are nonviable and show defects in neurogenesis and haematopoiesis. Nature 1992; 359:288–294.

46. Jacks T, Fazeli A, Schmitt EM, Bronson RT, Goodell MA, Weinberg RA. Effects of an Rb mutation in the mouse. Nature 1992; 359:295–300.

47. Clarke AR, Maandag ER, van Roon M, van der Lugt NM, van der Valk M, Hooper ML, Berns A, te Riele H. Requirement for a functional Rb-1 gene in murine development. Nature 1992; 359:328–330.

48. Morgenbesser SD, Williams BO, Jacks T, DePinho RA. p53-dependent apoptosis produced by Rb-deficiency in the developing mouse lens. Nature 1994; 371:72–74.

49. Zacksenhaus E, Jiang Z, Chung D, Marth JD, Phillips RA, Gallie BL. pRb controls proliferation, differentiation, and death of skeletal muscle cells and other lineages during embryogenesis. Genes Dev 1996; 10:3051–3064.

50. Chen PL, Riley DJ, Chen Y, Lee WH. Retinoblastoma protein positively regulates terminal adipocyte differentiation through direct interaction with C/EBPs. Genes Dev 1996; 10:2794–2804.

51. Chen PL, Riley DJ, Chen-Kiang S, Lee WH. Retinoblastoma protein directly interacts with and activates the transcription factor NF-IL6. Proc Natl Acad Sci USA 1996; 93:465–469.

52. Nead MA, Baglia LA, Antinore MJ, Ludlow JW, McCance DJ. Rb binds c-Jun and activates transcription. EMBO J 1998; 17:2342–2352.

53. Robanus-Maandag EC, van der Valk M, Vlaar M, Feltkamp C, O'Brien J, van Roon M, van der Lugt N, Berns A, te Riele H. Developmental rescue of an embryonic-lethal mutation in the retinoblastoma gene in chimeric mice. EMBO J 1994; 13:4260–4268.

54. Williams BO, Schmitt EM, Remington L, Bronson RT, Albert DM, Weinberg RA, Jacks T. Extensive contribution of Rb-deficient cells to adult chimeric mice with limited histopathological consequences. EMBO J 1994; 13:4251–4259.

55. Lipinski MM, Macleod KF, Williams BO, Mullaney TL, Crowley D, Jacks T. Cell-autonomous and non-cell-autonomous functions of the Rb tumor suppressor in developing central nervous system. EMBO J 2001; 20:3402–3413.

56. Hamel PA, Phillips RA, Muncaster M, Gallie BL. Speculations on the roles of RB1 in tissue-specific differentiation, tumor initiation, and tumor progression. FASEB J 1993; 7:846–854.

57. Lee WH, Shew JY, Hong FD, Sery TW, Donoso LA, Young LJ, Bookstein R, Lee EY. The retinoblastoma susceptibility gene encodes a nuclear phosphoprotein associated with DNA binding activity. Nature 1987; 329:642–645.

58. Hong FD, Huang HJ, To H, Young LJ, Oro A, Bookstein R, Lee EY, Lee WH. Structure of the human retinoblastoma gene. Proc Natl Acad Sci USA 1989; 86:5502–5506.

59. Toguchida J, McGee TL, Paterson JC, Eagle JR, Tucker S, Yandell DW, Dryja TP. Complete genomic sequence of the human retinoblastoma susceptibility gene. Genomics 1993; 17:535–543.

60. Mulligan G, Jacks T. The retinoblastoma gene family: Cousins with overlapping interests. Trends Genet 1998; 14:223–229.

61. Classon M, Dyson N. p107 and p130: versatile proteins with interesting pockets. Exp Cell Res 2001; 264:135–147.

62. Robanus-Maandag E, Dekker M, van der Valk M, Carrozza ML, Jeanny JC, Dannenberg JH, Berns A, te Riele H. p107 is a suppressor of retinoblastoma development in pRb-deficient mice. Genes Dev 1998; 12:1599–1609.

63. Takimoto H, Tsukuda K, Ichimura K, Hanafusa H, Nakamura A, Oda M, Harada M, Shimizu K. Genetic alterations in the retinoblastoma protein-related p107 gene in human hematologic malignancies. Biochem Biophys Res Commun 1998; 251:264–268.

64. Helin K, Holm K, Niebuhr A, Eiberg H, Tommerup N, Hougaard S, Poulsen HS, Spang-Thomsen M, Norgaard P. Loss of the retinoblastoma protein-related p130 protein in small cell lung carcinoma. Proc Natl Acad Sci USA 1997; 94:6933–6938.

65. Claudio PP, Howard CM, Fu Y, Cinti C, Califano L, Micheli P, Mercer EW, Caputi M, Giordano A. Mutations in the retinoblastoma-related gene RB2/p130 in primary nasopharyngeal carcinoma. Cancer Res 2000; 60:8–12.

66. Claudio PP, Howard CM, Pacilio C, Cinti C, Romano G, Minimo C, Maraldi NM, Minna JD, Gelbert L, Leoncini L, Tosi GM, Hicheli P, Caputi M, Giordano GG, Giordano A. Mutations in the retinoblastoma-related gene RB2/p130 in lung tumors and suppression of tumor growth in vivo by retrovirus-mediated gene transfer. Cancer Res 2000; 60:372–382.

67. Cinti C, Claudio PP, Howard CM, Neri LM, Fu Y, Leoncini L, Tosi GM, Maraldi NM, Giordano A. Genetic alterations disrupting the nuclear localization of the retinoblastoma-related gene RB2/p130 in human tumor cell lines and primary tumors. Cancer Res 2000; 60:383–389.

68. Cinti C, Leoncini L, Nyongo A, Ferrari F, Lazzi S, Bellan C, Vatti R, Zamparelli A, Cevenini G, Tosi GM, Claudio PP, Maraldi NM, Tosi P, Giordano A. Genetic alterations of the retinoblastoma-related gene RB2/p130 identify different pathogenetic mechanisms in and among Burkitt's lymphoma subtypes. Am J Pathol 2000; 156:751–760.

69. Paggi MG, Giordano A. Who is the boss in the retinoblastoma family? The point of view of Rb2/p130, the little brother. Cancer Res 2001; 61:4651–4654.

70. Morris EJ, Dyson NJ. Retinoblastoma protein partners. Adv Cancer Res 2001; 82:1–54.

71. Wu L, Timmers C, Maiti B, Saavedra HI, Sang L, Chong GT, Nuckolls F, Giangrande P, Wright FA, Field SJ, Greenberg ME, Orkin S, Nevins JR, Robinson ML, Leone G. The E2F1-3 transcription factors are essential for cellular proliferation. Nature 2001; 414:457–462.

72. Harbour JW, Luo RX, Dei Santi A, Postigo AA, Dean DC. Cdk phosphorylation triggers sequential intramolecular interactions that progressively block Rb functions as cells move through G1. Cell 1999; 98:859–869.

73. Knudsen ES, Wang JY. Differential regulation of retinoblastoma protein function by specific Cdk phosphorylation sites. J Biol Chem 1996; 271:8313–8320.

74. Lee JO, Russo AA, Pavletich NP. Structure of the retinoblastoma tumour-suppressor pocket domain bound to a peptide from HPV E7. Nature 1998; 391:859–865.

75. Brown VD, Gallie BL. The B-domain lysine patch of pRB is required for binding to large T antigen and release of E2F by phosphorylation. Mol Cell Biol 2002; 22:1390–1401.

76. Lin BT, Gruenwald S, Morla AO, Lee WH, Wang JY. Retinoblastoma cancer suppressor gene product is a substrate of the cell cycle regulator cdc2 kinase. EMBO J 1991; 10:857–864.

77. Lees JA, Buchkovich KJ, Marshak DR, Anderson CW, Harlow E. The retinoblastoma protein is phosphorylated on multiple sites by human cdc2. EMBO J 1991; 10:4279–4290.

78. Wang JY, Knudsen ES, Welch PJ. The retinoblastoma tumor suppressor protein. Adv Cancer Res 1994; 64:25–85.

79. Adams PD. Regulation of the retinoblastoma tumor suppressor protein by cyclin/cdks. Biochim Biophys Acta 2001; 1471:M123–133.

80. Sherr CJ, Roberts JM. CDK inhibitors: Positive and negative regulators of G1-phase progression. Genes Dev 1999; 13:1501–1512.

81. Wang JY, Naderi S, Chen TT. Role of retinoblastoma tumor suppressor protein in DNA damage response. Acta Oncol 2001; 40:689–695.

82. Lundberg AS, Hahn WC, Gupta P, Weinberg RA. Genes involved in senescence and immortalization. Curr Opin Cell Biol 2000; 12:705–709.

83. Zhang P. The cell cycle and development: Redundant roles of cell cycle regulators. Curr Opin Cell Biol 1999; 11:655–662.

84. Zhu L, Skoultchi AI. Coordinating cell proliferation and differentiation. Curr Opin Genet Dev 2001; 11:91–97.

85. Ravitz MJ, Wenner CE. Cyclin-dependent kinase regulation during G1 phase and cell cycle regulation by TGF-beta. Adv Cancer Res 1997; 71:165–207.

86. LaBaer J, Garrett MD, Stevenson LF, Slingerland JM, Sandhu C, Chou HS, Fattaey A, Harlow E. New functional activities for the p21 family of CDK inhibitors. Genes Dev 1997; 11:847–862.

87. Cheng M, Olivier P, Diehl JA, Fero M, Roussel MF, Roberts JM, Sherr CJ. The p21(Cip1) and p27(Kip1) CDK 'inhibitors' are essential activators of cyclin D-dependent kinases in murine fibroblasts. EMBO J 1999; 18:1571–1583.

88. Chen P-L, Scully P, Shew J-Y, Wang JYJ, Lee W-H. Phosphorylation of the retinoblastoma gene product is modulated during the cell cycle and cellular differentiation. Cell 1989; 58:1193–1198.

89. Knudson AG, Jr. Retinoblastoma: A prototypic hereditary neoplasm. Semin Oncol 1978; 5:57–60.

90. Whyte P, Buchkovich KJ, Horowitz JM, Friend SH, Raybuck M, Weinberg RA, Harlow E. Association between an oncogene and an anti-oncogene: The adenovirus E1A proteins bind to the retinoblastoma gene product. Nature 1988; 334:124–129.

91. Whyte P, Williamson NM, Harlow E. Cellular targets for transformation by the adenovirus E1A proteins. Cell 1989; 56:67–75.

92. DeCaprio JA, Ludlow JW, Figge J, Shew JY, Huang CM, Lee WH, Marsilio E, Paucha E, Livingston DM. SV40 large tumor antigen forms a specific complex with the product of the retinoblastoma susceptibility gene. Cell 1988; 54:275–283.

93. Ewen ME, Ludlow JW, Marsilio E, DeCaprio JA, Millikan RC, Cheng SH, Paucha E, Livingston DM. An N-terminal transformation-governing sequence of SV40 large T antigen contributes to the binding of both p110Rb and a second cellular protein, p120. Cell 1989; 58:257–267.

94. Dyson N, Howley PM, Munger K, Harlow E. The human papilloma virus-16 E7 onco-protein is able to bind to the retinoblastoma gene product. Science 1989; 243:934–937.

95. Munger K, Werness BA, Dyson N, Phelps WC, Harlow E, Howley PM. Complex formation of human papillomavirus E7 proteins with the retinoblastoma tumor suppressor gene product. EMBO J 1989; 8:4099–4105.

96. Bagchi S, Weinmann R, Raychaudhuri P. The retinoblastoma protein copurifies with E2F-I, an E1A-regulated inhibitor of the transcription factor E2F. Cell 1991; 65:1063–1072.

97. Bandara LR, La Thangue NB. Adenovirus E1a prevents the retinoblastoma gene product from complexing with a cellular transcription factor. Nature 1991; 351:494–497.

98. Chellappan SP, Hiebert S, Mudryj M, Horowitz JM, Nevins JR. The E2F transcription factor is a cellular target for the RB protein. Cell 1991; 65:1053–1061.

99. Chittenden T, Livingston DM, Kaelin WG, Jr. The T/E1A-binding domain of the retinoblastoma product can interact selectively with a sequence-specific DNA-binding protein. Cell 1991; 65:1073–1082.

100. Kovesdi I, Reichel R, Nevins JR. Identification of a cellular transcription factor involved in E1A trans- activation. Cell 1986; 45:219–228.

101. La Thangue NB, Rigby PW. An adenovirus E1A-like transcription factor is regulated during the differentiation of murine embryonal carcinoma stem cells. Cell 1987; 49:507–513.

102. Mudryj M, Hiebert SW, Nevins JR. A role for the adenovirus inducible E2F transcription factor in a proliferation dependent signal transduction pathway. EMBO J 1990; 9:2179–2184.

103. Shirodkar S, Ewen M, DeCaprio JA, Morgan J, Livingston DM, Chittenden T. The transcription factor E2F interacts with the retinoblastoma product and a p107-cyclin A complex in a cell cycle-regulated manner. Cell 1992; 68:157–166.

104. Schwarz JK, Devoto SH, Smith EJ, Chellappan SP, Jakoi L, Nevins JR. Interactions of the p107 and Rb proteins with E2F during the cell proliferation response. Embo J 1993; 12:1013–1020.

105. Hiebert SW, Chellappan SP, Horowitz JM, Nevins JR. The interaction of RB with E2F coincides with an inhibition of the transcriptional activity of E2F. Genes Dev 1992; 6:177–185.

106. Flemington EK, Speck SH, Kaelin WG, Jr. E2F-1-mediated transactivation is inhibited by complex formation with the retinoblastoma susceptibility gene product. Proc Natl Acad Sci USA 1993; 90:6914–6918.

107. Helin K, Harlow E, Fattaey A. Inhibition of E2F-1 transactivation by direct binding of the retinoblastoma protein. Mol Cell Biol 1993; 13:6501–6508.

108. Nevins JR. E2F: a link between the Rb tumor suppressor protein and viral oncoproteins. Science 1992; 258:424–429.

109. Dyson N. The regulation of E2F by pRB-family proteins. Genes Dev 1998; 12:2245–2262.

110. Müller H, Helin K. The E2F transcription factors: Key regulators of cell proliferation. Biochim Biophys Acta 2000; 1470:M1-M12.

111. Trimarchi JM, Lees JA. Sibling rivalry in the E2F family. Nat Rev Mol Cell Biol 2002; 3:11–20.

112. Lavia P, Jansen-Durr P. E2F target genes and cell-cycle checkpoint control. Bioessays 1999; 21:221–230.

113. Müller H, Bracken AP, Vernell R, Moroni MC, Christians F, Grassilli E, Prosperini E, Vigo E, Oliner JD, Helin K. E2Fs regulate the expression of genes involved in differentiation, development, proliferation, and apoptosis. Genes Dev 2001; 15:267–285.

114. Weintraub SJ, Prater CA, Dean DC. Retinoblastoma protein switches the E2F site from positive to negative element. Nature 1992; 358:259–261.

115. Weintraub SJ, Chow KN, Luo RX, Zhang SH, He S, Dean DC. Mechanism of active transcriptional repression by the retinoblastoma protein. Nature 1995; 375:812–815.

116. Zhang HS, Postigo AA, Dean DC. Active transcriptional repression by the Rb-E2F complex mediates G1 arrest triggered by p16INK4a, TGFbeta, and contact inhibition. Cell 1999; 97:53–61.

117. Zhang HS, Dean DC. Rb-mediated chromatin structure regulation and transcriptional repression. Oncogene 2001; 20:3134–3138.

118. Ayer DE. Histone deacetylases: transcriptional repression with SINers and NuRDs. Trends Cell Biol 1999; 9:193–198.

119. Kouzarides T. Histone acetylases and deacetylases in cell proliferation. Curr Opin Genet Dev 1999; 9:40–48.

120. Jones DO, Cowell IG, Singh PB. Mammalian chromodomain proteins: Their role in genome organisation and expression. Bioessays 2000; 22:124–137.

121. Kingston RE, Narlikar GJ. ATP-dependent remodeling and acetylation as regulators of chromatin fluidity. Genes Dev 1999; 13:2339–2352.

122. Tyler JK, Kadonaga JT. The "dark side" of chromatin remodeling: Repressive effects on transcription. Cell 1999; 99:443–446.

123. Brehm A, Miska EA, McCance DJ, Reid JL, Bannister AJ, Kouzarides T. Retinoblastoma protein recruits histone deacetylase to repress transcription. Nature 1998; 391:597–601.

124. Magnaghi-Jaulin L, Groisman R, Naguibneva I, Robin P, Lorain S, Le Villain JP, Troalen F, Trouche D, Harel-Bellan A. Retinoblastoma protein represses transcription by recruiting a histone deacetylase. Nature 1998; 391:601–605.

125. Luo RX, Postigo AA, Dean DC. Rb interacts with histone deacetylase to repress transcription. Cell 1998; 92:463–473.

126. Lai A, Lee JM, Yang WM, DeCaprio JA, Kaelin WG, Jr., Seto E, Branton PE. RBP1 recruits both histone deacetylase-dependent and -independent repression activities to retinoblastoma family proteins. Mol Cell Biol 1999; 19:6632–6641.

127. Zhang HS, Gavin M, Dahiya A, Postigo AA, Ma D, Luo RX, Harbour JW, Dean DC. Exit from G1 and S phase of the cell cycle is regulated by repressor complexes containing HDAC-Rb-hSWI/SNF and Rb-hSWI/SNF. Cell 2000; 101:79–89.

128. Lai A, Kennedy BK, Barbie DA, Bertos NR, Yang XJ, Theberge MC, Tsai SC, Seto E, Zhang Y, Kuzmichev A, Lane WS, Reinberg D, Harlow E, Branton PE. RBP1 recruits the mSIN3-histone deacetylase complex to the pocket of retinoblastoma tumor suppressor family proteins found in limited discrete regions of the nucleus at growth arrest. Mol Cell Biol 2001; 21:2918–2932.

129. Lai A, Marcellus RC, Corbeil HB, Branton PE. RBP1 induces growth arrest by repression of E2F-dependent transcription. Oncogene 1999; 18:2091–2100.

130. Nielsen SJ, Schneider R, Bauer UM, Bannister AJ, Morrison A, O'Carroll D, Firestein R, Cleary M, Jenuwein T, Herrera RE, Kouzarides T. Rb targets histone H3 methylation and HP1 to promoters. Nature 2001; 412:561–565.

131. Vandel L, Nicolas E, Vaute O, Ferreira R, Ait-Si-Ali S, Trouche D. Transcriptional repression by the retinoblastoma protein through the recruitment of a histone methyltransferase. Mol Cell Biol 2001; 21:6484–6494.

132. Rea S, Eisenhaber F, O'Carroll D, Strahl BD, Sun ZW, Schmid M, Opravil S, Mechtler K, Ponting CP, Allis CD, Jenuwein T. Regulation of chromatin structure by site-specific histone H3 methyltransferases. Nature 2000; 406:593–599.

133. Bannister AJ, Zegerman P, Partridge JF, Miska EA, Thomas JO, Allshire RC, Kouzarides T. Selective recognition of methylated lysine 9 on histone H3 by the HP1 chromo domain. Nature 2001; 410:120–124.

134. Lachner M, O'Carroll D, Rea S, Mechtler K, Jenuwein T. Methylation of histone H3 lysine 9 creates a binding site for HP1 proteins. Nature 2001; 410:116–120.

135. Dunaief JL, Strober BE, Guha S, Khavari PA, Alin K, Luban J, Begemann M, Crabtree GR, Goff SP. The retinoblastoma protein and BRG1 form a complex and cooperate to induce cell cycle arrest. Cell 1994; 79:119–130.

136. Singh P, Coe J, Hong W. A role for retinoblastoma protein in potentiating transcriptional activation by the glucocorticoid receptor. Nature 1995; 374:562–565.

137. Strober BE, Dunaief JL, Guha, Goff SP. Functional interactions between the hBRM/hBRG1 transcriptional activators and the pRB family of proteins. Mol Cell Biol 1996; 16:1576–1583.

138. Trouche D, Le Chalony C, Muchardt C, Yaniv M, Kouzarides T. RB and hbrm cooperate to repress the activation functions of E2F1. Proc Natl Acad Sci USA 1997; 94:11268–11273.

139. Strobeck MW, Knudsen KE, Fribourg AF, DeCristofaro MF, Weissman BE, Imbalzano AN, Knudsen ES. BRG-1 is required for RB-mediated cell cycle arrest. Proc Natl Acad Sci USA 2000; 97:7748–7753.

140. Wong AK, Shanahan F, Chen Y, Lian L, Ha P, Hendricks K, Ghaffari S, Iliev D, Penn B, Woodland AM, Smith R, Salada G, Carillo A, Laity K, Gupte J, Swedlund B, Tavtigian SV, Teng DH, Lees E. BRG1, a component of the SWI-SNF complex, is mutated in multiple human tumor cell lines. Cancer Res 2000; 60:6171–6177.

141. Harlow E. Retinoblastoma. For our eyes only. Nature 1992; 359:270–271.

142. Lee EY, Hu N, Yuan SS, Cox LA, Bradley A, Lee WH, Herrup K. Dual roles of the retinoblastoma protein in cell cycle regulation and neuron differentiation. Genes Dev 1994; 8:2008–2021.

143. Lin SC, Skapek SX, Papermaster DS, Hankin M, Lee EY. The proliferative and apoptotic activities of E2F1 in the mouse retina. Oncogene 2001; 20:7073–7084.

144. Jiang Z, Zacksenhaus E, Gallie BL, Phillips RA. The retinoblastoma gene family is differentially expressed during embryogenesis. Oncogene 1997; 14:1789–1797.

145. Charles A, Tang X, Crouch E, Brody JS, Xiao ZX. Retinoblastoma protein complexes with C/EBP proteins and activates C/EBP-mediated transcription. J Cell Biochem 2001; 83:414–425.

146. Yee AS, Shih HH, Tevosian SG. New perspectives on retinoblastoma family functions in differentiation. Front Biosci 1998; 3:D532–547.

147. Tevosian SG, Shih HH, Mendelson KG, Sheppard KA, Paulson KE, Yee AS. HBP1: A HMG box transcriptional repressor that is targeted by the retinoblastoma family. Genes Dev 1997; 11:383–396.

148. Sampson EM, Haque ZK, Ku MC, Tevosian SG, Albanese C, Pestell RG, Paulson KE, Yee AS. Negative regulation of the Wnt-beta-catenin pathway by the transcriptional repressor HBP1. EMBO J 2001; 20:4500–4511.

149. Shih HH, Xiu M, Berasi SP, Sampson EM, Leiter A, Paulson KE, Yee AS. HMG box transcriptional repressor HBP1 maintains a proliferation barrier in differentiated liver tissue. Mol Cell Biol 2001; 21:5723–5732.

150. Oppenheim RW. Cell death during development of the nervous system. Annu Rev Neurosci 1991; 14:453–501.

151. Raff MC, Barres BA, Burne JF, Coles HS, Ishizaki Y, Jacobson MD. Programmed cell death and the control of cell survival: Lessons from the nervous system. Science 1993; 262:695–700.

152. Burek MJ, Oppenheim RW. Programmed cell death in the developing nervous system. Brain Pathol 1996; 6:427–446.

153. Liu DX, Greene LA. Neuronal apoptosis at the G1/S cell cycle checkpoint. Cell Tissue Res 2001; 305:217–228.

154. Walsh K. Coordinate regulation of cell cycle and apoptosis during myogenesis. Prog Cell Cycle Res 1997; 3:53–58.

155. Schneider JW, Gu W, Zhu L, Mahdavi V, Nadal-Ginard B. Reversal of terminal differentiation mediated by p107 in Rb−/− muscle cells. Science 1994; 264:1467–1471.

156. Slack RS, El-Bizri H, Wong J, Belliveau DJ, Miller FD. A critical temporal requirement for the retinoblastoma protein family during neuronal determination. J Cell Biol 1998; 140:1497–1509.

157. Wang J, Guo K, Wills KN, Walsh K. Rb functions to inhibit apoptosis during myocyte differentiation. Cancer Res 1997; 57:351–354.

158. Ko LJ, Prives C. p53: Puzzle and paradigm. Genes Dev 1996; 10:1054–1072.

159. Levine AJ. p53, the cellular gatekeeper for growth and division. Cell 1997; 88:323–331.

160. Agarwal ML, Taylor WR, Chernov MV, Chernova OB, Stark GR. The p53 network. J Biol Chem 1998; 273:1–4.

161. Prives C, Hall PA. The p53 pathway. J Pathol 1999; 187:112–126.

162. Macleod KF, Hu Y, Jacks T. Loss of Rb activates both p53-dependent and independent cell death pathways in the developing mouse nervous system. Embo J 1996; 15:6178–6188.

163. Wu X, Levine AJ. p53 and E2F-1 cooperate to mediate apoptosis. Proc Natl Acad Sci USA 1994; 91:3602–3606.

164. Qin XQ, Livingston DM, Kaelin WG, Jr., Adams PD. Deregulated transcription factor E2F-1 expression leads to S-phase entry and p53-mediated apoptosis. Proc Natl Acad Sci USA 1994; 91:10918–10922.

165. Shan B, Lee WH. Deregulated expression of E2F-1 induces S-phase entry and leads to apoptosis. Mol Cell Biol 1994; 14:8166–8173.

166. Kowalik TF, DeGregori J, Schwarz JK, Nevins JR. E2F1 overexpression in quiescent fibroblasts leads to induction of cellular DNA synthesis and apoptosis. J Virol 1995; 69:2491–2500.

167. Hiebert SW, Packham G, Strom DK, Haffner R, Oren M, Zambetti G, Cleveland JL. E2F-1:DP-1 induces p53 and overrides survival factors to trigger apoptosis. Mol Cell Biol 1995; 15:6864–6874.

168. Hsieh JK, Fredersdorf S, Kouzarides T, Martin K, Lu X. E2F1-induced apoptosis requires DNA binding but not transactivation and is inhibited by the retinoblastoma protein through direct interaction. Genes Dev 1997; 11:1840–1852.

169. Phillips AC, Bates S, Ryan KM, Helin K, Vousden KH. Induction of DNA synthesis and apoptosis are separable functions of E2F-1. Genes Dev 1997; 11:1853–1863.

170. DeGregori J, Leone G, Miron A, Jakoi L, Nevins JR. Distinct roles for E2F proteins in cell growth control and apoptosis. Proc Natl Acad Sci USA 1997; 94:7245–7250.

171. Kowalik TF, DeGregori J, Leone G, Jakoi L, Nevins JR. E2F1-specific induction of apoptosis and p53 accumulation, which is blocked by Mdm2. Cell Growth Differ 1998; 9:113–118.

172. Tsai KY, Hu Y, Macleod KF, Crowley D, Yamasaki L, Jacks T. Mutation of E2f-1 suppresses apoptosis and inappropriate S-phase entry and extends survival of Rb-deficient mouse embryos. Mol Cell 1998; 2:293–304.

173. Phillips AC, Vousden KH. E2F-1 induced apoptosis. Apoptosis 2001; 6:173–182.

174. Vigo E, Muller H, Prosperini E, Hateboer G, Cartwright P, Moroni MC, Helin K. CDC25A phosphatase is a target of E2F and is required for efficient E2F- induced S phase. Mol Cell Biol 1999; 19:6379–6395.

175. Ziebold U, Reza T, Caron A, Lees JA. E2F3 contributes both to the inappropriate proliferation and to the apoptosis arising in Rb mutant embryos. Genes Dev 2001; 15:386–391.

176. Macleod K. pRb and E2f-1 in mouse development and tumorigenesis. Curr Opin Genet Dev 1999; 9:31–39.

177. Sherr CJ, Weber JD. The ARF/p53 pathway. Curr Opin Genet Dev 2000; 10:94–99.

178. Tsai KY, MacPherson D, Rubinson DA, Crowley D, Jacks T. ARF is not required for apoptosis in Rb mutant mouse embryos. Curr Biol 2002; 12:159–163.

179. Lasorella A, Noseda M, Beyna M, Yokota Y, Iavarone A. Id2 is a retinoblastoma protein target and mediates signalling by Myc oncoproteins. Nature 2000; 407:592–598.

180. Norton JD. ID helix-loop-helix proteins in cell growth, differentiation and tumorigenesis. J Cell Sci 2000; 113:3897–3905.

181. Zebedee Z, Hara E. Id proteins in cell cycle control and cellular senescence. Oncogene 2001; 20:8317–8325.

182. Yokota Y. Id and development. Oncogene 2001; 20:8290–8298.

183. Lasorella A, Uo T, Iavarone A. Id proteins at the cross-road of development and cancer. Oncogene 2001; 20:8326–8333.

184. Yokota Y, Mori S. Role of Id family proteins in growth control. J Cell Physiol 2002; 190:21–28.

185. Iavarone A, Garg P, Lasorella A, Hsu J, Israel MA. The helix-loop-helix protein Id-2 enhances cell proliferation and binds to the retinoblastoma protein. Genes Dev 1994; 8:1270–1284.

186. Novitch BG, Mulligan GJ, Jacks T, Lassar AB. Skeletal muscle cells lacking the retinoblastoma protein display defects in muscle gene expression and accumulate in S and G2 phases of the cell cycle. J Cell Biol 1996; 135:441–456.

187. Arnold HH, Winter B. Muscle differentiation: More complexity to the network of myogenic regulators. Curr Opin Genet Dev 1998; 8:539–544.

188. Gu W, Schneider JW, Condorelli G, Kaushal S, Mahdavi V, Nadal-Ginard B. Interaction of myogenic factors and the retinoblastoma protein mediates muscle cell commitment and differentiation. Cell 1993; 72:309–324.

189. Mal A, Sturniolo M, Schiltz RL, Ghosh MK, Harter ML. A role for histone deacetylase HDAC1 in modulating the transcriptional activity of MyoD: Inhibition of the myogenic program. EMBO J 2001; 20:1739–1753.

190. Puri PL, Iezzi S, Stiegler P, Chen TT, Schilta RL, Muscat GE, Giordano A, Kedes L, Wang JY, Sartorelli Y. Class I histone deacetylases sequentially interact with MyoD and pRb during skeletal myogenesis. Mol Cell 2001; 8:885–897.

191. Slack RS, Miller FD. Retinoblastoma gene in mouse neural development. Dev Genet 1996; 18:81–91.

192. Ferguson KL, Slack RS. The Rb pathway in neurogenesis. Neuroreport 2001; 12:A55–62.

193. Lee JE. Basic helix-loop-helix genes in neural development. Curr Opin Neurobiol 1997; 7:13–20.

194. Cepko CL. The roles of intrinsic and extrinsic cues and bHLH genes in the determination of retinal cell fates. Curr Opin Neurobiol 1999; 9:37–46.

195. Perron M, Harris WA. Determination of vertebrate retinal progenitor cell fate by the Notch pathway and basic helix-loop-helix transcription factors. Cell Mol Life Sci 2000; 57:215–223.

196. Vetter ML, Brown NL. The role of basic helix-loop-helix genes in vertebrate retinogenesis. Semin Cell Dev Biol 2001; 12:491–498.

197. Lin SC, Skapek SX, Lee EY. Genes in the RB pathway and their knockout in mice. Semin Cancer Biol 1996; 7:279–289.

198. Toma JG, El-Bizri H, Barnabe-Heider F, Aloyz R, Miller FD. Evidence that helix-loop-helix proteins collaborate with retinoblastoma tumor suppressor protein to regulate cortical neurogenesis. J Neurosci 2000; 20:7648–7656.

199. Lekstrom-Himes J, Xanthopoulos KG. Biological role of the CCAAT/enhancer-binding protein family of transcription factors. J Biol Chem 1998; 273:28545–28548.

200. Yamanaka R, Lekstrom-Himes J, Barlow C, Wynshaw-Boris A, Xanthopoulos KG. CCAAT/enhancer binding proteins are critical components of the transcriptional regulation of hematopoiesis. Int J Mol Med 1998; 1:213–221.

201. Darlington GJ, Ross SE, MacDougald OA. The role of C/EBP genes in adipocyte differentiation. J Biol Chem 1998; 273:30057–30060.

202. Cowherd RM, Lyle RE, McGehee RE, Jr. Molecular regulation of adipocyte differentiation. Semin Cell Dev Biol 1999; 10:3–10.

203. Diehl AM. Roles of CCAAT/enhancer-binding proteins in regulation of liver regenerative growth. J Biol Chem 1998; 273:30843–30846.

204. Classon M, Kennedy BK, Mulloy R, Harlow E. Opposing roles of pRB and p107 in adipocyte differentiation. Proc Natl Acad Sci USA 2000; 97:10826–10831.

205. Porse BT, Pedersen TA, Xiufeng X, Lindberg B, Wewer U, Friis-Hansen L, Nerlov C. E2F repression by C/EBPa is required for adipogenesis and granulopoiesis. Cell 2001; 107:247–258.

206. Ducy P. Cbfa1: a molecular switch in osteoblast biology. Dev Dyn 2000; 219:461–471.

207. Lemercier C, Duncliffe K, Boibessot I, Zhang H, Verdel A, Angelov D, Khochbin S. Involvement of retinoblastoma protein and HBP1 in histone H1(0) gene expression. Mol Cell Biol 2000; 20:6627–6637.

208. Bernards R, Schackleford GM, Gerber MR, Horowitz JM, Friend SH, Schartl M, Bogenmann E, Rapaport JM, McGee T, Dryja TP, et al. Structure and expression of the murine retinoblastoma gene and characterization of its encoded protein. Proc Natl Acad Sci USA 1989; 86:6474–6478.

209. Gallie BL, Campbell C, Devlin H, Duckett A, Squire JA. Developmental basis of retinal-specific induction of cancer by RB mutation. Cancer Res 1999; 59:1731s–1735s.

210. Partridge JF, La Thangue NB. A developmentally regulated and tissue-dependent transcription factor complexes with the retinoblastoma gene product. EMBO J 1991; 10:3819–3827.

211. Hu QJ, Dyson N, Harlow E. The regions of the retinoblastoma protein needed for binding to adenovirus E1A or SV40 large T antigen are common sites for mutations. EMBO J 1990; 9:1147–1155.

212. Kaelin WG, Jr., Ewen ME, Livingston DM. Definition of the minimal simian virus 40 large T antigen- and adenovirus E1A-binding domain in the retinoblastoma gene product. Mol Cell Biol 1990; 10:3761–3769.

213. Huang S, Wang NP, Tseng BY, Lee WH, Lee EH. Two distinct and frequently mutated regions of retinoblastoma protein are required for binding to SV40 T antigen. EMBO J 1990; 9:1815–1822.

214. Sellers WR, Rodgers JW, Kaelin WG, Jr. A potent transrepression domain in the retinoblastoma protein induces a cell cycle arrest when bound to E2F sites. Proc Natl Acad Sci USA 1995; 92:11544–11548.

215. Dahiya A, Gavin MR, Luo RX, Dean DC. Role of the LXCXE binding site in Rb function. Mol Cell Biol 2000; 20:6799–6805.

216. Hiebert SW. Regions of the retinoblastoma gene product required for its interaction with the E2F transcription factor are necessary for E2 promoter repression and pRb-mediated growth suppression. Mol Cell Biol 1993; 13:3384–3391.

217. Harbour JW. Overview of RB gene mutations in patients with retinoblastoma: implications for clinical genetic screening. Ophthalmology 1998; 105:1442–1447.

218. Welch PJ, Wang JY. A C-terminal protein-binding domain in the retinoblastoma protein regulates nuclear c-Abl tyrosine kinase in the cell cycle. Cell 1993; 75:779–790.

219. Whitaker LL, Su H, Baskaran R, Knudsen ES, Wang JY. Growth suppression by an E2F-binding-defective retinoblastoma protein (RB): Contribution from the RB C pocket. Mol Cell Biol 1998; 18:4032–4042.

220. Zacksenhaus E, Bremner R, Phillips RA, Gallie BL. A bipartite nuclear localization signal in the retinoblastoma gene product and its importance for biological activity. Mol Cell Biol 1993; 13:4588–4599.

221. Bremner R, Du DC, Connolly-Wilson MJ, Bridge P, Ahmad KF, Mostachfi H, Rushlow D, Dunn JM, Gallie BL. Deletion of RB exons 24 and 25 causes low-penetrance retinoblastoma. Am J Hum Genet 1997; 61:556–570.

222. Xiao ZX, Chen J, Levine AJ, Modjtahedi N, Xing J, Sellers WR, Livingston DM. Interaction between the retinoblastoma protein and the oncoprotein mdm2. Nature 1995; 375:694–698.

223. Yap DBS, Hsieh J-K, Chan FSG, Lu X. mdm2: A bridge over the two tumor suppressors, p53 and Rb. Oncogene 1999; 18:7681–7689.

224. Hsieh JK, Chan FS, O'Connor DJ, Mittnacht S, Zhong S, Lu X. RB regulates the stability and the apoptotic function of p53 via mdm2. Mol Cell 1999; 3:181–193.

225. Durfee T, Becherer K, Chen PL, Yeh SH, Yang Y, Kilburn AE, Lee WH, Elledge SJ. The retinoblastoma protein associates with the protein phosphatase type 1 catalytic subunit. Genes Dev 1993; 7:555–569.

226. Durfee T, Mancini MA, Jones D, Elledge SJ, Lee WH. The amino-terminal region of the retinoblastoma gene product binds a novel nuclear matrix protein that co-localizes to centers for RNA processing. J Cell Biol 1994; 127:609–622.

227. Sterner JM, Murata Y, Kim HG, Kennett SB, Templeton DJ, Horowitz JM. Detection of a novel cell cycle-regulated kinase activity that associates with the amino terminus of the retinoblastoma protein in G2/M phases. J Biol Chem 1995; 270:9281–9288.

228. Sterner JM, Dew-Knight S, Musahl C, Kornbluth S, Horowitz JM. Negative regulation of DNA replication by the retinoblastoma protein is mediated by its association with MCM7. Mol Cell Biol 1998; 18:2748–2757.

229. Choubey D, Lengyel P. Binding of an interferon-inducible protein (p202) to the retinoblastoma protein. J Biol Chem 1995; 270:6134–6140.

230. Choubey D, Li SJ, Datta B, Gutterman JU, Lengyel P. Inhibition of E2F-mediated transcription by p202. EMBO J 1996; 15:5668–5678.

231. Xin H, D'Souza S, Fang L, Lengyel P, Choubey D. p202, an interferon-inducible negative regulator of cell growth, is a target of the adenovirus E1A protein. Oncogene 2001; 20:6828–6839.

232. Qian Y, Luckey C, Horton L, Esser M, Templeton DJ. Biological function of the retinoblastoma protein requires distinct domains for hyperphosphorylation and transcription factor binding. Mol Cell Biol 1992; 12:5363–5372.

233. Riley DJ, Liu CY, Lee WH. Mutations of N-terminal regions render the retinoblastoma protein insufficient for functions in development and tumor suppression. Mol Cell Biol 1997; 17:7342–7352.

234. Dryja TP, Rapaport J, McGee TL, Nork TM, Schwartz TL. Molecular etiology of low-penetrance retinoblastoma in two pedigrees. Am J Hum Genet 1993; 52:1122–1128.

235. Otterson GA, Chen W, Coxon AB, Khleif SN, Kaye FJ. Incomplete penetrance of familial retinoblastoma linked to germ-line mutations that result in partial loss of RB function. Proc Natl Acad Sci USA 1997; 94:12036–12040.

236. Xu HJ, Xu K, Zhou Y, Li J, Benedict WF, Hu SX. Enhanced tumor cell growth suppression by an N-terminal truncated retinoblastoma protein. Proc Natl Acad Sci USA 1994; 91:9837–9841.

237. Xu HJ, Zhou Y, Seigne J, Perng GS, Mixon M, Zhang C, Li J, Benedict WF, Hu SX. Enhanced tumor suppressor gene therapy via replication-deficient adenovirus vectors expressing an N-terminal truncated retinoblastoma protein. Cancer Res 1996; 56:2245–2249.

238. Horowitz JM, Park SH, Bogenmann E, Cheng JC, Yandell DW, Kaye FJ, Minna JD, Dryja TP, Weinberg RA. Frequent inactivation of the retinoblastoma anti-oncogene is restricted to a subset of human tumor cells. Proc Natl Acad Sci USA 1990; 87:2775–2779.

239. Sakai T, Ohtani N, McGee TL, Robbins PD, Dryja TP. Oncogenic germ-line mutations in Sp1 and ATF sites in the human retinoblastoma gene. Nature 1991; 353:83–86.

240. Cowell JK, Bia B, Akoulitchev A. A novel mutation in the promotor region in a family with a mild form of retinoblastoma indicates the location of a new regulatory domain for the RB1 gene. Oncogene 1996; 12:431–436.

241. Schubert EL, Strong LC, Hansen MF. A splicing mutation in RB1 in low penetrance retinoblastoma. Hum Genet 1997; 100:557–563.

242. Scheffer H, Van Der Vlies P, Burton M, Verlind E, Moll AC, Imhof SM, Buys CH. Two novel germline mutations of the retinoblastoma gene (RB1) that show incomplete penetrance, one splice site and one missense. J Med Genet 2000; 37:E6.

243. Alonso J, García-Miguel P, Abelairas J, Mendiola M, Sarret E, Vendrell MT, Navajas A, Pestaña A. Spectrum of germline RB1 gene mutations in Spanish retinoblastoma patients: Phenotypic and molecular epidemiological implications. Hum Mutat 2001; 17:412–422.

244. Onadim Z, Hogg A, Baird PN, Cowell JK. Oncogenic point mutations in exon 20 of the RB1 gene in families showing incomplete penetrance and mild expression of the retinoblastoma phenotype. Proc Natl Acad Sci USA 1992; 89:6177–6181.

245. Lohmann DR, Brandt B, Höpping W, Passarge E, Horsthemke B. Distinct RB1 gene mutations with low penetrance in hereditary retinoblastoma. Hum Genet 1994; 94:349–354.

246. Kratzke RA, Otterson GA, Hogg A, Coxon AB, Geradts J, Cowell JK, Kaye FJ. Partial inactivation of the RB product in a family with incomplete penetrance of familial retinoblastoma and benign retinal tumors. Oncogene 1994; 9:1321–1326.

247. Cowell JK, Bia B. A novel missense mutation in patients from a retinoblastoma pedigree showing only mild expression of the tumor phenotype. Oncogene 1998; 16:3211–3213.

248. Otterson GA, Modi S, Nguyen K, Coxon AB, Kaye FJ. Temperature-sensitive RB mutations linked to incomplete penetrance of familial retinoblastoma in 12 families. Am J Hum Genet 1999; 65:1040–1046.

249. Ahmad NN, Barbosa de Melo MD, Singh AD, Donoso LA, Shields JA. A possible hot spot in exon 21 of the retinoblastoma gene predisposing to a low penetrant retinoblastoma phenotype? Ophthalmic Genet 1999; 20:225–231.

250. Harbour JW. Molecular basis of low-penetrance retinoblastoma. Arch Ophthalmol 2001; 119:1699–1704.

251. Strong LC, Riccardi VM, Ferrell RE, Sparkes RS. Familial retinoblastoma and chromosome 13 deletion transmitted via an insertional translocation. Science 1981; 213:1501–1503.

252. Lohmann D, Horsthemke B, Gillessen-Kaesbach G, Stefani FH, Höfler H. Detection of small RB1 gene deletions in retinoblastoma by multiplex PCR and high-resolution gel electrophoresis. Hum Genet 1992; 89:49–53.

253. Gallie BL, Squire JA, Goddard A, Dunn JM, Canton M, Hinton D, Zhu XP, Phillips RA. Mechanism of oncogenesis in retinoblastoma. Lab Invest 1990; 62:394–408.

254. Chen TT, Wang JY. Establishment of irreversible growth arrest in myogenic differentiation requires the RB LXCXE-binding function. Mol Cell Biol 2000; 20:5571–5580.

255. Morgan DO. Principles of CDK regulation. Nature 1995; 374:131–134.

256. Nigg EA. Cyclin-dependent protein kinases: Key regulators of the eukaryotic cell cycle. Bioessays 1995; 17:471–480.

257. DiCiommo D, Gallie BL, Bremner R. Retinoblastoma: The disease, gene and protein provide critical leads to understand cancer. Semin Cancer Biol 2000; 10:255–269.

258. Kerkhoff E, Rapp UR. Cell cycle targets of Ras/Raf signalling. Oncogene 1998; 17:1457–1462.

259. Crespo P, Leon J. Ras proteins in the control of the cell cycle and cell differentiation. Cell Mol Life Sci 2000; 57:1613–1636.

260. Takuwa N, Takuwa Y. Regulation of cell cycle molecules by the Ras effector system. Mol Cell Endocrinol 2001; 177:25–33.

261. Ekholm SV, Zickert P, Reed SI, Zetterberg A. Accumulation of cyclin E is not a prerequisite for passage through the restriction point. Mol Cell Biol 2001; 21:3256–3265.

262. Yen A, Sturgill R. Hypophosphorylation of the RB protein in S and G2 as well as G1 during growth arrest. Exp Cell Res 1998; 241:324–331.

263. Knudsen ES, Buckmaster C, Chen TT, Feramisco JR, Wang JY. Inhibition of DNA synthesis by RB: effects on G1/S transition and S- phase progression. Genes Dev 1998; 12:2278–2292.

264. Knudsen KE, Booth D, Naderi S, Sever-Chroneos Z, Fribourg AF, Hunton IC, Feramisco JR, Wang JY, Knudsen ES. RB-dependent S-phase response to DNA damage. Mol Cell Biol 2000; 20:7751–7763.

265. Lukas C, Sorensen CS, Kramer E, Santoni-Rugiu E, Lindeneg C, Peters JM, Bartek J, Lukas J. Accumulation of cyclin B1 requires E2F and cyclin-A-dependent rearrangement of the anaphase-promoting complex. Nature 1999; 401:815–818.

266. Harbour JW, Dean DC. The Rb/E2F pathway: Expanding roles and emerging paradigms. Genes Dev 2000; 14:2393–2409.

267. Zheng L, Lee WH. The retinoblastoma gene: A prototypic and multifunctional tumor suppressor. Exp Cell Res 2001; 264:2–18.
268. Ishida S, Huang E, Zuzan H, Spang R, Leone G, West M, Nevins JR. Role for E2F in control of both DNA replication and mitotic functions as revealed from DNA microarray analysis. Mol Cell Biol 2001; 21:4684–4699.
269. Dahiya A, Wong S, Gonzalo S, Gavin M, Dean DC. Linking the Rb and the polycomb pathways. Mol Cell 2001; 8:557–568.
270. Nelson DA, Krucher NA, Ludlow JW. High molecular weight protein phosphatase type 1 dephosphorylates the retinoblastoma protein. J Biol Chem 1997; 272:4528–4535.
271. Nelson DA, Ludlow JW. Characterization of the mitotic phase pRb-directed protein phosphatase activity. Oncogene 1997; 14:2407–2415.
272. Tamrakar S, Ludlow JW. The carboxyl-terminal region of the retinoblastoma protein binds non- competitively to protein phosphatase type 1alpha and inhibits catalytic activity. J Biol Chem 2000; 275:27784–27789.
273. Cooper S, Yu C, Shayman JA. Phosphorylation-dephosphorylation of retinoblastoma protein not necessary for passage through the mammalian cell division cycle. IUBMB Life 1999; 48:225–230.
274. Cooper S, Shayman JA. Revisiting retinoblastoma protein phosphorylation during the mammalian cell cycle. Cell Mol Life Sci 2001; 58:580–595.
275. Alexander K, Hinds PW. Requirement for p27Kip1 in retinoblastoma protein-mediated senescence. Mol Cell Biol 2001; 21:3616–3631.
276. Harrington EA, Bruce JL, Harlow E, Dyson N. pRB plays an essential role in cell cycle arrest induced by DNA damage. Proc Natl Acad Sci USA 1998; 95:11945–11950.
277. Brugarolas J, Moberg K, Boyd SD, Taya Y, Jacks T, Lees JA. Inhibition of cyclin-dependent kinase 2 by p21 is necessary for retinoblastoma protein-mediated G1 arrest after gamma-irradiation. Proc Natl Acad Sci USA 1999; 96:1002–1007.
278. Ohnuma S, Philpott A, Harris WA. Cell cycle and cell fate in the nervous system. Curr Opin Neurobiol 2001; 11:66–73.
279. Hanahan D, Weinberg RA. The hallmarks of cancer. Cell 2000; 100:57–70.
280. Ruas M, Peters G. The p16INK4a/CDKN2A tumor suppressor and its relatives. Biochim Biophys Acta 1998; 1378:F115–177.
281. Hall M, Peters G. Genetic alterations of cyclins, cyclin-dependent kinases, and Cdk inhibitors in human cancer. Adv Cancer Res 1996; 68:67–108.
282. Bruce JL, Hurford RK, Jr., Classon M, Koh J, Dyson N. Requirements for cell cycle arrest by p16Ink4a. Mol Cell 2000; 6:737–742.
283. Beijersbergen RL, Carlee L, Kerkhoven RM, Bernards R. Regulation of the retinoblastoma protein-related p107 by G1 cyclin complexes. Genes Dev 1995; 9:1340–1353.
284. Xiao ZX, Ginsberg D, Ewen M, Livingston DM. Regulation of the retinoblastoma protein-related protein p107 by G1 cyclin-associated kinases. Proc Natl Acad Sci USA 1996; 93:4633–4637.
285. Dong F, Cress WD, Jr., Agrawal D, Pledger WJ. The role of cyclin D3-dependent kinase in the phosphorylation of p130 in mouse BALB/c 3T3 fibroblasts. J Biol Chem 1998; 273:6190–6195.
286. Ashizawa S, Nishizawa H, Yamada M, Higashi H, Kondo T, Ozawa H, Kakita A, Hatakeyama M. Collective inhibition of pRB family proteins by phosphorylation in cells with p16INK4a loss or cyclin E overexpression. J Biol Chem 2001; 276:11362–11370.
287. Lasorella A, Iavarone A, Israel MA. Id2 specifically alters regulation of the cell cycle by tumor suppressor proteins. Mol Cell Biol 1996; 16:2570–2578.

288. Lasorella A, Boldrini R, Dominici C, Donfrancesco A, Yokota Y, Inserra A, Iavarone A. Id2 is critical for cellular proliferation and is the oncogenic effector of N-myc in human neuroblastoma. Cancer Res 2002; 62:301–306.

289. Friend SH, Horowitz JM, Gerber MR, Wang XF, Bogenmann E, Li FP, Weinberg RA. Deletions of a DNA sequence in retinoblastomas and mesenchymal tumors: Organization of the sequence and its encoded protein. Proc Natl Acad Sci USA 1987; 84:9059–9063.

290. Reissmann PT, Simon MA, Lee WH, Slamon DJ. Studies of the retinoblastoma gene in human sarcomas. Oncogene 1989; 4:839–843.

291. Wunder JS, Czitrom AA, Kandel R, Andrulis IL. Analysis of alterations in the retinoblastoma gene and tumor grade in bone and soft-tissue sarcomas. J Natl Cancer Inst 1991; 83:194–200.

292. Wadayama B, Toguchida J, Shimizu T, Ishizaki K, Sasaki MS, Kotoura Y, Yamamuro T. Mutation spectrum of the retinoblastoma gene in osteosarcomas. Cancer Res 1994; 54:3042–3048.

293. Weichselbaum RR, Beckett M, Diamond A. Some retinoblastomas, osteosarcomas, and soft tissue sarcomas may share a common etiology. Proc Natl Acad Sci USA 1988; 85:2106–2109.

294. Stratton MR, Williams S, Fisher C, Ball A, Westbury G, Gusterson BA, Fletcher CD, Knight JC, Fung YK, Reeves BR, et al. Structural alterations of the RB1 gene in human soft tissue tumours. Br J Cancer 1989; 60:202–205.

295. Chibon F, Mairal A, Freneaux P, Terrier P, Coindre JM, Sastre X, Aurias A. The RB1 gene is the target of chromosome 13 deletions in malignant fibrous histiocytoma. Cancer Res 2000; 60:6339–6345.

296. Lefevre SH, Vogt N, Dutrillaux AM, Chauveinc L, Stoppa-Lyonnet D, Doz F, Desjardins L, Dutrillaux B, Chevillard S, Malfoy B. Genome instability in secondary solid tumors developing after radiotherapy of bilateral retinoblastoma. Oncogene 2001; 20:8092–8099.

297. Karpeh MS, Brennan MF, Cance WG, Woodruff JM, Pollack D, Casper ES, Dudas ME, Latres E, Drobnjak M, Cordon-Cardo C. Altered patterns of retinoblastoma gene product expression in adult soft-tissue sarcomas. Br J Cancer 1995; 72:986–991.

298. Cohen JA, Geradts J. Loss of RB and MTS1/CDKN2 (p16) expression in human sarcomas. Hum Pathol 1997; 28:893–898.

299. Dei Tos AP, Maestro R, Doglioni C, Piccinin S, Libera DD, Boiocchi M, Fletcher CD. Tumor suppressor genes and related molecules in leiomyosarcoma. Am J Pathol 1996; 148:1037–1045.

300. Derre J, Lagace R, Nicolas A, Mairal A, Chibon F, Coindre JM, Terrier P, Sastre X, Aurias A. Leiomyosarcomas and most malignant fibrous histiocytomas share very similar comparative genomic hybridization imbalances: an analysis of a series of 27 leiomyosarcomas. Lab Invest 2001; 81:211–215.

301. Cairns P, Proctor AJ, Knowles MA. Loss of heterozygosity at the RB locus is frequent and correlates with muscle invasion in bladder carcinoma. Oncogene 1991; 6:2305–2309.

302. Xu HJ, Cairns P, Hu SX, Knowles MA, Benedict WF. Loss of RB protein expression in primary bladder cancer correlates with loss of heterozygosity at the RB locus and tumor progression. Int J Cancer 1993; 53:781–784.

303. Bataille V, Hiles R, Newton Bishop JA. Retinoblastoma, melanoma, and the atypical mole syndrome. Br J Dermatol 1995; 132:134–138.

304. Bartkova J, Lukas J, Guldberg P, Alsner J, Kirkin AF, Zeuthen J, Bartek J. The p16-cyclin D/Cdk4-pRb pathway as a functional unit frequently altered in melanoma pathogenesis. Cancer Res 1996; 56:5475–5483.

305. Maelandsmo GM, Florenes VA, Hovig E, Oyjord T, Engebraaten O, Holm R, Borresen AL, Fodstad O. Involvement of the pRb/p16/cdk4/cyclin D1 pathway in the tumorigenesis of sporadic malignant melanomas. Br J Cancer 1996; 73:909–916.

306. Walker GJ, Flores JF, Glendening JM, Lin AH, Markl ID, Fountain JW. Virtually 100% of melanoma cell lines harbor alterations at the DNA level within CDKN2A, CDKN2B, or one of their downstream targets. Genes Chromosomes Cancer 1998; 22:157–163.

307. Halaban R, Cheng E, Smicun Y, Germino J. Deregulated E2F transcriptional activity in autonomously growing melanoma cells. J Exp Med 2000; 191:1005–1016.

308. Halaban R. Melanoma cell autonomous growth: The Rb/E2F pathway. Cancer Metastasis Rev 1999; 18:333–343.

309. Tripathi BJ, Tripathi RC. Development of the human eye. In: Bron AJ, Tripathi RC, Tripathi BJ, eds. Wolff's anatomy of the eye and orbit. London: Chapman & Hall Medical, 1997.

310. Young RW. Cell differentiation in the retina of the mouse. Anat Rec 1985; 212:199–205.

311. Davis AA, Matzuk MM, Reh TA. Activin A promotes progenitor differentiation into photoreceptors in rodent retina. Mol Cell Neurosci 2000; 15:11–21.

312. Clarke AR. Murine models of neoplasia: Functional analysis of the tumour suppressor genes Rb-1 and p53. Cancer Metastasis Rev 1995; 14:125–148.

313. Jacks T. Tumor suppressor gene mutations in mice. Annu Rev Genet 1996; 30:603–636.

314. Vooijs M, Berns A. Developmental defects and tumor predisposition in Rb mutant mice. Oncogene 1999; 18:5293–5303.

315. Mills MD, Windle JJ, Albert DM. Retinoblastoma in transgenic mice: Models of hereditary retinoblastoma. Surv Ophthalmol 1999; 43:508–518.

316. Ali SH, DeCaprio JA. Cellular transformation by SV40 large T antigen: Interaction with host proteins. Semin Cancer Biol 2001; 11:15–23.

317. Mantovani F, Banks L. The human papillomavirus E6 protein and its contribution to malignant progression. Oncogene 2001; 20:7874–7887.

318. Zwerschke W, Jansen-Durr P. Cell transformation by the E7 oncoprotein of human papillomavirus type 16: interactions with nuclear and cytoplasmic target proteins. Adv Cancer Res 2000; 78:1–29.

319. Munger K, Basile JR, Duensing S, Eichten A, Gonzalez SL, Grace M, Zacny VL. Biological activities and molecular targets of the human papillomavirus E7 oncoprotein. Oncogene 2001; 20:7888–7898.

320. Windle JJ, Albert DM, O'Brien JM, Marcus DM, Disteche CM, Bernards R, Mellon PL. Retinoblastoma in transgenic mice. Nature 1990; 343:665–669.

321. O'Brien JM, Marcus DM, Niffenegger AS, Bernards R, Carpenter JL, Windle JJ, Mellon P, Albert DM. Trilateral retinoblastoma in transgenic mice. Trans Am Ophthalmol Soc 1989; 87:301–326.

322. O'Brien JM, Marcus DM, Bernards R, Carpenter JL, Windle JJ, Mellon P, Albert DM. A transgenic mouse model for trilateral retinoblastoma. Arch Ophthalmol 1990; 108:1145–1151.

323. Marcus DM, Carpenter JL, O'Brien JM, Kivela T, Brauner E, Tarkkanen A, Virtanen I, Albert DM. Primitive neuroectodermal tumor of the midbrain in a murine model of retinoblastoma. Invest Ophthalmol Vis Sci 1991; 32:293–301.

324. Kivelä T, Virtanen I, Marcus DM, O'Brien JM, Carpenter JL, Brauner E, Tarkkanen A, Albert DM. Neuronal and glial properties of a murine transgenic retinoblastoma model. Am J Pathol 1991; 138:1135–1148.

325. Marcus DM, O'Brien JM, Sahel J, Brauner E, Thor A, Roberts K, Barnstable C, Albert DM. The histogenesis of murine transgenic retinoblastoma (abstract). Invest Ophthalmol Vis Sci 1992; 33 (Suppl):875.

326. Nork TM, Schwartz TL, Doshi HM, Millecchia LL. Retinoblastoma. Cell of origin. Arch Ophthalmol 1995; 113:791–802.
327. Al-Ubaidi MR, Font RL, Quiambao AB, Keener MJ, Liou GI, Overbeek PA, Baehr W. Bilateral retinal and brain tumors in transgenic mice expressing simian virus 40 large T antigen under control of the human interphotoreceptor retinoid-binding protein promoter. J Cell Biol 1992; 119:1681–1687.
328. Howes KA, Lasudry JG, Albert DM, Windle JJ. Photoreceptor cell tumors in transgenic mice. Invest Ophthalmol Vis Sci 1994; 35:342–351.
329. Baetge EE, Behringer RR, Messing A, Brinster RL, Palmiter RD. Transgenic mice express the human phenylethanolamine N- methyltransferase gene in adrenal medulla and retina. Proc Natl Acad Sci USA 1988; 85:3648–3652.
330. Fung KM, Chikaraishi DM, Suri C, Theuring F, Messing A, Albert DM, Lee VM, Trojanowski JQ. Molecular phenotype of simian virus 40 large T antigen-induced primitive neuroectodermal tumors in four different lines of transgenic mice. Lab Invest 1994; 70:114–124.
331. Marcus DM, Lasudry JG, Carpenter JL, Windle J, Howes KA, al-Ubaidi MR, Baehr W, Overbeek PA, Font RL, Albert DM. Trilateral tumors in four lines of transgenic mice expressing SV-40 T-antigen. Invest Ophthalmol Vis Sci 1996; 37:392–396.
332. Al-Ubaidi MR, Hollyfield JG, Overbeek PA, Baehr W. Photoreceptor degeneration induced by the expression of simian virus 40 large tumor antigen in the retina of transgenic mice. Proc Natl Acad Sci USA 1992; 89:1194–1198.
333. Al-Ubaidi MR, Mangini NJ, Quiambao AB, Myers KM, Abler AS, Chang CJ, Tso MO, Butel JS, Hollyfield JG. Unscheduled DNA replication precedes apoptosis of photoreceptors expressing SV40 T antigen. Exp Eye Res 1997; 64:573–585.
334. Porrello K, Bhat SP, Bok D. Detection of interphotoreceptor retinoid binding protein (IRBP) mRNA in human and cone-dominant squirrel retinas by in situ hybridization. J Histochem Cytochem 1991; 39:171–176.
335. Carter-Dawson L, Alvarez RA, Fong SL, Liou GI, Sperling HG, Bridges CD. Rhodopsin, 11-cis vitamin A, and interstitial retinol-binding protein (IRBP) during retinal development in normal and rd mutant mice. Dev Biol 1986; 116:431–438.
336. Yokoyama T, Liou GI, Caldwell RB, Overbeek PA. Photoreceptor-specific activity of the human interphotoreceptor retinoid-binding protein (IRBP) promoter in transgenic mice. Exp Eye Res 1992; 55:225–233.
337. Hammang JP, Baetge EE, Behringer RR, Brinster RL, Palmiter RD, Messing A. Immortalized retinal neurons derived from SV40 T-antigen-induced tumors in transgenic mice. Neuron 1990; 4:775–782.
338. Hammang JP, Behringer RR, Baetge EE, Palmiter RD, Brinster RL, Messing A. Oncogene expression in retinal horizontal cells of transgenic mice results in a cascade of neurodegeneration. Neuron 1993; 10:1197–1209.
339. Cohen J. Postnatal development of phenylethanolamine N-methyltransferase activity of rat retina. Neurosci Lett 1987; 83:138–142.
340. Sidman RL. Histogenesis of mouse retina studied with thymidine-H3. In: Smelser GK, ed. The Structure of the Eye. New York: Academic Press, 1961:487–506.
341. Polley EH, Zimmerman RP, Fortney RL. Neurogenesis and maturation of cell morphology in the development of the mammalian retina. In: Finlay BL, Sengelaub DR, eds. Development of the Vertebrate Retina. New York: Plenum Press, 1987:3–29.
342. Griep AE, Krawcek J, Lee D, Liem A, Albert DM, Carabeo R, Drinkwater N, McCall M, Sattler C, Lasudry JG, Lambert PF. Multiple genetic loci modify risk for retinoblastoma in transgenic mice. Invest Ophthalmol Vis Sci 1998; 39:2723–2732.
343. Howes KA, Ransom N, Papermaster DS, Lasudry JG, Albert DM, Windle JJ. Apoptosis or retinoblastoma: alternative fates of photoreceptors expressing the HPV-16 E7 gene in the presence or absence of p53. Genes Dev 1994; 8:1300–1310.

344. Papermaster DS, Howes K, Ransom N, Windle JJ. Apoptosis of photoreceptors and lens fiber cells with cataract and multiple tumor formation in the eyes of transgenic mice lacking the p53 gene and expressing the HPV 16 E7 gene under the control of the IRBP promoter. In: Anderson RE, LaVail MM, Hollyfield JG, eds. Degenerative Diseases of the Retina. New York: Plenum Press, 1995:39–49.

345. Pan H, Griep AE. Temporally distinct patterns of p53-dependent and p53-independent apoptosis during mouse lens development. Genes Dev 1995; 9:2157–2169.

346. Bischoff FZ, Yim SO, Pathak S, Grant G, Siciliano MJ, Giovanella BC, Strong LC, Tainsky MA. Spontaneous abnormalities in normal fibroblasts from patients with Li-Fraumeni cancer syndrome: Aneuploidy and immortalization. Cancer Res 1990; 50:7979–7984.

347. Livingstone LR, White A, Sprouse J, Livanos E, Jacks T, Tlsty TD. Altered cell cycle arrest and gene amplification potential accompany loss of wild-type p53. Cell 1992; 70:923–935.

348. Yin Y, Tainsky MA, Bischoff FZ, Strong LC, Wahl GM. Wild-type p53 restores cell cycle control and inhibits gene amplification in cells with mutant p53 alleles. Cell 1992; 70:937–948.

349. Harvey M, Sands AT, Weiss RS, Hegi ME, Wiseman RW, Pantazis P, Giovanella BC, Tainsky MA, Bradley A, Donehower LA. In vitro growth characteristics of embryo fibroblasts isolated from p53- deficient mice. Oncogene 1993; 8:2457–2467.

350. Bouffler SD, Kemp CJ, Balmain A, Cox R. Spontaneous and ionizing radiation-induced chromosomal abnormalities in p53-deficient mice. Cancer Res 1995; 55:3883–3889.

351. Donehower LA, Godley LA, Aldaz CM, Pyle R, Shi YP, Pinkel D, Gray J, Bradley A, Medina D, Varmus HE. Deficiency of p53 accelerates mammary tumorigenesis in Wnt-1 transgenic mice and promotes chromosomal instability. Genes Dev 1995; 9:882–895.

352. Venkatachalam S, Shi YP, Jones SN, Vogel H, Bradley A, Pinkel D, Donehower LA. Retention of wild-type p53 in tumors from p53 heterozygous mice: Reduction of p53 dosage can promote cancer formation. EMBO J 1998; 17:4657–4667.

353. Jones JM, Attardi L, Godley LA, Laucirica R, Medina D, Jacks T, Varmus HE, Donehower LA. Absence of p53 in a mouse mammary tumor model promotes tumor cell proliferation without affecting apoptosis. Cell Growth Differ 1997; 8:829–838.

354. Hu N, Gutsmann A, Herbert DC, Bradley A, Lee WH, Lee EY. Heterozygous Rb-1 delta 20/ + mice are predisposed to tumors of the pituitary gland with a nearly complete penetrance. Oncogene 1994; 9:1021–1027.

355. Lee MH, Williams BO, Mulligan G, Mukai S, Bronson RT, Dyson N, Harlow E, Jacks T. Targeted disruption of p107: Functional overlap between p107 and Rb. Genes Dev 1996; 10:1621–1632.

356. Cobrinik D, Lee MH, Hannon G, Mulligan G, Bronson RT, Dyson N, Harlow E, Beach D, Weinberg RA, Jacks T. Shared role of the pRB-related p130 and p107 proteins in limb development. Genes Dev 1996; 10:1633–1644.

357. Donehower LA, Godley LA, Aldaz CM, Pyle R, Shi Y-P, Pinkel D, Gray J, Bradley A, Demina D, Varmus HE. Mice deficient for p53 are developmentally normal but susceptible to spontaneous tumours. Nature 1992; 356:215–221.

358. Williams BO, Remington L, Albert DM, Mukai S, Bronson RT, Jacks T. Cooperative tumorigenic effects of germline mutations in Rb and p53. Nat Genet 1994; 7:480–484.

359. Bowman T, Symonds H, Gu L, Yin C, Oren M, Van Dyke T. Tissue-specific inactivation of p53 tumor suppression in the mouse. Genes Dev 1996; 10:826–835.

360. Albert DM, Hogan RN. Does retinoblastoma occur in animals? Prog Vet Comp Ophthalmol 1991; 1991:73–82.

361. Syed NA, Nork TM, Poulsen GL, Riis RC, George C, Albert DM. Retinoblastoma in a dog. Arch Ophthalmol 1997; 115:758–763.

362. Oliveros O, Yunis E. Chromosome evolution in retinoblastoma. Cancer Genet Cytogenet 1995; 82:155–160.
363. Chen D, Gallie BL, Squire JA. Minimal regions of chromosomal imbalance in retinoblastoma detected by comparative genomic hybridization. Cancer Genet Cytogenet 2001; 129:57–63.
364. Cano J, Oliveros O, Yunis E. Phenotype variants, malignancy, and additional copies of 6p in retinoblastoma. Cancer Genet Cytogenet 1994; 76:112–115.
365. Mairal A, Pinglier E, Gilbert E, Peter M, Validire P, Desjardins L, Doz F, Aurias A, Couturier J. Detection of chromosome imbalances in retinoblastoma by parallel karyotype and CGH analyses. Genes Chromosomes Cancer 2000; 28:370–379.
366. Douglass EC, Green AA, Hayes FA, Etcubanas E, Horowitz M, Wilimas JA. Chromosome 1 abnormalities: a common feature of pediatric solid tumors. J Natl Cancer Inst 1985; 75:51–54.
367. Atkin NB. Chromosome 1 aberrations in cancer. Cancer Genet Cytogenet 1986; 21:279–285.
368. Heim S, Mitelman F. Cancer cytogenetics. New York: Wiley-Liss, 1995.
369. Gardner HA, Gallie BL, Knight LA, Phillips RA. Multiple karyotypic changes in retinoblastoma tumor cells: presence of normal chromosome No. 13 in most tumors. Cancer Genet Cytogenet 1982; 6:201–211.
370. Herzog S, Lohmann DR, Buiting K, Schuler A, Horsthemke B, Rehder H, Rieder H. Marked differences in unilateral isolated retinoblastomas from young and older children studied by comparative genomic hybridization. Hum Genet 2001; 108:98–104.
371. Almeida A, Zhu XX, Vogt N, Tyagi R, Muleris M, Dutrillaux AM, Dutrillaux B, Ross D, Malfoy B, Hanash S. GAC1, a new member of the leucine-rich repeat superfamily on chromosome band 1q32.1, is amplified and overexpressed in malignant gliomas. Oncogene 1998; 16:2997–3002.
372. Kusnetsova LE, Prigogina EL, Pogosianz HE, Belkina BM. Similar chromosomal abnormalities in several retinoblastomas. Hum Genet 1982; 61:201–204.
373. Squire J, Phillips RA, Boyce S, Godbout R, Rogers B, Gallie BL. Isochromosome 6p, a unique chromosomal abnormality in retinoblastoma: verification by standard staining techniques, new densitometric methods, and somatic cell hybridization. Hum Genet 1984; 66:46–53.
374. Potluri VR, Helson L, Ellsworth RM, Reid T, Gilbert F. Chromosomal abnormalities in human retinoblastoma. A review. Cancer 1986; 58:663–671.
375. Horsthemke B, Greger V, Becher R, Passarge E. Mechanism of i(6p) formation in retinoblastoma tumor cells. Cancer Genet Cytogenet 1989; 37:95–102.
376. Mertens F, Johansson B, Mitelman F. Isochromosomes in neoplasia. Genes Chromosomes Cancer 1994; 10:221–230.
377. Bruch J, Schulz WA, Haussler J, Melzner I, Bruderlein S, Moller P, Kemmerling R, Vogel W, Hameister H. Delineation of the 6p22 amplification unit in urinary bladder carcinoma cell lines. Cancer Res 2000; 60:4526–4530.
378. Ishikawa J, Xu HJ, Hu SX, Yandell DW, Maeda S, Kamidono S, Benedict WF, Takahashi R. Inactivation of the retinoblastoma gene in human bladder and renal cell carcinomas. Cancer Res 1991; 51:5736–5743.
379. Miyamoto H, Shuin T, Torigoe S, Iwasaki Y, Kubota Y. Retinoblastoma gene mutations in primary human bladder cancer. Br J Cancer 1995; 71:831–835.
380. Richter J, Wagner U, Schraml P, Maurer R, Alund G, Knonagel H, Moch H, Mihatsch MJ, Gasser TC, Sauter G. Chromosomal imbalances are associated with a high risk of progression in early invasive (pT1) urinary bladder cancer. Cancer Res 1999; 59:5687–5691.
381. Tomovska S, Richter J, Suess K, Wagner U, Rozenblum E, Gasser TC, Moch H, Mihatsch MJ, Sauter G, Schraml P. Molecular cytogenetic alterations associated with

rapid tumor cell proliferation in advanced urinary bladder cancer. Int J Oncol 2001; 18:1239–1244.

382. Chen D, Pajovic S, Duckett A, Brown VD, Squire JA, Gallie BL. Genomic amplification in retinoblastoma narrowed to 0.6 megabase on chromosome 6p containing a kinesin-like gene, RBKIN. Cancer Res 2002; 62:967–971.

383. Manning BD, Snyder M. Drivers and passengers wanted! the role of kinesin-associated proteins. Trends Cell Biol 2000; 10:281–289.

384. Nakagawa T, Setou M, Seog D, Ogasawara K, Dohmae N, Takio K, Hirokawa N. A novel motor, KIF13A, transports mannose-6-phosphate receptor to plasma membrane through direct interaction with AP-1 complex. Cell 2000; 103:569–581.

385. De Souza AT, Yamada T, Mills JJ, Jirtle RL. Imprinted genes in liver carcinogenesis. FASEB J 1997; 11:60–67.

386. Fero ML, Randel E, Gurley KE, Roberts JM, Kemp CJ. The murine gene p27Kip1 is haplo-insufficient for tumour suppression. Nature 1998; 396:177–180.

387. Yagi T, Takeichi M. Cadherin superfamily genes: Functions, genomic organization, and neurologic diversity. Genes Dev 2000; 14:1169–1180.

388. Steinberg MS, McNutt PM. Cadherins and their connections: Adhesion junctions have broader functions. Curr Opin Cell Biol 1999; 11:554–560.

389. Cavallaro U, Schaffhauser B, Christofori G. Cadherins and the tumour progression: Is it all in a switch? Cancer Lett 2002; 176:123–128.

390. Newsham I, Kindler-Rohrborn A, Daub D, Cavenee W. A constitutional BWS-related t(11;16) chromosome translocation occurring in the same region of chromosome 16 implicated in Wilms' tumors. Genes Chromosomes Cancer 1995; 12:1–7.

391. Austruy E, Candon S, Henry I, Gyapay G, Tournade MF, Mannens M, Callen D, Junien C, Jeanpierre C. Characterization of regions of chromosomes 12 and 16 involved in nephroblastoma tumorigenesis. Genes Chromosomes Cancer 1995; 14:285–294.

392. Sato T, Saito H, Morita R, Koi S, Lee JH, Nakamura Y. Allelotype of human ovarian cancer. Cancer Res 1991; 51:5118–5122.

393. Kaye FJ. Can p53 status resolve paradoxes between human and non-human retinoblastoma models? J Natl Cancer Inst 1997; 89:1476–1477.

394. Schlamp CL, Poulsen GL, Nork TM, Nickells RW. Nuclear exclusion of wild-type p53 in immortalized human retinoblastoma cells. J Natl Cancer Inst 1997; 89:1530–1536.

395. Hollstein M, Sidransky D, Vogelstein B, Harris CC. p53 mutations in human cancers. Science 1991; 253:49–53.

396. Hainaut P, Hollstein M. p53 and human cancer: the first ten thousand mutations. Adv Cancer Res 2000; 77:81–137.

397. Kato MV, Shimizu T, Ishizaki K, Kaneko A, Yandell DW, Toguchida J, Sasaki MS. Loss of heterozygosity on chromosome 17 and mutation of the p53 gene in retinoblastoma. Cancer Lett 1996; 106:75–82.

398. Nork TM, Poulsen GL, Millecchia LL, Jantz RG, Nickells RW. p53 regulates apoptosis in human retinoblastoma. Arch Ophthalmol 1997; 115:213–219.

399. Doz F, Peter M, Schleiermacher G, Vielh P, Validire P, Putterman M, Blanquet V, Desjardins L, Dufier JL, Zucker JM, Mosseri V, Thomas G, Magdelenat H, Delattre O. N-MYC amplification, loss of heterozygosity on the short arm of chromosome 1 and DNA ploidy in retinoblastoma. Eur J Cancer 1996; 32A:645–649.

400. Lee WH, Murphree AL, Benedict WF. Expression and amplification of the N-myc gene in primary retinoblastoma. Nature 1984; 309:458–460.

401. Sakai K, Kanda N, Shiloh Y, Donlon T, Schreck R, Shipley J, Dryja T, Chaum E, Chaganti RS, Latt S. Molecular and cytologic analysis of DNA amplification in retinoblastoma. Cancer Genet Cytogenet 1985; 17:95–112.

402. Squire J, Goddard AD, Canton M, Becker A, Phillips RA, Gallie BL. Tumour induction by the retinoblastoma mutation is independent of N-myc expression. Nature 1986; 322:555–557.

403. Seshadri R, Matthews C, Norris MD, Brian MJ. N-myc amplified in retinoblastoma cell line FMC-RB1. Cancer Genet Cytogenet 1988; 33:25–27.

404. Gupta J, Han LP, Wang P, Gallie BL, Bacchetti S. Development of retinoblastoma in the absence of telomerase activity. J Natl Cancer Inst 1996; 88:1152–1157.

405. Ewen ME, Xing YG, Lawrence JB, Livingston DM. Molecular cloning, chromosomal mapping, and expression of the cDNA for p107, a retinoblastoma gene product-related protein. Cell 1991; 66:1155–1164.

406. Egan C, Bayley ST, Branton PE. Binding of the Rb1 protein to E1A products is required for adenovirus transformation. Oncogene 1989; 4:383–388.

407. Brantley MA, Jr., Harbour JW. The molecular biology of retinoblastoma. Ocul Immunol Inflamm 2001; 9:1–8.

408. Margo C, Hidayat A, Kopelman J, Zimmerman LE. Retinocytoma. A benign variant of retinoblastoma. Arch Ophthalmol 1983; 101:1519–1531.

409. Balaban G, Gilbert F, Nichols W, Meadows AT, Shields J. Abnormalities of chromosome #13 in retinoblastomas from individuals with normal constitutional karyotypes. Cancer Genet Cytogenet 1982; 6:213–221.

410. Benedict WF, Banerjee A, Mark C, Murphree AL. Nonrandom chromosomal changes in untreated retinoblastomas. Cancer Genet Cytogenet 1983; 10:311–333.

411. Workman ML, Soukup SW. Chromosome features of two retinoblastomas. Cancer Genet Cytogenet 1984; 12:365–370.

412. Chaum E, Ellsworth RM, Abramson DH, Haik BG, Kitchin FD, Chaganti RS. Cytogenetic analysis of retinoblastoma: Evidence for multifocal origin and in vivo gene amplification. Cytogenet Cell Genet 1984; 38:82–91.

413. Squire J, Gallie BL, Phillips RA. A detailed analysis of chromosomal changes in heritable and non- heritable retinoblastoma. Hum Genet 1985; 70:291–301.

414. Yan Y, Dunkel IJ, Guan X, Abramson DH, Jhanwar SC, O'Reilly RJ. Engraftment and growth of patient-derived retinoblastoma tumour in severe combined immunode-ficiency mice. Eur J Cancer 2000; 36:221–228.

415. Naumova A, Hansen M, Strong L, Jones PA, Hadjistilianou D, Mastrangelo D, Griegel S, Rajewsky MF, Shields J, Donoso L, et al. Concordance between parental origin of chromosome 13q loss and chromosome 6p duplication in sporadic retinoblastoma. Am J Hum Genet 1994; 54:274–281.

416. Balaban-Malenbaum G, Gilbert F, Nichols WW, Hill R, Shields J, Meadows AT. A deleted chromosome no. 13 in human retinoblastoma cells: Relevance to tumorigenesis. Cancer Genet Cytogenet 1981; 3:243–250.

9

Biochemical Pathways: Differential Gene Expression and Cellular Pathways Determining Tumor Phenotype Comparison of Uveal Melanocytes and Uveal Melanoma Cells In Vitro

DAN-NING HU and STEVEN A. MCCORMICK

The New York Eye and Ear Infirmary and New York Medical College, New York, New York, U.S.A.

I. NORMAL UVEAL MELANOCYTES

Uveal melanocytes are embryonically derived from nonpigmented precursor cells, melanoblasts, which originate from neural crest cells that migrate to the uveal tract. Uveal melanocytes are well established in the uveal tract at birth, dispersed throughout the stroma. In the iris, uveal melanocytes are present throughout the stroma and form a dense layer at the anterior surface of the iris just under a layer of fibroblasts. In the ciliary body, uveal melanocytes can be less dendritic (at the base) or dendritic (in the ciliary processes). In the choroid, uveal melanocytes are present in the stroma, especially gathered around the blood vessels. A large number of uveal melanocytes appear in the suprachoroidal lamellae [1].

Uveal melanocytes are dendritic in shape (with two or more processes) and possess prominent oval nuclei. The cytoplasm is heavily filled with oval melanosomes, predominately in terminal maturation stage IV. The cytoplasm also contains other cellular organelles, e.g., endoplasmic reticulum, Golgi apparatus, and mitochondria.

Iris color is determined by the melanin content of the melanocytes. Melanin is synthesized and stored in melanosomes located in the cytoplasm of uveal melanocytes. In the past, it was supposed that the color of the iris varied with the number of uveal melanocytes. However, quantitative studies have demonstrated that the number of melanocytes does not differ with iris color. Density and the size of melanosomes in the melanocytes do vary with iris color [2–4]. Recently, we found that the type of melanin in the uveal melanocytes differs from that in the iris pigment epithelial cells [5]. There are at least two different types of melanin in the eye, eumelanin and pheomelanin. Eumelanin predominates in the skin and hair of people with dark hair (black or dark brown), whereas pheomelanin is predominate in people with light hair (red or blonde) [6]. The iris pigment epithelial cells contain mainly eumelanin. In contrast, uveal melanocytes contain both eumelanin and pheomelanin, and the eumelanin/pheomelanin ratio varies with iris color [5]. Therefore, iris color is determined by the quantity and quality of melanin located in the uveal melanocytes.

In vivo, uveal melanocytes (UM) are very stable in adulthood. Mitotic figures are not seen in the uveal melanocytes in normal eyes. Except from neoplastic proliferation (melanoma), uveal melanocytes do not show growth activity even in pathological conditions, such as injury or inflammation. These stimuli often lead to growth of other cell types (e.g., retinal pigment epithelium) [7–9]. The only exceptions are proliferation of UM on the posterior surface of cornea (retrocorneal melanin pigmentation), on the trabecular meshwork (iris melanocytization of the anterior chamber angle), and in pupillary membranes (pigmented pupillary membranes) [10–12]. These changes appear to be stimulated by surgical or accidental trauma.

II. CELL CULTURE OF UVEAL MELANOCYTES

In the past, in vitro study of the pathogenesis of malignant melanoma was limited by the difficulties in establishing pure cell cultures of UM, which could be a useful comparative control. Culture of UM has been hampered by their low proliferative potential and the tendency for contamination by other cell types under usual culture conditions. We have developed a method for isolation and cultivation of pure cultures of human UM [13]. The contaminating cells can be eliminated by the use of geneticin, which has a selectively toxic effect on the contaminating cells, such as fibroblasts and pigment epithelial cells, but does not adversely affect the UM at moderate concentrations. UM can be cultured for long periods of time in a special medium (containing serum, growth factors, and cAMP-elevating agents) with a doubling time of 2–3 days and dividing 30–50 times. Cultured UM produce melanin and express tyrosinase activity in vitro. Uveal melanocytes isolated from eyes of different iris color maintained their inherent capacity for melanogenesis in vitro [14]. We have established many cell lines of UM from human donor eyes. Therefore it is now possible to use these cultured UM to study the factors regulating growth and differentiation of UM and also to study the pathogenesis of malignant melanoma cells at the cellular level. However, the application of this information to the in vivo circumstances should be cautious because the difference of in vitro and in vivo situations.

III. METHODS FOR ISOLATION AND CULTIVATION OF UVEAL MELANOCYTES

Uveal melanocytes can be isolated and cultured using our trypsin-collagenase sequential method, as described previously [13]. Briefly, the iris pigment epithelium, ciliary pigment, and nonpigment epithelium and the retinal pigment epithelium are separated from the stroma after trypsin treatment. The uveal stroma is placed in trypsin solution at $4°C$ for 18 hr, followed by incubation at $37°C$ for 1 hr. The isolated cells are collected and the trypsin solution is replaced by collagenase solution, followed by incubation at $37°C$. The collagenase solution is replaced and the cells collected, centrifuged, resuspended, and plated each hour for 3 hr [13].

The isolated UM are cultured in flasks with F12 medium supplemented with 10% fetal bovine serum, 20 ng/mL bFGF, 0.1 mM IBMX, 10 ng/mL cholera toxin (CT), 2 mM glutamine, and 50 µg/mL gentamicin. The culture dishes were incubated in a CO_2-regulated incubator in a humidified 95% air and 5% CO_2 atmosphere. The medium is changed three times weekly. Geneticin, a cytotoxic agent, is added (100 µg/mL) for 3–7 days when necessary to eliminate contaminating cells. Fibroblasts and pigment epithelial cells are sensitive to geneticin, while UM are much less so. After confluence, the UM are detached by trypsin-EDTA solution, diluted 1:3–1:4 and plated into culture dishes for subculture [13].

Several other media have been used for the culture of uveal melanocytes, such as TIC medium, which uses the 12-O-tetradecanoyl-phorbol-13-acetate (TPA) as a substitute for bFGF in the FIC medium; or the TI medium, which is the TIC medium with deletion of cholera toxin. A comparative study for testing the effects of three media (FIC, TIC, or TI medium) showed that cells cultured with FIC medium grew better than those in other media [15]. In comparing TPA and bFGF, it should be noted that TPA is not a natural substance like bFGF. It is a tumor promoter; therefore caution should be used to avoid potential hazards to the culturists. TPA is less stable than the bFGF, requiring fresh preparation from the stock solution and addition to the culture medium once or twice a week. TPA has a downregulating effect on the TPA receptor, and growth stimulation may decrease after long-term treatment. The only advantage of TPA is that its cost is lower than that of bFGF. Cholera toxin induces uveal melanocytes to spread to a disk-like morphology in senescence. However, cells cultured in cholera toxin–deleted medium (TI medium) do not grow after senescence, although they retain dendritic morphology. Therefore, the deletion of cholera toxin only changes the morphology of cultured melanocytes but does not improve growth capacity. IBMX raises intracellular cAMP by inhibiting cAMP phosphodiesterase and cholera toxin raises cAMP level by activating adenylate cyclase. The combination of both compounds are additive. Therefore it is suggested to use FIC medium for routine culture of UM.

Cultured UM have prominent but small nuclei, surrounded by a thin rim of cytoplasm, and two or more dendritic processes. Ultrastructurally, the cytoplasm of cultured UM contains melanosomes, mitochondria, Golgi apparati, endoplasmic reticulum, and free ribosomes. Many immature melanosomes and numerous mitochondria are present in the cultured cells, in contrast to melanocytes in vivo, indicating that cultured cells are active in growth and melanogenesis. In the UM of late passages, lipofuscin is also present in the cytoplasm [13].

Morphologically, UM cultured with TPA are different from cells cultured with bFGF. The dendrites of TPA-cultured melanocytes are straight and narrow and have a uniform diameter throughout the whole length of the dendrites. TPA-cultured melanocytes are also characterized by less perinuclear cytoplasm and a more

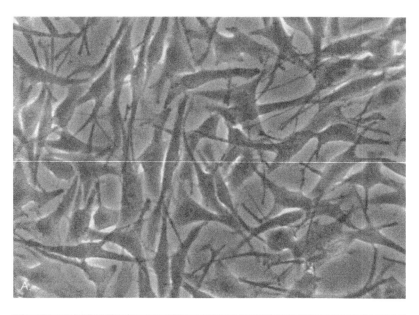

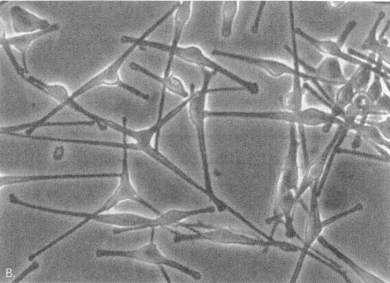

Figure 1 Phase contrast microscopy of cultured human uveal melanocytes. A, Cells cultured with FIC medium; B, cells cultured with TIC medium; C, cells cultured with TIC medium (near confluence); D, senescent uveal melanocytes.

refractile and three-dimensional appearance as compared to cells cultured with bFGF (Fig. 1).

UM cultured with FIC medium grow well, have a doubling time of 2–3 days, and can divide 30–50 times over 3–6 months. Cultured UM never transformed to a continuous cell line. At senescence, the cell growth ceases and the cells become large and disk-like, with an increase of pigmentation [13,15].

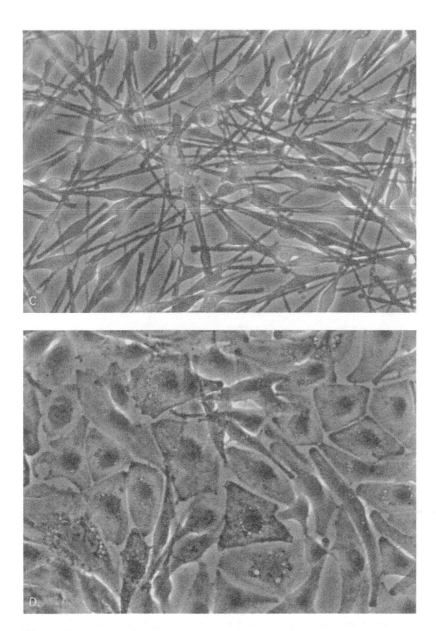

Figure 1 Continued.

Cultured malignant melanoma cells can be epithelium-like or spindle-shaped. They typically display prominent nucleoli and show various degrees of pigmentation (Fig. 2). Cells from amelanotic melanoma can be amelanotic in the initial stage of culture and may then become pigmented after several generations, a result accomplished by a decrease in growth capacity. Noncontinuous melanoma cells

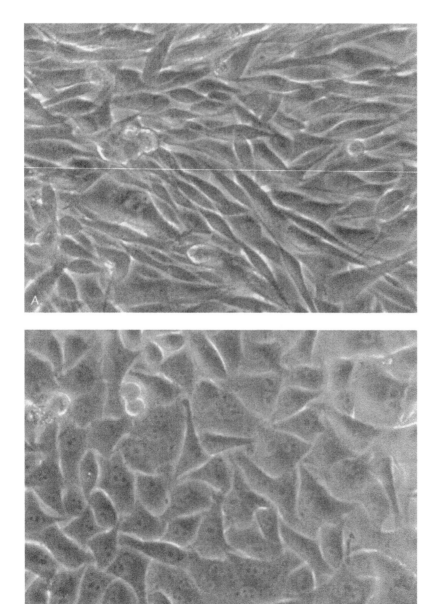

Figure 2   Phase contrast microscopy of cultured human uveal melanoma cells. A, Spindle type; B, epithelioid type; C, mixed type.

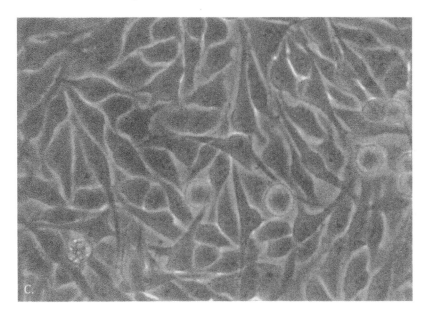

Figure 2   Continued.

have a limited growth capacity and readily become terminally differentiated, showing increased dendrites and pigmentation, cessation of growth, and gradual detachment from the culture dish. A few cell lines of cultured UM have spontaneously transformed into continuous (immortal) cell lines. The continuous cell lines grow faster, have a doubling time of 1.5–2.5 days, maintain melanogenic activity and a certain level of melanin per cell, and can be passaged indefinitely. Three continuous lines of melanoma cells have been established in our lab from cultures isolated from 39 uveal melanomas (most of them primary choroidal melanomas). The incidence of spontaneous transformation is approximately 1 in 10–15 cell lines of uveal melanoma cells.

IV.   GROWTH REQUIREMENTS OF NORMAL UVEAL MELANOCYTES AND MELANOMA CELLS IN VITRO

We have compared the growth requirements of cultured UM to human uveal melanoma cells. Three continuous human uveal melanoma cell lines were established in our lab (M 17, M 21, M 23), and three cell lines (SP6.5, SP8.0, and TP31) were obtained from Dr. Pelletier (Quebec, Canada). All of these cell lines were isolated from primary choroidal melanoma, and have been cultured for more than 3 years with more than 100 cell divisions.

The most striking difference between melanoma cells and UM in vitro is the latter's requirement of a growth stimulator. There are two important groups of growth stimulator in addition to serum, (1) cAMP-elevating agents and (2) bFGF or TPA. UM do not grow in the absence of these factors. In fact, cultured UM cannot survive without these factors [15–17]. UM cultured with culture medium without the bFGF (or TPA) first cease to grow, gradually accumulate pigment, then gradually degenerate, detaching from the culture dish within 7–15 days. In the absence of cAMP-elevating agents (IBMX and cholera toxin), cultured UM lose their dendrites, become bipolar in shape, and grow slowly. They then cease to grow and finally detach from the dish and degenerate within 7–14 days. In contrast, melanoma cells survive and grow well in the culture medium without any growth stimulators (Table 1). The only growth requirement of cultured melanoma cells is serum, which is also required by normal UM. Cultured melanoma cells grow well in the regular culture medium (F12 medium or DMEM medium) with 5–10% serum. Noncontinuous melanoma cell lines grow irregularly but can also survive and grow in serum containing culture medium without bFGF, TPA, and cAMP-elevating agents. Addition of insulin, hydrocortisone, and transferrin to the serum-free medium may prolong the life span of cultured UM and uveal melanoma cells, but these cells eventually lose their growth capacity and viability, indicating that serum contains some undetermined factors that are essential for the survival and growth of UM and melanoma cells in vitro.

The independence of melanoma cells from growth stimulators and the unlimited growth potential of melanoma cells in vivo may be due to the following:

1. The production of growth stimulators by the melanoma cells (autocrine mechanism) to meet the requirements of growth stimulation for the survival and growth of these cells. Cutaneous melanoma cells can produce bFGF and continuously activate the bFGF-receptor kinase [18–20].
2. The response of melanoma cells to some growth stimulators that normally do not affect the growth of uveal melanocytes.
3. Gene mutations that causes constitutive activation of the receptors for these growth stimulators or activation of other components of the signal tranduction pathway [19].

Anchorage independence is a character of malignant cells in vitro. It has been reported that cultured normal uveal melanocytes fail to grow in soft agar, while continuous cell lines of uveal melanoma cells can grow to large colonies in soft agar, indicating that uveal melanoma cells lines possess the ability to grow in an anchorage-independent manner [21].

In cutaneous melanoma, the growth requirements and independence from growth stimulators of melanoma cells are different in various stages of tumor progression. Normal melanocytes require insulin-like growth factor (IGF-1) (one of the main components of the serum for stimulating of growth of melanocytes), bFGF, TPA, and cAMP-elevating agents. Nevus cells can produce bFGF to stimulate the

Table 1   Growth Requirement of Uveal Melanocytes and Melanoma Cells In Vitro

	bFGF/TPA	cAMP-elevating agents	Serum	Anchorage-dependent
Uveal melanocytes	+	+	+	+
Uveal melanoma cells	−	−	+	−

+, requirement for growth and survival; −, not required.

growth of tumor cells (autocrine) and the neovascularization (paracrine). Primary melanoma cells require only IGF-1, and metastatic melanoma cells may not even require IGF-1 [22,23].

V. SIGNAL TRANSDUCTION PATHWAYS OF NORMAL UVEAL MELANOCYTES AND MELANOMA CELLS

We have studied the various signal transduction pathways of the normal uveal melanocytes and compared with those of uveal melanoma cells (Table 2).

A. Cyclic Adenosine Monophosphate (cAMP) System

The effects of cAMP-elevating agents on the growth and differentiation of uveal melanocytes have been tested in vitro. Three different cAMP-elevating agents were selected to represent three different mechanisms for increasing intracellular cAMP level. dbcAMP is capable of penetrating the cell membrane and raising the intracellular cAMP level directly. IBMX raises the intracellular cAMP level by inhibiting cAMP phosphodiesterase. Cholera toxin raises the cAMP level by activating adenylate cyclase, which catalyzes the synthesis of cAMP from intracellular ATP. All three substances show a dose-dependent stimulation of growth and melanogenesis of cultured uveal melanocytes within a certain range, indicating that elevated intracellular cAMP stimulates uveal melanocytes. Concentrations higher than the optimal levels (dbcAMP, 1.0 mM; IBMX, 0.3 mM; and cholera toxin, 100 ng/mL) inhibit growth but not melanogenesis, indicating that a very high level of cAMP may be growth-inhibitory (Fig. 3) [15–17].

At concentrations that stimulate UM, none of the cAMP-elevating agents showed significant effects on the growth of continuous cell lines of uveal melanoma. At the levels slightly higher than those used for culturing UM, cAMP-elevating agents inhibit the growth but stimulate melanogenesis of cultured uveal melanoma cells. The different responses could result from several scenarios. First, a higher basal level of cAMP could be present in melanoma cells as compared to normal melanocytes. Further increasing cAMP level could result in a very high level of cAMP that leads to growth inhibition, Secondarily, the effect of the cAMP elevation after using cAMP-elevating agents is greater in melanoma cells than in melanocytes,

Table 2 Effect of Activation of Signal Transduction Pathways on the Growth of Uveal Melanocytes and Melanoma Cells In Vitro

	cAMP	Tyrosine kinase	PKC	Serine/ Threonine
Uveal melanocytes	++	++	++	−
Uveal melanoma cells	0	+	−	−

++, marked stimulating effects; +, stimulating effects; 0, no effects; −, inhibiting effects.

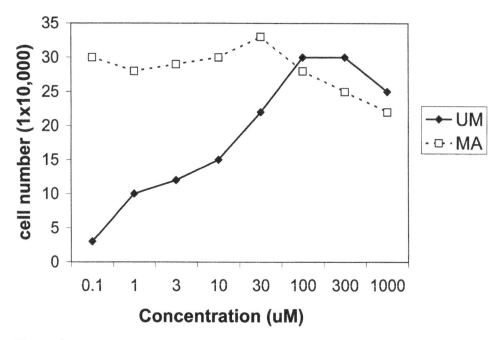

Figure 3 Effect of cAMP-elevating agents on the growth of uveal melanocytes and melanoma cells. Cells were cultured in culture medium with various concentrations of cAMP-elevating agents (IBMX). Number of cells after 6 days of culture were plotted against the concentrations (micromoles) of IBMX.

likewise leading to growth inhibition. Lastly, melanoma cells might intrinsically differ from their normal counterparts in their response to elevation of cAMP levels. Study of the basal level of cAMP and level of cAMP after use of cAMP-elevating agents in UM and melanoma cells may be helpful in elucidating the differing responses of these cells to activation of the cAMP system.

B. Tyrosine Kinase System

bFGF was selected as a representative tyrosine kinase activator. bFGF significantly stimulates the growth of cultured UM. It also stimulates the growth of cultured uveal melanoma cells to a much lesser degree (Fig. 4). Other growth factors, which activate the tyrosine kinase system, such as hepatocyte growth factor (HGF), and fibroblast growth factor-6 (FGF-6), have similar results on both cultured UM and melanoma cells [15]. These results indicate that activation of the tyrosine kinase system has a growth-stimulating effect on both normal and malignant melanocytes in vitro.

C. Protein Kinase C (PKC) System

TPA is a PKC activator; it stimulates growth and melanogenesis of cultured UM [15–17]. In contrast, TPA inhibits the growth of all six continuous cell lines of uveal melanoma cells (also all noncontinous cell lines) in our lab (Fig. 5). Therefore,

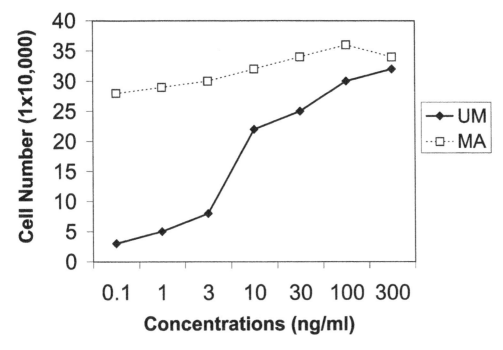

Figure 4 Effect of bFGF on the growth of uveal melanocytes and melanoma cells. Cells were cultured in culture medium with various concentrations of bFGF. Number of cells after 6 days of culture were plotted against the concentrations (nanograms per milliliter) of bFGF.

activation of the PKC system seems to have the opposite effect on the growth of UM and melanoma cells in vitro. Further investigation of the levels of various PKC isozymes in UM and uveal melanoma cells and the interaction between the isozymes and other proteins or growth factor receptors may be helpful in elucidating the role of the PKC system in the uveal melanoma cells.

D. Serine/Threonine Kinase System

The receptors of transforming growth factor (TGF-β) have intrinsic serine/threonine kinase activity. TGF-β inhibits the growth of both cultured normal uveal melanocytes and continuous cell lines of uveal melanoma (15,24).

E. Calcium Channel System

Many effects of calcium as a second messenger are mediated by calcium-binding proteins. The expression of various calcium-binding proteins in the normal uveal melanocytes and melanoma cells will be discussed later.

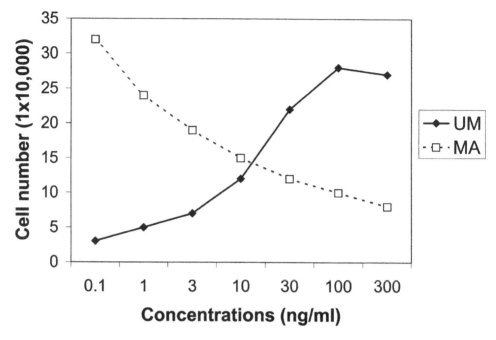

Figure 5   Effect of TPA on the growth of uveal melanocytes and melanoma cells. Cells were cultured in culture medium with various concentrations of TPA. Number of cells after 6 days of culture were plotted against the concentrations of TPA (nanograms per milliliter).

VI.   EFFECTS OF VARIOUS SUBSTANCES ON UVEAL MELANOCYTES AND UVEAL MELANOMA CELLS

The effects of various growth factors, hormones, neurotransmitters and prostaglandins have been studied by us and others (Table 3).

A.   Growth Factors

bFGF and HGF stimulate the growth of cultured human UM. HGF has a potent stimulating effect on the migration of UM. Fibroblast growth factor-6 (FGF-6) and keratinocyte growth factor (KGF) show similar but less stimulatory effects [15].

Table 3   Effects of Various Substances on the Growth of Uveal Melanocytes and Melanoma Cells In Vitro

	bFGF	HGF	EGF	TNF-α	α-MSH	Melatonin	PGE	PGF$_{2\alpha}$
Uveal melanocytes	++	+	0	−	0	0	+	0
Melanoma cells	+	+	+	−	0	−	+	0

++, marked stimulating effects; +, stimulating effects; 0, no effects; −, inhibiting effects.

Other growth factors, such as epidermal growth factor (EGF), nerve growth factor (NGF), platelet-derived growth factor AB (PDGF), vascular endothelial growth factor (VEGF), and acidic fibroblast growth factor (aFGF), do not have any effect on growth and melanogenesis in uveal melanocytes in vitro [15,16].

bFGF also stimulates the growth of both continuous and noncontinuous cell lines of uveal melanoma cells, but to a lesser degree. In addition to the direct effects on the uveal melanoma cells, bFGF is a potent stimulator for neovascularization.

HGF stimulates the growth and migration of cultured uveal melanoma cells. This effect is very peculiar, because in most malignant tumors, HGF does not stimulate the growth of tumor cells but only stimulates neovascularization. The direct growth-stimulation effect and the strong chemoattraction effect of HGF on uveal melanoma cells may provide an explanation for the observation that melanoma most commonly metastasizes to the liver.

EGF stimulated the growth of two of three continuous cell lines of uveal melanoma in our lab, whereas it did not have any growth stimulating effects on cultured normal UM. This may be an example of a malignant cell's ability to respond to some growth factors that do not normally stimulate its normal, nonneoplastic counterpart.

TGF-β2 shows marked inhibitory effects on the growth of UM [24]. The cause of unlimited growth of melanoma cells may be due to the loss of response of melanoma cells to growth-inhibiting factors that normally limit the growth of UM. TGF-β2 can be one of the candidates of these growth-inhibiting factors. It has been reported that loss of TGF-β2 receptor expression occurs in some cases of uveal melanoma. However, TGF-β2 does have a potent growth inhibiting effects on all five tested continuous cell lines of uveal melanoma cells in our lab. Therefore, the role of TGF-β2 in the occurrence of uveal melanoma still requires further investigation. TGF-β2 not only has a direct effect on the uveal melanoma cells but may also inhibit neovascularization and the immune response to the melanoma and influence the susceptibility of uveal melanoma cells to natural killer cell-mediated cytotoxic effects [26,27]. Therefore the effect of TGF-β2 on uveal melanoma is a complicated one and requires further study.

B. Cytokines

Both interleukin-l (IL-1) and tumor necrosis factor alpha (TNF-α) inhibit the growth and melanogenesis of cultured UM and uveal melanoma cells. Interleukin-6 (IL-6) had mild inhibitory effects on growth and melanogenesis of UM and uveal melanoma cells [15].

C. Hormones

Melatonin is an endogenous neurohormone produced in the pineal gland, the hypothalamus, and the eye. Melatonin has been found to inhibit the growth of a variety of malignant cell lines in vitro, including malignant dermal melanoma [28–30]. In human cells, melatonin can act through two membrane receptors (Mel$_{1a}$ and Mel$_{1b}$) and perhaps a putative nuclear receptor [31]. We found that melatonin and its membrane receptor agonists do not have effects on growth and melanogenesis of UM in vitro. However, reverse-transcribed PCR studies detected the presence of melatonin membrane receptors (Mel_{1b}) in UM [31]. It is not known whether these receptors are functionless or have effects on functions other than those we have tested.

We have studied the effects of melatonin, its precursors, and derivatives on the growth of several continuous cell lines of uveal melanoma cells [31–33]. Melatonin and its membrane receptor agonists (6-chloromelatonin, the Mel_{1a}-$_{1b}$ receptor agonist, and S-20098, the Mel_{1b} receptor agonist) inhibit the growth of cultured uveal melanoma cells [31]. The precursors of melatonin (tryptophan and serotonin) and the abnormal metabolites of tryptophan (kynurenine) do not inhibit the growth of uveal melanoma cells [33]. RNA encoding the Mel_{1b} receptor is also expressed in uveal melanoma cells [31]. These findings indicate that changes in the metabolic processes of melatonin may play a role in the pathogenesis of uveal melanoma. The antiproliferative effect of melatonin on uveal melanoma cells occurs in the range of nM–pM, which is comparable to the reported levels of melatonin in the aqueous humor (2 nM) [31]. The decrease of melatonin in the body fluid in aged individual may play a role in the occurrence of several types of malignant tumors. In the clinical treatment of metastatic cancer, a synergistic oncostatic effect between IL-2 immunotherapy and melatonin has been reported. This effect may be explained by the therapeutic replacement of depleted melatonin [34,35].

Endothelin 1 stimulates growth and melanogenesis of UM [15]. The effect of endothelin on cultured melanoma cells has not been studied.

Controversy still exists concerning the existence of melanocortin-1 receptors in uveal melanocytes [36,37]. We have studied the effect of α-melanocyte-stimulating hormone (α-MSH) and ACTH on the UM in cAMP-deleted medium in 12 cell lines and could not find significant effects on growth and melanogenesis of cultured UM [15], while they usually showed stimulating effects on cultured epidermal melanocytes. α-MSH also does not affect the growth and differentiation of cultured uveal melanoma cells.

Progesterone and estradiol does not have significant effects on growth and melanogenesis of cultured UM [15].

D. Neurotransmitters

The effect of neurotransmitters on melanocytes was studied extensively and systematically first in the UM [38]. The adrenergic agonist epinephrine, which activates both α- and β-adrenergic receptors, stimulates growth and melanogenesis of cultured UM in cAMP-depleted medium. Methoxamine and clonidine, which activate α_1- and α_2-adrenergic receptors, show no effects. Isoproterenol, which activates β_1- and β_2-receptors, stimulates growth and melanogenesis of cultured UM in cAMP-depleted medium. The β_2 receptor agonists, metaproterenol and salbutamol also show stimulating effects; but the β_1 and β_3 receptor agonists (metaproterenol and D-7114), do not have any effects. These results indicate that adrenergic agonists stimulate growth and melanogenesis of UM in vitro. This effect is mainly through the adrenergic β_2 receptors [38].

The cholinergic agonist muscarine inhibits growth and melanogenesis of UM. These studies indicate that the growth and melanogenesis of UM are modulated by reciprocal innervation. Adrenergic agonists stimulate and cholinergic agonists inhibit the growth and melanogenesis of UM [38].

The effects of neurotransmitters on the uveal melanoma cells require further investigation.

E. Prostaglandins (PGs)

The effect of PGs on uveal melanocytes has been studied extensively and systematically because of the side effect of iris pigmentation caused by several PGs used in the treatment of glaucoma. PGE_2, PGE_1, and PGA_2 stimulate the growth and melanogenesis of cultured UM in cAMP-deleted medium [39,40]. The EP_2 receptor agonist AH13205 causes stimulation, but the EP_1 and EP_3 receptor agonist (sulprostone) and EP_4 receptor agonist (ONO-AE1–329) do not have any effect. Therefore, the PGEs and PGA_2 may stimulate the UM through activation of EP_2 receptors [40]. This result is consistent with the known function of EP_2 receptors [41] and the increase in iris pigmentation of monkey eyes following local application of PGE_2, a natural EP_2 agonist [42]. PGD_2 stimulates growth and melanogenesis of cultured UM at relatively high concentrations, but a DP receptor agonist (BW 245C) does not have stimulatory effect. Furthermore, the PGD_2 stimulatory effect cannot be blocked by a DP receptor antagonist (BW A868C), indicating that the effect of PGD_2 may involve receptors other than the DP receptor subtype [40]. One of the TP receptor agonists (AGN 192093) stimulates growth and melanogenesis of cultured uveal melanocytes; however, another TP receptor agonists (U-46619) does not have any effect. Therefore, the mechanism of action of AGN 192093 needs further investigation [40]. The IP receptor agonists (cicaprost and iloprost) do not have stimulating effects [40].

Latanoprost, a $PGF_{2\alpha}$ analogue and antiglaucoma drug, causes iris pigmentation in about 10% of glaucoma patients [43]. But $PGF_{2\alpha}$, latanoprost, and PhXA85 (the active form of latanoprost) do not stimulate melanogenesis and growth of cultured iridal melanocytes from blue, green, and brown irides and one cell line from mixed-colored iris in various tested media [15,39]. Clinical observations indicate latanoprost-induced iris pigmentation mainly occurs in patients with mixed colored irides [43]. It is possible that latanoprost only selectively stimulates the iridal melanocytes from mixed colored irides. In another series of studies we found that latanoprost increased transcription of the tyrosinase gene in iridal melanocytes from the mixed color iris but not in those from blue and brown irides [44]. Another possibility is that the effect of $PGF_{2\alpha}$ may be indirect. For example, it may stimulate other types of cells to produce some substances that stimulate melanogenesis in UM, or it activates uveal melanocytes to respond to some substances that normally do not have melanogenic activity.

It has been reported that $PGF_{2\alpha}$, latanoprost, and PhXA85 have no effect on the cell number and mitotic activity of cultured human uveal or cutaneous melanoma cells [45,46]. PGE_1 and PGE_2 induce tyrosinase activity of murine melanoma cell lines, whereas they produce only little if any increase in tyrosinase activity in continuous human uveal melanoma cells [46]. The effects of $PGF_{2\alpha}$ and latanoprost on melanogenesis of human or murine melanoma cell lines are conflicting. Some authors reported that $PGF_{2\alpha}$ and latanoprost increase tyrosinase activity in murine melanoma cells lines (S91 and B16) [46]; other groups have reported that these PGs do not stimulate melanogenesis of S91 cell lines [47]. It has been suggested that the in vivo iris pigmentation side effect of latanoprost is not related to an increase in cell growth but results from elevated tyrosinase activity [46].

VII. EXPRESSION OF VARIOUS SUBSTANCES IN UVEAL MELANOCYTES AND MELANOMA CELLS

Uveal melanoma cells may produce (1) various substances that stimulate their own growth (autocrine) or the growth of other cells, such as vascular endothelial cells (paracrine) or (2) various substances that can faciliate their invasive and metastatic potential. The expression of several growth factors and cytokines has been studied in uveal melanoma cells [26]. However, without the comparative quantitative studies in of uveal melanocytes, it would not be known whether this expression is common to both normal and malignant melanocytes or truly a feature of malignant cells.

Here, we summarized the results of several comparative studies of UM and uveal melanoma cells in vitro (Table 4).

A. Vascular Endothelial Growth Factor (VEGF)

VEGF stimulates the growth of vascular endothelial cells, enhances the permeability of blood vessels, and induces angiogenesis. It may therefore play an important role in the pathogenesis of melanoma.

We have studied the production of VEGF by cultured UM using the ELISA method and found that a relatively high amount of VEGF is present in the conditioned medium of UM. VEGF mRNA is also detected in the cultured UM by RT-PCR methods. VEGF levels in the conditioned medium of human uveal melanoma cells and the expression of VEGF mRNA in melanoma cells are 30–40 times higher than that of normal UM. Increased production of VEGF by melanoma cells can stimulate angiogenesis and may play a role in the development, invasion, and metastasis of uveal melanoma.

Expression of VEGF by uveal melanoma cells has been demonstrated in six other continuous cell lines of human primary uveal melanoma (92–1, Mel-202, OCM-1, OCM-3, OCM-8, and EOM-3) and one cell line from a human metastatic uveal melanoma [26]. Therefore virtually all known continuous cell lines of human uveal melanoma express VEGF.

Table 4   Expression of Various Genes of Uveal Melanocytes and Uveal Melanoma Cells In Vitro

	VEGF	t-PA	MMP	Integrin $\alpha 5$	Cell invasion
Uveal melanocytes	+	+	+	+	0
Uveal melanoma cells	++	++	++	0–+	+

++, marked expression; +, expression; 0, no expression.

B. Tissue Plasminogen Activator (t-PA)

t-PA is a serine protease that catalyzes the conversion of plaminogen to plasmin. Plasmin degrades various matrix proteins, activates matrix metalloproteinases, and may induce the invasion and metastasis of malignant cells.

We have studied free plasminogen activity of cultured UM and compared it to that of the continuous cell lines of uveal melanoma cells. We also determined the plasminogen activator type by fibrinography and antibody blocking (anti-t-PA and u-PA antibodies). Free PA activity is found in the conditioned medium of both UM and uveal melanoma cells. The predominant PA activity is t-PA. Normal uveal melanocytes produce t-PA ($3.23\,IU/10^5$ cells per 24 hr), which is significantly less than that of uveal melanoma cells ($11.0\,IU/10^5$ cells per 24 hr). Western blot studies revealed that the majority of t-PA in conditioned media is one chain t-PA.

PA plays a role in the development, invasion and metastasis of malignant tumors. The increased levels of PA are usually present as u-PA in most types of malignant tumors [48,49]. However, melanoma is an exception. A number of studies indicate that the t-PA level is increased in the dermal melanoma cells in vivo and in vitro [48,49]. t-PA can be isolated from cultured melanoma cells, and melanoma cells in vitro make more t-PA than other tumors, enabling the cells to degrade extracellular matrix and to migrate through reconstituted matrix [49]. This increase in t-PA expression has also been demonstrated in pathological specimens of human uveal melanoma, in cultured human uveal melanoma cells, and in experimental animal melanoma models [49–52]. It has also been reported that t-PA is involved in the metastasis of murine uveal melanomas [50]. t-PA is found more abundantly in uveal melanomas with a less favorable prognosis [51]. In our in vitro study, cultured uveal melanoma cells produced more t-PA than UM. The increased production of t-PA may play a role in the invasion and metastasis of uveal melanoma.

C. Calcium-Binding Proteins

Several calcium-binding proteins are involved in the cellular pathways that endow tumor cells with special properties related to their malignant and metastatic phenotypes [53]. For example, S100A6 is a cell cycle-related gene that is overexpressed in several human tumors. Cap g regulates actin polymerization in response to changes in the level of calcium or PIP2. Changes in cell shape associated with growth and migration are essential events during tumorigenesis and require the regulation of the cytoskeleton. S100A11 is associated with cytoskeletal elements and may function by inhibiting PKC. A comparative study of expression of various calcium-binding proteins in cultured normal UM and cutaneous and uveal melanoma cell lines using immunobloting method revealed that these calcium-binding proteins are differently expressed in these cell lines [53]. Normal UM express significantly lower levels of each of the calcium-binding proteins (annexin VI, cap g, S100A6, and S100A11) when compared to uveal melanoma cells; only the level of annexinV is comparable. Cap g is expressed in all melanoma cell lines but not in normal UM. Both cap g and S100A11 are expressed at lower levels in the cutaneous melanoma cells as compared to uveal melanoma cells. S100A6 is expressed at higher levels in the two melanoma cell lines with the shortest doubling times. Western blot analysis showed that S100B is expressed in melanoma cell lines, while S100A is not detected. All calcium-binding proteins identified in cultured cells could be detected in ocular melanoma specimens by immunoblotting methods. Based on these results, it has been suggested that the expression of S100A6 may correlate with the malignant properties of the tumor [53].

D. Cell Invasion Ability

Cell invasion ability of cultured normal and malignant cells can be determined by culturing the cells in the Boyden chamber. This consists of two chambers separated by a filter that can be coated with basement membrane extracellular matrix (ECM). Cells with culture medium are added to the upper chamber, and the bottom chamber is filled with culture medium. After culture for a certain period of time, cells are fixed and examined. The cells that have penetrated to the bottom side of the filter are counted and used for evaluating the invasive and migratory capacities of cells in vitro [21].

Beliveau and others compared the invasive capacity of cultured uveal melanocytes and four continuous cell lines of human uveal melanoma cells (SP6.5, SP.81, TP31, and TP17) and found that only a small number of cultured UM can migrate through the filter. Melanoma cell lines migrate through the filter better than UM. TP17, which is the most malignant cell line, has an epithelioid morphology and the shortest doubling time. It was the most invasive cell line in this study [21].

E. Matrix Metalloproteinases (MMPs)

MMPs are a group of enzymes that degrade the ECM. MMP-2 and MMP-9, also known as gelatinase A and B, respectively, or type IV collagenase of 72 and 92 kDa, can degrade collagen type IV and V, which are the essential components of the basal membrane. Increased expression of these proteolytic enzymes can lead to degradation of the ECM, accelerate angiogenesis, and enhance the invasion and metastasis of malignant tumors. Studies in pathological specimens of uveal melanoma showed that uveal melanoma cells expressed MMP-2 and /or MMP-9. The expression of MMP-2 and MMP-9 is associated with a poor prognosis [54,55].

A comparative study of expression of MMPs in cultured UM and uveal melanoma cells using gelatine zymography revealed that MMP-2 can be detected in the culture medium of UM and uveal melanoma cells. In addition, the most malignant cell line of melanoma (TP17) also expressed an MMP with an apparent molecular weight of 117 kDa, which is not detected in the medium from other melanoma cell lines or normal UM.

F. Integrins

Integrins are receptor proteins that bind the cell to the ECM (e.g., fibronectin). Integrin consists of two subunits (α and β). Downregulation of $\alpha 5 \beta 1$ integrin has been observed in several malignant cell lines [21].

Expression of integrin $\alpha 5$ has been studied in cultured UM and uveal melanoma cells by antibody inhibition of cell adhesion and flow cytometry. A moderate level of the $\alpha 5$ integrin subunit is detected in cultured UM. A low level of the $\alpha 5$ integrin subunit is detected in several less malignant melanoma cell lines. No expression of this integrin subunit is detected in the highly tumorigenic and invasive TP17 cells. RT-PCR analysis revealed a moderate level of $\alpha5$ mRNA in the least tumorigenic melanoma cell line (SP65), whereas the most malignant melanoma cell line (TP17) expressed the lowest level of $\alpha5$ in all four cell lines tested. These results indicate that expression of the $\alpha5$ subunit inversely correlates with the tumorigenic abilities of all the uveal melanoma cell lines tested [21].

VIII. SUMMARY

1. The development of methods for cultivation and in vitro study of human UM and uveal melanoma cells has provided an invaluable model system for comparing these cell types and understanding their cell biology. This is critical for the elucidation of the pathogenesis of uveal melanoma.

2. The most striking difference between UM and melanoma cells in vitro is the UM's requirement of the growth stimulators. Two groups of growth stimulators, bFGF (or TPA) and cAMP-elevating agents, are essential for the survival and growth of UM. These are not required by melanoma cells. This independence from growth stimulators may lead to the unlimited growth of melanoma cells in vivo. This may be due to (1) intrinsic production of growth stimulators by melanoma cells; (2) the response of melanoma cells to some growth stimulators that normally do not affect the growth of UM; or (3) gene mutations cause constitutive activation of the receptors for these growth stimulators or activation of other components of the signal tranduction pathway.

3. Although the effects of activation of several signal transduction pathways (such as the tyrosine kinase system) on the growth and differentiation of melanocytes and melanoma cells are similar, differences are present in several other signal transduction pathways, such as the cAMP system and the PKC system. The mechanism and significance of these differences will require further investigation.

4. An important difference in the response to various biological substances by UM and melanoma cells in vitro is that the melanoma cells respond to some growth stimulators that normally do not affect the growth of UM (e.g., EGF). This may be one of the causes for the unlimited growth of melanoma cells in vivo. Many factors that have been tested in cultured UM have not been tested in melanoma cells. Further study of the effects of these factors on cultured uveal melanoma cells may provide important clues to its pathogenesis. The most striking difference between uveal melanoma cells and other malignant cells in vitro is that HGF is a potent growth stimulator and chemoattractant for uveal melanoma cell. This may help explain why liver metastasis is common in this tumor.

5. The expression of several genes in melanoma cells contrasts with their expression in UM. Uveal melanoma cells produce more growth factors (VEGF) to stimulate the growth of vascular endothelial cells and to induce angiogenesis or to produce a greater amount of factors (t-PA and MMPs) that degrade the ECM, generating a microenvironment favorable for

tumor invasion and metastasis. This correlates with the invasive and metastatic properties of the uveal melanoma in vivo.

6. Although comparative studies of UM and melanoma cells in vitro during the past decade have led to a better understanding of the difference between these cells, many aspects of the cell biology of these cells still require further study. For example, cutaneous melanoma cells produce many growth factors and their receptors to stimulate their own growth (autocrine) or the growth of other cells (paracrine), which allows their expansion, invasion, and metastasis. Very little is known about the production of growth factors by cultured UM and uveal melanoma cells. Studies in this field may be helpful in elucidating the pathogenesis of uveal melanoma.

REFERENCES

1. Jakobiec FA. Ocular Anatomy, Embryology and Tetratology. New York: Harper & Row, 1982.
2. Eagle RC. Iris pigmentation and pigmented lesions: An ultrastructural study. Trans Am Ophthalmol Soc 1988; 84:579–687.
3. Wilkerson CL, Syed NA, Fisher MR, Robinson NL, Wallow IHL, Albert DM. Melanocytes and iris color: Light microscopy findings, Arch Ophthalmol 1996; 114:437–442.
4. Imesch PD, Bindley CD, Khademian Z, Ladd B, Gangnon R, Albert DM, Wallow IHL. Melanocytes and iris color: Electron microscopy findings. Arch Ophthalmol 1996; 114:443–447.
5. Prota G, Hu DN, Vincensi MR, McCormick SA, Napolitano A. Characterization of melanins in human irides and cultured uveal melanocytes from eyes of different colors. Exp Eye Res 1998; 67:293–299.
6. Prota G. Melanins and Melanogenesis. San Diego, CA: Academic Press, 1992.
7. Green WR. Uveal tract. In: Spencer WH, eds. Ophthalmic Pathology: An Atlas and Textbook, Vol. 3, 3rd ed. Philadelphia: Saunders, 1986:1375–1414, 1527, 2024–2025.
8. Yanoff M, Fine BS. Ocular Pathology, 4th ed. London: Mosby-Wolfe, 1996.
9. Proia AD. Inflammation. In: Garner A, Klintworth GK, eds. Pathobiology of Ocular Diseases. 2nd ed. New York: Marcel Dekker, 1994, pp 89–90.
10. Kampik A, Patrinely JR, Green WR. Morphologic and clinical feature of retrocorneal melanin pigmentation and pigmented pupillary membranes: Review of 225 cases. Surv Ophthalmol 1982; 27:161–180.
11. Weiss DI, Krohn DL. Benign melanocytic glaucoma complicating oculodermal melanocytosis. Ann Ophthalmol 1971; 3:958–963.
12. Snip RC, Green WR, Kreutzer, Hirst LW, Kenyon KR. Posterior corneal pigmentation and fibrous proliferation by iris melanocytes. Arch Ophthalmol 1981; 99:1232–1238.
13. Hu DN, McCormick SA, Ritch R, Pelton-Henrion K. Studies of human uveal melanocytes in vitro: Isolation, purification and cultivation of human uveal melanocytes, Invest Ophthalmol Vis Sci 1993; 33:2210–2219.
14. Hu DN, McCormick SA, Orlow SJ, Rosemblat S, Lin AY, Wo K. Melanogenesis in cultured human uveal melanocytes, Invest Ophthalmol Vis Sci 1995; 36:931–938.
15. Hu DN. Regulation of growth and melanogenesis of uveal melanocytes. Pigment Cell Res 2000; 13 (Suppl 8):81–86.

16. Hu DN, McCormick SA, Ritch R. Studies of human uveal melanocytes in vitro: Growth regulation of cultured human uveal melanocytes. Invest Ophthalmol Vis Sci 1993; 34:2220–2227.

17. Hu DN, McCormick SA, Orlow SJ, Rosemblat S, Lin AY. Regulation of melanogenesis by human uveal melanocytes in vitro. Exp Eye Res 1997; 64:397–404.

18. Herlyn M, Shih IM. Interaction of melanocytes and melanoma cells with the microenvironment. Pigment Cell Res 1994; 7:81–88.

19. Halbban R, Moellmann G. Proliferation and malignant transformation of melanocytes. Crit Rev Oncogen 1990; 2:247–258.

20. Rodeck U, Melber K, Kath R, Menssen HD, Varello M, Atkinson B, Herlyn M. Constitutive expression of multiple growth factor genes by melanoma cells but not normal melanocytes. J Invest Dermatol 1991; 97:20–26.

21. Beliveau A, Berube M, Rousseau A, Pelletier G, Guerin SL. Expression of integrin $\alpha 5\beta 1$ and MMPs associated with epithelioid morphology and malignancy of uveal melanoma. Invest Ophthalmol Vis Sci 2000; 41:2363–2372.

22. Shih IM, Herlyn M. Role of growth factors and their receptors in the development and progression of melanoma. J Invest Dermatol 1993; 100:196S–203S.

23. Mancianti S, Gyorfi T, Shih IM, Valyi-Nagy I, Levengood G, Menssen HD, Halpern AC, Elder DE, Herlyn M. Growth regulation of cultured human nevus cells. J Invest Dermatol 1993; 100:281S–287S.

24. Hu DN, McCormick SA, Lin AY, Lin JY. TGF-β2 inhibits growth of uveal melanocytes at physiological concentrations. Exp Eye Res 1998; 67:143–150.

25. Myatt N, Aristodemou P, Neale MH, Foss AJ, Hungerford JL, Bhattacharya S, Cree IA. Abnormalities of the transforming growth factor-beta pathway in ocular melanoma. J Pathol 2000; 192:511–518.

26. Ijland SA, Jager MJ, Heijdra BM, Westphal JR, Peek R. Expression of angiogenic and immunosuppressive factors by uveal melanoma cell lines. Melanoma Res 1999; 9:445–450.

27. Ma D, Niederkorn JY. Transforming growth factor-β down-regulates major histocompatibility complex class I antigen expression and increase the susceptibility of uveal melanoma cells to natural killer cell–mediated cytolysis. Immunology 1995; 86:263–269.

28. Sze SF, Ng TB, Liu WK. Antiproliferative effect of pineal indoles on cultured tumor cell lines. J Pineal Res 1993; 14:27–33.

29. Shellare SA, Whelan RDH, Hill BT. Growth inhibitory and cytotoxic effects of melatonin and its metabolites on human tumour cell lines in vitro. Br J Cancer 1989; 60:288–290.

30. Slominski A, Pruski D. Melatonin inhibits proliferation and melanogenesis in rodent melanoma cells. Exp Cell Res 1993; 206:189–194.

31. Roberts JE, Wiechmann AF, Hu DN. Melatonin receptors in human uveal melanocytes and melanoma cells. J Pineal Res 2000; 28:165–171.

32. Hu DN, Roberts JE. Melatonin inhibits growth of cultured human uveal melanoma cells. Melanoma Res 1997; 7:27–31.

33. Hu DN, McCormick SA, Roberts JE. Effects of melatonin, its precursors and derivatives on the growth of cultured human uveal melanoma cells. Melanoma Res 1998; 8:201–210.

34. Lissoni P, Barni S, Cattaneo G. Clinical results with the pineal hormone melatonin in advanced cancer resistant to standard antitumor therapies. Oncology 1991; 48:448–450.

35. Lissoni P, Barni S, Tancini G. A randomized study with subcutaneous low-dose interleukin 2 alone vs interleukin 2 plus the pineal neurohormone melatonin in advanced solid neoplasms other than renal cancer and melanoma. Br J Cancer 1994; 69:196–199.

36. Zhao H, Li L, Boissy RE, Nordlund JJ. Ocular melanocytes express beta-adrenergic receptor and respond to autonomic neurotransmitters. Pigment Cell Res 1997; 10:119–120.

37. Mac Neil S, Hay D, Wagner M, Morandini R, Ghanem. Dual signaling by human melanocortin-1 (MC-1) receptor in melanocytes and melanoma cells. Pigment Cell Res 1999; 12(Suppl 7):37.

38. Hu DN, Woodward DF, McCormick SA. Influence of autonomic neurotransmitters on human uveal melanocytes in vitro. Exp Eye Res 2000; 71:217–224.

39. Hu DN, Stjernschantz J, McCormick SA. Effect of prostaglandin A_2, E_1, $F_{2\alpha}$, and latanoprost on cultured human iridal melanocytes. Exp Eye Res 2000; 70:113–120.

40. Hu, DN, McCormick SA, Woodward DF. A functional study of prostanoid receptors involved in cultured human iridal melanocyte stimulation. Exp Eye Res 2001; 73:93–100.

41. Coleman RA, Smith WL, Narumiya S. Classification of prostanoid receptors: Properties, distribution, and structure of the receptors and their subtypes. Pharmacol Rev 1994; 46:205–229.

42. Selen G, Stjernschantz J, Resul B. Prostaglandin-induced iridial pigmentation in primates. Surv Ophthalmol 1997; 41:S125–S128.

43. Wistrand PJ, Stjernschantz J, Olsson K. The incidence and time-course of latanoprost-induced iridal pigmentation as a function of eye color. Surv Ophthalmol 1997; 41:S129–S138.

44. Stjernschantz J, Ocklind A, Wentzel P, Lake S, Hu DN. Latanoprost-induced increase of tyrosinase transcription in iridial melanocyte. Acta Ophthalmol Scand. 2000; 78:618–622.

45. Imesch PD, Wallow IHL, Albert DM. The color of the human eye: A review of morphologic correlates and of some conditions that affect iridial pigmentation. Surv Ophthalmol 1997; 41:S117–S123.

46. Dutkiewicz R, Albert DM, Levin LA. Effects of latanoprost on tyrosinase activity and mitotic index of cultured melanoma lines. Exp Eye Res 2000; 70:563–569.

47. Krauss AHP, Shi L, Spada CS, Regan JW, Woodward DF. S91 cells stably transfected with prostaglandin FP receptors fail to respond to PGF2α. Pigment Cell Res 1999; 12(suppl 7):68–69.

48. Duffy MJ. Plasminogen activators and cancer. Blood Coagul Fibrinolysis 1990; 1:681–687.

49. De Vries TJ, van Muijen GN, Ruiter DJ. The plasminogen activation system in tumour invasion and metastasis. Pathol Res Pract 1996; 192:718–733.

50. Alizadeh H, Ma D, Berman M, Bellingham D, Comerford A, Gething MJ, Sambrook JE, Niederkorn JY. Tissue plasminogen activator-induced invasion and metastasis of murine melanomas. Curr Eye Res 1995; 14:449–458.

51. De Vries TJ, Mooy CM, Balken MR, Luyten GP, Quax PH, Verspaget HW, Weidle UH, Ruiter DJ, van Muijen GN. Components of the plasminogen activation system in uveal melanoma—A clinico-pathological study. J Pathol 1995; 175:59–67.

52. Park SS, Korn TS, Mitra MM. Niederkorn JY. Effect of transforming growth factor-beta on plasminogen activator production of cultured human uveal melanoma cells. Curr Eye Res 1996; 15:755–763.

53. Van Ginkel PR, Gee RL, Walker TM, Hu DN, Heizmann CW, Polans AS. The identification and differential expression of calcium-binding proteins associated with ocular melanoma. Biochem Biophy Acta 1998; 1448:290–297.

54. Vaisanen A, Kallioinen M, von Dichoff K, Laatikainen L, Hoyhtya M, Turpeenniemi-Hujanen T. Matrix metalloproteinase-2 (MMP-2) immunoreactive protein—A new prognostic marker in uveal melanoma? J Pathol 1999; 188:56–62.

55. El-Shabrawi Y, Ardjomand N, Radner H, Ardjomand N. MMP-9 is predominantly expressed in epithelioid and not spindle cell uveal melanoma. J Pathol 2001; 194(pt.3A):201–206.

10

p53 and the Molecular Regulation of Cell Fate in Retinoblastoma

ROBERT W. NICKELLS and CASSANDRA L. SCHLAMP

University of Wisconsin, Madison, Wisconsin, U.S.A.

I. THE MOLECULAR ETIOLOGY OF RETINOBLASTOMA—TWO HITS OR THREE?

Retinoblastoma is the most common ocular cancer of children. Several years ago, Knudson noted that the incidence of retinoblastoma followed a statistical pattern of inheritance suggesting the acquisition of two mutations [1]. He proposed the "two-hit" mutation hypothesis as a mechanism of at least initially developing this form of cancer. Comings elaborated on this model shortly thereafter and proposed that the two mutations were actually affecting the two alleles of the same gene [2]. This theory lead to the concept of tumor suppressor proteins and ultimately to the cloning of the retinoblastoma susceptibility gene (*Rb1*) and the characterization of its protein product (pRB) [3–5]. Mutations in both alleles of the *Rb1* gene that lead to protein dysfunction, improper expression, or loss of heterozygosity have been identified in all human retinoblastomas to date.

The 110-kDa pRB protein plays a role in regulating cell growth and differentiation. It is present in a nonphosphorylated state in G0 and G1 and binds to a variety of transcription factors, particularly the E2F family of proteins [6]. This interaction prevents transcription of genes required for DNA synthesis and effectively arrests the cell cycle at the G1/S interface. Phosphorylation of pRB by cyclin-dependent kinases causes the release of E2F and subsequent progression of the cell cycle [7–9].

Several lines of experimental evidence suggest that the function of pRB is important for neuronal differentiation [10]. The levels of pRB rise dramatically in differentiating neuroectoderm of mouse embryos [11] and in tissue culture cells differentiating into neuronal phenotypes [12]. Loss of *Rb1* function, either by the introduction of pRB inactivating viral oncoproteins [13] or by directed mutagenesis in knockout mice, results in the activation of neuronal cell death during the period when these cells would normally be differentiating. It is not clear how loss of pRB activity leads to cell death, but this signal may be associated with elevated levels of free E2F transcription factors [10]. Independent studies indicate that overexpression of E2F1 is sufficient to activate cell death in postmitotic neurons [14,15]. In addition, studies involving chimeric mice indicate that the function of pRB in regulating cell cycle progression is cell-autonomous, but its role in differentiation is cell nonautonomous [6,16]. In chimeric embryos, *Rb1* mutant neuroectoderm cells still exhibit ectopic entry into S phase, like *Rb1*$^{-/-}$ embryos, but—unlike the cells in the knockout animals—they survive and differentiate into neurons. Therefore activation of cell death is likely to be modulated by several factors, such as elevated E2F concentration within the mutant cell and the level of exposure to survival (antideath) signals from neighboring wild-type cells.

Why is loss of pRB function in the developing human eye sufficient to stimulate tumorigenesis? Gallie and colleagues [17] proposed a model that encompasses many of the characteristics observed for pRB function. In their model, a developing retinoblast expresses pRB at the point of their terminal mitosis in the outer (ventricular) region of the neuroblast layer. These cells then migrate to the differentiating ganglion cell and inner nuclear layers, where extensive remodeling of the tissue is regulated by the activation of programmed cell death. *Rb1*$^{-/-}$ mutant cells do not achieve terminal mitosis and are targeted for cell death through a mechanism such as that proposed above. Some cells are able to escape this signal and continue to proliferate exponentially. This model argues that a third genetic hit that disrupts the cell death signaling mechanism is required for retinoblastoma formation. One candidate is a gene with similarity to a mouse kinesin-like protein (termed RBKIN). This gene was recently cloned from a region of chromosome 6p22 that undergoes low-level amplification in a large proportion of tumors [18]. At present, however, it is not known how this gene contributes to the etiology of retinoblastoma.

II. FORMATION OF RETINOBLASTOMA TUMORS—THE CELL OF ORIGIN

Retinoblastomas occur in the developing retina, but the cell of origin is not clear. Histological analyses suggest that tumor masses can form in nearly all layers of the retina, although recent studies suggest that the majority of tumors arise from the inner nuclear layer [17]. Tumors likely develop early in the life of the patient [19–21] and the events leading to a malignancy may occur well before final specification and differentiation of either the photoreceptors or the neurons of the inner nuclear layer, leaving open the possibility that any cell in the retinal neuroblastic layer may be potentially susceptible to Knudson's two hits and/or Gallie's third hit. It is clear, however, that once neuroblasts acquire the *Rb1* null phenotype, they have the potential to differentiate into photoreceptors. Several studies showing either morphological [22], immunogenic [23–25], or molecular [26–28] features of photoreceptor cells have prompted several investigators to suggest that retinoblastomas most frequently arise from precursors of photoreceptor cells. Although this may be the case, it is also plausible that the molecular events leading to retinoblastoma occur so early in the development of the retina that affected cells are stimulated to activate a default pathway of differentiation in the absence of other clear regulatory signals. Specification of the cone cell lineage is one of the first to occur in the embryonic retina and also appears to be one of the least restricted with respect to developmental signals [29,30]. This pathway is consistent with the characteristics of the majority of differentiated retinoblastoma cells [24,26]. The incidence and consequences of differentiation of retinoblastoma cells are discussed further in the following section.

III. CELL FATE IN RETINOBLASTOMA TUMORS

Retinoblastoma tumors are composed of transformed neuroblasts and support cells. Support cells consist primarily of blood vessels derived from the retinal vasculature, and there is evidence that these tumors signal increased growth of vessels. Tumors also contain Müller-like glial cells, particularly in areas of differentiation [19]. Some observers have suggested that this glial cell type is a second form of differentiated tumor cell, based on evidence that immortalized retinoblastoma cells in culture have been found to express glial markers such as glial fibrillary acidic protein [31]. Others have refuted this speculation [19] and suggested that glial cells are derived from nonmalignant cells recruited to regions of differentiated tumor.

Tumor cells have four basic phenotypes. The primary tumor cell type contains variably sized basophilic nuclei and scanty cytoplasm [19] (Figs. 1 and 2). It is likely that these cells represent the direct progeny of the initial neuroblast that developed defects in both alleles of the *Rb1* gene. There are three general fates of these cells in most retinoblastoma tumors (Figs. 1 and 2). The dominant fate is cell death [32]. In a majority of tumors, dying cells or regions of complete cell death make up more than 50% of the tumor mass. Recent studies [32] indicate that the primary mechanism of cell death is through a form of programmed cell death known as apoptosis (Fig. 3), although these regions are classically referred to as necrosis in most pathological descriptions of retinoblastoma [19]. Areas of tumors with features of necrosis are likely the result of secondary necrosis [33]. In these cases, there is such widespread apoptotic death that cellular debris is not effectively cleared by surrogate macrophage activity, leaving it to break down by a more necrotic-like mechanism.

The signal that initiates apoptosis in the primary tumor cell is not known. Some histological features of retinoblastoma suggest that cell death results from nutrient starvation. A compelling example of this is seen in the cuffs of cells that surround a central blood vessel (Fig. 3). These cuffs are sometimes referred to as "pseudorosettes" from their appearance in histological sections. Cells at the center of the cuff have the morphology of the primary tumor cell, while cells at the edges are actively undergoing apoptosis [32]. Burnier and colleagues [34] conducted a morphometric study of these structures and found that cell death occurred at a uniform distance from the central blood vessel ($98.7 \pm 11.9\,\mu m$), suggesting that the reduction in nutrient supply at this region was sufficient to send cells into crisis. Although reduced access to vascular nutrition may be one of the signals that can precipitate apoptosis, there are clearly exceptions to the distance rule, and dying cells

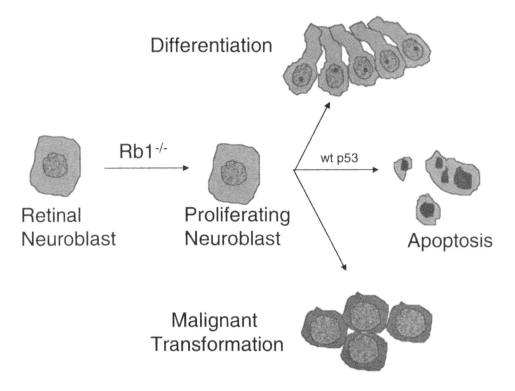

Differentiation

Rb1$^{-/-}$

wt p53

Retinal
Neuroblast

Proliferating
Neuroblast

Apoptosis

Malignant
Transformation

Figure 1   Cell fates in human retinoblastoma. A flow diagram showing the potential fates of immature retinoblasts that have acquired abnormalities in both alleles of the retinoblastoma susceptibility gene (*Rb1*). Once these cells lose pRB function, they enter a period of unregulated division, consistent with the cell-autonomous function of pRB (16). The primary fate of proliferating *Rb1*$^{-/-}$ retinoblasts is to undergo cell death (apoptosis). Studies show that this process is regulated by activation of the p53 tumor suppressor protein. Some cells escape this fate and attempt to differentiate. Morphological, immunohistochemical, and molecular studies indicate that the preferred pathway of differentiation is into a photoreceptor cone phenotype, although some differentiated tumor cells have been found to express rod photoreceptor antigens. On occasion, especially if left untreated, *Rb1*$^{-/-}$ cells become invasive. This third fate may be associated with an additional malignant transformation, perhaps involving another cell cycle regulatory gene or part of the apoptotic signaling pathway. There is some evidence to suggest that this process also involves the immortalization of tumor cells.

can often be found directly adjacent to blood vessels (Fig. 3). Retinoblastoma tumor cells are already primed for cell death because of the lack of functional pRB and their inability to differentiate properly. It is possible that, after a certain number of divisions, tumor cells must make the decision to differentiate or execute the apoptotic program. In the case of the latter, cell death may be a favored fate in cells with abnormally high levels of E2Fs [10].

The second most likely fate of the primary tumor cell is differentiation (Figs. 1 and 2). A majority of retinoblastoma tumors examined in the United States exhibit some degree of differentiation, although the percentage of tumors showing extensive

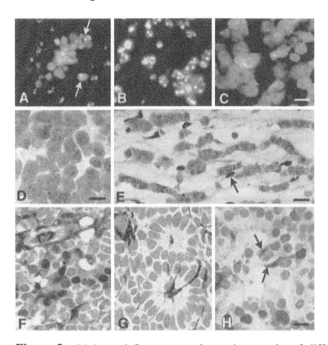

Figure 2 Light and fluorescent photomicrographs of different cell phenotypes in human retinoblastoma tumors. Panels A–C are sections taken from a single tumor and stained with 4,6-diamidino-2-phenylindole (DAPI) to highlight their nuclear morphology. All micrographs are shown at the same magnification. (A) A small cluster of the primary cell type found in retinoblastoma tumors. The nuclear diameter of these cells is typically around 10 μm. Some dying cells are also evident (arrows). (B) Dying tumor cells, with brightly staining nuclear fragments. This morphology is typical of apoptosis, which is associated with nuclear condensation and subsequent fragmentation. (C) Tumor cells that have invaded the choroid. The nuclei of these cells are typically larger than the primary cell type (between 15–20 μm in diameter). No evidence of dying cells is detected. Size bar of A–C = 10 μm. (D) A section stained with hematoxylin and eosin (H&E) showing the primary cell type. The cells have plump nuclei and scanty cytoplasm. Size bar = 10 μm. (E) An H&E-stained section of rows of invading cells found in the choroid. These cells are tightly packed together and have a high nuclear-to-cytoplasm ratio. Pigmented cells (arrow) are choroidal melanocytes. Size bar = 20 μm. (F) A section from a tumor showing cells in early stages of differentiation. The section has been stained for carbonic anhydrase activity (toluidine blue counterstain), which is present in glial cells (dark filamentous structures) and red and green cone photoreceptors (darkly stained nuclei). Unstained cells may represent primary cells that are in early stages of differentiation. It is also noteable that a high proportion of cells contain nucleoli, which are often not seen in cells undergoing rapid mitosis. (G) A section through two Flexner-Wintersteiner rosettes showing the organization typically found in differentiated tumors. The cellular structures pointing toward the interior of the rosette have features of photoreceptor outer segments. In addition, these structures are often associated with glial cells that send processes around the differentiated cells, as evidenced by the dark immunohisto-chemical staining for glial fibrillary acid protein (hematoxylin counterstain). (H) A section through a fleurette. These structures are often considered to represent the most highly differentiated state of cells in tumors. This section has been immunostained for a variant of S antigen (hematoxylin counterstain), which is expressed in rod and blue cone photoreceptors (arrows). Size bar (F–H) = 10 μm. (D–F courtesy of Dr. T. M. Nork, University of Wisconsin. G and H, from Ref. 24.)

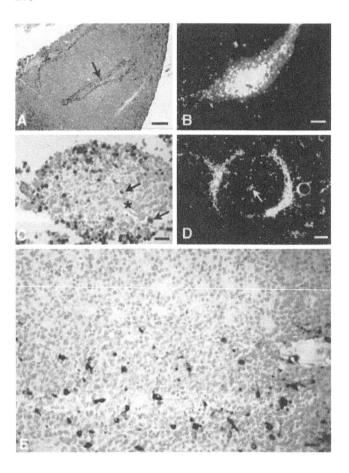

Figure 3 Cell death in retinoblastoma. Dying cells undergo DNA fragmentation. In apoptotic cells, these fragments form multiples of 180 base pairs that can be visualized by gel electrophoresis. Analysis of human retinoblastoma tumors shows clear evidence of these DNA "ladders" [32]. DNA fragmentation can also be detected histologically using methods that attach labels to the ends of fragmented sequences. (A) An H&E-stained section through a tumor showing a region of differentiated cells (note the circular structures indicative of Flexner-Wintersteiner rosettes) that contains a small pocket of "necrosis" (arrow). Size bar = 120 μm. (B) A fluorescent micrograph of an adjacent section taken from the same region shown in (A), stained for DNA fragmentation using a method specific for apoptotic cells (3′ OH overhand ligation [88]). The area of "necrosis" is actually a patch of cells actively undergoing apoptosis. Size bar = 60 μm. (C) A section through a cuff of cells surrounding a central blood vessel (asterisk), commonly referred to as a pseudorosette. The section has been stained for DNA fragmentation using the terminal transferase deoxyUTP end-labeling method (TUNEL) [89]. Dying cells are concentrated around the edge of the cuff, although dying cells can be found throughout the mass, including directly adjacent to the central blood vessel (arrows). Size bar = 30 μm. (D) A fluorescent micrograph of a pseudorosette stained with the 3′ overhang method. As with TUNEL staining, dying cells are concentrated at the periphery of the cuff of cells surrounding a central vessel (arrow). Size bar = 100 μm. (E). A section taken from a tumor showing a clear demarcation between differentiated cells (upper) and undifferentiated primary cells. TUNEL staining shows that dying cells are restricted to the region of primary cells. Size bar = 40 μm. (C and E from Ref. 32.)

differentiation is quite small (studies in the literature, which have not been controlled for bias, range from 10–25%). Differentiated cells appear benign, with smaller, less basophilic nuclei and more cytoplasm [19]. There is little evidence of mitotic figures or the expression of proliferating antigens associated with areas of differentiated cells, and they rarely exhibit signs of cell death (Fig. 3), although regions of differentiation may contain pockets of undifferentiated and apoptotic cells. As indicated above, differentiated cells exhibit morphological and molecular features of photoreceptors, particularly cone cells. Areas of differentiated cells form either rosettes (Flexner-Wintersteiner rosettes) or fleurettes and are distinguished by cytoplasmic structures that resemble photoreceptor outer segments (Fig. 2). The level of tumor differentiation is a primary diagnostic of prognosis, with a higher survival rate being directly related to the degree of differentiation [19,20]. Interestingly, well-differentiated tumors are more resistant to radiation therapy [19] and chemotherapeutic drugs [35]. The molecular basis for this is discussed below.

The third fate of the primary tumor cell is to undergo an additional transformation and become invasive and/or metastatic (Figs. 1 and 2). A finding of invasion is a very poor indicator of survival [19,20] and is associated with the formation of secondary metastatic tumors [36]. It is likely that some cells in nearly all retinoblastoma tumors (with the exception of highly differentiated ones) would undergo this additional transformation if left untreated. The basis for this speculation comes from several studies showing that tumors with invading cells are predominantly associated with delayed diagnosis and treatment. One study, for example, found a strong association between the misdiagnosis of retinoblastoma and an increase in mortality [37], while another found that cellular invasion was significantly higher in referral centers in rural third-world countries, where the average age of diagnosis was over a year later than at centers in developed countries [38]. Invasive tumor cells exhibit the basic morphological features of the primary cell type, although there is evidence that they have even larger nuclei and less cytoplasm (Fig. 2). These cells show no signs of either cell death or differentiation [32]. Recent evidence has linked the molecular events leading to invasion of tumor cells to a process of immortalization [39] and suggests that this fate of the primary tumor cell is associated with an additional genetic hit.

IV. THE MOLECULAR BIOLOGY OF APOPTOSIS IN RETINOBLASTOMA TUMORS—THE ROLE OF p53

As indicated earlier, cell death, in the form of apoptosis, is the dominant fate of the primary undifferentiated cell type found in retinoblastoma tumors. Several lines of evidence suggest that p53, the tumor suppressor protein, plays an important role in regulating this process [32,40,41]. p53 is a transcription factor and one of the most important molecules found in cells, acting as a check point that controls their ability to progress through the cell cycle or enter the apoptotic pathway [42]. In many cells, sensor proteins can detect strand breaks or abnormalities in the nuclear DNA and activate latent p53 [43]. For cell cycle control, p53 directly activates the expression of at least two genes, $p21^{WAF-1/Cip-1}$ and $14-3-3\sigma$, that function to arrest the cell cycle at the G1/S and G2/M interfaces, respectively [7,8,44–47]. $p21^{WAF-1/Cip-1}$ is well known as an inhibitor of cyclin-dependent kinases. These same kinases are involved in the phosphorylation of pRB, precipitating the release of the E2F transcription complex and progression of the cell cycle into S phase. Not surprisingly, p21$^{WAF-1/Cip-1}$ has no effect on arresting cell division in retinoblastoma tumors, presumably because there is no pRB/E2F complex present on which to exert its effect. In fact, *p21$^{WAF-1/Cip-1}$* expression has been correlated with cell survival and continued growth in these tumors (Figs. 4 and 5) [32,41]. Conversely, *p21$^{WAF-1/Cip-1}$* has been shown to

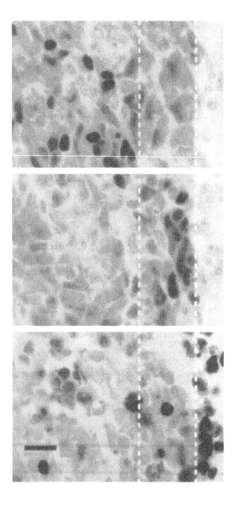

Figure 4   Comparison of p21$^{WAF-1/Cip-1}$, p53, and TUNEL staining in adjacent sections of a pseudorosette. High-magnification images from adjacent sections show three distinct zones that distinguish the relationship between the expression of these proteins and dying (TUNEL-labeled) cells. Top: p21$^{WAF-1/Cip-1}$ staining is most prevalent in the central regions of the pseudorosette (zone I). Middle: p53 immunoreactivity is strongest in the layer of cells adjacent to dying cells at the edge of the pseudorosette (zone II). Bottom: TUNEL-labeled cells are predominantly restricted to the layer of cells at the very edge of the pseudorosette. This region of TUNEL labeling defines zone III. The region outside of the pseudorosette is composed mostly of cellular debris or is completely devoid of cells. Size bar = 10 μm. (From Ref. 32.)

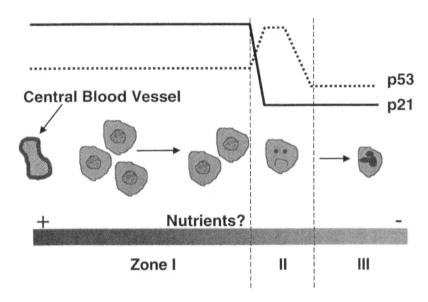

Figure 5 A diagram showing the relationship between p21$^{\text{WAF-1/Cip-1}}$ and p53 expression in cells of the pseudorosette. Cells in zone I express high levels of p21$^{\text{WAF-1/Cip-1}}$ and low levels of p53. This may be indicative of efforts by the cells to restrict uncontrolled proliferation in this zone. Since p21$^{\text{WAF-1/Cip-1}}$ is unable to affect cell division in the absence of pRb function, the cells continue to proliferate until they reach a point of crisis (zone II). The actual signal for crisis is not well understood but may be related to the distance these cells get from the central blood vessel leading to a lack of vascular nutrients. It may also be related to the accumulation of unbound E2Fs (see text) and thus a function of the number of divisions the cells have undergone. Whatever the signal, cells in crisis downregulate p21$^{\text{WAF-1/Cip-1}}$ and upregulate p53 expression, which leads to apoptotic cell death (zone III).

activate cell death of an immortalized retinoblastoma cell line in gene transfer experiments [40], underlying the molecular differences between these two cell phenotypes.

The other role of *p53* is to stimulate cell death, which it can do by directly activating the expression of a gene called *Bax* [48]. *Bax* is a member of the Bcl2 gene family and plays a crucial role in the committed step of apoptosis [49]. Its actual function is not known, but there is strong evidence that it accelerates mitochondrial dysfunction leading to the activation of cysteine proteases called caspases [50–55]. In the sequence of events associated with apoptotic cell death, caspases participate in an activation cascade that marks one of the last steps in this cellular suicide program [56,57]. Their role is to systematically digest the dying cell from within, leaving little or no cellular debris that could otherwise elicit an inflammatory response in the affected organ or tissue. Recent evidence indicates that caspases play an important role in retinoblastoma cell death, both in vitro [58] and in vivo (G. Poulsen and R. Nickells, unpublished results).

Because one of the principal mechanisms of activating *p53* is the formation of DNA strand breaks, treatments that elicit DNA damage, such as ionizing radiation or chemotherapy with alkylating agents, invariably stimulate *p53*-dependent cell death. Conversely, tumor cells that carry a *p53* mutation and/or a loss of heterozygosity of the *p53* allele are much more resistant to these treatments [59,60]. Retinoblastoma tumor cells likely fall into the former category. Cells of these tumors are wild-type for *p53* (see below), and immunocytochemical studies indicate that the p53 protein is expressed at varying levels in the primary cell type of most tumors [32,39]. These same studies have also noted that cells appear to accumulate higher levels of p53 just prior to cell death [32]. This phenomenon is particularly evident in cells surrounding blood vessels (pseudorosettes), in a zone just adjacent to dying cells present at the periphery of the cuff [32,41] (Figs 4 and 5). More direct evidence of p53-mediated cell death has come from the study of immortalized retinoblastoma cell lines. Transfection of WERI-Rb1 cells with a temperature-sensitive variant of *p53* activated cell death, but only at the permissive temperature [32] (Fig. 6). Similarly, Kondo and coworkers [40] found that Y79 cells were sensitive

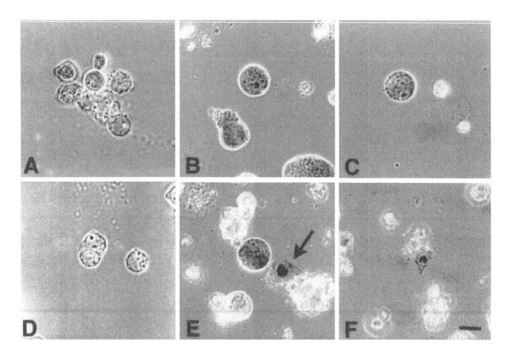

Figure 6 Activation of cell death in immortalized retinoblastoma cells by deregulated expression of an exogenous p53 gene. (A–C) Phase contrast photomicrographs of WERI-Rb1 cells transfected with a control plasmid (pBK·CMV). (D–F) A plasmid containing a temperature sensitive mutant of mouse p53 (pCMV·XV-Δ). Transfected cells were selected for antibiotic resistance (G418) for 8 days at 38°C, the temperature at which mouse p53 exhibits a mutant phenotype. After this period, transfected cells in both conditions appear relatively normal (A, D). After 6 days at 32.5°C (B, E), at which the mouse p53 assumes a wild-type phenotype, cells transfected with pCMV·XV-Δ show signs of dying that are consistent with apoptosis, such as the formation of pyknotic nuclei (arrow in E). After 11 days at 32.5°C (C, F), cells transfected with pBK·CMV still appear normal. Cells transfected with pCMV·XV-Δ are almost all dead. Size bar = 10 μm. (Modified from Ref. 32.)

to ionizing gamma irradiation, which stimulated an increase in both *p53* and *p53*-dependent gene expression, while ultimately leading to cell death.

It is noteworthy that *p53* expression has not been detected in differentiated cells of retinoblastoma tumors [32]. This is consistent with the evidence that apoptotic cells are only rarely found in differentiated regions (Fig. 3) and the observation that these cells are resistant to therapies that primarily stimulate cell death by the activation of *p53*.

V. THE ROLE OF p53 IN THE DEVELOPMENT OF INVASIVE RETINOBLASTOMA

As discussed above, *p53* plays a role in regulating cell death in retinoblastoma tumors. Ironically, some of the best tools for studying this phenomenon are immortalized retinoblastoma cell lines, raising the question of why these cells are not susceptible to the expression of their endogenous *p53* genes. One possible explanation is that the immortalization process of retinoblastoma cells is associated with a third mutation that disables either *p53* or the *p53* response pathway. The fact that these cells are receptive to exogenous *p53* expression or treatments that upregulate endogenous p53 indicates that immortalized cells have a functional response pathway. Examination of the *p53* genes in both tumor specimens and a variety of tumor derived immortalized cell lines have invariably revealed wild type alleles for this tumor suppressor gene [17,39,41,61,62]. Immunocytochemical analyses of six different lines, however, showed that the majority of them had abnormal localization of wild-type protein, with it being concentrated in the cytoplasm [39] (Fig. 7). Nuclear exclusion of *p53* is not uncommon in neuroblastoma cells [42,63,64]. Since the primary function of *p53* is to act as a transcription factor, it is not unreasonable to assume that cells with this localization pattern have a *p53*-null phenotype and are thus more likely to exhibit aggressive malignant behavior. In neuroblastomas, nuclear exclusion of *p53* is found only in poorly differentiated cells rather than differentiated ones [63], while this localization pattern for *p53* is associated with a reduced survival rate of individuals with either colorectal adenocarcinoma or stage II breast cancer [65,66]. Nuclear exclusion of *p53* is only rarely observed in retinoblastoma cells found within an ocular tumor mass, but it has been detected more frequently in cells that have invaded other ocular tissues such as the choroid and ciliary body [39] (Fig. 7). Based on their similarities of *p53* immunolocalization, invasive cells may be the most likely source of cells for developing cell lines, possibly because they have already acquired a genetic makeup that effectively immortalizes them.

The mechanism of nuclear exclusion is not yet defined, but a study using murine erythroleukemia cells suggested that increased expression of both c-*myc* and *Bcl2* genes can alter the subcellular trafficking of p53 leading to cytoplasmic accumulation [67]. Similar molecular conditions have been reported in retinoblastoma cells. Immortalized culture cells express high levels of the Bcl2 homologue, BclX [39], while very little of this gene product is detected in primary tumors themselves (Fig. 8). In addition, several observations of elevated N-*myc* expression, including amplification of this gene, have been reported in both immortalized cells

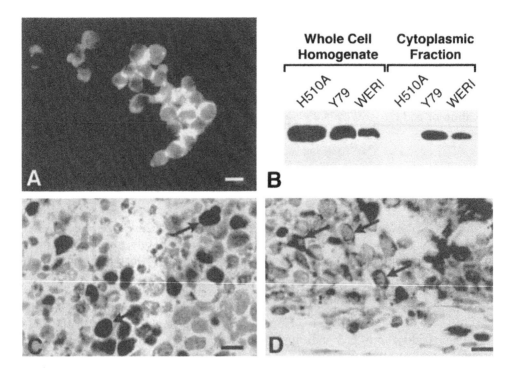

Figure 7   Nuclear exclusion of p53 in retinoblastoma. (A) Immunofluorescent localization of p53 in the Y79 immortalized retinoblastoma cell line. The majority of the p53 in these cells is in the cytoplasm ringing the nuclei. Several other retinoblastoma cell lines exhibit a similar pattern of localization [39]. Size bar = 10 μm. (B) Western blot analysis of p53 levels in whole-cell lysates and soluble cytosolic fractions of Y79 and WERI-Rb1 cells. As a control, cells from a small cell lung carcinoma (H510A cells), which exhibit nuclear accumulation of a mutant form of p53, were included in this fractionation experiment. All three cell lines contain p53 in the whole-cell lysates, but only the retinoblastoma cell lines have soluble p53 in the cytoplasmic fraction. (C, D) Immunohistochemical localization of p53 in a human tumor specimen. (C) Cells in the tumor mass found inside the globe exhibit nuclear localization of p53 (arrows). (D) In a region from the same eye, cells that have invaded the choroid exhibit cytoplasmic localization of p53 (arrows). Size bar (C, D) = 10 μm. (C and D from Ref. 39.)

and primary tumors [68–70]. Both BCL-X and N-*myc* proteins have functions similar to BCL-2 and c-*myc*, respectively.

Nuclear exclusion may not be the only mechanism of *p53* inactivation leading to metastasis. In a study of 25 retinoblastoma tumors (23 primary, 1 recurring, and 1 that had metastasized to the lung), loss of heterozygosity for the chromosomal location of the *p53* allele was detected in only 1 primary tumor and the single recurring tumor, while the metastatic tumor showed both a loss of heterozygosity and a mutation in *p53* [62]. Whether the loss of *p53* function is common for all invasive/metastatic retinoblastomas is a question that remains to be examined.

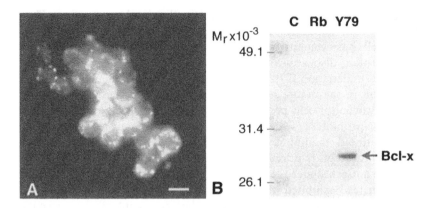

Figure 8 BCL-X is highly expressed in immortalized retinoblastoma. (A) Immunofluor-escent photomicrograph of BCL-X localization in Y79 cells. BCL-X is normally localized to mitochondria and exhibits a typical punctate staining pattern as seen in these cells. Size bar $= 10\,\mu m$. (B) Western blot of equal amounts ($50\,\mu g$) of total protein lysates isolated from control retina (C), whole retinoblastoma tumors tissue taken from inside the globe of an affected eye (Rb), and Y79 cells. The Western blot membrane was challenged with a polyclonal antibody against human BCL-X. Y79 cells contain significantly more BCL-X than either the normal retina or an ocular retinoblastoma tumor.

VI. WHAT TRANSGENIC MOUSE MODELS OF RETINOBLASTOMA TELL US ABOUT THE MOLECULAR BIOLOGY OF THE HUMAN DISEASE?

A dramatic surge in the study of retinoblastoma has come from the development of transgenic mouse models of this ocular tumor. A detailed description of the various mouse models is found in Chap. 6 of this volume. Essentially, these models have revealed information on both the developmental timing of tumor formation and the molecular events associated with malignant transformation and possibly the evolution of the invasive cell phenotype.

Like all other mammals, mice do not naturally develop retinoblastoma tumors [71,72]. The reason for this phenomenon has not yet been elucidated. Knockout mice, completely lacking a functional *Rb1* gene, are unable to survive beyond 13–15 days of gestation because of abnormalities in both erythroid and neuronal development [73,74]. Complete loss of pRB throughout the organism, however, is not analogous to the development of Knudson's two hits in the human eye. A more accurate model comes from the study of chimeric mice, composed of both wild-type and *Rb1⁻/⁻* cells. These studies have shown that pRB.-deficient cells do not form tumors but instead survive and differentiate normally when surrounded by cells with a normal genotype [16,75]. Similarly, mouse cells that are heterozygous for *Rb1* (*Rb1⁺/⁻*) do not exhibit an increased incidence of eye tumors, although they are significantly more susceptible to acquiring pituitary and thyroid tumors [76].

More aggressive strategies have been employed to stimulate retinoblastoma tumor growth in mice, and all of them require inactivation of both Rb1 and *p53*. These strategies have utilized the expression of viral oncoproteins in select target cells in transgenic mice. The primary models employ the simian virus 40 (SV40) large T-antigen controlled by promoters that are expressed in the developing retina. This oncoprotein binds to and inactivates both pRB and p53 [77,78], so typically its ability to transform cells has been attributed to this dual role. It is important to note, however, that this protein also appears to have a variety of other transforming functions not yet fully understood [79].

Tumor formation in the mouse eye using the SV40 T antigen requires early expression in retinal progenitor cells present in the developing neuroblast layer. One of the most useful promoters for this requirement is from the gene for interphotoreceptor retinoid binding protein (IRBP) [80], which is expressed in developing mouse photoreceptors prior to postnatal day 5 [81]. A similar transgenic line, with the SV40 T antigen under the control of the rod opsin promoter failed to develop tumors and instead exhibited widespread cell death [82]. The reason for this failure is likely due to the timing of expression of the opsin-controlled transgene, which is activated quite late in the differentiation sequence of photoreceptors [81]. A second successful line expressing the SV40 T antigen was fortuitously generated using the promoter for lutenizing hormone β (LHβ) [83]. These mice, which were originally developed for the study of pituitary gonadotropin-derived tumors, showed ectopic expression in a cell lineage present in the retinal inner nuclear layer, making these tumors possibly more analogous to human retinoblastoma with respect to the actual cell of origin [17]. In similar experiments, ectopic expression of the human papillomavirus (HPV) E7 and E6 oncoproteins in presumptive bipolor neurons (these genes were being expressed by the lens α-A crystalline promoter) also caused the formation of a retinoblastoma tumor, but only in certain genetic backgrounds [84]. The E7 protein binds to and inactivates pRB and the E6 protein binds to p53 and targets it for degradation [85]. Subsequent lines generated by using HPV E7 under the control of the IRBP promoter to specifically inactivate pRB did not develop tumors but instead exhibited pronounced cell death at the period coinciding with the rod photoreceptor terminal differentiation [86]. Conversely, some retinal cells in the IRBP-HPV E7 transgenic mice were able to give rise to retinoblastoma tumors when placed on a p53-null genetic background.

VII. SUMMARY

$Rb1^{-/-}$ cells in both mice and men appear to activate a p53-dependent pathway of cell death, but tumors can arise in mice only if both pRB and p53 are disabled. This is in direct contrast to findings in humans, in which wild-type p53 is always detected in these tumors, leading some to question whether these mice represent an accurate model of this eye tumor [87]. Rather than being contradictory, however, it is possible that tumor cells in mice are more similar to the immortalized retinoblastoma cells found in some human tumors. Mouse tumors never exhibit signs of differentiation and only seldom show histological evidence of cell death [72]. Typically, cells in these tumors initially organize into Homer-Wright rosettes, which in human tumors are composed of undifferentiated primary cells and have been associated with cytoplasmic localization of p53 (T. M. Nork, C. L. Schlamp, and R. W. Nickells, unpublished observations). Lastly, mouse tumor cells are also highly aggressive and often metastasize within a few months [72,80]. In this context, mouse models argue that more aggressive behavior of cells in human tumors is associated with additional genetic damage involving p53.

ACKNOWLEDGMENTS

The authors would like to thank Dr. T. Michael Nork for helpful discussions and for providing several photomicrographs used in this chapter and Dr. Isabelle Audo for her help in researching the literature. Some of this work was supported by funding from Research to Prevent Blindness and by an institutional grant from the American Cancer Society to the University of Wisconsin.

REFERENCES

1. Knudson AJ. Mutation and childhood cancer: Statistical study of retinoblastoma. Proc Natl Acad Sci USA 1971;68:820–823.
2. Comings DE. A general theory of carcinogenesis. Proc Natl Acad Sci USA 1973;70:3324–3328.
3. Friend SH, Bernards R, Rogelj S, Weinberg RA, Rapaport JM, Albert DM, et al. A human DNA segment with properties of the gene that predisposes to retinoblastoma and osteosarcoma. Nature 1986;323:643–646.
4. Lee WH, Bookstein R, Hong F, Young LJ, Shew JY, Lee EY. Human retinoblastoma susceptibility gene: Cloning, identification, and sequence. Science 1987;235:1394–1399.
5. Fung YKT, Murphree AL, T'Ang A, Qian J, Hinrichs SH, Benedict WF. Structural evidence for the authenticity of the human retinoblastoma gene. Science 1987;236:1657–1661.
6. Whyatt DFG, Grosveld F. Cell-nonautonomous function of the retinoblastoma tumor supressor protein: New interpretations of old phenotypes. EMBO Rep 2002;3:130–135.
7. Harper JW, Adami GR, Wei N, Keyomarsi K, Elledge SJ. The p21 Cdk-interacting protein Cip1 is a potent inhibitor of G1 cyclin-dependent kinases. Cell 1993;75:805–816.
8. Xiong Y, Hannon GJ, Zhang H, Casso D, Kobayashi R, Beach D. p21 is a universal inhibitor of cyclin kinases. Nature 1993;366:701–704.
9. Gartel AL, Serfas MS, Tyner AL. p21-negative regulator of the cell cycle. Proc Soc Exp Biol Med 1996;213:138–149.
10. Ferguson KL, Slack RS. The Rb pathway in neurogenesis. Neuroreport 2001;12:A55–A62.
11. Bernards R, Schackleford GM, Gerber MR, Horowitz JM, Friend SH, Schartl M, et al. Structure and expression of the murine retinoblastoma gene and characterization of its encoded protein. Proc Natl Acad Sci USA 1989;86:6474–6478.
12. Slack RS, Hamel PA, Bladon TS, Gill RM, McBurney MW. Regulated expression of the retinoblastoma gene in differentiating embryonal carcinoma cells. Oncogene 1993;8:1585–1591.
13. Slack RS, Skerjanc IS, Lach B, Craig J, Jardine K, McBurney MW. Cells differentiating into neuroectoderm undergo apoptosis in the absence of functional retinoblastoma family proteins. J Cell Biol 1995;129:779–788.
14. Azuma-Hara M, Taniura H, Uetsuki T, et al. Regulation and deregulation of E2F1 in postmitotic neurons differentiated from embryonal carcinoma P19 cells. Exp Cell Res 1999;251:442–451.
15. Hou ST, Callaghan D, Fournier MC, et al. The transcription factor E2F1 modulates apoptosis of neurons. J Neurochem 2000;75:91–100.

16. Lipinski MM, Macleod KF, Williams BO, Mullaney TL, Crowley D, Jacks T. Cell-autonomous and non-cell-autonomous functions of the Rb tumor supressor in developing central nervous system. EMBO J 2001;20:3402–3413.

17. Gallie BL, Campbell C, Devlin H, Duckett A, Squire JA. Developmental basis of retinal-specific induction of cancer by RB mutation. Can Res 1999;59(Suppl):1731s–1735s.

18. Chen D, Pajovic S, Duckett A, Brown VD, Squire JA, Gallie BL. Genomic amplification in retinoblastoma narrowed to 0.6 megabase on chromosome 6p containing a kinesin-like gene, RBKIN. Can Res 2002;62:967–971.

19. Zimmerman LE. Retinoblastoma and retinocytoma. In: Spencer WH, ed. Ophthalmic Pathology, 3rd ed. San Francisco: Saunders, 1985, pp 1292–1351.

20. Murphree AL, Clark RD. Retinoblastoma. In: Rimion DL, Connor JM, Pyeritz RE, Korf BR, eds. Principles and Practice of Medical Genetics, 4th ed. London: Churchill Livingstone, 2002, pp 3604–3634.

21. Abramson DH, Du TT, Beaverson KL. (Neonatal) retinoblastoma in the first month of life. Arch Ophthalmol 2002;120:138–142.

22. Tso MO, Fine BS, Zimmerman LE. The nature of retinoblastoma. II. Photoreceptor differentiation: an electron microscopic study. Am J Ophthalmol 1970;69:350–359.

23. Gonzalez-Fernandez F, Lopes MB, Garcia-Fernandez JM, Foster RG, De Grip WJ, Rosemberg S, et al. Expression of developmentally defined rctinal phenotypes in the histogenesis of retinoblastoma. Am J Pathol 1992;141:363–375.

24. Nork TM, Schwartz TL, Doshi HM, Millecchia LL. Retinoblastoma: Cell of origin. Arch Ophthalmol 1995;113:791–802.

25. Tsuji M, Goto M, Uehara F, Kaneko A, Sawai J, Yonezawa S, et al. Photoreceptor cell differentiation in retinoblastoma demonstrated by a new immunohistochemical marker mucin-like glycoprotein associated with photoreceptor cells (MLGAPC). Histopathology 2002;40:180–186.

26. Bogenmann E, Lochrie MA, Simon MI. Cone cell-specific genes expressed in retinoblastoma. Science 1988;240:76–78.

27. Hurwitz RL, Bogenmann E, Font RL, Holcombe V, Clark D. Expression of the functional cone phototransduction cascade in retinoblastoma. J Clin Invest 1990;85:1872–1878.

28. Di Polo A, Farber DB. Rod photoreceptor-specific gene expression in human retinoblastoma cells. Proc Natl Acad Sci USA 1995;92:4016–4020.

29. Cepko CL, Austin CP, Yang X, Alexiades M, Ezzeddine D. Cell fate determination in the vertebrate retina. Proc Natl Acad Sci USA 1996;93:589–595.

30. Alexiades M, Cepko CL. Subsets of retinal progenitors display temporally regulated and distinct biases in the fates of their progeny. Development 1997;124:1119–1131.

31. Kyritsis AP, Tsokos M, Triche TJ, Chader GJ. Retinoblastoma—Origin from a primitive neuroectodermal cell? Nature 1984;307:471–473.

32. Nork TM, Poulsen G, Millecchia LL, Jantz RG, Nickells RW. p53 regulates apoptosis in human retinoblastoma. Arch Ophthalmol 1997;115:213–219.

33. Majno G, Joris I. Apoptosis, oncosis, and necrosis. An overview of cell death. Am J Pathol 1995;146:3–15.

34. Burnier MN, McLean IW, Zimmerman LE, Rosenberg SH. Retinoblastoma. The relationship of proliferating cells to blood vessels. Invest Ophthalmol Vis Sci 1990;31:2037–2040.

35. Schouten-van Meeteren AYN, van der Valk P, van der Linden HC, Moll AC, Imhof SM, Huismans DR, et al. Histopathologic features of retinoblastoma and its relation with in vitro drug resistance measured by means of the MTT assay. Cancer 2001;92:2933–2940.

36. Shields CL, Shields JA, Baez KA, Cater J, De Potter PV. Choroidal invasion of retinoblastoma: Metastatic potential and clinical risk factors. Br J Ophthalmol 1993;77:544–548.

37. Stafford WR, Yanoff M, Parnell B. Retinoblastoma initially misdiagnosed as primary ocular inflammation. Arch Ophthalmol 1969;82:771–773.

38. Schultz KR, Ranade S, Neglia JP, Ravindranath Y. An increased relative frequency of retinoblastoma at a rural regional referral hospital in Miraj, Maharashtra, India. Cancer 1993;72:282–286.

39. Schlamp CL, Poulsen GL, Nork TM, Nickells RW. Nuclear exclusion of wild-type p53 in immortalized human retinoblastoma cells. J Natl Can Inst 1997;89:1530–1536.

40. Kondo Y, Kondo S, Liu JB, Haqqi T, Barnett GH, Barna BP. Involvement of p53 and waf1/cip1 in gamma-irradiation-induced apoptosis of retinoblastoma cells. Exp Cell Res 1997;236:51–56.

41. Divan A, Lawry J, Dunsmore IR, Parsons MA, Royds JA. p53 and p21/waf-1 expression correlates with apoptosis or cell survival in poorly differentiated, but not well-differentiated, retinoblastomas. Can Res 2001;61:3157–3163.

42. Levine AJ. p53, the cellular gatekeeper for growth and division. Cell 1997;88:323–332.

43. Agarwal ML, Taylor WR, Chernov MV, Chernova OB, Stark GR. The p53 network. J Biol Chem 1998;273:1–4.

44. El-Deiry WS, Kern SE, Pietenpol JA, Kinzler KW, Vogelstein B. Definition of a consensus binding site for p53. Nat Genet 1992;1:45–49.

45. El-Deiry W, Tokino T, Velculescu VE, Levy DB, Parsons R, Trent JM, et al. WAF1, a potential mediator of p53 tumor suppression. Cell 1993;75:817–825.

46. El-Deiry WS, Harper JW, O'Connor PM, Velculescu VE, Canman CE, Jackman J, et al. *WAF1/CIP1* is induced in p53-mediated G_1 arrest and apoptosis. Cancer Res 1994;54:1169–1174.

47. Hermeking H, Lengauer C, Polyak K, He T-C, Zhang L, Thiagalingam S, et al. 14–3–3σ is a p53-regulated inhibitor of G2/M progression. Mol Cell 1997;1:3–11.

48. Miyashita T, Reed JC. Tumor supressor p53 is a direct transcriptional activator of the human *bax* gene. Cell 1995;80:293–299.

49. Oltvai Z, Milliman C, Korsmeyer SJ. Bcl-2 heterodimerizes *in vivo* with a conserved homolog, Bax, that accelerates programmed cell death. Cell 1993;74:609–619.

50. Antonsson B, Montessuit S, Lauper S, Eskes R, Martinou JC. Bax oligomerization is required for channel-forming activity in liposomes and to trigger cytochrome c release from mitochondria. Biochem 2000;345:271–278.

51. Crompton M. Mitochondrial intermembrane junctional complexes and their role in cell death. J Physiol 2000;529:11–21.

52. Finkel E. The mitochondrian: Is it central to apoptosis? Science 2001;292:624–626.

53. Marzo I, Brenner C, Zamzami N, Jurgensmeier JM, Susin SA, Vieira HLA, et al. Bax and adenine nucleotide translocator cooperate in the mitochondrial control of apoptosis. Science 1998;281:2027–2031.

54. Reed JC. Cytochrome c: Can't live with it—Can't live without it. Cell 1997;91:559–562.

55. Jurgensmeier JM, Xie ZH, Deveraux Q, Ellerby L, Bredesen D, Reed JC. Bax directly induces release of cytochrome c from isolated mitochondria. Proc Natl Acad Sci USA 1998;95:4997–5002.

56. Salvesen GS, Dixit VM. Caspases: intracellular signaling by proteolysis. Cell 1997;91:443–446.

57. Slee EA, Harte MT, Kluck RM, Wolf BB, Casiano CA, Newmeyer DD, et al. Ordering the cytochrome c-initiated caspase cascade: Hierarchical activation of caspases-2, −3, −6, −7, −8, and −10 in a caspase-9-dependent manner. J Cell Biol 1999;144:281–292.

58. Kondo Y, Liu J, Haqqi T, Barna BP, Kondo S. Involvement of interleukin-1beta-converting enzyme in apoptosis of irradiated retinoblastomas. Invest Ophthalmol Vis Sci 1998;39:2769–2774.

59. Lee JM, Bernstein A. p53 mutations increase resistance to ionizing radiation. Proc Natl Acad Sci USA 1993;90:5742–5746.

60. Lee JM, Bernstein A. Apoptosis, cancer and the p53 tumour suppressor gene. Can Metastasis Rev 1995;14:149–161.

61. Hamel PA, Phillips RA, Muncaster M, Gallie BL. Speculations on the roles of RB1 in tissue-specific differentiation, tumor initiation, and tumor progression. FASEB J 1993;7:846–854.

62. Kato MV, Shimizu T, Ishizaki K, Kaneko A, Yandell DW, Toguchida J, et al. Loss of heterozygosity on chromosome 17 and mutation of the *p53* gene in retinoblastoma. Cancer Lett 1996;106:75–82.

63. Moll UM, LaQuaglia M, Benard J, Riou G. Wild-type p53 protein undergoes cytoplasmic sequestration in undifferentiated neuroblastomas but not in differentiated tumors. Proc Natl Acad Sci USA 1995;92:4407–4411.

64. Goldman SC, Chen C-Y, Lansing TJ, Gilmer TM, Kastan MB. The p53 signal transduction pathway is intact in human neuroblastoma despite cytoplasmic localization. Am J Pathol 1996;148:1381–1385.

65. Sun X-F, Carstensen JM, Zhang H, Stål O, Wingren S, Hatschek T, et al. Prognostic significance of cytoplasmic p53 oncoprotein in colorectal adenocarcinoma. Lancet 1992;340:1369–1373.

66. Stenmark-Askmalm M, Stål O, Sullivan S, Ferraud L, Sun X-F, Carstensen J, et al. Cellular accumulation of p53 protein: An independent prognostic factor in stage II breast cancer. Eur J Cancer 1994;30A:175–180.

67. Ryan JJ, Prochownik E, Gottlieb CA, Apel IJ, Merino R, Nuñez G, et al. *c-myc* and *bcl-2* modulate p53 function by altering p53 subcellular trafficking during the cell cycle. Proc Natl Acad Sci USA 1994;91:5878–5882.

68. Lee W-H, Murphree AL, Benedict WF. Expression and amplification of the N-myc gene in primary retinoblastoma. Nature 1984;309:458–460.

69. Choi SW, Lee TW, Ynag SW, Hong WS, Kim CM, Lee JO. Loss of retinoblastoma gene and amplification of N-myc in retinoblastoma. J Korean Med Sci 1993;8:73–77.

70. Mairal A, Pinglier E, Gilbert E, Peter M, Validire P, Desjardins L, et al. Detection of chromosome imbalances in retinoblastoma by parallel karyotype and CGH analyses. Genes Chromosomes Cancer 2000;28:370–379.

71. Hogan RN, Albert DM. Does Rb occur in animals? Prog Vet Comp Ophthalmol 1991;1:73–82.

72. Albert DM, Griep AE, Lambert PF, Howes KA, Windle JJ, Lasudry JGH. Transgenic models of retinoblastoma: What they tell us about its cause and treatment. Trans Am Ophthalmol Soc 1994;92:385–401.

73. Lee EY, Chang CY, Hu N, Wang YC, Lai CC, Herrup K, et al. Mice deficient for Rb are nonviable and show defecs in neurogenesis and haematopoiesis. Nature 1994;359:288–295.

74. Lipinski MM, Jacks T. The retinoblastoma gene family in differentiation and development. Oncogene 1999;18:7873–7882.

75. Williams BO, Schmitt EM, Remington L, Bronson RT, Albert DM, Weinberg RA, et al. Extensive contribution of Rb-deficient cells to adult chimeric mice with limited histopathological consequences. EMBO J 1994;13:4251–4259.

76. Williams BO, Remington L, Albert DM, Shizou M, Bronson RT, Jacks T. Cooperative tumerogenic effects of germline mutations in Rb and p53. Nat Genet 1994;7:480–484.

77. DeCaprio JA, Ludlow JW, Figge J, et al. SV40 large tumor antigen forms a specific complex with the product of the retinoblastoma suceptibility gene. Cell 1988;54:275–283.

78. Levine AJ. The p53 protein and its interactions with the oncogene products of the small DNA tumor viruses. Virology 1990;177:419–426.

79. Ali SH, DeCaprio JA. Cellular transformation by SV40 large T antigen: Interaction with host proteins. Semin Cancer Biol 2001;11:15–23.

80. Al-Ubaidi MR, Font RL, Quiambao AB, Keener MJ, Liou GI, Overbeek PA, et al. Bilateral retinal and brain tumors in transgenic mice expressing simian virus 40 large T-antigen under control of the human interphotoreceptor retinoid-binding protein promoter. J Cell Biol 1992;119:1681–1687.

81. Gonzalez-Fernandez F, Van Niel E, Edmonds C, Beaver H, Nickerson JM, Garcia-Fernandez JM, et al. Differential expression of interphotoreceptor retinoid-binding protein, opsin, cellular retinaldehyde-binding protein, and basic fibroblast growth factor. Exp Eye Res 1993;56:411–427.

82. Al-Ubaidi MR, Mangini NJ, Quiambao AB, Myers KM, Abler AS, Chang CJ, et al. Unscheduled DNA replication precedes apoptosis of photoreceptors expressing SV40 T antigen. Exp Eye Res 1997;64:573–585.

83. Windle JJ, Albert DM, O'Brien JM, Marcus DM, Disteche CM, Bernards R, et al. Retinoblastoma in transgenic mice. Nature 1990;343:665–669.

84. Griep AE, Krawcek J, Lee D, Liem A, Albert DM, Carabeo R, et al. Multiple genetic loci modify risk for retinoblastoma in transgenic mice. Invest Ophthalmol Vis Sci 1998;39:2723–2732.

85. Munger K, Scheffner M, Huibregtse JM, Howley PM. Interactions of HPV E6 and E7 oncoproteins with tumor suppressor gene products. Cancer Surv 1992;12:197–217.

86. Howes KA, Ransom N, Papermaster DS, Lasudry JGH, Albert DM, Windle JJ. Apoptosis or retinoblastoma: Alternative fates of photoreceptors expressing the HPV-16 E7 gene in the presence or absence of p53. Genes Dev 1994;8:1300–1310.

87. Kaye FJ. Can p53 status resolve paradoxes between human and non-human retinoblastoma models? J Natl Can Inst 1997;89:1530–1536.

88. Didenko VV, Hornsby PJ. Presence of double-strand breaks with single-base 3′ overhangs in cells undergoing apoptosis but not necrosis. J Cell Biol 1996;135:1369–1376.

89. Gavrieli Y, Sherman Y, Ben-Sasson SA. Identification of programmed cell death in situ via specific labeling of nuclear DNA fragmentation. J Cell Biol 1992;119:493–501.

11

Immunology of Uveal Melanoma: Adaptive Antitumor Immunity and the Basis for Immunotherapy

JACOBUS J. BOSCH and BRUCE R. KSANDER

Harvard Medical School and Schepens Eye Research Institute, Boston, Massachusetts, U.S.A.

I. INTRODUCTION

During the past decade, tumor immunologists have been extremely productive, resulting in many important advances that have been critical in improving cancer immunotherapies. Two seminal discoveries that sparked this remarkable progress were (1) the discovery of genes encoding tumor antigens and (2) the discovery of genes encoding costimulatory molecules. Together, these provided immunologists with the tools needed to initiate a T-cell response directed at antigens expressed on spontaneous human tumors. Terry Boon and coworkers at the Ludwig Cancer Institute in Belgium were the first to identify the MAGE-1 gene, which encodes an antigen expressed on metastatic skin melanomas [1]. This was the first report of a gene defining a target antigen that was expressed on tumor cells and recognized by antigen-specific T cells; it has led to the discovery of many other tumor antigens.

T cells that recognize tumor antigens need two separate activation signals: the tumor antigen provides the first signal and costimulatory signals expressed on antigen-presenting cells provide the second. One of the first costimulatory genes identified was *CD80* (B7.1) [2]. There is now a whole family of different costimulatory signals that are involved in activating and regulating the development of antigen-specific T cells. Thus, immunologists now have a better understanding of the two critical components in activating tumor-specific T cells. With this information, a variety of new and novel cancer immunotherapies were developed, leading to the successful treatment of cancer patients with progressively growing tumors. The best results have been reported for patients with metastatic skin melanoma. In spite of this progress, many significant obstacles remain for cancer immunotherapies: (1) the frequency of patients responding to these new treatments is extremely low; (2) the cost of the treatments is enormous—they are also time-consuming, and technically very demanding; and (3) there is no direct correlation between the response to therapy and the markers of immunity [3]. This last problem is particularly troubling. Many patients receiving therapy generate a vigorous tumor-specific T-cell response directed against a tumor antigen expressed on the tumor, but the T-cell response fails to control tumor growth. In addition, a few patients with partial or complete tumor responses fail to display any detectable specific antitumor immunity. For these reasons, immunologists are currently focusing on determining why the current cancer immunotherapies are not more effective.

There are a number of reasons why few if any of the current immunotherapies have been attempted on uveal melanoma patients: (1) the number of patients is relatively low; (2) there is no large source of tumor tissue available for immunological studies; (3) the immune response has not been characterized extensively; (4) patients with metastatic disease are highly resistant to chemotherapy, giving oncologists the impression these patients will respond poorly to immunotherapy; and (5) the immune-privileged environment of the eye, as compared with other anatomical sites, will decrease the effectiveness of immunotherapy. Although this last issue may be a potent critical barrier for immunotherapeutic treatment of uveal melanomas, the difficulties associated with eliminating tumors from an immune-privileged site may reveal important insights into why cancer immunotherapies in general are not more effective. We propose that *the reason cancer immunotherapies fail is also the reason that the eye succeeds at maintaining immune privilege*. If we can learn how to terminate immune privilege in the eye, we will know how to make cancer immunotherapies succeed.

This chapter outlines a strategy for the development of a tumor cell vaccine for uveal melanomas that utilizes a unique characteristic of these tumors. In order to fully appreciate this strategy, a preliminary review of the research and background that form the basis for this approach is in order.

II. EFFECTOR T CELLS IN ADAPTIVE IMMUNITY

The principle behind adaptive antitumor immunity is deceptively simple. Tumors express specific antigens recognized by antigen-specific immune effector cells that eliminate only the malignant tumor and leave the normal tissue intact. It is now well established that tumors express specific antigens found on malignant cells but absent from normal cells. There are variations of this scenario, such as the following: tumor antigens may be expressed on normal cells at low levels, but at much higher levels on tumor cells. However, the important issue is that the tumor cells display a target antigen that allows the immune system to recognize and differentiate between normal and malignant cells. Since tumors express these antigens but still grow progressively, it is obvious that these antigens are unable to elicit protective immunity. Immunologists distinguish between "antigenic" and "immunogenic." An antigen is anything that can be recognized by the immune system, but not all antigens are capable of eliciting an immune response. Only immunogenic antigens induce immunity. Essentially all of the antigens identified to date on spontaneous human tumors are *not* immunogenic. Therefore the goal of adaptive antitumor immunotherapy is to manipulate the immune response so that effective immunity is directed against the tumor antigens, resulting in elimination of the tumor. How to manipulate the tumor-specific immune response to produce protective immunity is a complicated issue, in which some but not all of the important mechanisms have been identified.

There are two components to the immune response, the *innate* phase and the *adaptive* phase. This chapter focuses on the role of adaptive immunity in immunotherapy. There are many excellent reviews on the role of innate immunity in tumor immunology [4,5]. Innate immunity (1) is immediate, (2) is nonspecific, and (3) has no memory. The main cellular components are natural killer (NK) cells, natural killer T (NKT) cells, macrophages, dendritic cells, and neutrophils. Although these cells are nonspecific, they display a limited level of specificity. They respond to certain groups of pathogens or "danger" signals through the expression of Toll receptors and pathogen-associated molecular patterns (PAMPS).

By contrast, adaptive immunity (1) is delayed, (2) is antigen-specific, and (3) has long-term memory. The main effector cells are T cells and B cells. In the past, B cells were not believed to participate effectively in antitumor immunity. However, this idea is beginning to change [6]. Tumor immunologists have focused almost exclusively on antigen-specific T cells in the past decade due to their antigen specificity and memory. Specificity is required to prevent destruction of normal tissue and memory is required to prevent recurrences of primary and metastatic tumors. Although T cells are clearly important in antitumor immunotherapy, it is becoming more obvious that innate immunity also plays a critical role in the development of a sustained antitumor T-cell response. The problems associated with current tumor immunotherapies may stem from the failure to include strategies to activate innate immunity.

Experiments from laboratories that study viral immunity indicate that protective immunity requires both innate and adaptive responses. Innate immunity alone is unable to control viral infections, and activation of adaptive immunity does not occur without an initial innate response. In addition, experimental animal models that study activation of antigen-specific T cells require that animals be immunized with antigen in conjunction with a potent adjuvant. If the animal is exposed to the antigen *without* the adjuvant, no T-cell response occurs. A major function of the adjuvant is to stimulate a local inflammatory response; it is therefore similar to the early innate immune response induced by most pathogens. It may not be surprising that recent studies suggest tumors go to great lengths to prevent local inflammation and activation of innate immunity [7].

The following section describes antigen-specific T-cell subpopulations, the tumor antigens expressed on human tumors, the antigen processing pathways used to express tumor antigens, and how specific T cells are normally activated. This information is important to understand how the current forms of cancer immunotherapy attempt to manipulate the immune response to generate protective antitumor immunity.

III. CD8z+ CYTOTOXIC T CELLS

There are two major T-cell subpopulations, CD8+ T cells and CD4+ T cells, that recognize distinct antigens and display distinct effector functions. CD8+ cytotoxic T cells (CTLs) display T-cell receptors (TcRs) that recognize small peptide antigens displayed by class I molecules. CD8 on T cells binds a nonpolymorphic region of class I that stabilizes the TcR-antigen complex (Fig. 1A). Two signals are required to successfully activate CD8+ T cells: (1) signal one is provided by TcR recognition of antigen in the context of class I and (2) signal two is provided by CD80 (B7.1) costimulatory molecules that are also expressed on antigen presenting cells (APCs). Successful activation of CD8+ T cells occurs only when both signal one and signal two are received. CTL activation proceeds through a series of distinct stages, starting with the clonal expansion of precursor T cells, differentiation into cells that acquire cytolytic capacity, and ending with fully mature CTLs. The mechanism of CTL-mediated tumor cell lysis is rapid and involves several consecutive steps. It starts with the formation of the TcR antigen–class I complex, which is reinforced by ligation of adhesion molecules and colocalization of additional TcR. Signal transduction pathways trigger migration of intracellular vesicles that contain cytolytic factors to the site where the T cells bind the tumor cell. Cytolytic factors are then released from the T cell into the tumor cell membrane, causing cell death. CTLs are resistant to their own cytolytic factors and therefore are able to survive and proceed rapidly to bind and kill another tumor target cell. By this recycling mechanism, a small number of CTLs can eliminate a much larger tumor burden.

IV. CD4+ HELPER T CELLS

Helper T cells are restricted by MHC class II molecules, express CD4, and secrete a vast array of cytokines. These cytokines drive the differentiation and proliferation of other T helper cells to become $CD4^+$ Th1 and $CD4^+$ Th2 cells. The distinction between Th1 and Th2 cells is based on the cytokine secretion profile [8]. Th1 cells stimulate growth and proliferation of other T cells (cell-mediated immunity). Th2 cells activate B cells to differentiate into antibody-secreting plasma cells (humoral immunity). Tumor immunologists have focused on the Th1 subpopulation due to its important role in activating cytotoxic T cells.

CD4+ T cells display receptors (TcRs) that recognize peptide antigens that are presented by MHC class II (Fig. 1B). Class II expression is highly regulated and restricted mainly to professional APCs responsible for activating naïve CD4+ T cells. As was the case with CD8+ T cells, two signals are required to activate CD4+ T cells successfully: (1) signal one is provided by TcR recognition of antigen in the context of class II and (2) signal two is provided by CD80 costimulatory molecules that are also expressed on APCs. Primed CD4+ T cells display three effector functions in antitumor immunity: (1) secretion of "helper" lymphokines (such as IL-2 and IFN-γ), required to induce proliferation and differentiation of CD8+ T cells (Fig. 2); (2) indirect activation of CD8+ T cells via induction of costimulatory signals in APC (Fig. 3A and B); and (3) indirect killing of tumor cells via activation of macrophages to secrete cytokines (TNF-α and nitric oxide) that lyse tumor cells (Fig. 4). The second function is achieved through expression of CD40 ligand on activated CD4+ T cells. This ligand triggers CD40 receptors found on APCs,

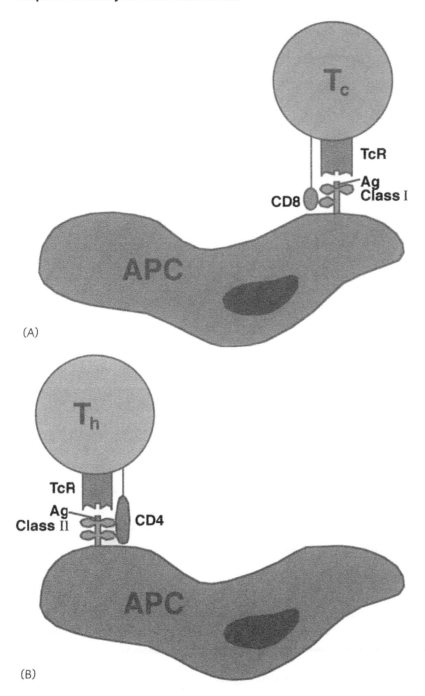

Figure 1 Activation of tumor-specific T cells. Cytotoxic T cells (CD8+T cells) are activated when T-cell receptors (TcR) recognize small peptide tumor antigens presented by class I. CD8 binds class I and stabilizes the TcR/antigen complex (A). T-helper cells (CD4+ T cells) are activated when TcR recognize peptide tumor antigens presented by class II. CD4 binds Class II and stabilizes the TcR/antigen complex (B).

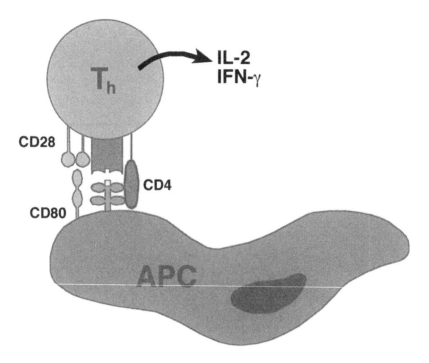

Figure 2   Effector functions of CD4+ T cells—secretion of lymphokines. T-helper cells that are activated by antigen and costimulatory signals secrete lymphokines, such as IL-2 and IFN-γ, that induce proliferation and activation of CD8+ cytotoxic T cells.

resulting in upregulation of other costimulatory receptors on the APC, such as CD137 (BB-1), that preferentially activates CD8+ CTL.

V. GEOGRAPHIC SPECIFICITY OF CD4+ T-HELPER CELLS

One of the criticisms against CD4+ T cells as effector T cells in antitumor immunotherapy is the lack of specificity. Although CD4+ T cells are triggered by specific antigens expressed on APCs, they activate APCs, to release TNF-α and nitric oxide, *nonspecific* cytokines that lack any specificity for malignant tumor cells. Once APCs release these cytokines into the surrounding environment, tumor cells and normal cells are equally vulnerable and can be destroyed. However, even though the effector cytokines are nonspecific, there is a "geographic" specificity to this response that may allow this type of immunity to work even within the eye (Fig. 5). In order for primed CD4+ T cells to be activated in peripheral tissues, they must recognize their specific antigen presented by class II. For uveal melanomas that rarely express class II, this occurs only when APCs infiltrate the tumor site and reprocess tumor antigens. Therefore CD4+ T cells and APCs are activated within the tumor site only when they are both within close proximity. This limits the release of nonspecific cytokines to a small geographic location within the tumor, diminishing the extent of nonspecific destruction of surrounding normal tissues.

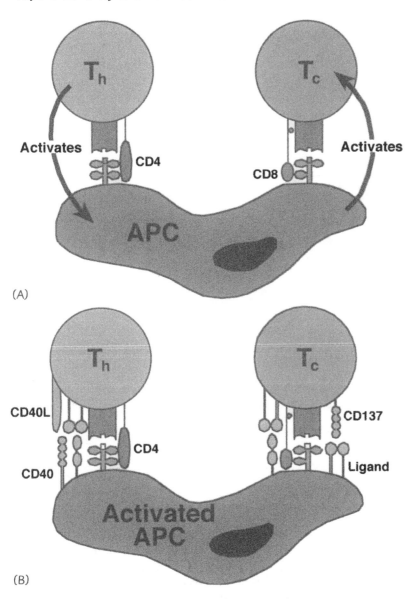

Figure 3 Effector functions of CD4+ T cells—activation of APC. T-helper cells activate APC to express costimulatory signals that stimulate CD8+ T cells (A). CD40 ligand on T-helper cells triggers CD40 receptors on APC, resulting in activation of APC and upregulation of other costimulatory signals, such as CD137 ligand. CD8+ T cells preferentially express CD137 receptors that are triggered by activated APC, resulting in activation of CD8+ cytotoxic T cells (B).

VI. COSTIMULATORY MOLECULES

As mentioned above, naïve CD4+ T cells and CD8+ T cells need to recognize antigen plus a second costimulatory signal to induce proliferation and differentiation

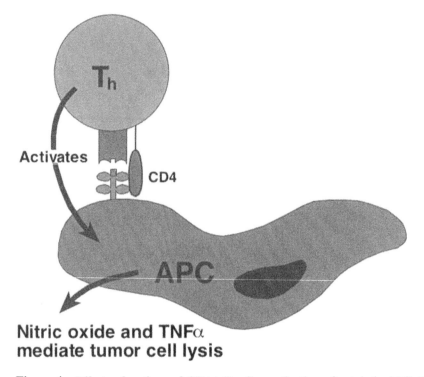

**Nitric oxide and TNFα
mediate tumor cell lysis**

Figure 4 Effector functions of CD4+ T cells—activation of cytolytic APC. T-helper cells indirectly lyse tumor cells via activation of APC to secrete cytokines, such as TNF-α and nitric oxide, that nonspecifically lyse tumor cells.

into armed effector T cells. The best-characterized costimulatory molecules are the closely related B7 molecules B7.1 (CD80) and B7.2 (CD86). CD80 is a cell-surface protein that triggers CD28 receptors on T cells [9]. An important issue for antitumor immunity is that recognition of antigen in the *absence* of costimulation not only fails to stimulate naïve T cells but also induces anergy—a form of unresponsiveness that makes T cells resistant to future activation [10]. Anergized T cells fail to respond even when triggered by professional APCs that present signals one and two. This is an important mechanism that could allow tumors to prevent activation of specific T cells.

 T cells activated in the lymph node by APCs expressing both signals are "primed" and migrate into the periphery where they mediate their effector function when triggered by their specific antigen. Once T cells are successfully primed to an antigen, a second costimulatory signal is no longer required [11]. In recent years the number of costimulatory signals identified has increased dramatically. Now there are a number of positive and negative costimulatory signals that function during different stages of T-cell activation (reviewed in Ref. 12). This new information will clearly be important in future studies that refine our methods of activating tumor-specific T cells.

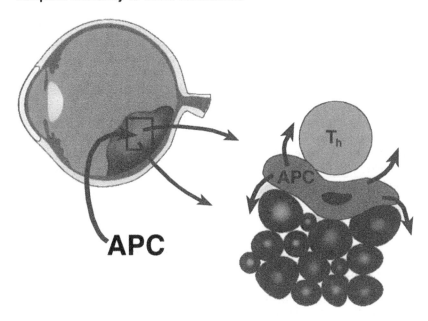

Figure 5 Geographic specificity of T-helper cells. APCs that infiltrate into tumors are activated only when they come into contact with CD4+ T-helper cells specific for antigens expressed on the APCs. This limits the release of nonspecific cytokines from APCs and CD4+ T-helper cells to a small geographical area within the tumor, resulting in limited destruction of normal tissue.

VII. TUMOR ANTIGENS

There are four general categories of tumor antigens (reviewed in Ref. 13): (1) tissue-specific differentiation antigens expressed on melanomas and normal melanocytes, (2) tumor-selective antigens that are expressed in fetal tissues but not found on adult tissues (except the testis), (3) antigens derived from mutated proteins found only in tumors and not normal tissues, and (4) viral antigens found in virus-associated cancers. Uveal melanomas express tissue-specific tumor antigens that are found on skin melanomas, such as Mart-1, and tumor selective antigens, such as MAGE-1 [14]. Unfortunately, there has not been an extensive analysis of tumor antigens expressed on either primary uveal melanomas or liver metastases. Furthermore, it is unknown whether uveal melanomas express *unique* tumor antigens that are not found on skin melanomas. Considering the extensive differences in the clinical pattern of disease progression between skin and uveal melanomas and the functional differences between normal skin and choroidal melanocytes, it seems likely that unique tumor antigens will be expressed on uveal melanomas. Much more work is needed in this area if immunotherapies are to be used for treating patients with uveal melanomas.

Tumor immunologists have focused almost exclusively on the activation of CTLs for several reasons. First, tumor-specific CD8+ T cells can be recovered from cancer patients and activated in vitro. Second, almost all of the tumor antigens identified to date are recognized by CTLs. Third, the highest degree of specificity for tumor target cells is displayed by CTLs. Fourth, numerous animal models demonstrate that CTLs are highly effective in eliminating progressively growing tumors. Finally, it was predicted that excessive amounts of costimulation plus tumor antigens would bypass the need for CD4+ T helper cells. In spite of these observations, immunotherapies utilizing CD8+ T cells are not as effective as originally predicted. Even though tumor-specific CD8+ CTLs are activated, in many cases they are unable to prevent continued progressive tumor growth. Although there are many potential reasons for the failure of CD8+ T-cell therapy, the lack of a sustained T-cell response is currently a primary focus of many immunologists. Therefore many researchers have begun to focus their attention on the activation of tumor-specific CD4+ T-helper cells.

VIII. ANTIGEN PROCESSING AND PRESENTATION PATHWAYS— MAJOR HISTOCOMPATIBILITY COMPLEX (MHC)

As a defense against foreign pathogens, mammals have evolved a sophisticated system that enables them to distinguish self from non-self. This was first demonstrated by the rejection of foreign tissue grafts in mice [15–17]. The genetic loci involved in graft rejection were subsequently mapped to a region on chromosome 17 [17], which became known as the major histocompatibility complex (MHC). The human MHC, also known as the human leukocyte antigen (HLA) system, is located on the short arm of chromosome 6 [18,19].

The MHC complex is divided into three different classes of genes: I, II, and III. There are a variety of class I genes, but three loci are typically identified in humans: HLA-A, HLA-B, and HLA-C. Class II genes are located in the HLA-D region and consist of at least three loci: HLA-DR, HLA-DQ, and HLA-DP [20,21]. The class III genes encode components of the complement system and a diverse collection of at least 20 other genes [22–24].

In order to detect and eliminate pathogens from different anatomical sites, the immune system has developed a mechanism to recognize foreign antigens derived from two different cellular sources. CD8+ T cells recognize antigens derived from *intracellular/endogenous* proteins presented by class I. By contrast, CD4+ T cells recognize antigens derived from *extracellular/exogenous* proteins presented by class II. The class I and class II pathways of antigen processing have evolved in order to present small peptide fragments of degraded proteins derived from these two different sources.

It is believed that there is a strong selective pressure to develop an immune system which can protect the host during the childbearing years from bacterial and viral infections threatening the propagation of the species. This selective advantage is absent for pathogens that threaten only older adults that are past the childbearing stage. Since cancer is mainly a disease of old age, it is frequently hypothesized that the immune system is *not* specifically designed to protect the host from malignant transformation. For this reason, it is important to understand the class I and class II pathways of antigen processing and how these pathways are used or not used to process and present tumor antigens. This is critical for understanding how these pathways can be manipulated in cancer immunotherapies.

IX. THE CLASS I ANTIGEN-PROCESSING PATHWAY

MHC class I molecules present endogenous peptide antigens. Proteins present in the cytoplasm are degraded by proteasomes into short peptide fragments that are transported across the membrane of the endoplasmic reticulum (ER) by the transporter associated with antigen presentation (TAP) proteins (Fig. 6). In the ER, peptide antigens are bound by preassembled class I heterodimers synthesized within the ER and composed of a heavy chain and $\beta 2$ microglobulin ($\beta 2m$). This trimolecular complex of peptide, class I heavy chain, and $\beta 2m$ is then transported via the exocytic pathway to the cell surface (Golgi complex and post-Golgi vesicles). By this mechanism, antigens derived from endogenous proteins within the cell are processed and presented on the cell surface. This is necessary because viral pathogens infect cells and express viral proteins within the cell. The immune system can sample the array of intracellular proteins via class I on the cell surface and determine whether the cell is healthy or infected. During malignant transformation, a cascade of mutations occurs in the proteins that regulate cellular proliferation. Mutations in normal proteins can be recognized as tumor antigens by specific T cells. Therefore the class I pathway is critical in detecting tumor antigens.

Endogenous Pathway

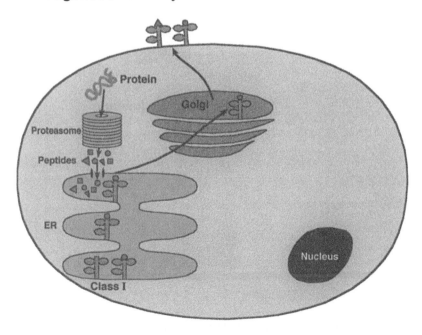

Figure 6 Class I pathway of antigen processing. The class I pathway processes endogenous antigens present within the cytoplasm of the cell. Proteins are broken down into small peptide fragments that enter the endoplasmic reticulum, where they bind class I molecules. The endogenous peptide antigens are then shuttled to the cell surface via the Golgi apparatus.

X. THE CLASS II ANTIGEN-PROCESSING PATHWAY

MHC class II molecules predominantly present antigens derived from extracellular sources, such as bacteria. Exogenous proteins first gain access to the class II pathway when they are either endocytosed or phagocytosed by APCs. These proteins are then broken down into small peptide fragments within the endosome after it fuses with a lysosome [25,26]. The formation of MHC class II–peptide complexes is a complicated, multistep process (Fig. 7). It starts with the transcription of the MHC class II alpha (α) and beta (β) chains and accessory molecules (invariant chain and DM). This transcription is under the control of a variety of transcription factors that are ultimately controlled by a master regulator, called CIITA (class II transactivator). In general, activation of CIITA initiates transcription of all genes involved in the class II pathway. Many proinflammatory cytokines, such as IFN-γ, activate CIITA. For this reason, there is a close association between inflammation and induction of class II.

MHC class II α and β chains, along with the associated invariant chain (Ii), are assembled in the endoplasmic reticulum (ER) [27,28]. Ii association has three major functions: (1) it stabilizes the $\alpha\beta$ complexes, (2) it prevents an antigenic peptide (endogenously synthesized) from binding to the $\alpha\beta$ dimers in the ER, and (3) it provides a guiding signal for transport of the $\alpha\beta$ complex through the MHC class II antigen-processing pathway. Binding of Ii chain to class II is critical in preventing the loading of endogenous peptides in the ER [29–31]. The fragment of Ii chain that

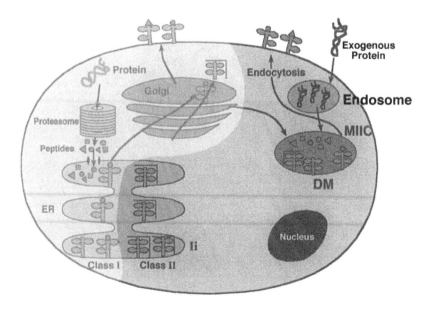

Figure 7   Class II pathway of antigen processing. The class II pathway processes exogenous antigens, since the class II molecules within the endoplasmic reticulum are bound by invariant chain (Ii). Exogenous proteins are endocytosed and digested into small peptides within the endosome. Class II molecules are loaded with exogenous antigens within the MIIC compartment when the last fragments of Ii chain are removed from class II. Antigen-loaded class II molecules are then shuttled to the cell surface.

is stably associated with class II is called CLIP [32–34]. Synthetic peptides corresponding to the CLIP region of Ii chain bind with high avidity to class II and compete with antigenic peptides for class II binding [35,36]. Following dissociation of the Ii chain from the class II α/β chains, the class II binding site becomes open for loading with peptides [37].

After migration through the Golgi system, the class II–Ii complex is transported into specialized endosomal compartments (MIIC). This MIIC is similar to late endosomes [38]. In these compartments, Ii chain undergoes proteolysis and dissociation from class II. If Ii chain degradation is blocked and remains bound to class II, then class II–Ii complexes are retained within the cell and fail to present antigen [39–41]. A potent additional cofactor necessary to promote class II–Ii dissociation, through the removal of CLIP, is DM [42]. Once CLIP is removed from the class II–peptide binding site, class II encounters antigen that binds the peptide-binding groove. Loaded class II–peptide complexes are now ready to travel to the cell surface where they are expressed and can be recognized by specific CD4+ T cells.

XI. CROSS-PRIMING VERSUS DIRECT RECOGNITION

Understanding how tumor antigens enter the class I and class II pathways is critical for the successful activation of tumor- specific CD4+ T cells and CD8+ T cells. For

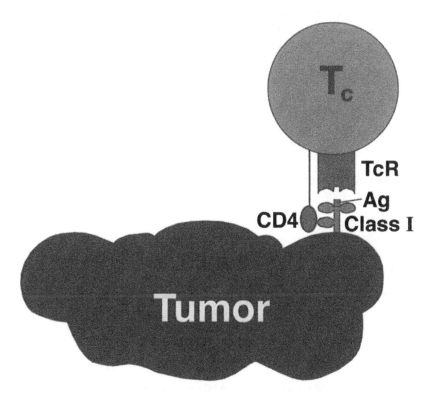

Figure 8 Direct recognition of tumor antigens. CD8+ cytotoxic T cells recognize directly endogenous tumor antigens presented by class I on the surface of tumor cells.

this reason, this has been an area of intense research and controversy among tumor immunologists. Currently there are three possible pathways tumor antigens are presented to the immune system: (1) tumor antigens derived from endogenous proteins are presented on the cell surface of class I positive tumor cells (direct pathway) (Fig. 8); (2) APCs migrate into the tumor site, phagocytize tumor cell fragments, and present tumor antigens via class II on the cell surface (indirect pathway) (Fig. 9); and (3) cross-priming occurs when APCs infiltrate into the tumor site and process and present tumor antigens on both class I and class II (Fig. 10). The latter mechanism does not fit the antigen-processing pathways described earlier, since endogenous tumor proteins are *not* present within APCs and therefore should not enter the class I pathway. For this reason, immunologists originally did not think that cross-priming occurred. However, recent evidence suggests that cross-priming of tumor antigens *does* occur, suggesting that there must be an unknown link between the endocytic pathway and the endoplasmic reticulum allowing endogenous peptide antigens access to class II molecules [43].

XII. CURRENT IMMUNOTHERAPIES AND BARRIERS TO THEIR SUCCESS

Since the current immunotherapies result in a very low, but significant response, an important question is: What is the mechanism that prevents activation of successful antitumor immunity in patients with progressively growing malignancies? In a "normal" immune response to a foreign pathogen, host APCs migrate into the site of infection, phagocytize infected cells, and return to the draining lymph node, where

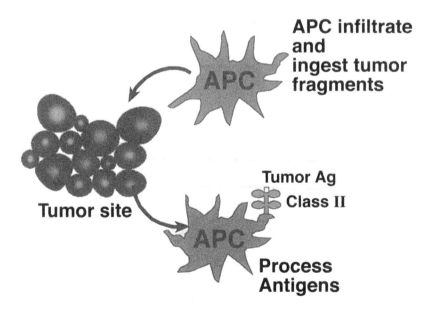

Figure 9 Indirect recognition of tumor antigens. APCs infiltrate the tumor site and digest tumor cell fragments. Exogenous antigens are reprocessed and expressed on the cell surface by class II. CD4+ T-helper cells indirectly recognize tumor antigens presented on APCs.

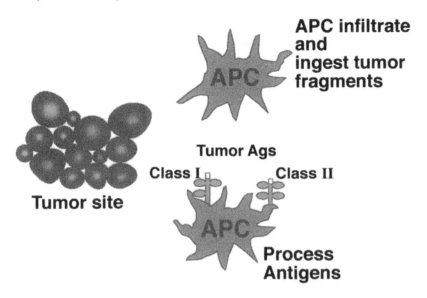

Figure 10   Cross-priming of tumor antigens. Cross-priming occurs when APC infiltrate the tumor site and process and present tumor antigens on both class I and class II. APCs that use this route of antigen presentation activate CD4+ T cells and CD8+ T cells.

they process and present the antigens to responding naïve T cells. This results in proliferation, differentiation, and clonal expansion of antigen-specific effector T cells that migrate systemically and eliminate infected cells. This same mechanism should also successfully eliminate spontaneous human tumors expressing tumor antigens. Although animal models demonstrate that cross-priming of tumor antigens *can* occur, there is hardly any evidence that host APCs in cancer patients successfully present tumor antigens. Several mechanisms used by tumors to escape immune detection and destruction have been identified (reviewed in Ref. 44). One important escape mechanism is blocking the activation of CD4+ T-helper cells.

Extensive studies using animal models indicate that, although either CD8+ or CD4+ T cells alone can independently mediate tumor rejection, the most *effective and long-lasting protective immunity* occurs when *both* CD4+ and CD8+ T cells are activated. For this reason, the current lack of tumor antigens presented by class II and recognized by CD4+ T cells is an obvious important deficiency. It has been proposed that tumor cells block APC activation of CD4+ T cells by releasing either (1) suppressive factors that block APC antigen processing or (2) factors that block APC maturation. For example, vascular endothelial growth factor (VEGF) secreted by tumor cells has been shown to inhibit tumor antigen presentation by APCs [45]. Together with other reports, this evidence suggests that tumor cells create a local microenvironment that is hostile to infiltrating APCs and activation of tumor-specific CD4+ T cells.

Some approaches of experimental immunotherapy aim to modify host APCs in an attempt to increase antigen presentation to CD4+ T helper cells. The most widely studied host APCs are dendritic cells (DC). Mature DCs induce specific T-cell immunity and resistance to tumors in several different animal models. However, since the inflammatory and microbial stimuli required for DC maturation are frequently absent in tumors, it is likely that tumor-infiltrating DCs fail to mature. Immature DCs downregulate adaptive T-cell responses by inducing regulatory T cells [46,47]. In an effort to avoid this, some cancer immunotherapy strategies use mature DCs that are pulsed with tumor antigens or transduced with genes encoding tumor antigens in vitro prior to injection into tumor-bearing patients. This strategy successfully generated APCs that were highly effective at inducing antitumor immunity in animal models [48–51]. Whether this strategy will be successful in patients is still unclear.

XIII. SUCCESSFUL ACTIVATION OF CTL REQUIRES T-HELPER CELLS

Primed tumor-specific CTIs can be found among peripheral blood lymphocytes and lymphocytes that infiltrate the tumor site [52–54]. In vitro, these primed T cells can be activated to become cytolytic cells by addition of exogenous lymphokines; however, there is little evidence that mature cytolytic T cells develop in situ. Because $CD8^+$ T cells are capable of responding to lymphokines in vitro and it has been very difficult to detect tumor-specific $CD4^+$ T cells in vivo, it seems that stimulation of specific cytotoxic T cells to differentiate into functional killer cells requires the presence of helper lymphokines. Many immunotherapy approaches have attempted to bypass the requirement for T helper cells and directly stimulate cytotoxic T cells. Tumor cells were genetically modified to express a variety of different cytokine genes: IL-2, IL-4, IL-7, TNF-α, IFN-γ, and GM-CSF [55]. This approach was successful in activating antitumor lymphocytes with cytolytic activity. However, this antitumor immunity was time-limited and ineffective against progressive, growing tumors. Expression of cell membrane–bound costimulatory molecules was also attempted by expressing CD80 on tumor cells. This strategy induced significant antitumor immune responses and generated protection against a challenge from wild-type tumors at a distant site [56]. However, further analysis suggested that this approach was *not* successful for weakly immunogenic tumor antigens [57].

Increasing evidence from animal studies and clinical trials indicates that $CD4^+$ T cells are indispensable in inducing host immunity against tumors [58–61]. Compared to the high number of reports on the role of specific cytotoxic T cells in antitumor immunity, much less attention has been given to activation of $CD4^+$ T cells. There are at least two reasons for this: (1) most tumor cells express MHC class I but not MHC class II molecules and (2) few MHC class II–restricted tumor antigens have been identified. With increasing evidence supporting the hypothesis that $CD4^+$ T cells play a central role in a successful antitumor immunity, it is necessary to develop strategies for the identification of MHC class II-restricted tumor antigens and activation of tumor-specific $CD4^+$ T cells. For a number of reasons described below, human uveal melanomas are an ideal tumor to study the activation of tumor specific CD4+ T cells and may provide important information on the activation of this critical subpopulation of T cells.

XIV. HOW TO OPEN THE MHC CLASS II PATHWAY FOR TUMOR ANTIGENS

Tumor antigens are derived from *endogenous* proteins found within tumor cells. Thus, class II positive tumor cells *fail* to express tumor antigens, since this pathway is generally reserved for *exogenous* peptide antigens. As described earlier, invariant chain plays a pivotal role in blocking endogenously synthesized peptides from binding class II molecules in the ER. In order to open the class II pathway for endogenous peptides, it is necessary to eliminate Ii. Creating class II positive tumor cells by inducing class II expression with IFN-γ treatment or introducing CIITA genes will fail, because this also upregulates Ii chain expression [62–64]. Tumor cells that express class II in the absence of Ii chain would be ideal for presenting endogenous tumor antigens by MHC class II molecules [Fig. 11].

During the past decade Dr. S. Ostrand-Rosenberg has developed tumor vaccines in several different animal models that directly activate tumor-specific CD4$^+$ T cells, eliminate primary tumors, and provide long-term protection from metastases. The vaccine strategy was based on the hypothesis that genetically modified tumor cells can be APCs for endogenously synthesized tumor antigens. These vaccines used autologous tumor cells transfected with syngeneic MHC class II and the costimulatory molecule CD80 (B7.1) genes. For a number of reasons discussed later, uveal melanomas are among the few human spontaneous tumors that can utilize this vaccine strategy. Therefore it is important to summarize the in

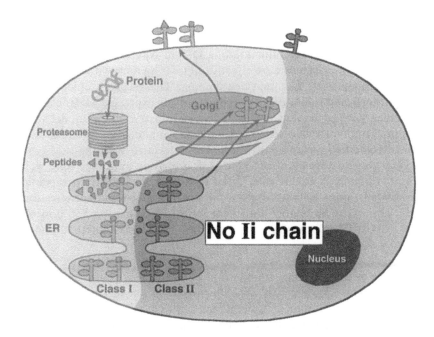

Figure 11 Opening the class II pathway to endogenous tumor antigens. Tumor cells are normally unable to present endogenous tumor antigens via the class II pathway. However, tumor cells that express class II in the absence of Ii chain acquire the ability to present endogenous tumor antigens via class II and activate CD4+ T-helper cells.

vivo studies with tumor-bearing mice that demonstrate the significant activity of
these vaccines as therapeutic agents for the treatment of established primary tumors
and progressive metastatic disease. The experiments were performed in three animal
models: sarcoma, melanoma, and mammary carcinoma.

The first-generation tumor cell vaccine was produced over a decade ago and
protected naïve animals from a subsequent challenge of wild-type tumor cells. This
initial approach was based on the hypothesis that tumor cells expressing syngeneic
MHC class II molecules would directly present tumor antigens to CD4$^+$ T cells and
thereby facilitate antitumor immunity. This hypothesis was tested by transfecting
mouse SaI sarcomas (H-2^a) with syngeneic MHC class II genes (Aa^k + Ab^k genes;
SaI/A^k tumor cells) and using the tumor cells to vaccinate syngeneic A/J mice. Mice
immunized with several clones of this vaccine were completely protected against the
wild-type tumor [65]. In vivo antibody depletion studies confirmed that CD4$^+$ T cells
were required for protection.

At the time of these initial studies 10 years ago, the role of costimulation was
not understood. In several studies, it was demonstrated that antigen presentation by
MHC class II molecules required the cytoplasmic domain of the class II heterodimer
[66]. Since, in the above described experiments, the hypothesis was that class II-
transfected tumor cells functioned as APCs, SaI tumor cells transfected with MHC
class II genes truncated for their cytoplasmic domains (SaI/A^k/tr) were generated.
These transfectants were not effective vaccines and were tumorigeneic themselves
[67]. However, the vaccine effect was restored if the SaI/A^k/tr cells were further
transfected with the gene encoding the CD80 (B7.1) costimulatory molecule (SaI/
A^{k}tr/B7.1) [68]. These experiments, along with two other studies [69,70], provided
the first evidence that tumor cell expression of costimulatory molecules enhanced
antitumor immunity. They also suggested that one of the functions of MHC class II
molecules in antigen presentation is induction of CD80 in APCs.

The second-generation vaccines were effective in treating mice with established
primary sarcoma and metastatic mammary carcinoma. The vaccine's efficacy was
increased by using transfected tumor cells that constitutively expressed MHC class II
plus CD80. Vaccines were generated and tested in a primary tumor model (SaI
sarcoma) and in metastatic models (BALB/c-derived 4T1 mammary carcinoma and
C57BL/6-derived B16melF10 melanoma). Mice were inoculated with the wild-type
tumor cells and the tumors were allowed to grow progressively until they were well
vascularized (approximately 3 weeks after initial inoculation). Weekly therapeutic
injections of irradiated tumor cells were given for 3 weeks and tumor progression
was monitored. The most dramatic antitumor effect was observed following
vaccination with class II/CD80 transfectants in the SaI, 4T1, and B16melF10 tumor
systems [71–72].

The third-generation vaccines were more effective in treating mice with
established metastatic disease. The enterotoxin B of *Staphylococcus aureus* (SEB) is a
potent activator of CD4$^+$ T cells [73]. The third-generation vaccines therefore
consisted of SEB-transfected tumor cells combined with class II/B7 transfectants.
This strategy was tested in the BALB/c-derived 4T1 mammary carcinoma model.
Mice treated with this combination vaccine had significantly fewer lung metastases.

Together, these results support the hypothesis that MHC class II and CD80-
transfected tumor cell vaccines induce antitumor immunity because they directly
present endogenously synthesized tumor antigens to CD4$^+$ T cells [74]. If this MHC

class II–positive tumor cell vaccine strategy is to be applied clinically, convenient methods for generating class II$^+$ tumor cells are necessary. Class II expression is upregulated by treatment with either gamma interferon (IFN-γ), or transduction of the class II transactivator (CIITA) gene. However, these treatments also upregulate the expression of the class II-associated accessory molecules, invariant chain and DM. To investigate whether tumor cells treated with either IFN-γ or CIITA to express class II could be used as tumor cell vaccines, the following experiments were performed. Sarcoma tumor cells that expressed combinations of class II, Ii, or DM were tested for their effectiveness as vaccines. Sarcoma cells that expressed class II *without* coexpression of Ii were effective vaccines, while tumor cells coexpressing class II plus Ii, or class II/Ii/DM failed. These results suggest that if tumor cells coexpress MHC class II, Ii, and DM, then presentation of endogenously synthesized tumor antigens is blocked and transfectants do not function as effective vaccines.

Overall, these data demonstrate that genetically modified tumor cells are efficacious vaccines for the treatment of primary and metastatic cancers in experimental animal models. It is likely these vaccines work by activating directly CD4$^+$ tumor-specific T cells. Success of these vaccines requires that tumor cells *express MHC class II and not invariant chain*. The next step is to translate this vaccine strategy to the treatment of human tumors.

XV. HUMAN MODEL: UVEAL MELANOMA

Uveal melanomas are attractive targets for the tumor cell vaccine discovered by Dr. Sue Ostrand-Rosenberg. Preliminary studies indicate that a significant number of cultured tumor cells derived from ocular melanomas *do not* express MHC class II. Most importantly, they fail to express invariant chain and DM. Moreover, treatment of uveal melanoma cells with INF-γ *fails* to induce expression of either class II or accessory molecules. The failure to respond to IFN-γ coincides with the absence of CIITA. Therefore uveal melanomas are among the few human tumors fitting the criteria for a tumor cell vaccine that will activate CD4+ T cells. If these tumors are transfected with MHC class II, then tumor antigens that activate protective immunity should be expressed. Currently, our group and the Ostrand-Rosenberg Laboratory are constructing MHC class II$^+$/CD80$^+$/tetanus toxoid-positive uveal melanoma cells using a retroviral vector. The efficacy of these genetically modified tumor cells will be assessed in activating tumor-specific CD4$^+$ T cells in the first step toward determining whether this vaccine strategy is successful in activating protective immunity against uveal melanomas.

REFERENCES

1. Boon T. Cancer tumor antigens. Curr Opin Immunol 9:681–683, 1997.
2. June CH, Bluestone JA, Nadler LM, Thompson CB. The B7 and CD28 receptor families. *Immunol Today* 15:321–331, 1994.
3. Rosenberg SA. Progress in human tumor immunology and immunotherapy. Nature 411:380–384, 2001.
4. Medzhitov R, Janeway C. Innate immune recognition: Mechanisms and pathways. Immunol Rev 173:89–97, 2000.

5. Symth MJ, et al. Differential tumor surveillance by natural killer and NKT cells. J Exp Med 191:661–668, 2000.

6. Chen YT, Scanlan MJ, Sahin U, Tureci O, Gure AO, Tsang S, Williamson B, Stockert E, Pfreundschuh M, Old LJ. A testicular antigen aberrantly expressed in human cancers detected by autologous antibody screening. Proc Natl Acad Sci USA 94:1914–1918, 1997.

7. Smyth MJ, Godfrey DI, Trapani JA. A fresh look at tumor or immunosurveillance and immunotherapy. Nat Immunol 2:293–299, 2001.

8. Morel PA, Oriss TB. Cross regulation between Th1 and Th2 cells. Crit Rev Immunol 18:275–303, 1998.

9. June CH, Bluestone JA, Nadler LM, Thompson CB. The B7 and CD28 receptor families. Immunol Today 15:321–331, 1994.

10. Boussiotis VA, Freeman GJ, Gribben JC, Nadler LM. The role of B7-1/B7-2;CD28/ CTLA-4 pathways in the induction of protective immunity and downregulation of the immune response. Immunol Rev 153:5–26, 1996.

11. Gause WC, Mitro V, Via C, Linsley P, Urban JF, Greenwald RJ. Do effector and memory T helper cells also need B7 ligand costimulation? J Immunol. 159:1055–1058, 1997.

12. Pardoll D. Spinning molecular immunology into successful immunotherapy. Nat Immunol Rev 2:227–238, 2002.

13. Wang R, Rosenberg SA. Human tumor antigens for cancer vaccine development. Immunol Rev 170:85–100, 1999.

14. Chen P, Murray TG, Salgaller ML, and Ksander BR. Expression of MAGE genes in ocular melanoma cell lines. J Immunother 20:265–275, 1997.

15. Gorer PA. The detection of antigenic differences in mouse erythrocytes by the employment of immune sera. Br J Exp Pathol 17:42–50, 1936.

16. Snell GD. Histocompatibility genes of the mouse. II. Production and analysis of isogenic resistant lines. J Natl Cancer Inst 21:843–877, 1958.

17. Klein J. Biology of the Mouse Histocompatibility-2 Complex: Principles of Immuno-genetics Applied to a Single System. Berlin: Springer-Verlag. 1975.

18. Van Someren H, Westerveld A, Hagemeijer A, Mees JR, Meera Khan P, Zaalberg OB. Human antigen and enzyme markers in man—Chinese hamster somatic cell hybrids: Evidence for synteny between the HLA-A, PGM_3, ME_1 and IPO-B loci. Proc Natl Acad Sci USA 71:962–965, 1974.

19. Breuning MH, Berg-Loonen van den EM, Bernini LF, Bijlsma JB, Loghem van E, Meera Khan P, Nijenhuis LE. Localization of HLA on the short arm of chromosome 6 Hum Genet 37:131–139, 1977.

20. Benacerraf B, Paul WE, Green L. The immune response of guinea pigs to haptenpoly-L-lysine conjugates as example of the genetic control of the recognition of antigenicity. Cold Spring Harbor Symp Quant Biol 32:569–574, 1967.

21. McDevitt HO, Chinitz A. Genetic control of the antibody response: Relationship between immune response and histocompatibility (H-2) type. Science 254:1788–1791, 1972.

22. Bird A. CpG islands as gene markers in the vertebrate nucleus. Trends Genet 3:342–347, 1987.

23. Sargent CA, Dunham I, Campbell RD. Identification of multiple HTF-islands associated genes in the human major histocompatibility complex class II region. EMBO J 8:2305–2312, 1989.

24. Spies T, Bresnahan M, Strominger JL. Human major histocompatibility complex contains a minimum of 19 genes between the complement cluster and HLA-B. Proc Natl Acad Sci USA 86:8955–8958, 1989.

25. Loss G, Sant A. Invariant chain retains MHC class II molecules in the endocytic pathway. J Immunol 150:3187–3197, 1993.
26. Germain RN, Margulies DH. The biochemistry and cell biology of antigen processing and presentation. Annu Rev Immunol 11:403–450, 1993.
27. Germain RN. MHC-dependent antigen processing and peptide presentation: providing ligands for T lymphocyte activation. Cell, 76:287–299, 1994.
28. Cresswell P. Invariant chain structure and MHC class II function. Cell 84:505–507, 1996.
29. Roche PA, Cresswell P. Invariant chain association with HLA-DR molecules inhibits immunogenic peptide binding. Nature (London) 345:615–618, 1990.
30. Teyton L, O'Sullivan D, Dickson PW, Lotteau V, Sette A, Fink P, Peterson PA. Invariant chain distinguishes between the exogenous and endogenous antigen presentation pathways. Nature (London), 348:39–44, 1990.
31. Newcomb J, Cresswell P. Characterization of endogenous peptides bound to purified HLA-DR molecules and their absence from invariant chain-associated $\alpha\beta$ dimers. J Immunol 150(2):499–507, 1993.
32. Rudensky A, Preston-Hurlburt P, Hong S, Barlow A, Janeway C. Sequence analysis of peptides bound to MHC class II molecules. Nature 353:622–627, 1991.
33. Hunt D, Michel H, Dickinson T, Shabanowitz J, Cox A, Sakaguchi K, Appella E, Grey H, Sette A. Peptides presented to the immune system by the murine class II major histocompatibility complex molecule I-Ad. Science 256:1817–1820, 1992.
34. Chicz R, Urban R, Gorga J, Vignali D, Lane W, Strominger J. Specificity and promiscuity among naturally processed peptides bound to HLA-DR molecules. J Exp Med 178(1):27–47, 1993.
35. Sette A, Ceman S, Kubo R, Sakaguchi K, Apella E, Hunt D, Davis T, Michel H, Shabanowitz J, Rudersdorf R, Grey H, Demars R. Invariant chain peptides in most HLA-DR molecules of an antigen processing mutant. Science 258:1801–1804, 1992.
36. Riberdy J, Cresswell P. The antigen processing mutant T2 suggests a role for MHC-linked genes in class II antigen presentation. J Immunol 148(8):2586–2590, 1992.
37. Roche PA, Cresswell P. Proteolysis of the class II associated invariant chain generates a peptide binding site in intracellular HLA-DR molecules. Proc Natl Acad Sci USA 88:3150–3154, 1991.
38. Peters P, Neefjes J, Oorschot V, Ploegh H, Geuze H. Segregation of MHC class II molecules from MHC class I molecules in the Golgi complex for transport to lysosomal compartments. Nature 349:669–676, 1991.
39. Neefjes JJ and Ploegh HL. Inhibition of endosomal proteolytic activity by leupeptin blocks surface expression of MHC class II molecules and their conversion to SDS resistant $\alpha\beta$ heterodimers in endosomes. EMBO J 11(2):411–416, 1992.
40. Loss G, Sant A. Invariant chain retains MHC class II molecules in the endocytic pathway. J Immunol 150:3187–3197, 1993.
41. Mellins E, Smith L, Arp B, Cotner T, Celis E, Pious D. Defective processing and presentation of exogenous antigens in mutants with normal HLA class II genes. Nature 343:71–74, 1990.
42. Cresswell P. Invariant chain structure and MHC class II function. Cell 84:505–507, 1996.
43. Levitsky HI, Lazenby A, Hayashi RJ, Pardoll DM. In vivo priming of two distinct effector populations: The role of MHC class I expression. J Exp Med 179:1215–1224, 1994.
44. Marincola FM, Jaffee EM, Hicklin DJ, Ferrone S. Escape of human solid tumors from T cell recognition: Molecular mechanisms and functional significance. Adv Immunol 74:181–273, 2000.
45. Gabrilovich DI, Chen HL, Girgis KR, Cunningham HT, Meny GM, Nadaf S, Kavanaugh D, Carbone DP. Production of vascular endothelial growth factor by human

tumors inhibits the functional maturation of dendritic cells. Nat Med 2(10):1096–1103, 1996.

46.   Jonuleit H, Schmitt E, Schuler G, Knop J, Enk AH. Induction of human IL-10-producing, non-proliferating CD4+ T cells with regulatory properties by repetitive stimulation with allogeneic immature dendritic cells. J Exp Med 193:233–238, 2001.

47.   Dhodapkar MV, Steinman RM, Krasovsky J, Munz C, Bhardwaj N. Antigen specific inhibition of effector T cell function in humans after injection of immature dendritic cells. J Exp Med 192:1213–1222, 2001.

48.   Young JW, Inaba K. Dendritic cells as adjuvants for class I major histocompatibility complex-restricted antitumor immunity. J Exp Med 183(1):7–11, 1996.

49.   Schuler G, Steinman RM. Dendritic cells as adjuvants for immune-mediated resistance to tumors. J Exp Med 186(8):1183–1187, 1997.

50.   Song W, Kong HL, Carpenter H, Torii H, Granstein R, Rafii S, Moore MA, Crystal RG. Dendritic cells genetically modified with an adenovirus vector encoding the cDNA for a model antigen induce protective and therapeutic antitumor immunity. J Exp Med. 186(8):1247–1256, 1997.

51.   Nestle FO, Alijagic S, Gilliet M, Sun Y, Grabbe S, Dummer R, Burg G, Schadendorf D. Vaccination of melanoma patients with peptide- or tumor lysate-pulsed dendritic cells. Nat Med 4:382–332, 1998.

52.   Itoh K, Platsoucas CD, Balch CM. Autologous tumor-specific cytotoxic T lymphocytes in the infiltrate of human metastatic melanomas. Activation by interleukin 2 and autologous tumor cells, and involvement of the T cell receptor. J Exp Med 168(4):1419–1441, 1988.

53.   Mukherji B, Guha A, Chakraborty NG, Sivanandham M, Nashed AL, Sporn JR, Ergin MT. Clonal analysis of cytotoxic and regulatory T cell responses against human melanoma. J Exp Med 169(6):1961–1976, 1989.

54.   Topalian SL, Solomon D, Rosenberg SA. Tumor specific cytolysis by lymphocytes infiltrating human melanomas. J Immunol 142(10):3714–3725, 1989.

55.   Hock H, Dorsch M, Richter G, Kunzendorf U, Kruger-Krasagakes S, Blankenstein T, Qin Z, Diamantstein T. Tumor cell targeted cytokine gene transfer in animal models for cancer therapy. Nat Immunol 13(2–3):85–92, 1994.

56.   Townsend SE and Allison JP. Tumor rejection after direct costimulation of CD8+ T cells by B7-transfected melanoma cells. Science 259:368–370, 1993.

57.   Chen L, McGowan P, Ashe S, Johnston J, Li, Hellstrom K. Tumor immunogenicity determines the effect of B7 costimulation on T cell-mediated tumor immunity. J Exp Med 179:523–532, 1994.

58.   Cohen PA, Peng L, Plautz GE, Kim JA, Weng DE, Shu S. CD4+ T cells in adoptive immunotherapy and the indirect mechanism of tumor rejection. Crit Rev Immunol 20(1):17–56, 2000.

59.   Toes RE, Ossendorp, F, Offringa R, Melief CJ. CD4+ T cells and their role in anti-tumor immune responses. J Exp Med 189(5):753–756, 1999.

60.   Pardoll DM, Topalian SL. The role of CD4+ T cell responses in antitumor immunity. Curr Opin Immunol 10(5):58–594, 1998.

61.   Kalams SA and Walker BD. The critical need for CD4 help in maintaining effective cytotoxic T lymphocyte responses. J Exp Med 188(12):2199–2204, 1998.

62.   Cresswell P. Invariant chain structure and MHC class II function. Cell, 84:505–507, 1996.

63.   Denzin LK and Cresswell P. HLA-DM induces clip dissociation from MHC class II alpha-beta dimers and facilitates peptide loading. Cell 82:155–165, 1995.

64.   Sloan VS, Cameron P, Porter G, Gammon M, Amaya M, Mellins E, Zaller D. Mediation by HLA-DM of dissociation of peptides from HLA-DR. Nature 375:802–806, 1995.

65. Ostrand-Rosenberg S, Thakur A, Clements VK. Rejection of mouse sarcoma cells after transfection of MHC class II genes. J Immunol 144:4068–4071, 1990.
66. Nabavi N, Freeman GJ, Gault A, Godfrey D, Nadler LM, Glimcher LH. Signaling through the MHC class II cytoplasmic domain is required for antigen presentation and induces B7 expression. Nature 360:266–268, 1992.
67. Ostrand-Rosenberg S, Roby CA, Clements VK. Abrogation of tumorigenicity by MHC Class II antigen expression requires the cytoplasmic domain of the class II molecule. J Immunol 147:2419–2422, 1991.
68. Baskar S, Ostrand-Rosenberg S, Nabavi N, Nadler LM, Freeman GJ, Glimcher LH. Constitutive expression of B7 restores immunogenicity of tumor cells expressing truncated major histocompatibility complex class II molecules. Proc Natl Acad Sci USA 90:5687–5690, 1993.
69. Chen L, Ashe S, Brady WA, Hellstrom I, Hellstrom KE, Ledbetter JA, McGowan P, Linsley PS. Costimulation of antitumor immunity by the B7 counterreceptor for the T lymphocyte molecules CD28 and CTLA-4. Cell 71:1093–1102, 1992.
70. Townsend SE, Allison JP. Tumor rejection after direct costimulation of CD8+ T cells by B7-transfected melanoma cells. Science 259:368–370, 1993.
71. Pulaski B, Ostrand-Rosenberg S. MHC Class II and B7.1 immunotherapeutic cell based vaccine reduces spontaneous mammary carcinoma metastases without affecting primary tumor growth. Cancer Res 58:1486–1493, 1998.
72. Armstrong T, Clements V, Ostrand-Rosenberg S. Class II transfected tumor cells directly present endogenous antigen to CD4+ T cells in vitro and are APC for tumor-encoded antigens in vivo. J Immunother 21(3):218–224, 1998.
73. Marrack P, Kappler J. The staphylococcal enterotoxins and their relatives. Science 248:705–711, 1990.
74. Ostrand-Rosenberg S, Thakur A, Clements VK. Rejection of mouse sarcoma cells after transfection of MHC class II genes. J Immunol 144:4068–4071, 1990.

12

Immunology of Uveal Melanoma: Immunosuppressive Factors and the Basis for Immunotherapy

JERRY Y. NIEDERKORN

University of Texas Southwestern Medical Center, Dallas, Texas, U.S.A.

I. OCULAR IMMUNE PRIVILEGE

Evidence that the body's immune apparatus is capable of responding to neoplasms in a favorable manner was recognized in the century before last when William Coley used extracts of pyogenic bacteria [presumably rich sources of tumor necrosis factor alpha (TNF-α)] to elicit spontaneous albeit inconsistent tumor resolution [1]. The notion that the immune system might attack tumors in an antigen-specific manner was first articulated by Burnet, who coined the term "immune surveillance" in 1967 [2]. In the decades following the birth of the immune surveillance theory, thousands of studies have explored the possibility of activating the immune system as a means of treating neoplasms. Although results from early studies were disappointing, recent insights into the immunobiology of antigen-presenting cells, the cloning of tumor-specific antigens, and a more sophisticated appreciation about the dialogue between the innate and adaptive immune responses have led to guarded optimism that immunosurveillance and immunotherapy hold promise for controlling a variety of neoplasms. However, if immunotherapy of uveal melanoma is to succeed, it must negotiate the immune privilege of the intraocular milieu.

It has been recognized for over 100 years that the anterior chamber of the eye is endowed with remarkable qualities that permit the long-term survival of foreign tissue and tumor grafts [3]. The capacity of immunogenic tumor and tissue grafts to survive in the anterior chamber (AC) but not at other sites suggested that a state of immune privilege was extended to alien tissues placed into this compartment of the eye. In the 1940s, Greene and Lund took advantage of this property and used the AC as a site for propagating various human and animal tumors and as an assay for evaluating the metastatic potential of tumor biopsy specimens [4]. The conspicuous absence of patent lymphatic vessels draining the AC of the eye led to the conclusion that tissue and tumor grafts were sequestered from the peripheral lymphoid apparatus and thereby escaped immunological recognition.

It was not until the late 1970s that this perception was revised, when Kaplan and Streilein demonstrated that alloantigenic cells placed into the AC were not only perceived by the systemic immune apparatus but, in fact, elicited antigen-specific downregulation of cell-mediated immune responses [5,6]. Although AC priming with alloantigens inhibited the generation of cell-mediated immunity, it concomitantly activated the humoral immune response. This deviant form of immune response is termed anterior chamber–associated immune deviation (ACAID) and has since been confirmed in numerous laboratories using a multitude of antigens, including tumor antigens [7,8].

ACAID is a dynamic immunoregulatory phenomenon that manifests itself as an antigen-specific downregulation of delayed-type hypersensitivity (DTH) and the concomitant generation of non-complement-fixing IgG1 antibodies (in the mouse) and cytotoxic T lymphocytes (CTL) [8–10]. The pivotal role of suppressed DTH in ocular immune privilege was shown in experiments utilizing immunogenic tumor allografts placed into the eyes of mice. P815 mastocytoma, which arose in DBA/2 mice and expresses the full array of DBA/2 minor histocompatibility (H) antigens, is briskly rejected when transplanted subcutaneously into allogeneic BALB/c mice. However, if P815 mastocytoma cells are transplanted into the eyes of BALB/c mice, the intraocular tumor cells induce ACAID, which is manifest by the systemic suppression of DTH responses to the antigens expressed on the intraocular tumors. As a consequence, the suppression of DTH promotes the progressive intraocular growth of the P815 mastocytomas. However, ACAID is malleable and can be circumvented. The induction of ACAID begins with the transmission of an antigen-specific signal from the eye to the spleen, where immunoregulatory T cells are generated. If either the eye or the spleen is removed prematurely, ACAID is not induced [8,9,11,12]. Accordingly, splenectomy prevents the induction of ACAID and, coincidentally, induces the spontaneous immune rejection of P815 mastocytomas in the eyes of BALB/c mice [11]. Thus, by simply disrupting the induction of ACAID, it is possible to profoundly alter the growth of immunogenic intraocular tumors and, in some cases, induce their immune rejection.

Although ACAID plays a pivotal role in suppressing T cell-mediated processes in the eye, additional factors contribute to ocular immune privilege (Table 1). The aqueous humor (AH) that fills the anterior chamber of the eye is a potpourri of immunosuppressive and anti-inflammatory cytokines. These include transforming growth factor beta (TGF-β), alpha-melanocyte stimulating hormone (α-MSH), calcitonin gene-related protein (CGRP), vasoactive intestinal peptide (VIP), macrophage migration inhibitory factor (MIF), and somatostatin [8,13]. The immunosuppressive factors in the AH conspire to impair both the induction and expression of cell-mediated immune responses. TGF-β, VIP, and somatostatin inhibit T-cell proliferative responses to mitogens and antigens, while VIP, α-MSH, TGF-β, and CGRP suppress the production of proinflammatory factors such as

Table 1 Factors That Support Immune Privilege in the Eye

Contribution to immune privilege	Factor
Exclusion of inflammatory cells	Blood ocular barrier
Inhibition of T-cell proliferation	TGF-β
	VIP
	α-MSH
Inhibition of proinflammatory cytokine secretion	TGF-β
	α-MSH
	CGRP
Inhibition of NK-cell activity	MIF
	TGF-β
Inhibition of delayed-type hypersensitivity	ACAID
	α-MSH
	CGRP
	TGF-β
Apoptotic deletion of activated inflammatory cells	FasL
Inhibition of complement activation	Complement regulatory proteins

interferon gamma [IFN-γ] and nitric oxide [13]. AH also contains MIF and TGF-β, which are potent inhibitors of natural killer (NK) cell activity [14–17].

Humoral immune mechanisms are also suppressed by AH-borne factors. The complement system serves as an important link between the innate and the adaptive immune responses. The complement cascade can be activated by either bacterial products (alternative pathway) or by antibodies following binding to their respective epitopes (classical pathway). Activation of the complement cascade culminates in the generation of a membrane attack complex that lyses bacteria and mammalian cells. Although complement proteins have been detected in various ocular tissues and fluids [18–20], activation of the complement cascade is restrained in the eye by complement-regulatory proteins [21–23]. The AH contains multiple soluble factors that have the capacity to suppress C3 cleavage, a critical step in the alternative pathway of complement activation [23–25]. The corneal endothelial cells that line a portion of the anterior segment of the eye express complement-regulatory proteins on their cell membranes, thereby providing additional protection against capricious activation of the complement cascade within the eye [21,22]. In addition to ocular fluids and tissues thwarting the complement cascade, uveal melanoma cells themselves express complement-regulatory proteins that protect the tumor cells from complement-mediated lysis [26].

Ocular immune privilege is also sustained by cell membrane-bound factors expressed on cells within the eye. The most prominent of these is the apoptosis-inducing molecule FasL (CD95L), which is widely expressed on ocular cells and purges the eye of inflammatory cells [27]. Moreover, expression of FasL on corneal cells contributes to the immune privilege and survival of corneal allografts [28,29]. Some uveal melanoma cells are decorated with FasL [30] and, as such, might be shielded from immunological attack in a manner similar to the protection conferred to corneal allografts. In addition to their presence in the AH, complement-regulatory proteins are also expressed on the cell membranes of cells within the uveal tract [27].

II. CIRCUMVENTION OF IMMUNE PRIVILEGE AND INTRAOCULAR TUMOR IMMUNITY

In spite of the elaborate and redundant mechanisms that sustain ocular immune privilege, immune inflammation can occur in the eye. The development of idiopathic uveitis and corneal allograft rejection are reminders of the limitations of immune privilege. There is considerable evidence that intraocular tumors are vulnerable to immune control. Although relatively rare, spontaneous regressions of uveal melanomas and retinoblastomas have been reported [31–34]. The expression of the melanoma-specific MAGE antigens and melanoma-associated antigens gp100 and tyrosinase on uveal melanomas suggests that intraocular melanomas are potentially susceptible to immunological attack [35–37]. Moreover, antigen-specific cytolysis of uveal melanoma cells by $CD8^+$ T cells from the peripheral blood and by CTLs isolated from primary uveal melanomas is tangible evidence that uveal melanomas are capable of eliciting melanoma-specific cell-mediated immunity and succumbing to T cell-mediated immunological attack [38–40].

Prospective studies in animal models have demonstrated that the adaptive immune system, namely T cell–mediated immunity, is capable of circumventing ocular immune privilege and attacking immunogenic intraocular tumors. Investigations using the P815 intraocular tumor model have shown that removal of the spleen before or shortly after intraocular tumor implantation results in the abrogation of ACAID, the appearance of tumor-specific DTH, and the immune rejection of intraocular P815 tumors [11]. Interestingly, intraocular tumor rejection takes on the appearance of a DTH lesion and is characterized by ischemic necrosis of the tumor en masse, followed by extensive damage to innocent bystander cells in the eye. However, not all tumors induce ACAID. A highly immunogenic mutant of P815 mastocytoma, designated P91, expresses potent tumor-specific antigens that induce strong DTH responses following intraocular transplantation in syngeneic DBA/2 mice, even in the presence of an intact spleen [41]. The P91 tumors grow transiently in the DBA/2 mouse eye and induce DTH responses to the tumor-specific antigens. The acquisition of DTH coincides with the onset of tumor resolution. The histopathological features of intraocular P91 tumor resolution strongly resemble those found in P815 tumors undergoing immune rejection when ACAID is abrogated in splenectomized BALB/c mice. In both cases, tumor regression culminates in ischemic necrosis and phthisis of the affected eye.

The immune rejection of intraocular tumors can also occur via a T cell-mediated mechanism that does not culminate in phthisis. Studies in mice have shown that some highly immunogenic, syngeneic tumors (e.g., UV5C25 fibrosarcoma) undergo immune rejection following intraocular transplantation in syngeneic hosts [42,43]. The resolving tumor lesions display a moth-eaten appearance and are characterized by the presence of tumor-infiltrating lymphocytes (TILs) and piecemeal necrosis of the intraocular tumors [42,43]. Prospective studies using a "Koch's postulates-like" approach have demonstrated that this form of intraocular tumor regression is mediated by tumor-specific CTLs [43]. In situ immunohistochemical staining has confirmed that the TILs express the CD8 molecule, the most common surface marker for CTLs. TILs isolated from the intraocular tumors kill the tumor cells in an antigen-specific manner in vitro. Adoptive transfer of the TILs has demonstrated that they are able to recapitulate the regression of intraocular tumors in third party hosts. That is, TILs expanded in vitro and coinjected with tumor cells into the eyes of immunoincompetent hosts produced intraocular tumor resolution that mimicked the original phenotype, both clinically and histopathologically.

Results from two other studies lend support to the hypothesis that T cell–dependent immune mechanisms can mediate intraocular tumor rejection without jeopardizing the anatomical and functional integrity of the eye [44–46]. Using an adenovirus-induced tumor model in syngeneic C57BL/6 mice, Schurmans and coworkers demonstrated that intravenously injected tumor-specific CTLs entered the intraocular tumors and produced tumor resolution in a manner reminiscent of the aforementioned UV5C25 tumor rejection [45]. That is, tumor resolution occurred in a nonnecrotizing manner that culminated in tumor rejection and minimal damage to normal ocular tissues. An almost identical pattern of intraocular tumor resolution was observed in an SV40 large-T-antigen transgenic retinal pigmented epithelial (RPE) tumor model in FVB/N mice [44]. Tumor resolution was accompanied by infiltration of $CD8^+$ TILs that displayed tumor-specific cytolytic activity in vitro and produced intraocular tumor rejection following adoptive transfer to third-party hosts. However, further examination of the aforementioned adenovirus-induced intraocular tumor model in syngeneic C57BL/6 mice indicated that, in contrast to the rejection induced by adoptively transferred immune lymphocytes, spontaneous immune rejection proceeded unabatedly in hosts who were depleted of $CD8^+$ T cells. By contrast, intraocular tumors grew progressively in either C57BL/6 mice depleted of $CD4^+$ T cells or in MHC class II-deficient C57BL/6 mice [46]. Intraocular tumor rejection did not require TNF-α, Fas ligand, perforin, transporters associated with antigen processing (TAP), or B cells, as mice with disruptions of the respective genes encoding these molecules were able to reject their intraocular tumors in a manner that was indistinguishable from that seen in wild-type C57BL/6 mice. These results indicate that syngeneic intraocular tumors can undergo immune rejection by a CD4-dependent mechanism that (1) does not involve $CD8^+$ T cells; (2) does not bear the hallmarks of a DTH response in situ; and (3) does not culminate in damage to innocent bystander cells. Thus, immunogenic intraocular tumors can undergo immune rejection in the eye by two distinct patterns. In one pattern, the mechanism involves ischemic necrosis by a DTH-like process that carries a heavy burden of innocent bystander damage. A second pattern is characterized by piecemeal necrosis of the tumor cells and culminates in the preservation of the normal ocular architecture. This nonnecrotizing pattern of rejection can be mediated by classical $CD8^+$ CTL or by an unconventional CD4-dependent process that does not require either perforin, MHC class I antigen expression or the participation of $CD8^+$ T cells. Understanding the immunoregulatory processes that determine which pathway is invoked could have enormous clinical applications in devising immunotherapeutic strategies for managing intraocular tumors without jeopardizing vision.

III. THE ROLE OF THE INNATE IMMUNE SYSTEM IN UVEAL MELANOMA

In addition to T cell-mediated tumor immunity, natural resistance mechanisms may also be important in the immune response to neoplasms [47]. Natural resistance mechanisms involve macrophages, NK cells, and granulocytes. NK cells seem particularly suited for the surveillance of neoplasms, as these cells do not require priming or clonal expansion in order to exert antitumor effects. Like T cells, NK cells produce cell-mediated cytotoxicity and secrete a diverse array of cytokines and chemokines. However, unlike those of B and T cells, the development and function of NK cells do not require gene rearrangement [47]. Results from animal studies over the past two decades have provided compelling evidence that NK cells play an important role in limiting the growth and metastasis of various rodent tumors, especially skin melanomas. The importance of NK cells in the surveillance of human tumors is less clear. Human melanoma cell lines are susceptible to NK cell-mediated cytolysis in vitro and in vivo [48]. NK cells have been detected within skin melanoma lesions [49], and a positive correlation between NK cell activity and disease-free survival time in cutaneous melanoma patients has been observed [50].

The significance of NK cells in uveal melanomas is just emerging. Preliminary findings suggest that the innate immune system, especially the NK-cell arm, may play an important role in controlling metastases arising from uveal melanomas. Human uveal melanoma cells display varying degrees of susceptibility to NK cell-mediated lysis in vitro [51,52]. Moreover, there is a close correlation between the expression of the MHC class I antigen on uveal melanoma cells and a reduced susceptibility to NK cell-mediated cytolysis [51,52]. These findings are in keeping with the "missing self" hypothesis, which proposes that MHC class I molecules on a potential target cell transmit an inhibitory signal to NK cells and thereby prevent cytolysis [53]. However, cells failing to express MHC class I molecules do not send an "off" signal to NK cells; as a result, they are killed. Unlike skin melanomas, intraocular melanomas reside in an environment containing a myriad of factors that might influence MHC class I expression. The AH in particular is richly endowed with TGF-β [54,55], a cytokine noted for its capacity to downregulate MHC class I expression [56,57]. Uveal melanoma cells incubated in TGF-β display significantly reduced levels of MHC class I molecules and a proportional increased susceptibility to NK cell-mediated lysis in vitro [51]. Analogous effects have been reported with uveal melanomas that constitutively express low levels of MHC class I molecules. Stimulation of class I antigen expression by incubation with IFN-γ results in a sharp increase in MHC class I expression and a comparable diminution in NK cell-mediated lysis [51]. Thus it appears that human uveal melanomas are indeed susceptible to NK cell-mediated lysis in vitro. The capacity of TGF-β, an intraocular cytokine, to downregulate class I expression and thereby increase the vulnerability of melanoma cells to NK-mediated cytotoxicity suggests that melanomas within the eye might be particularly susceptible to NK cell-mediated surveillance. This begs the question as to whether cells of the immune system, especially NK cells, can enter the eye and penetrate intraocular tumors.

There is considerable evidence that lymphocytes enter tumor-containing eyes. Lymphocytes have been found infiltrating 7–20% of the uveal melanomas examined [58–60]. However, whether the lymphocyte population infiltrating uveal melanomas displays antigen-specificity is uncertain. Nitta and coworkers demonstrated that TILs present in 7 of 8 human uveal melanomas expressed the same Va T cell receptor (TCR) gene, which is suggestive of a melanoma-specific T-cell response [60]. By contrast, others have reported that TIL populations from uveal melanomas express a diversity of TCR $V\beta$ genes [61]. Thus it is not clear whether the lymphocytes that infiltrate uveal melanomas are oligoclonal in nature or represent a random array of lymphocytes. The former proposition is supported by in vitro studies demonstrating that TILs from uveal melanoma patients can mediate uveal melanoma–specific cytolysis [39,40]. Much less is known about the presence and functional capacities of NK cells that infiltrate uveal melanomas. In two studies, less than 10% of the TILs in uveal melanomas expressed surface markers indicative of NK cells [62,63]. However, Ksander and coworkers reported that 41% of the TIL population from a choroidal melanoma expressed the CD16 NK-cell marker and lysed NK-sensitive K562 target cells in vitro [40].

Once NK cells enter the eye, they must negotiate the multiple layers of immune privilege. Until only recently, it was not known whether ocular immune privilege affected NK cell-mediated immune mechanisms. An important contributor to the immune privilege in the eye is TGF-β, a cytokine present within both the anterior and posterior compartments of the eye. TGF-β is a pleiotropic molecule, and among its many functions is its capacity to inhibit T- and B-cell proliferation and NK cell-mediated cytotoxicity [17]. Macrophage migration inhibitory factor (MIF) is another potent inhibitor of NK cell-mediated cytotoxicity, which is produced by many cells within the eye, including those of the uveal tract [64]. Importantly, both of these molecules are present in ocular tissues at concentrations known to inhibit NK activity in vitro [15–17]. The in vivo significance of TGF-β and MIF in influencing the fate of NK cell-sensitive uveal melanoma cells has been confirmed in a nude mouse model of intraocular melanoma [14]. Although nude mice are deficient in T cell-mediated and T cell-dependent immune responses, they exhibit above normal NK cell-mediated immunity. NK-sensitive human uveal melanomas are promptly rejected following subcutaneous transplantation in nude mice. The rejection of the subcutaneous tumors by nude mice is mediated by NK cells, as the same tumors grow progressively in nude mice whose NK-cell populations have been depleted by systemic treatment with antibodies specific for murine NK cells [14]. By contrast, NK-sensitive tumors, which are rejected at subcutaneous sites, grow progressively in the eyes of nude mice, even at doses 50-fold lower than those that are rejected following subcutaneous transplantation [14]. Thus, NK cells can enter at least some intraocular melanomas. However, the intraocular milieu stifles the NK cell-mediated cytolytic machinery and allows the tumors to grow progressively.

Although the intraocular milieu provides relief from NK cell-mediated attack, once metastatic uveal melanoma cells leave the eye, they must evade NK cells within the bloodstream and the parenchyma of the liver—two sites of intense NK activity. Studies in mice have shown that in vivo depletion of NK cells results in a 200-fold increase in liver metastases in hosts challenged intravenously with B16 skin melanoma cells [65]. If NK cell-mediated immune surveillance plays a significant role in controlling uveal melanoma metastases, one might predict that successful metastases must be equipped with properties that inhibit NK-cell activity outside of the immunologically privileged confines of the eye. Two possibilities come to mind. First, the expression of MHC class I molecules is known to protect tumor cells from

NK cell-mediated lysis and might be an effective strategy for metastases to escape destruction in the bloodstream and liver. A second strategy is for the melanoma cells to create their own immune-privileged nidus by secreting NK-inhibitory factors such as TGF-β and MIF. Two studies on human melanoma patients offer support for the hypothesis that MHC class I antigen expression favors the development of uveal melanoma metastases. Verbik and coworkers demonstrated that only 4% of the tumor cells from a primary uveal melanoma expressed MHC class I molecules. By contrast, expression of MHC class I was nine times higher in melanoma cells isolated from four different liver metastases in the same patient [66]. Further support for this hypothesis comes from studies by Blom and coworkers, who examined 30 primary uveal melanomas and found a significant correlation between the expression of MHC class I molecules on primary uveal melanomas and poor prognosis [67].

Some cell lines from uveal melanomas and their metastases escape NK cell-mediated lysis by producing MIF [68]. In a recent study, it was reported that the uveal melanoma cell lines that produced the most MIF were those that were isolated from metastases [68]. The capacity of uveal melanoma cells to express MHC class I antigens or to secrete MIF spontaneously suggests that metastases might arise from subpopulations of cells within primary uveal melanomas that are preadapted to escape NK cell-mediated assault once they leave the sanctuary of the eye.

One can only speculate as to whether activation of NK cells will be an effective adjunct therapy for uveal melanoma patients. The profound inhibitory effect of TGF-β and MIF within the eye casts doubt on the feasibility of activating NK cells as a means of eradicating primary uveal melanomas. Likewise, NK cells might be faced with an insurmountable task if liver metastases express high MHC class I antigens and secrete MIF (and perhaps other inhibitor molecules such as TGF-β). Efforts to utilize NK cells to treat liver metastases should consider strategies for dismantling these barriers, thereby allowing NK cells to perform their role in immune surveillance.

IV. CONCLUSIONS

The immune privilege of the eye gives uveal melanomas sanctuary from some forms of immunological attack. However, once uveal melanomas depart from the eye and begin their metastatic journey, they are confronted with a full array of immunological defense mechanisms. Metastatic uveal melanoma cells must evade the watchful eye of NK cells in the bloodstream and in the liver—two sites of the most intense NK activity in the body [69–71]. Uveal melanomas express melanoma-specific and melanoma-associated antigens that are potential targets of CTLs and antibody [35–37]. However, uveal melanoma metastases employ strategies that serve to thwart both antibody-mediated and CTL-mediated immune surveillance. Goslings and coworkers [26] reported that all 10 human uveal melanoma cell lines tested expressed at least one of the complement regulatory proteins and, as a result, resisted complement-mediated lysis. Uveal melanoma cells are also able to evade immune surveillance mediated by CD8$^+$ CTLs. CTL-mediated lysis of target cells can occur only if the relevant antigens are displayed in the groove of MHC class I molecules. Expression of melanoma-specific antigens is reduced or absent in many uveal melanomas. Moreover, uveal melanoma cells express little or no MHC class I molecules; as a result, they are invisible to CTL-mediated surveillance. The absence of MHC class I molecules, however, renders uveal melanoma cells potentially vulnerable to NK cell-mediated attack. Some uveal melanoma metastases appear to overcome this vulnerability by secreting TGF-β [72] and MIF [68], two cytokines that strongly inhibit NK cell-mediated cytolysis [15–17].

Although there has been a rebirth of interest in tumor immunotherapy, it might be worthwhile to ponder the other side of the coin and reconsider an iconoclastic hypothesis proposed by Richmond Prehn over 30 years ago [73]. Prehn raised the disconcerting proposition that, under certain circumstances, the immune system enhanced rather than hindered tumor progression. Two observations regarding the behavior of uveal melanomas are consistent with the Prehn "immune stimulation" hypothesis of tumor development. The first observation is that the presence of TILs carries a poor prognosis in uveal melanoma patients [58]. If confirmed, this conclusion is counterintuitive and contradicts the immune surveillance theory. What benefit can TILs convey to uveal melanoma cells? Two possibilities come to mind. The first is that TILs produce cytokines, such as IFN-γ, that upregulate MHC class I molecules and thereby protect uveal melanoma cells from NK cell-mediated attack once the tumor cells metastasize from the eye. The second explanation is that TILs produce IL-2, which serves as a growth factor for the uveal melanoma cells. Importantly, human uveal melanoma cells and murine skin melanoma cells express IL-2 receptors [74] (Niederkorn et al., unpublished findings). Studies in mice have shown that IL-2 stimulates the proliferation of murine skin melanoma cells and increases their resistance to NK cell-mediated lysis in vitro [74,75]. Moreover, murine skin melanoma cells incubated in IL-2 and injected intravenously produced three times as many liver metastases as untreated melanoma cells [75]. It remains to be determined whether uveal melanoma cells behave in a similar manner. If they do, it would explain the paradoxical association between TILs and a poor prognosis in uveal melanoma patients.

A second paradoxical observation is the correlation between the presence of tumor-infiltrating macrophages and increased malignancy in uveal melanoma patients [76]. It has been recognized for over three decades that activated macrophages are capable of killing a wide variety of tumor cells in vitro, and maneuvers that activate macrophages in vivo often produce favorable results in controlling the growth and metastasis of murine tumors. However, in the case of intraocular tumors, the macrophages that infiltrate uveal melanomas may unwittingly contribute to the generation of an aberrant immune response that hinders the expression of conventional tumor immunity, including the generation of tumoricidal macrophages. One of the unique features of the intraocular milieu is the abundance of immunosuppressive cytokines, especially TGF-β. This cytokine is expressed throughout the eye and is also produced by uveal melanoma cells [13,68]. Several studies have demonstrated that macrophages exposed to antigens in the presence of TGF-β present antigens to T cells in a manner that leads the development of ACAID [77–80]. Moreover, TGF-β acts in an autocrine fashion to induce macrophages to secrete additional TGF-β [81] and IL-10 [78]. In addition to facilitating the induction of ACAID, TGF-β and IL-10 are potent anti-inflammatory molecules that inhibit Th1 immune responses to tumors. Thus, uveal melanomas have the capacity to coerce tumor-infiltrating macrophages to promote systemic downregulation of Th1 immune responses (i.e., ACAID) and thereby to paralyze the immune surveillance apparatus.

It is not surprising that in spite of three decades of intense investigation, the immunology of uveal melanoma remains a conundrum. Unraveling which immunological modalities are effective against uveal melanomas and—equally important—identifying those immune elements that betray the immune surveillance machinery is daunting but remain important goals.

REFERENCES

1. Coley WB. The treatment of malignant tumors by repeated inoculations of erysipelas: With a report of ten original cases. Am J Med Sci 1893; 105:487–511.
2. Burnet FM. Immunological aspects of malignant diseases. Lancet 1967; 1:1171–1174.
3. van Dooremaal JC. Die Entwicklung der in fremden Grund versetzten lebenden Gewebe. Graefes Arch Ophthalmol 1873; 19:358–373.
4. Greene HSN LP. The heterologous transplantation of human cancers. Cancer Res 1944; 4:352–363.
5. Kaplan HJ, Streilein JW. Immune response to immunization via the anterior chamber of the eye. I. F lymphocyte-induced immune deviation. J Immunol 1977; 118:809–814.
6. Kaplan HJ, Streilein JW, Stevens TR. Transplantation immunology of the anterior chamber of the eye. II. Immune response to allogeneic cells. J Immunol 1975; 115:805–810.
7. Niederkorn JY. Anterior chamber-associated immune deviation. Chem Immunol 1999; 73:59–71.
8. Niederkorn JY. Ocular Immune Privilege. Crit Rev Immunol 2002. In press.
9. Niederkorn JY. Immune privilege and immune regulation in the eye. Adv Immunol 1990; 48:191–226.
10. Streilein JW. Immune privilege as the result of local tissue barriers and immunosuppressive microenvironments. Curr Opin Immunol 1993; 5:428–432.
11. Streilein JW, Niederkorn JY. Induction of anterior chamber-associated immune deviation requires an intact, functional spleen. J Exp Med 1981; 153:1058–1067.
12. Ferguson TA, Griffith TS. A vision of cell death: insights into immune privilege. Immunol Rev 1997; 156:167–184.
13. Taylor AW. Ocular immunosuppressive microenvironment. Chem Immunol 1999; 73:72–89.
14. Apte RS, Mayhew E, Niederkorn JY. Local inhibition of natural killer cell activity promotes the progressive growth of intraocular tumors. Invest Ophthalmol Vis Sci 1997; 38:1277–1282.
15. Apte RS, Niederkorn JY. Isolation and characterization of a unique natural killer cell inhibitory factor present in the anterior chamber of the eye. J Immunol 1996; 156:2667–2673.
16. Apte RS, Sinha D, Mayhew E, Wistow GJ, Niederkorn JY. Cutting edge: Role of macrophage migration inhibitory factor in inhibiting NK cell activity and preserving immune privilege. J Immunol 1998; 160:5693–5696.
17. Rook AH, Kehrl JH, Wakefield LM, Roberts AB, Sporn MB, Burlington DB, Lane HC, Fauci AS. Effects of transforming growth factor beta on the functions of natural killer cells: Depressed cytolytic activity and blunting of interferon responsiveness. J Immunol 1986; 136:3916–3920.
18. Mondino BJ, Rao H. Complement levels in normal and inflamed aqueous humor. Invest Ophthalmol Vis Sci 1983; 24:380–384.

19. Mondino BJ, Ratajczak HV, Goldberg DB, Schanzlin DJ, Brown SI. Alternate and classical pathway components of complement in the normal cornea. Arch Ophthalmol 1980; 98:346–349.

20. Chandler JW, Leder R, Kaufman HE, Caldwell JR. Quantitative determinations of complement components and immunoglobulins in tears and aqueous humor. Invest Ophthalmol 1974; 13:151–153.

21. Lass JH, Walter EI, Burris TE, Grossniklaus HE, Roat MI, Skelnik DL, Needham L, Singer M, Medof ME. Expression of two molecular forms of the complement decay-accelerating factor in the eye and lacrimal gland. Invest Ophthalmol Vis Sci 1990; 31:1136–1148.

22. Bora NS, Gobleman CL, Atkinson JP, Pepose JS, Kaplan HJ. Differential expression of the complement regulatory proteins in the human eye. Invest Ophthalmol Vis Sci 1993; 34:3579–3584.

23. Goslings WR, Prodeus AP, Streilein JW, Carroll MC, Jager MJ, Taylor AW. A small molecular weight factor in aqueous humor acts on C1q to prevent antibody-dependent complement activation. Invest Ophthalmol Vis Sci 1998; 39:989–995.

24. Sohn JH, Kaplan HJ, Suk HJ, Bora PS, Bora NS. Complement regulatory activity of normal human intraocular fluid is mediated by MCP, DAF, and CD59. Invest Ophthalmol Vis Sci 2000; 41:4195–4202.

25. Sohn JH, Kaplan HJ, Suk HJ, Bora PS, Bora NS. Chronic low level complement activation within the eye is controlled by intraocular complement regulatory proteins. Invest Ophthalmol Vis Sci 2000; 41:3492–3502.

26. Goslings WR, Blom DJ, de Waard-Siebinga I, van Beelen E, Claas FH, Jager MJ, Gorter A. Membrane-bound regulators of complement activation in uveal melanomas. CD46, CD55, and CD59 in uveal melanomas. Invest Ophthalmol Vis Sci 1996; 37:1884–1891.

27. Griffith TS, Brunner T, Fletcher SM, Green DR, Ferguson TA. Fas ligand-induced apoptosis as a mechanism of immune privilege. Science 1995; 270:1189–1192.

28. Stuart PM, Griffith TS, Usui N, Pepose J, Yu X, Ferguson TA. CD95 ligand (FasL)-induced apoptosis is necessary for corneal allograft survival. J Clin Invest 1997; 99:396–402.

29. Yamagami S, Kawashima H, Tsuru T, Yamagami H, Kayagaki N, Yagita H, Okumura K, Gregerson DS. Role of Fas-Fas ligand interactions in the immunorejection of allogeneic mouse corneal transplants. Transplantation 1997; 64:1107–1111.

30. Repp AC, Mayhew ES, Howard K, Alizadeh H, Niederkorn JY. Role of Fas ligand in uveal melanoma-induced liver damage. Graefes Arch Clin Exp Ophthalmol 2001; 239:752–758.

31. Jensen OA, Anderson SR. Spontaneous regression of malignant melanoma of the choroid. Acta Ophthalmol (Copenh) 1974; 173–182.

32. Khodadoust AA, Roozitalab HM, Smith RE, Green WR. Spontaneous regression of retinoblastoma. Surv Ophthalmol 1977; 21:467–478.

33. Ashton N. Primary tumors of the iris. Br J Ophthalmol 1964; 48:650–668.

34. Reese AB. Precancerous and cancerous melanosis. Am J Ophthalmol 1766; 61:1272–1277.

35. Luyten GP, van der Spek CW, Brand I, Sintnicolaas K, de Waard-Siebinga I, Jager MJ, de Jong PT, Schrier PI, Luider TM. Expression of MAGE, gp100 and tyrosinase genes in uveal melanoma cell lines. Melanoma Res 1998; 8:11–16.

36. Chen PW, Murray TG, Salgaller ML, Ksander BR. Expression of MAGE genes in ocular melanoma cell lines. J Immunother 1997; 20:265–275.

37. Mulcahy KA, Rimoldi D, Brasseur F, Rodgers S, Lienard D, Marchand M, Rennie IG, Murray AK, McIntyre CA, Platts KE, Leyvraz S, Boon T, Rees RC. Infrequent expression of the MAGE gene family in uveal melanomas. Int J Cancer 1996; 66:738–742.

38. Kan-Mitchell J, Liggett PE, Harel W, Steinman L, Nitta T, Oksenberg JR, Posner MR, Mitchell MS. Lymphocytes cytotoxic to uveal and skin melanoma cells from peripheral blood of ocular melanoma patients. Cancer Immunol Immunother 1991; 33:333–340.

39. Ksander BR, Geer DC, Chen PW, Salgaller ML, Rubsamen P, Murray TG. Uveal melanomas contain antigenically specific and non-specific infiltrating lymphocytes. Curr Eye Res 1998; 17:165–173.

40. Ksander BR, Rubsamen PE, Olsen KR, Cousins SW, Streilein JW. Studies of tumor-infiltrating lymphocytes from a human choroidal melanoma. Invest Ophthalmol Vis Sci 1991; 32:3198–3208.

41. Niederkorn JY, Meunier PC. Spontaneous immune rejection of intraocular tumors in mice. Invest Ophthalmol Vis Sci 1985; 26:877–884.

42. Knisely TL, Luckenbach MW, Fischer BJ, Niederkorn JY. Destructive and non-destructive patterns of immune rejection of syngeneic intraocular tumors. J Immunol 1987; 138:4515–4523.

43. Knisely TL, Niederkorn JY. Emergence of a dominant cytotoxic T lymphocyte antitumor effector from tumor-infiltrating cells in the anterior chamber of the eye. Cancer Immunol Immunother 1990; 30:323–330.

44. Ma D, Alizadeh H, Comerford SA, Gething MJ, Sambrook JF, Anand R, Niederkorn JY. Rejection of intraocular tumors from transgenic mice by tumor-infiltrating lymphocytes. Curr Eye Res 1994; 13:361–369.

45. Schurmans LR, den Boer AT, Diehl L, van der Voort EI, Kast WM, Melief CJ, Toes RE, Jager MJ. Successful immunotherapy of an intraocular tumor in mice. Cancer Res 1999; 59:5250–5254.

46. Schurmans LR, Diehl L, den Boer AT, Sutmuller RP, Boonman ZF, Medema JP, van der Voort EI, Laman J, Melief CJ, Jager MJ, Toes RE. Rejection of intraocular tumors by CD4(+) T cells without induction of phthisis. J Immunol 2001; 167:5832–5837.

47. Ortaldo JR, Longo DL. Human natural lymphocyte effector cells: definition, analysis of activity, and clinical effectiveness. J Natl Cancer Inst 1988; 80:999–1010.

48. Hill LL, Perussia B, McCue PA, Korngold R. Effect of human natural killer cells on the metastatic growth of human melanoma xenografts in mice with severe combined immunodeficiency. Cancer Res 1994; 54:763–770.

49. Kornstein MJ, Stewart R, Elder DE. Natural killer cells in the host response to melanoma. Cancer Res 1987; 47:1411–1412.

50. Brittenden J, Heys SD, Ross J, Eremin O. Natural killer cells and cancer. Cancer 1996; 77:1226–1243.

51. Ma D, Niederkorn JY. Transforming growth factor-beta down-regulates major histocompatibility complex class I antigen expression and increases the susceptibility of uveal melanoma cells to natural killer cell-mediated cytolysis. Immunology 1995; 86:263–269.

52. Ma D, Luyten GP, Luider TM, Niederkorn JY. Relationship between natural killer cell susceptibility and metastasis of human uveal melanoma cells in a murine model. Invest Ophthalmol Vis Sci 1995; 36:435–441.

53. Ljunggren HG, Ohlen C, Hoglund P, Franksson L, Karre K. The RMA-S lymphoma mutant: Consequences of a peptide loading defect on immunological recognition and graft rejection. Int J Cancer Suppl 1991; 6:38–44.

54. Jampel HD, Roche N, Stark WJ, Roberts AB. Transforming growth factor-beta in human aqueous humor. Curr Eye Res 1990; 9:963–969.

55. Cousins SW, McCabe MM, Danielpour D, Streilein JW. Identification of transforming growth factor-beta as an immunosuppressive factor in aqueous humor. Invest Ophthalmol Vis Sci 1991; 32:2201–2211.

56. Orcel P, Bielakoff J, De Vernejoul MC. Effects of transforming growth factor-beta on long-term human cord blood monocyte cultures. J Cell Physiol 1990; 142:293–298.

57. Krueger JG, Krane JF, Carter DM, Gottlieb AB. Role of growth factors, cytokines, and their receptors in the pathogenesis of psoriasis. J Invest Dermatol 1990; 94:135S–140S.
58. de la Cruz PO, Jr., Specht CS, McLean IW. Lymphocytic infiltration in uveal malignant melanoma. Cancer 1990; 65:112–115.
59. Durie FH, Campbell AM, Lee WR, Damato BE. Analysis of lymphocytic infiltration in uveal melanoma. Invest Ophthalmol Vis Sci 1990; 31:2106–2110.
60. Nitta T, Oksenberg JR, Rao NA, Steinman L. Predominant expression of T cell receptor V alpha 7 in tumor-infiltrating lymphocytes of uveal melanoma. Science 1990; 249:672–674.
61. Durie FH, George WD, Campbell AM, Damato BE. Analysis of clonality of tumour infiltrating lymphocytes in breast cancer and uveal melanoma. Immunol Lett 1992; 33:263–269.
62. Meecham WJ, Char DH, Kaleta-Michaels S. Infiltrating lymphocytes and antigen expression in uveal melanoma. Ophthalm Res 1992; 24:20–26.
63. de Waard-Siebinga I, Hilders CG, Hansen BE, van Delft JL, Jager MJ. HLA expression and tumor-infiltrating immune cells in uveal melanoma. Graefes Arch Clin Exp Ophthalmol 1996; 234:34–42.
64. Matsuda A, Kotake, S., Tagawa, Y, Matsuda, H., and Nishihira, J. Detection and localization of macrophage migration inhibitory factor in rat iris and ciliary epithelium. Immunol Lett 1996; 53:1–5.
65. Wiltrout RH, Santoni A, Peterson ES, Knott DC, Overton WR, Herberman RB, Holden HT. Reactivity of anti-asialo GM1 serum with tumoricidal and non- tumoricidal mouse macrophages. J Leukoc Biol 1985; 37:597–614.
66. Verbik DJ, Murray TG, Tran JM, Ksander BR. Melanomas that develop within the eye inhibit lymphocyte proliferation. Int J Cancer 1997; 73:470–478.
67. Blom DJ, Luyten GP, Mooy C, Kerkvliet S, Zwinderman AH, Jager MJ. Human leukocyte antigen class I expression. Marker of poor prognosis in uveal melanoma. Invest Ophthalmol Vis Sci 1997; 38:1865–1872.
68. Repp AC, Mayhew ES, Apte S, Niederkorn JY. Human uveal melanoma cells produce macrophage migration-inhibitory factor to prevent lysis by NK cells. J Immunol 2000; 165:710–715.
69. O'Farrelly C, Crispe IN. Prometheus through the looking glass: Reflections on the hepatic immune system. Immunol Today 1999; 20:394–398.
70. Roh MS, Kahky MP, Oyedeji C, Klostergaard J, Wang L, Curley SA, Lotzova E. Murine Kupffer cells and hepatic natural killer cells regulate tumor growth in a quantitative model of colorectal liver metastases. Clin Exp Metastasis 1992; 10:317–327.
71. Scott P, Trinchieri G. The role of natural killer cells in host-parasite interactions. Curr Opin Immunol 1995; 7:34–40.
72. Park SS, Li L, Korn TS, Mitra MM, Niederkorn JY. Effect of transforming growth factor-beta on plasminogen activator production of cultured human uveal melanoma cells. Curr Eye Res 1996; 15:755–763.
73. Prehn RT, Lappe MA. An immunostimulation theory of tumor development. Transplant Rev 1971; 7:26–54.
74. Garcia de Galdeano A, Boyano MD, Smith-Zubiaga I, Canavate ML. B16F10 murine melanoma cells express interleukin-2 and a functional interleukin-2 receptor. Tumour Biol 1996; 17:155–167.
75. Boyano MD, Garcia de Galdeano A, Smith-Zubiaga I, Canavate ML. IL-2 treatment of B16F10 melanoma cells stimulates metastatic colonization in the liver. Anticancer Res 1997; 17:1135–1141.
76. Makitie T, Summanen P, Tarkkanen A, Kivela T. Tumor-infiltrating macrophages (CD68(+) cells) and prognosis in malignant uveal melanoma. Invest Ophthalmol Vis Sci 2001; 42:1414–1421.

77. Wilbanks GA, Strelien, JW. Macrophages capable of inducing anterior chamber associated immune deviation demonstrate spleen-seeking migratory properties. Reg Immunol 1992; 4:130–137.

78. D'Orazio TJ, Niederkorn JY. A novel role for TGF-beta and IL-10 in the induction of immune privilege. J Immunol 1998; 160:2089–2098.

79. Wilbanks GA, Mammolenti M, Streilein JW. Studies on the induction of anterior chamber-associated immune deviation (ACAID): III. Induction of ACAID depends upon intraocular transforming growth factor-beta. Eur J Immunol 1992; 22:165–173.

80. Wilbanks GA, Streilein JW. Fluids from immune privileged sites endow macrophages with the capacity to induce antigen-specific immune deviation via a mechanism involving transforming growth factor-beta. Eur J Immunol 1992; 22:1031–1036.

81. Takeuchi M, Kosiewicz MM, Alard P, Streilein JW. On the mechanisms by which transforming growth factor-beta 2 alters antigen-presenting abilities of macrophages on T cell activation. Eur J Immunol 1997; 27:1648–1656.

13

Models of Uveal Melanoma: Characterization of Transgenic Mice and Other Animal Models for Melanoma

STEFAN DITHMAR

University of Heidelberg, Heidelberg, Germany

HANS E. GROSSNIKLAUS

Emory University, Atlanta, Georgia, U.S.A.

I. INTRODUCTION

The study of experimental animal models of human ocular disease comprises an important area of research in ophthalmology and the visual sciences. As early as 1882, animal models were being developed for human diseases [1]. Although investigators have been attempting to develop animal models of human cancer over the past century, the availability of relevant animal models of human ocular melanoma is relatively recent. An animal model for the study of intraocular melanoma should ideally exhibit tumors that have similarities in their pathogenesis, morphology, and molecular biology to human uveal melanoma. In this review, we summarize what is currently known about animal models of human uveal melanoma [2].

II. TRANSGENIC MICE

Transgenic mice have recently been described as potentially useful models of human ocular melanoma. These models are based on using the promoter region of the tyrosinase gene to target expression of oncogenes in pigment-producing cells. The tyrosinase promoter was chosen because it drives the expression of downstream genes in melanocytes [3]. Pigmented intraocular tumors that arise in transgenic mice strains represent a spectrum of proliferations of uveal melanocytes and retinal pigment epithelium (RPE) [4–9]. Tanaka and coworkers introduced the murine tyrosinase minigene mg-Tyrs-J into fertilized eggs of albino Balb/c mice and found increased pigment production in the choroid [3]. Bradl and associates reported the regular occurrence of intraocular melanomas in mice expressing a transgene constructed by fusion of the simian virus 40 (SV40) early region, including the coding sequences of the transforming large tumor and small tumor antigens, with a mouse tyrosinase promoter [5]. These transgenic mice developed primary cutaneous melanomas and spontaneous bilateral pigmented tumors of the posterior segment of the eye. A majority of these appeared to originate in the RPE, some were distinctly in the choroid, and some were at the RPE-choroid interface. It is unclear using immunostaining and histologic analysis if these tumors represent a melanoma or a retinal pigment epithelium adenocarcinoma. Distant metastases were reported in lymph nodes, lung, bone, muscle, brain, salivary gland, thymus and subcutaneous tissue, but not in the liver [5].

Similarly, another intraocular tumor from FVB/N mice, which have the SV40 oncogene, has features that suggest an RPE tumor [4]. This tumor, if inoculated into the AC of FVB/N and athymic nude Balb/c mice, does metastasize to the liver [11,12].

Syed and associates characterized Tyr TagA and Tyr TagB, two similar lines of transgenic mice that express the SV40 T antigen, under the control of the tyrosinase promoter. These mice develop spontaneous, bilateral, pigmented intraocular tumors in the absence of primary cutaneous tumors. These tumors were found to arise from the RPE and were composed primarily of epithelioid cells with a variable spindle cell component. Metastases were reported in the subcutaneous tissue, lungs and brain [8].

Another transgenic mouse model was produced by a tyrosinase promoter that targeted expression of the mutated human T24 Ha-*ras* oncogene [7]. Alterations or activation of the *ras* oncogene have been studied regarding cutaneous neoplasms; in studies of human cutaneous melanoma, activated *ras* genes were found in 15–25% of tumors [13]. The T24 Ha-*ras* gene itself increases proliferation but does not transform primary cultures of melanocytes or rat embryo fibroblasts in tissue culture [14]. Furthermore, in vivo expression of T24 Ha-*ras* cause functional activation of melanocytes [7]. The resulting transgenic mice exhibited abnormal behavior and morphology, including abnormal movements soon after birth and deafness. Several abnormalities were observed in sections of the eyes and the eyelids. These tissues contained enlarged cells with intracytoplasmic melanin. The uveal tissue was thickened and heavily pigmented [7]. Kramer and associates studied 8 transgenic TP-*ras* mice with bilateral pigmented combined uveal melanocytic/RPE proliferations and found benign cytological characteristics in six of the mice (Figs. 1 and 2). The two remaining mice had cytologically malignant, bilateral melanocytic proliferations

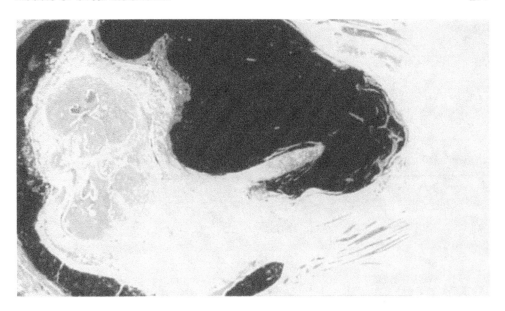

Figure 1 TPras transgenic mouse eye with diffuse, heavily pigmented uveal proliferation. (H&E, × 10.)

of the uveal tract, which was morphologically consistent with melanoma (Figs. 3 and 4) [15]. It is difficult to ascertain the reason for the alterations in the primary pigmented cells in these various transgenic models. The expression of the SV40 gene and the Ha-*ras* gene might occur at times during embryological development, not consistent with the production of pigment and proliferation of uveal melanocytes and retinal pigment epithelium. It is possible that expression of different genes at different embryological stages allows for the partially selective proliferation of melanocytes or retinal pigment epithelium [15].

III. SPONTANEOUSLY OCCURRING UVEAL TUMORS IN ANIMALS

A. Ocular Melanoma in Dogs

Tumors of melanocytic origin are the most common form of primary ocular neoplasia in dogs [16,17]. The first melanotic sarcoma (melanoma) of the dog choroid was described in 1919 by Petit [18]. Since then, several cases of uveal melanoma have been described in different breeds of dog [19]. The iris and ciliary body are the most common sites of origin for both benign and malignant ocular melanocytic proliferations in dogs [20–22]. There are only a few reported primary melanocytic tumors of the choroid [16,19,23]. The Callender classification and its modification [24], including the veterinary adaptation [25], are inappropriate for canine tumors, since most canine primary intraocular melanocytic neoplasms are histologically benign and contain a large proportion of plump cells that are not found in human uveal melanoma [17]. There is some indication that, as in humans, tumors with epithelioid-like cells are more locally aggressive than spindle cell tumors

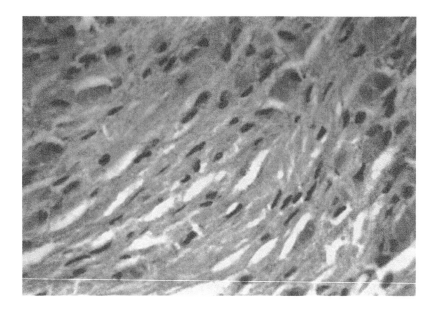

Figure 2 The cytological features of the uveal proliferation shown in Fig. 1 reveal cells with bland features, consistent with a benign melanocytic proliferation. (H&E, bleached, ×160.)

[20]. The literature suggests that the behavior of canine choroidal melanoma is relatively benign and that these tumors have features consistent with melanocytoma and other forms of uveal melanocytic nevi that occur in humans.

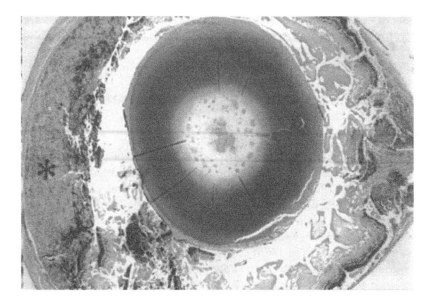

Figure 3 TPras transgenic mouse eye with melanocytic proliferation confined to the anterior chamber (*). (H&E, ×10.)

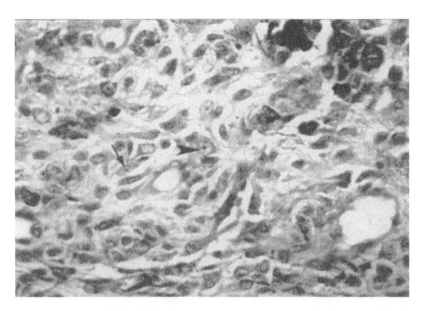

Figure 4   The cytological features of the anterior uveal proliferation shown in Fig. 3 depicting cells with malignant cytological features, including epithelioid-like cells (arrowhead) and spindle cells (arrow). (H&E, × 160.)

B.   Ocular Melanoma in Cats

Melanoma is the most frequently reported primary ocular neoplasm in cats [26]. Feline ocular melanoma usually arises on the anterior surface of the iris, and there is usually a diffuse darkening of the entire iris (Fig. 5) [21,27]. The neoplastic melanocytes in diffuse iris melanoma of the cat tend to be large, rounded cells with abundant cytoplasm and centrally positioned, round nuclei. Bizarre, enlarged nuclear forms are commonly encountered in these tumors. A smaller percentage of tumors have localized areas of pigmented spindle cells, and a few are predominantly composed of spindle cells. There is no evidence to suggest that the morphology of the tumor cells is related to prognosis, and long-term follow-up is limited. Intraocular melanomas in cats have been suggested to have a greater malignant potential than those in dogs [21]. There have been reported cases of metastatic disease in cats following enucleation for diffuse iris melanoma [21,28]. Feline ocular melanomas metastasize to the abdominal viscera and particularly the liver [21,27]. The lung is the second most common site of visceral metastasis [21].

C.   Pigmented Ocular Tumors in Other Animals

Primary pigmented intraocular tumors—which may represent adenoma, adenocarcinoma—or uveal melanoma, have also been reported in the horse, sheep, fish, and

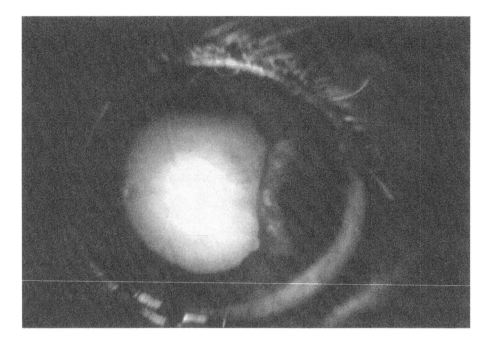

Figure 5   Feline ocular melanoma arising on the anterior iris surface.

chicken [19]. Spontaneously occurring cutaneous melanomas in animals, which are utilized in animal models of ocular melanoma, are described further on.

IV.   CHEMICAL AND RADIATION INDUCED UVEAL PROLIFERATIONS

Uveal proliferations have been induced in laboratory animals with various chemical agents. Bensen and Hill reported intraocular tumor development in a rat after intraperitoneal injections of ethione and oral administration of N-2-fluorenylacetamide [29]. The tumor was found after 339 days in one of 25 study rats. The tumor arose in and extended around the iris, contained no visible pigment, did not metastasize, and was found to closely resemble a human spindle A type melanocytic proliferation [29]. Patz and collaborators reported experimental production of ocular tumors in mice [30]. Sutures impregnated with methylcholantrene and cholesterol were drawn through and fixed within the anterior chamber (AC) or posterior segment. The resulting iris tumors were not found to be identical to any specific cell type of human ocular melanoma, although they did resemble malignant melanoma of the iris. Tumors in the posterior segment were markedly anaplastic and undifferentiated. The possibility that these tumors originated from the retina or retinal pigment epithelium could not be excluded. No metastases were detected from these tumors [30]. Pigmented intraocular tumors have been produced with radium in dogs [31]. Beagles intravenously injected with 226Ra showed the presence of this material in melanin granules. The lesions induced by the intraocular retention of radium were dose-dependent and characterized by loss of pigment at high dose levels and melanosis at lower levels. Induction of presumed intraocular melanoma occurred in both eyes in approximately 20% of the affected dogs and arose in the ciliary body. The cell of origin of the radiation-induced tumors was uncertain, although several features supported an origin from the ciliary body pigment epithelium. The tumors were microscopically characterized as consisting of clusters of large, round, densely pigmented cells separated by spindle-shaped cells. The incidence of mitotic figures was low and the tumor grew slowly. Widespread metastases were observed in two cases [31]. Secondary glaucoma occurred in a high percentage of the dogs with melanoma.

Albert and coworkers reported intraocular tumors in rats 6 to 9 months following injections of nickel subsulfide (Ni3S3), a potent carcinogen, into the vitreous cavity. Histologically, these tumors were composed of spindle and epithelioid cells; electron microscopy revealed premelanosomes in tumor cells [32].

An animal model of conjunctival primary acquired melanosis has been induced by the chronic topical application of the chemical carcinogen 7,12-dimethylbenz[a]-anthracene (DMBA) [33]. Chronic topical application of DMBA directly to the rabbit's sclera is capable of inducing hyperplastic melanocytic lesions of the choroid [34]. Pe'er and coworkers induced primary uveal melanocytic lesions in Dutch (pigmented) rabbits using a two-stage carcinogenesis protocol involving initiation with four weekly topical applications of DMBA in acetone, followed by 12 weekly topical applications of croton oil in acetone. Exposure to DMBA followed by promotion with croton oil was effective in inducing clinically detectable fundus lesions. Lesions that showed unrestricted growth or metastasis were not detected. Clinical regression of the fundus lesions was noted after promotion was discontinued [35].

V. VIRAL-INDUCED UVEAL PROLIFERATIONS

A. Feline Uveal Melanoma Induced by Gardner Strain of Feline Sarcoma Virus

McCullough and coworkers determined that feline sarcoma virus can induce malignant melanoma associated with fibrosarcoma in nonocular tissues of the cat [36]. Additionally, feline leukemia virus injected into the eyes of newborn kittens or into fetal kittens resulted in severe developmental abnormalities and the production of a retinal tumor resembling retinoblastoma [37]. Albert and coworkers injected the Gardner strain of feline sarcoma virus into the inferior iris root of kittens [38,39]. Tumors were clinically detectable in approximately 80% of the injected eyes, were typically present by 40 days after injection, and were always recognizable by 60 days [38,40]. Two types of lesion were observed: (1) discrete areas of increased pigmentation of the iris or a mass enlarging within the iris and ciliary body and (2) diffuse tumors, clinically characterized by thickening of the iris. Both the discrete and diffuse types continued to enlarge and eventually filled the anterior chamber and, in some cases, extended beyond the sclera [38]. Hypertrophy and hyperplasia of uveal melanocytes were histologically noted as early as 14 days after injection. In progressively enlarging tumors, pigmented epithelioid and pigmented or nonpigmented spindle-shaped cells invaded the iris stroma. In the large tumors, epithelioid cells were common and often predominated. The ultrastructural appearance of the melanoma cells was similar to that described for human ocular melanoma. A significant difference from human melanoma was the constant finding of virus particles budding from the cell membrane [38].

There are several advantages of this model of virally induced uveal proliferations. It uses a virus that is among the most thoroughly studied of the tumor viruses [41,42]. Transformation of normal melanocytes into tumor cells occurs in this model and may be studied. Disadvantages include the high mortality among infected animals as a result of feline infectious peritonitis. The presence of easily identifiable virus within most tumor cells is in striking contrast to human uveal melanoma. Injected animals develop disseminated viral infections, and secondary tumors produced are second primary tumors induced by virus shed from the primary intraocular melanoma, not metastases [43]. Most of the second primary tumors, ultrastructurally and in tissue culture, resemble fibrosarcoma [43]. Additionally, caution must be used in working with oncogenic viruses.

B. Uveal Melanoma Induced by SV40

In 1962, the simian virus 40 (SV40), a papovavirus found as a contaminant in rhesus monkey kidney tissue culture, was noted to induce neoplastic transformation in hamster kidney in vitro [44]. In 1968, Albert and coworkers introduced SV40 to hamster retina, choroid, and iris tissue grown in vitro [45]. These transformed tissue culture cells were subcutaneously injected into hamsters, resulting in firm, white neoplasms. Spindle and epithelioid cell types were observed [45]. SV40 tumors derived from retina, iris, and choroid tissue were similar in histological appearance, which was not unexpected, since an oncogenic virus may produce tumors with similar morphology in many different tissues [46]. The tumor cells observed by Albert and coworkers gradually lost their pigmentation and lacked ultrastructural evidence of premelanosomes.

VI. INTRAOCULAR INOCULATION OF TISSUE CULTURE MELANOMA CELLS IN ANIMAL EYES

A. Ocular Immune Privilege

The value of the anterior chamber (AC) of the animal eye as a privileged environment for heterologous tumor implantation was studied by Greene in 1949 [47–49]. He succeeded in transplantating rabbit tumors and several human tumors into the AC of animals of various species, including rabbit, mouse, rat, hamster, guinea pig, pig, sheep, and goat. It has subsequently been found that, after preliminary transfer of a new species of tumor cells into the AC, the tumor cells grown in the AC may be successfully transferred to and grown in different body regions of naive animals [48]. Investigators have found that introduction of tumor cells [50] or viruses [51] into the AC induces antigen-specific suppressor T cells that suppress cellular immunity to that antigen [52].

The immune privilege of the AC has been termed anterior chamber-associated immune deviation (ACAID) and has been confirmed in many studies [52]. In ACAID, T-suppressor cells cause suppression of delayed-type hypersensitivity (DTH), whereas humoral immunity is preserved. This explains long-term survival of the allograft in the AC, although destruction of tumor in the AC after a prior subcutaneous graft indicates that some antigenicity exists. It is possible that a humoral response plays a role in this form of AC tumor destruction [53]. The posterior segment of the eye, especially the subretinal space and vitreous, contains many immunomodulatory factors that maintain immune privilege [54]. The ocular milieu may thus provide immunological privilege for uveal melanoma [55].

B. Cell Lines

1. Greene Melanoma

In 1958, Greene isolated a spontaneous cutaneous hamster melanoma [56]. Homologous subcutaneous transfer of this tumor tissue resulted in a 100% growth rate. All the transplanted tumors grew progressively, and all the recipient animals died within 5 months of diffuse metastases.

The histological features of the tumor had changed after the tumor had been maintained by serial transfer through six generations over a 2-year period. A variation in pigment content was noted in one animal after the third passage; transfer of this tumor resulted in growth varying in color from the original black to pale white. The white tumors differed from the parental cell line with respect to pigment content and biological behavior [56]. The most distinctive biological changes associated with the amelanotic transformation consisted of an enhancement in heterologous transplantability and the attainment of the ability to metastasize [57].

In 1966, Greene and Harvey described another method of producing amelanotic melanomas in the hamster [57]. This new method was derived from the observation that intra-aortic inoculation of cells from melanotic melanoma produced amelanotic metastases, whereas intravenous inoculation of melanotic melanoma or vascular invasion from subcutaneous transplants resulted in pigmented metastases, similar to the primary tumor. Ultrastructurally, the cells in the amelanotic metastases were primitive and could not be differentiated from other anaplastic tumors [57]. The pigmented parental melanoma is rarely transplantable in foreign species and does not grow if placed into the AC of the rabbit eye. In contrast, amelanotic metastases readily grow in foreign species. The amelanotic variant fills the AC of the rabbit eye in less than 2 weeks, and large, widespread metastases involving the skin, contralateral eye, brain, pituitary, mammary tissue, skeletal muscle, liver, kidney, spleen, ovaries, adrenals, gastric and intestinal mucosa, diaphragm, lungs, heart, and thymus are observed within 1 month [57]. With continued passages of tissue culture cells, tumor growth in the AC and metastases are enhanced.

An advantage of using the hamster Greene melanoma model is that light and electron microscopic features of the amelanotic Greene melanoma are similar to human uveal melanoma, especially the epithelioid cell type [58]. Although Greene melanoma is a popular model for ophthalmic researchers, it has shortcomings. At least one retrovirus associated with Greene melanoma is apparently able to transform adjacent ocular tissues—for instance, the retinal pigment epithelium [59]. This retrovirus may cause distant viral infection and neoplasia, which may be confused with metastases [59], similar to what occurs in the feline leukemia-sarcoma virus model. Another disadvantage of this model is that the biological behavior of Greene melanoma differs from human uveal melanoma. Even without therapy, Greene melanoma exhibits necrosis and hemorrhage 8–10 days after inoculation into the AC of the rabbit eye [53]. These changes could interfere with interpretation of the results of experimental therapies.

2. B16 Melanoma

The B16 melanoma arose spontaneously in 1954 in skin at the base of the ear of a C57BL mouse at the Jackson Laboratory [60]. Since its origin, it has been carried continuously in mice and used in many investigations. Pigmented cell strains were established in vitro from this tumor in the early 1960s [61]. Fidler developed a system of animal transplantation and tissue culture to select B16 tumor lines that possess enhanced metastatic properties [62]. The original cell line was designated as line number 26 (Fidler's melanoma clone 26), and its daughter lines designated as lines 27, 28, 29, and 30. Later, Fidler renamed them to be B16 line F1 for the first passage line and then numbered them consecutively (i.e., lines F2, F3, etc.) [63]. Subcultures of B16 cells with different metastatic rates, such as the B16-F10, B16-F10 Queens [62–64], B16-LS8, and B16-LS9 [65,66] cell lines were developed after serial passages and isolation of metastatic tumors.

The B16 melanoma cell line has been used extensively for investigating the metastatic process and the immunological parameters that influence metastatic tumor development in mice [67]. The B16 melanoma model, although not ideal, offers several important advantages over other animal models. The origin and genetic background of the tumor is well documented [67]. Intraocular B16 melanoma metastasizes spontaneously in a predictable time frame [64,68]. B16 melanoma has been used extensively in a wide variety of studies of the biology and immunology of tumor metastasis and is among the most commonly used tumors in metastasis research [67].

3. Human Uveal Melanoma

In 1969, the discovery that the mutant athymic nude mouse was unable to reject a heterotransplant of human tumor tissue (human adenocarcinoma) [69] opened a new area for experimental study of human tumors, including the analysis of metastatic properties [70]. In contrast to human cutaneous melanoma, human uveal melanoma cells do not readily grow in tissue culture [71]. Culturing of uveal melanoma was first attempted in 1929 by Kirby [72]. Kirby's studies as well as subsequent observations of in vitro growth of uveal melanoma consisted of relatively short-term experiments [73–76]. It was demonstrated that uveal melanoma cells can survive in culture for periods of several months or longer if transfer of the cells is not attempted. Although, until recently, no continuous cell lines of uveal melanoma have been established, some interesting features of this tumor were observed, including the spontaneous transformation of spindle cells to epithelioid cells and vice versa [74]. The first continuous cell lines of human uveal melanoma were reported by Albert and coworkers in 1984 [71]. Several cell lines from primary uveal melanoma [77–81] and metastatic uveal melanoma [81] have been described. Some of these cell lines have been growing for several years without morphological change [81]. It has become apparent that there is no single universal grwoth medium for human uveal melanoma and that a particular cell type may grow well in one medium but not another.

Human uveal melanomas transferred to the eyes of animals are termed *orthotopic* transplantations, whereas cutaneous melanomas like the Greene or the B16 melanoma transferred to the eye are termed *heterotopic* transplantations. It is becoming evident that tumors transplanted to heterotopic sites often do not display metastatic behavior consistent with the original tumor. Many tumors do not metastasize from heterotopic sites in nude mice but will form metastases after orthotopic transplantation [82]. For these reasons, orthotopic transplantations of human uveal melanoma constitute an important model. The effect of orthotopic transplantation may be due at least in part to the influence of local organ-specific factors [83].

C. Hamster Model

In 1961, Burns and Fraunfelder described establishment of an ocular melanoma model using suspensions of Greene melanoma cells [84]. Those investigators injected tumor cell suspensions into the AC of Syrian golden hamsters. Tumors grew and extended into the eyelids, orbit, and cranial cavity. Posterior auricular, cervical, and thoracic cage lymph nodes were involved by lymphatic spread. Metastases to lungs, liver, thoracic wall, and diaphragm were observed [84]. Fournier and associates inserted pieces of melanotic Greene melanoma onto the surface of the iris in Syrian golden hamsters [85]. In 1974, Albert and collaborators injected Greene melanoma cells into the choroid of the Syrian hamster [86]. Those investigators found histological evidence of development of choroidal melanomas in most injected eyes. Two weeks after injection, the eyes showed tumor growth and extension through Bruch's membrane in most instances. Some 3–4 weeks after injection, the tumor within the globe was often necrotic, and perforation of the sclera had occurred, resulting in extensive orbital invasion. Necropsy revealed evidence of extensive metastases by the sixth week [32].

D. Murine Model

1. Murine Model Using Greene Melanoma Cells

In 1966, Greene and Harvey transferred amelanotic Greene melanoma into the AC and brain of a few mice of the DBA or BDF strain and found that the tumor survived the transfer to both transplantation sites [57].

2. Murine Model Using B16 Melanoma Cells

B16 melanoma cell lines have been successfully inoculated into the AC of syngeneic murine eyes (Figs. 6 to 8), resulting in tumor growth and pulmonary metastases [6,50,68,87–89]. Different AC inoculation techniques have been described, including

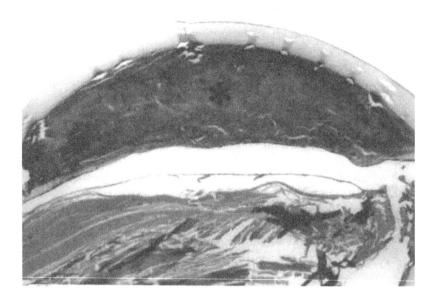

Figure 6   Human eye with anterior chamber (AC) filled with melanoma (*) arising in the iris.
(H&E, × 4.)

quantitative techniques for depositing a defined number of tumor cells into the AC
[50]. Various cell concentrations and cell suspension volumes have been used [87,89].
Although ocular tumor growth depends on concentration of inoculum, there are
only slight differences in metastatic rate provided that there is intraocular tumor
growth [87,89].

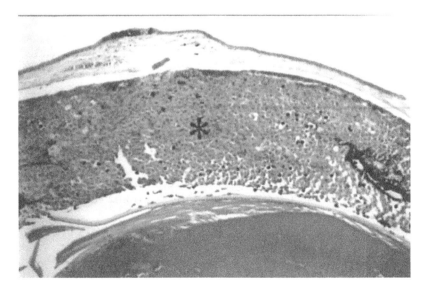

Figure 7   Murine AC filled with tissue culture B16 melanoma (*). (H&E, × 25.)

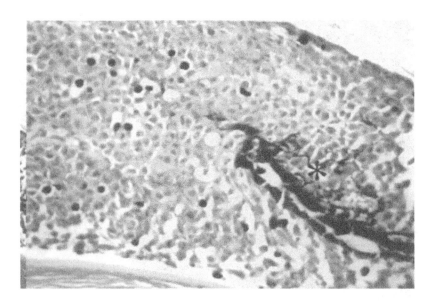

Figure 8   The AC melanoma shown in Fig. 2 is present in the iris. (H&E, × 63.)

Enucleation performed 8 to 12 days after AC inoculation of B16-F10 melanoma cell suspensions and necropsies approximately 4 weeks after inoculation have shown a pulmonary metastatic rate of 0–33% [68,87,88]. B16-F10 cells derived in vivo differ from cultured B16-F10 cells with regard to the metastatic rate to the lung. When B16-F10 cells are passaged five times in culture and inoculated into the AC, a marked decrease in the frequency and extent of metastases, and an increase in survival are observed as compared to inoculation of B16-F10 tumors cells maintained in vivo [64].

Successful inoculation of tissue culture B16 melanoma cells into the posterior compartment (PC) of murine eyes has been described by Grossniklaus and coworkers [87,88,90]. The PC includes the ciliary body, choroid, subretinal space and vitreous. There is evidence that the PC provides a unique immune-privileged environment. The PC model is analogous to human intraocular melanoma, which arises in the choroid and metastasizes hematogenously. B16-F10 melanoma cells inoculated into the PC of C57BL/6 mice were found to metastasize to the lung in 89% of the mice [88]. This higher metastatic rate in the PC compared to the AC model is comparable to the higher metastatic rate of choroidal melanoma compared to iris melanoma. The metastatic rate correlated with tumor vascular pattern and vascular density [90]. One difficulty with the inoculation of melanoma cells into the murine PC was that tumor cells frequently reflux into the subconjunctival space, resulting in subconjunctival melanoma. The primary extraocular tumor growth does not reflect the human situation, in which uveal melanoma is confined to the inside of the eye. A transcorneal inoculation technique that results in intraocular confinement of the inoculated melanoma cells has recently been developed (Figs. 9 and 10) [91]. Hematogenous metastases develop from intraocular melanoma. It appears that extraocular extension of tumor and invasion of conjunctival lymphatics in either the

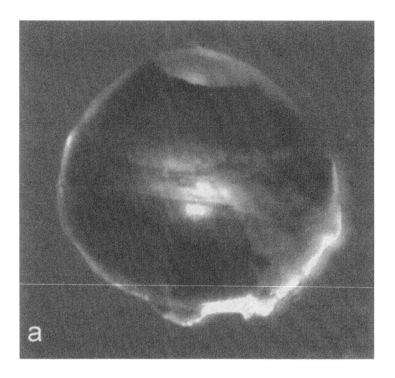

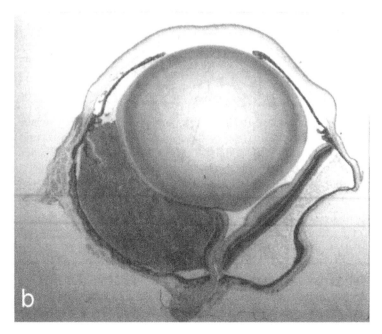

Figure 9   Transcorneal inoculation of B16 melanoma cells. a, The enucleated murine eye exhibits no extraocular melanoma after 7 days of intraocular tumor growth. b and c, A corresponding secton displays melanoma in the vitreous, subretinal space, and choroid. (H&E. b, ×4; c, ×63.)

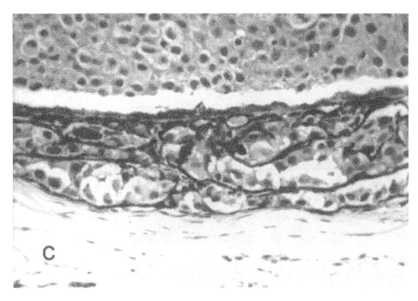

Figure 9 Continued.

AC or PC model results in lymph node metastasis (Fig. 11). A subculture of the B16 melanoma cell line, the B16-LS9 line, has been developed after repetitive intrasplenic inoculation of B16 melanoma cells and recovery of the cells from the liver [66]. In subsequent experiments, these cells metastasized from the eye to the liver of immune competent mice and there was a positive correlation between the number of pulmonary and liver metastases [65]. B16-LS9 melanoma cells show low MHC class I expression, suggesting that they are susceptible to NK cell-mediated lysis [92]. B16-LS9 cells inoculated into the PC of C57BL6 mice, which have been rendered NK cell-deficient by treatment with antiasialo GM1, results in a significant increase in hepatic micrometastases and growth of the hepatic micrometastases compared with controls (Fig. 12) [92,93].

3. Murine Model Using Human Uveal Melanoma Cells

Human uveal melanoma cells have been successfully transplanted into the AC of athymic "nude" mice [94]. Albert and coworkers were able to culture human uveal melanoma experimentally in nude mice by transplanting fresh human uveal melanoma into the AC and vitreous [32]. Niederkorn and collaborators inoculated human uveal melanoma cells into the AC of nude Balb/c mice and found tumor growth and liver lesions characterized by necrosis, mild neutrophilic infiltration, and karyorrhexis. Tumor cells in these lesions diffusely stained with a monoclonal antibody that specifically reacted to human nuclear membrane antigens. The authors concluded that human ocular melanoma cells may metastasize to the liver in nude mice but fail to grow progressively [94]. Ma and collaborators found the human

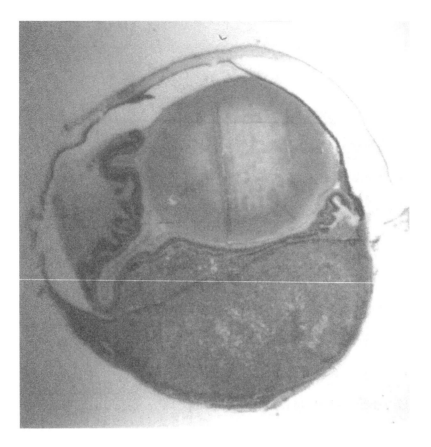

Figure 10   Transcorneal inoculation of B16 melanoma cells shows intrachoroidal melanoma (*) infiltrating the sclera.

uveal cell line OCM3 to be susceptible to NK cell-mediated cytolysis [95]. These investigators inoculated the OCM3 cell line into the AC of athymic nude mice and in vivo disruption of NK function resulted in the increased severity of metastatic hepatic foci [95]. Injection of human uveal melanoma cells into the PC of beige nude x-linked immune deficient (BNX) mice has been performed (Figs. 13 to 16) [96]. Tumor growth and liver micrometastases were found when different primary and metastatic uveal melanomas were inoculated into the PC of BNX mice [96].

E.   Rabbit Model

The rabbit eye is suitable because of its relatively large size, permitting funduscopy and fundus photography, the relatively low cost of procuring and maintaining rabbits compared with other animals with comparably sized eyes, the relatively long life span of the rabbit, and the well-known anatomy and physiology of the rabbit eye [97].

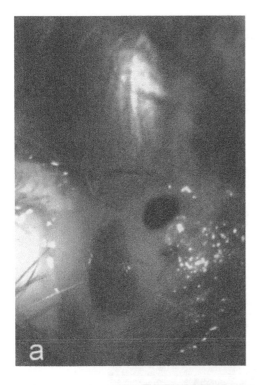

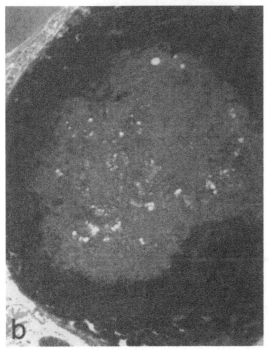

Figure 11 Lymph node metastasis of melanoma in murine model shown grossly (a) and microscopically (b). (H&E, × 10.)

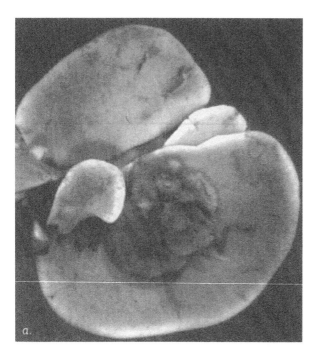

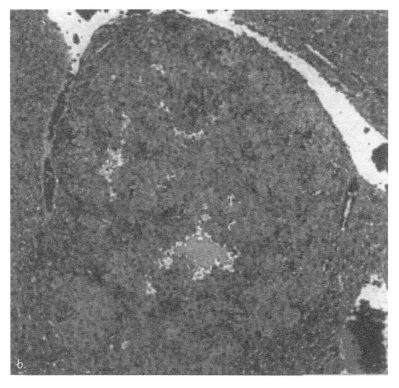

Figure 12   Liver metastasis of melanoma in murine model with B16-LS9 cell line shown grossly (a) and microscopically (b). (H&E, ×10.)

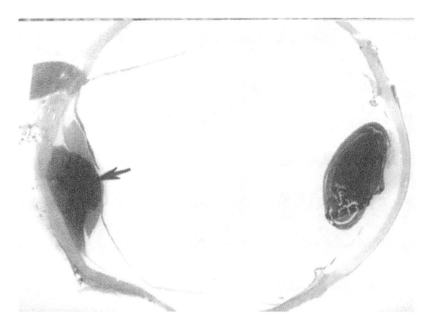

Figure 13 Human eye with posterior compartment (PC) melanoma arising in choroid and breaking through Bruch's membrane, forming a collarbutton-shaped mass. (H&E, ×2.)

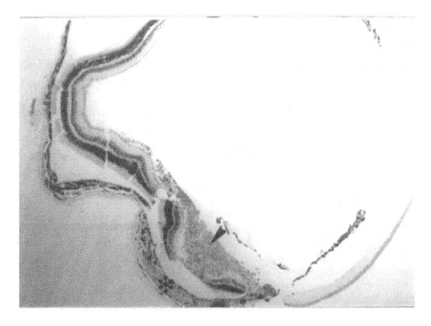

Figure 14 Murine eye with PC tissue culture human uveal melanoma in choroid (arrowhead) and extending through retina into vitreous (*). (H&E, ×10.)

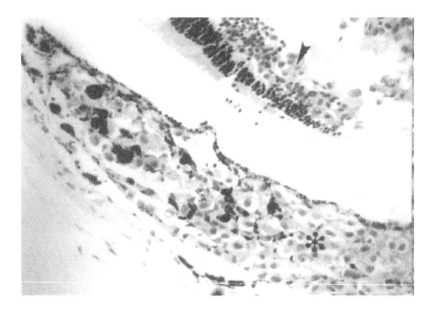

Figure 15 The PC melanoma shown in Fig. 13 is present in the choroid and has extended into the retina and vitreous. (H&E, × 63.)

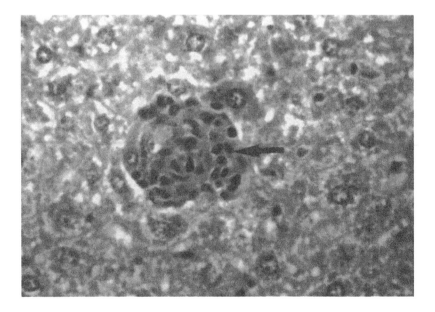

Figure 16 The PC murine melanoma shown in Figs. 14 and 15 has metastasized to the liver (arrow). (H&E, × 160.)

1. Rabbit Model Using Greene Melanoma Cells

Krohn and collaborators described the successful transplantation of Greene melanoma cells into the posterior ocular segment of rabbits in 1970 [98]. These investigators used amelanotic Greene melanoma that was maintained in the AC of rabbits [98]. After AC implantation, the tumor grew rapidly and ruptured the globe within 12 to 14 days. Pieces of this tumor were then transplanted into the subchoroidal space of New Zealand albino rabbit eyes. Tumor growth occurred in most of the animals and was ophthalmoscopically detectable within 16 days [98]. In 1982, Liu and collaborators used a rabbit model with implanted hamster Greene melanoma grown in the choroid of the eye [99], using the implantation procedure of Krohn and collaborators [98]. The tumor grew and was clinically recognizable 4 to 6 weeks after implantation. After an additional 6 to 8 weeks, the tumor-bearing eye perforated, and at the 10th week after implantation, the rabbits exhibited weakness and loss of body weight. Necropsies revealed widespread metastases, including metastases in the liver [99]. The histopathological appearance of the metastatic tumor was identical to that of the primary choroidal Greene melanoma. Most tumor cells in the metastatic lesion appeared to be epithelioid and showed marked pleomorphism [100]. Other techniques for subchoroidal implantation of Greene melanoma were subsequently developed [101]. Lambrou and collaborators used a transvitreal approach to deposit a tumor fragment into the subchoroidal space of rabbits [102].

Greene melanoma transplanted into the eyes of rabbits has been used for evaluation of treatment effects on intraocular tumor. These studies have included anticancer agents [103,104], ionizing radiation [105,106], ferromagnetic hyperthermia combined with iodine-125 brachytherapy [107], hyperthermia [108], photodynamic therapy on choroidal tumors [109,110], photoradiation treatment [111], fluorouracil therapy [112], indocyanine green–enhanced diode laser treatment [113], and phototherapy of AC tumors [114].

2. Rabbit Model Using B16 Melanoma Cells

Inoculation of B16 melanoma into the rabbit requires immunosuppression in order to enable tumor growth. Inoculation of B16F10 melanoma into the subchoroidal space in rabbits treated with cyclosporin A results in tumor growth [115,116]. These globes are usually half filled with tumor by the third week and totally filled with tumor by the fourth week after implantation [115]. Grossly visible metastatic lesions are present only in the lung, consistent with the metastatic pattern seen with B16F10 melanoma when grown in the syngeneic host [115]. In a study using murine cutaneous B16F10 melanoma cells, hamster cutaneous melanoma, and human uveal melanoma cell lines transplanted into the subchoroidal space of the rabbit eyes, the B16F10 line was the only source that consistently generated heavily pigmented choroidal tumors [115]. A rabbit model of extrascleral extension of ocular melanoma has also been established [116].

A major disadvantage of this rabbit model is the requirement of daily injections, of cyclosporin A, which limits the time the animal can be kept for observation. Cyclosporin-treated rabbits usually die within 6 to 10 weeks. To date, the only melanoma cell line successfully implanted in the rabbit eye without immunosuppression is the amelanotic Greene hamster melanoma.

3. Rabbit Model Using Human Uveal Melanoma

Kann-Mitchel and coworkers observed that the addition of cyclosporin A improves the growth and survival of human uveal melanoma cell lines in the AC of rabbit eyes [80]. Ligget and collaborators successfully established human uveal melanoma xenografts in the choroid of immunosuppressed rabbits [117]. These authors noted spontaneous disappearance of the tumor over a 2-week period when the immunosuppression was discontinued.

F. Chick Embryo Model

Luyten and coworkers injected cultured human uveal melanoma cells into the chicken embryonal eye at a stage when the immune system was not mature. The melanoma cells were accepted as part of the organism by the host. Tumors were found in 20% of the embryos injected with uveal melanoma. The eyes were removed on the 19th embryonal day and did not exhibit abnormal development as a result of the injection [118].

VII. SUMMARY

Various animal models of human uveal melanoma have been studied. Each of these models has unique advantages and disadvantages. Spontaneous uveal melanoma rarely occurs in dogs and cats. The occurrence of these tumors is unpredictable. Chemical- or radiation-induced intraocular pigmented tumors may be of RPE. Feline leukemia-sarcoma virus-and simian virus 40-induced uveal proliferations fail to metastasize. The biological behavior of Greene and B16 melanoma cell lines after intraocular injection into various animal species is predictable, allowing for study of mechanisms of growth and metastasis. The pathogenesis of intraocular pigmented tumors in transgenic mice is beginning to be understood and offers promise as a model for studying growth and metastasis, with the potential for developing more effective treatments.

REFERENCES

1. Fischer E. Dtsch Ztschr Chir 1882;17:61–92, cited in Blake EM. Cultivation of human tumor in the anterior chamber of guinea pig's eye. Am J Ophthalmol 1946;29:1098–1106.
2. Dithmar S, Albert DM, Grossniklaus HE. Animal models of uveal melanoma. Melanoma Res 2000;10:195–211.
3. Tanaka S, Yamamoto H, Takeuchi S, et al. Melanization in albino mice transformed by introducing cloned mouse tyrosinase gene. Development 1990;108:223–227.
4. Anand R, Ma D, Alizadeh H, Comerford SA, Sambrook JF, Gefhing MJH, McLean IW, Niederkorn JY. Characterization of intraocular tumors arising in trt transgenic mice. Invest Ophthalmol Vis Sci 1994;35:3533–3539.
5. Bradl M, Klein-Szanto A, Porter S. Malignant melanoma in transgenic mice. Proc Nat Acad Sci USA 1991;88:164–168.
6. Knisely TL, Niederkorn JY. Immunologic evaluation of spontaneous regression of an intraocular murine melanoma. Invest Ophthalmol Vis Sci 1990;31:247–257.

7. Powell MB, Hyman P, Bell OD, et al. Hyperpigmentation and melanocytic hyperplasia in transgenic mice expressing the human T24 Ha-ras gene regulated by a mouse tyrosinase promoter. Mol Carcinog 1995;12:82–90.
8. Syed NA, Windle JA, Darjatmoko SR, et al.Transgenic mice with pigmented intraocular tumors: Tissue of origin and treatment. Invest Ophthalmol Vis Sci 1998;39:2800–2805.
9. Zhu H, Reuhl K, Zhang X, et al. Development of heritable melanoma in transgenic mice. J Invest Dermatol 1998;110:247–252.
10. Andriole GL, Mule JJ, Hansen CT, et al. Evidence that lymphokine-activated killer cells and natural killer cells are distinct on an analysis of congenitally immunodeficient mice. J Immunol 1985;135:2911–2913.
11. Ma D, Alizadeh H, Comerford SA, et al. Rejection of intraocular tumors from transgenic mice by tumor infiltrating lymphocytes. Curr Eye Res 1994;13:361–369.
12. Ma D, Niederkorn JY. Efficacy of tumor-infiltrating lymphocytes in the treatment of hepatic metastases arising from transgenic intraocular tumors in mice. Invest Ophthalmol Vis Sci 1995;36:1067–1075.
13. Albino AP, Nanus DM, Mentle JR, et al. Analysis of ras oncogenes in malignant melanoma and precursor lesions: Correlation of point mutations with differentiation phenotype. Oncogene 1989;4:1363–1374.
14. Land H, Chen AC, Morgenstern JP. Behavior of myc and ras oncogenes in transformation of rat embryo fibroblasts. Mol Cell Biol 1986;6:1917–1925.
15. Kramer TR, Powell MB, Wilson MM, Salvatore J, Grossniklaus HE. Pigmented uveal tumours in a transgenic mouse model. Br J Ophthalmol 1998;82:953–960.
16. Dubielzig RR, Aguirre GD, Gross SL, et al. Choroidal melanomas in dogs. Vet Pathol 1985;22:582–585.
17. Wilcock BP, Pfeiffer RL. Morphology and behaviour of primary ocular melanomas in 91 dogs. Vet Pathol 1986;23:418–424.
18. Petit G. La mécanisme de la pigmentation dans le sarcome mélanique. Rec Med Vet 1919;95:121–125.
19. Saunders LZ, Barron CN. Primary pigmented intraocular tumors in animals. Cancer Res 1958;18:234–245.
20. Diters RW, Dubielzig RR, Aguirre GD, et al. Primary ocular melanoma in dogs. Vet Pathol 1983;20:379–395.
21. Dubielzig RR. Ocular neoplasia in small animals. Vet Clin North Am 1990;20:840–841.
22. Ryan AM, Diters RW. Clinical and pathologic features of canine ocular melanomas. J Am Vet Med Assoc 1984;184:60–67.
23. Schoster JV, Dubielzig RR, Sullivan L. Choroidal melanoma in a dog. J Am Vet Med Assoc 1993;203:89–91.
24. McLean IW, Zimmerman LE, Evans RM. Reappraisal of Callender's spindle A type of malignant melanoma of choroid and ciliary body. Am J Ophthalmol 1978;86:557–564.
25. Kircher CH, Garner FM, Robinson FR. International histological classification of tumors in domestic animals. X. Tumors of the eye and adnexa. Bull WHO 1974;50:135–142.
26. Acland GM, McLean IW, Aguirre GD, et al. Diffuse iris melanoma in cats. J Am Vet Med Assoc 1980;176:52–56.
27. Schäffer EH, Gordon S. Feline ocular melanoma. Clinical and pathologico-anatomic findings in 37 cases. Tierärztl Prax 1993;21:255–264.
28. Bertoy RW, Brightman AH, Regan K. Intraocular melanoma with multiple metastases in a cat. J Am Vet Med Assoc 1988;192:87–89.
29. Benson WR, Hill C. Intraocular tumor after ethionine and N-2-fluorenylacetamide. Arch Pathol 1962;73:404–406.

30. Patz A, Wulff LB, Rogers SW. Experimental production of ocular tumors. Am J Ophthalmol 1959;48:98–117.

31. Taylor GN, Dougherty TF, Mays CW, et al. Radium-induced eye melanoma in dogs. Radiat Res 1972;5:361–373.

32. Albert DM, Shadduck JA, Liu HA, et al. Animal models for the study of uveal melanoma. Int Ophthalmol Clin 1980;2012:143–160.

33. Folberg R, Baron J, Reeves RD, et al. Animal model of conjunctival primary acquired melanosis. Ophthalmology 1989;96:1006–1013.

34. Folberg R, Baron J, Reeves RD, et al. Primary melanocytic lesions of the rabbit choroid following topical application of 7,12-dimethylbenz[a]-anthracene: preliminary observations. J Toxicol Cutaneous Ocul Toxicol 1990;9:313–334.

35. Pe'er J, Folberg R, Massicotte SJ, et al. Clinicopathologic spectrum of primary uveal melanocytic lesions in an animal model. Ophthalmology 1992;99:977–986.

36. McCullough B, Schaller J, Shadduck JA, Yohn DS. Brief communication. Induction of malignant melanomas associated with fibrosarcomas in gnotobiotic cats inoculated with Gardner feline sarcoma virus. J Natl Cancer In 1972;48:1893–1895.

37. Albert DM, Lahav M, Colby ED, et al. Retinal neoplasia and dysplasia: I.Induction by feline leukemia virus. Invest Ophthalmol Vis Sci 1977;16:325–337.

38. Albert DM, Shadduck JA, Craft JL, Niederkorn JY. Feline uveal melanoma induced with feline sarcoma virus. Invest Ophthalmol Vis Sci 1981;20:606–624.

39. Shadduck JA, Albert DM, Niederkorn JY. Feline uveal melanomas induced with feline sarcoma virus: Potential model of the human counterpart. J Natl Cancer Inst 1981;24:733–738.

40. Albert DM. The association of viruses with uveal melanoma. Trans Am Ophthalmol Soc 1979;77:367–421.

41. Francis DP, Essex M, Hardy WD. Excretion of feline leukemia viruses by naturally infected pet cats. Nature 1977;269:252.

42. Sarma PS, Log T, Skuntz S, et al. Experimental horizontal transmission of feline leukemia viruses of subgroups A,B and C. J Natl Cancer Inst 1978;60:871–874.

43. Niederkorn JY, Shadduck JA, Albert DA. Enucleation and the appearance of second primary tumors in cats bearing virally induced intraocular tumors. Invest Ophthalmol Vis Sci 1982;23:719–725.

44. Rabson AS, Kirschstein RL. Induction of malignancy in vitro in newborn haster kidney tissue infected with simian vacuolating virus (SV40). Proc Soc Exp Biol Med 1962;111:323–330.

45. Albert DM, Rabson AS, Dalton AJ. In vitro neoplastic transformation of uveal and retinal tissue by oncogenic DNA viruses. Invest Ophthalmol 1968;7:357–365.

46. Strohl WA, Rabson AS, Rouse H. Adenovirus tumorigenesis: The role of the viral genome in determining tumor morphology. Science 1967;156:1631–1633.

47. Green HSN. Heterologous transplantation of mammalian tumors. II. The transfer of human tumors to alien species. J Exp Med 1941;73:475–489.

48. Greene HSN. Heterologous transplantation of the Brown-Pearce tumor. Cancer Res 1949;9:728–735.

49. Greene HSN. The heterologous transplantation of human melanomas. Yale J Biol Med 1950;22:611–620.

50. Niederkorn JY, Streilein JW, Shadduck JA. Deviant immune response to allogeneic tumors injected intracamerally and subcutaneously in mice. Invest Ophthalmol Vis Sci 1981;20:355–363.

51. Whittum RP, Niederkorn JY, McCulley J, Streilein JW. Suppressor T cell induction by intracameral presentation of HSV-1. Invest Ophthalmol Vis Sci 1983 (Suppl): 213.

52. Ferguson TA, Waldrep JC, Kaplan HJ. The immune response and the eye. II. The nature of T suppressor cell induction in anterior chamber-associated immune deviation (ACAID). J Immunol 1987;139:352–357.
53. Römer TJ, Van Delft JL, De Wolff-Rouendaal D, Jager MJ. Hamster Greene melanoma implanted in the anterior chamber of a rabbit eye: A reliable tumor model? Ophthalmic Res 1992;24:119–124.
54. Streilein JW. Immune privilege of local tissue barriers and immunosuppressive microenvironments. Curr Opin Immunol 1993;5:428–432.
55. Apte RS, Mayhew E, Niederkorn JY. Local inhibition of natural killer cell activity promotes the progressive growth of intraocular tumors. Invest Ophthalmol Vis Sci 1997;38:1277–1282.
56. Greene HSN. A spontaneous melanoma in the hamster with a propensity for amelanotic alteration and sarcomatous transformation during transplantation. Cancer Res 1958;18:422–425.
57. Greene HSN, Harvey EK. The growth and metastasis of amelanotic melanomas in heterologous hosts. Cancer Res 1966;26:706–714.
58. Hahn I, Spitznas M. The morphology of the amelanotic Greene melanoma. Graefes Arch Clin Ophthalmol 1981;216:1–15.
59. Russell P, Gregerson DS, Albert DM, Reid TW. Characteristics of a retrovirus associated with a hamster melanoma. J Gen Virol 1979;43:317.
60. Green EL, ed. Handbook on Genetically Standardized JAX Mice. Bar Harbor, ME: Jackson Laboratory, 1962.
61. Hu F, Lesney PF. The isolation and cytology of two pigment cell strains from B16 mouse melanomas. Cancer Res 1964;24:1634–1643.
62. Fidler IJ. Selection of successive tumour lines for metastasis. Nature (New Biol) 1973;242:148–149.
63. Fidler IJ. Biological behavior of malignant melanoma cells correlated to their survival in vivo. Cancer Res 1975;35:218–224.
64. Harning R, Szalay J. Ocular metastasis in vivo and in vitro derived syngeneic murine melanoma. Invest Ophthalmol Vis Sci 1987;28:1599–1604.
65. Diaz CE, Rusciano D, Dithmar S, Grossniklaus HE. B16LS9 melanoma cells spread to the liver from murine posterior compartment (PC) intraocular melanoma. Curr Eye Res 1999;18:125–129.
66. Rusciano D, Lorenzoni P, Burger MM. Murine model of liver metastasis. Invas Metast 1994–95;14:349–361.
67. Poste G, Fidler IJ. The pathogenesis of cancer metastasis. Nature 1980;283:139–146.
68. Niederkorn JY. Enucleation in consort with immunological impairment promotes metastasis of intraocular melanomas in mice. Invest Ophthalmol Vis Sci 1984;25:1080–1086.
69. Rygaard J, Povlsen CO. Heterotransplantation of a human malignant tumor to nude mice. Acta Pathol Microbiol Scand 1969;76(1):146–148.
70. Giovanella BC, Fogh J. The nude mouse in cancer research. Adv Cancer Res 1985;44:69–120.
71. Albert DM, Ruzzo MA, McLaughlin MA, Robinson NL, Craft JL, Epstein J. Establishment of cell lines of uveal melanoma. Invest Ophthalmol Vis Sci 1984;25:1284–1299.
72. Kirby DB. Tissue culture in ophthalmic research. Trans Am Ophthalmol Soc 1929;27:334–383.
73. Barishak YR, Vanherick W, Yoneda C. Tissue culture of uveal melanomas. Arch Opthalmol 1960;64:352.
74. Irvine AR, Mahhagh J, Arya DV. Change in cell type of human choroidal malignant melanoma in tissue culture. Am J Ophthalmol 1975;80:418–424.

75. Oettgen HF, Aoki T, Old LJ, et al. Suspension culture of a pigment producing cell line derived from a human malignant melanoma. J Natl Cancer Inst 1968;41:827–843.

76. Toshima S, Moore GE, Sandberg AA. Ultastructure of human melanoma in cell culture. Electron microscopic studies. Cancer 1968;21:202–216.

77. Aubert C, Rouge F, Reillaudou M, Metge P. Establishment and characterization of human ocular melanoma cell lines. Int J Cancer 1993;54:784–792.

78. DeWaard-Siebinga I, Blom DJR, Griffioen M, et al. Establishment and characterization of an uveal melanoma cell line. Int J Cancer 1995;62:155–161.

79. Hu DN, McCormick SA, Paka K, et al. Establishment of three cell lines of uveal melanoma. Invest Ophthalmol Vis Sci 1997;38(Suppl):S802.

80. Kan-Mitchell J, Mitchell MS, Rao N, Liggett PE. Characterization of uveal melanoma cell lines that grow as xenografts in rabbit eyes. Invest Ophthalmol Vis Sci 1989;30:829–843.

81. Luyten GPM, Naus NC, Mooy CM, et al. Establishment and characterization of primary and metastatic uveal melanoma cell lines. Int J Cancer 1996;66:380–387.

82. Gohji K, Nakajima M, Dinney CPN, et al. The importance of orthotopic implantation to the isolation and biological characterization of a metastatic human clear cell renal carcinoma in nude mice. In J Oncol 1993;2:23–32.

83. Fidler IJ. Orthotopic implantation of human colon carcinomas into nude mice provides a valuable model for the biology and therapy of metastasis. Cancer Metast Rev 1991;10:229–243.

84. Burns RP, Frauenfelder FT. Experimental intraocular malignant melanoma in the Syrian golden hamster. Am J Ophtalmol 1961;51:977–993.

85. Fournier G, Saulanas A, Seddon J, et al. The effects of pre-enucleation irradiation on the development of metastases from intraocular Greene melanoma in hamsters. Am J Ophthalmol 1985;100:669–677.

86. Albert DM, Lahav M, Packer S, Yimoyines D. Histogenesis of malignant melanomas of the uvea: Occurence of nevus-like structures in experimental choroidal tumors. Arch Ophthalmol 1974;92:318–323.

87. Grossniklaus HE, Barron BC, Wilson MW. Murine model of anterior and posterior ocular melanoma. Curr Eye Res 1995; 14:399–404.

88. Grossniklaus HE, Wilson MW, Barron BC, Lynn MJ. Anterior vs posterior intraocular melanoma. Metastatic differences in a murine model. Arch Ophthalmol 1996; 114:1116–1120.

89. Harning R, Koo GC, Szalay J. Regulation of the metastasis of murine ocular melanoma by natural killer cells. Invest Ophthalmol Vis Sci 1989;30:1909–1915.

90. Grossniklaus HE. Tumor vascularity and hematogenous metastasis in experimental murine intraocular melanoma. Trans Am Ophthalmol Soc 1998;96:721–752.

91. Dithmar S, Rusciano D, Grossniklaus HE. A new technique for implantation of tissue culture melanoma cells in a murine model of metastatic ocular melanoma. Melanoma Res 2000;10:2–8.

92. Dithmar S, Rusciano D, Armstrong CA, et al. Depletion of NK cell activity results in growth of hepatic micrometastases in a murine ocular melanoma model. Curr Eye Res 1999;19:426–431.

93. Dithmar S, Rusciano D, Lynn MJ, Lawson DH, Armstrong CA, Grossniklaus HE. Neoadjuvant interferon alfa-2b treatment in a murine model for metastatic ocular melanoma: a preliminary study. Arch Ophthalmol 2000;118:1085–1089.

94. Niederkorn JY, Mellon J, Pidherney M, et al. Effect of anti-ganglioside antibodies on the metastatic spread of intraocular melanomas in a nude mouse model of human uveal melanoma. Curr Eye Res 1993;12(4):347–358.

95. Ma D, Luyten GP, Luider TM, Niederkorn JY. Relationship between natural killer cell susceptibility and metastasis of human uveal melanoma cells in a murine model. Invest Ophthalmol Vis Sci 1995;36:435–441.

96. Dithmar S, Diaz CE, Wallace AI, Kapp LM, Armstrong CA, Grossniklaus HE. Liver micrometastases in a murine ocular melanoma model. Invest Ophthalmol Vis Sci (Suppl) 1999;40:S247.

97. Prince JH, ed. The Rabbit Eye in Research. Springfield, IL: Charles C. Thomas, 1964.

98. Krohn DL, Brandt R, Morris DA, Keston AS. Subchoroidal transplantation of experimental malignant melanoma. Am J Ophthalmol 1970;70:753–756.

99. Liu LHS, Albert DM, Dohlman HG, Ni C. Metastasis in a rabbit choroidal melanoma model. Invest Ophthalmol Vis Sci 1982;22:115–118.

100. Liu LHS, Ni C. Rabbit model of uveal Greene melanoma: Morphologic studies of metastatic lesions. Graefes Arch Chir Exp Opthalmol 1983;220:179–183.

101. Riedel KG, Svittra PP, Albert DM, Finger PT, Packer S. Subchoroidal implanted Greene melanoma: An animal experiment model for malignant choroid melanoma. Klin Montsbl Augenheilk 1990;197:128–132.

102. Lambrou FH, Chilbert M, Mieler WF, Williams GA, Olsen K. A new technique for subchoroidal implantation of experimental malignant melanoma. Invest Ophthalmol Vis Sci 1988;29:995–998.

103. Liu HS, Refojo MF, Albert DM. Experimental combined systemic and local chemotherapy for intraocular malignancy. Arch Ophthalmol 1980;98:905–908.

104. Liu HS, Refojo MF, Perry HD, Albert DM. Sustained release of BCNU for treatment of intraocular malignancies in animal models. Invest Ophthalmol Vis Sci 1978;17(Suppl):202.

105. Packer S, Rotman M, Fairchild R, et al. Radiotherapy of ocular melanoma with I-125. Invest Optalmol Vis Sci 1978;17(Suppl):160.

106. Packer S, Rotman M, Fairchild RG, et al. Irradiation of choroidal melanoma with iodine 125 ophthalmic plaque. Arch Ophthalmol 1980;98:1453–1457.

107. Mieler WF, Jaffe GJ, Steeves RA. Ferromagnetic hyperthermia and iodine 125 brachytherapy in the treatment of choroidal melanoma in a rabbit model. Arch Ophthalmol 1989;107:1524–1528.

108. Finger PT, Packer S, Svitia PP, et al. Hyperthermic treatment of intraocular tumors. Arch Ophthalmol 1984;102:1477–1481.

109. Hill RA, Reddi S, Kenney ME, et al. Photodynamic therapy of ocular melanoma with bis silicon 2,3-naphthalocyanine in a rabbit model. Invest Ophthalmol Vis Sci 1995;36:2476–2481.

110. Schmidt-Erfurth U, Baumann W, Gragoudas E, et al. Photodynamic therapy of experimental choroidal melanoma using lipoprotein-delivered benzoporphyrin. Ophthalmology 1994;101:89–99.

111. Franken NAP, van Delft JL, Dubelman TMAR, et al. Hematoporphyrin derivate photoradiation treatment of experimental malignant melanoma in the anterior chamber of the rabbit. Curr Eye Res 1985;4:641–654.

112. Olsen KR, Blumenkranz M, Hernandez E, et al. Fluorouracil therapy of intraocular Greene melanoma in the rabbit. Arch Ophthalmol 1988;106:812–815.

113. Chong LP, Özler SA, De Queiroz JM, Liggett PE. Indocyanine green-enhanced diode laser treatment of melanoma in a rabbit model. Retina 1993;13:251–259.

114. Liu LH, Ni C. Hematoporphyrin phototherapy for experimental intraocular malignant melanoma. Arch Ophthalmol 1983;101:901–903.

115. Hu LK, Huh K, Gragoudas ES, Young LHY. Establishment of pigmented choroidal melanomas in a rabbit model. Retina 1994;14:264–268.

116. Pineda II R, Theodossiadis PG, Gonzalez VH, et al. Establishment of a rabbit model of extrascleral extension of ocular melanoma. Retina 1998;18:368–372.

117. Liggett PE, Lo G, Pince KJ, et al. Heterotransplantation of human uveal melanoma. Graefes Arch Clin Exp Ophthalmol 1993;231:15–20.
118. Luyten GPM, Mooy CM, De Jong PTVM, Hoogeveen AT, Luider TM. A chicken embryo model to study the growth of human uveal melanoma. Biochem Biophy Res Commun 1993;192:22–29.

14

Using Retinoblastoma Models to Develop New Treatment: Vitamin D Analogues

DANIEL M. ALBERT, ROBERT W. NICKELLS, and SOESIAWATI R. DARJATMOKO

University of Wisconsin, Madison, Wisconsin, U.S.A.

ISABELLE AUDO

Hôpital Saint Antoine, Paris, France

I. INTRODUCTION

Until recently, external-beam radiation was the principal means of treatment of retinoblastoma (RB); through it, survival rates of better than 90% were achieved [1]. This treatment, however, was associated with a 35% or higher risk of secondary cancers in patients with bilateral RB during a 30-year period [2–4]. In the 1990s, traditional chemotherapies were employed more extensively, but many of these are also mutagenic and pose an increased risk of secondary cancers [1,5]. Hence there remains a need for improved methods of treatment for RB.

In 1966, Frederick C. Verhoeff suggested the possibility that RB cells may be sensitive to vitamin D, because this tumor sometimes undergoes calcification and spontaneous regression [6]. Due to the toxicity that such treatment would have caused and because there were no clinical or experimental data at the time to indicate a role for vitamin D therapy in the treatment of any human malignancy, implementation of Verhoeff's suggestion was deferred. Until the 1970s, all therapeutic studies involving RB were carried out in patients. With our establishment of the Y-79 human cell line of RB in 1974, tissue culture studies could be utilized for drug-response and other investigations [7]. Heterotransplantation of RB into the athymic "nude" mouse provided an animal model that still is extremely useful [8]. In 1990, we demonstrated that transgenic mice expressing the SV40 large tumor antigen (Tag) gene in the retina developed RB [9]. This model resembles human RB in its morphology and clinical behavior [10].

The two predominant natural forms of vitamin D are vitamin D_2 (ergocalciferol) and vitamin D_3 (cholecalciferol). Vitamin D_2 comes strictly from diet and vitamin D_3 both from diet and synthesis in the skin via a photochemical reaction [11]. As vitamin D_2 and D_3 are hydroxylated, first in the liver and again in the kidney, they become more potent [12]. In our experiments, we used the hydroxylated form of vitamin D_3, calcitriol (1,25-dihydroxycholecalciferol); nonhydroxylated vitamin D_2 (ergocalciferol); a synthetic analogue of calcitriol, 1,25-dihdyroxy-16-ene-23-yne-vitamin D_3 (16,23-D_3); and a synthetic analogue of vitamin D_2, 1α-hydroxyvitamin D_2 (1α-OH-D_2) (Fig. 1). The availability of the Y-79 cell line and the xenograft and transgenic models of RB have made possible the systematic study of these compounds as a treatment for RB and have enabled us to investigate their mechanism of action.

II. EXPERIMENTAL PROCEDURES

A. Reverse Transcription PCR of VDR cDNA

In our laboratory experiments, human RB samples were collected from tumor-containing eyes following enucleation. Whole kidneys grossly free of tumor were obtained from the LHβ-Tag mice to serve as controls for the murine vitamin D receptor (VDR) polymerase chain reaction (PCR) experiments. HL60 human leukemia cells were propagated to serve as a control for the human VDR PCR experiments.

Total RNA was isolated using the method of Chomczynski and Sacchi [13]. Contaminating genomic DNA was eliminated. Complementary DNA (cDNA) was synthesized from messenger RNA (mRNA) using reverse transcriptase along with random oligonucleotide primers and the required deoxynucleosides triphosphates. Afterwards, the samples were incubated with RNase to digest the RNA templates.

Complementary DNA strands encoding the human or murine VDR were specifically amplified using species-specific sets of oligonucleotide primers recognizing either the human or mouse VDR coding sequence, respectively. To control for genomic DNA contamination, these primer pairs were specifically chosen to amplify sequence regions that span an intron.

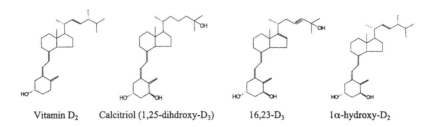

Vitamin D$_2$ Calcitriol (1,25-dihdroxy-D$_3$)   16,23-D$_3$ 1α-hydroxy-D$_2$

Figure 1   Vitamin D compounds and analogues.

Quantitative measurement of VDR was made using a tritiated calcitriol binding technique, described elsewhere [14].

B. Xenograft and Transgenic Models

In the xenograft model treatment, athymic "nude" mice (4 to 6 weeks old) were injected subcutaneously with human RB cells, as previously described [14–16]. Five days later, they were randomized into treatment and control groups. Animals receiving calcitriol, vitamin D_2, and 16,23-D_3 received intraperitoneal injections of the vitamin D compound in mineral oil five times a week; control animals received mineral oil alone administered intraperitoneally five times a week. Animals receiving 1α-OH-D_2 were given the compound dissolved in 0.1 mL coconut oil by oral gavage, while the control animals received coconut oil alone. Administration was continued for 5 weeks, during which tumor size was measured using calipers and individual mouse weights were recorded three times per week. Toxicity was assessed by survival, animal body weight, and clinical appearance. The mice were then killed and the size, tumor volume, and tumor weight were determined. Serum calcium was measured in blood taken from the subclavian artery just prior to time of death. From representative animals in each group, kidneys were evaluated for calcification. These techniques are described in detail elsewhere [15,16].

The transgenic model treatment was as follows: LHβ-Tag mice, a well-characterized model of RB [9], were used to determine drug effectiveness in inhibiting tumor growth. Eight- to ten-week-old mice were randomized by sex and litter into treatment groups and control groups. The presence of the transgene was confirmed by PCR [9]. Animals receiving calcitriol, vitamin D_2, and 16,23-D_3 received intraperitoneal injections of the vitamin D compound in mineral oil, while control animals received intraperitoneal injections of mineral oil (vehicle) alone. Treatment was administered five times per week. Animals receiving 1α-OH-D_2 were given the compound dissolved in 0.1 mL coconut oil by oral gavage, and control animals received coconut oil alone. The treatment schedule was 5 weeks. Toxicity was assessed and serum calcium determined in the manner described for the xenograft model. At the termination of the treatment period, animals were killed and the eyes were enucleated, fixed in 10% neutral buffered formalin, and subjected to routine histological processing. Tumor area and volume measurements for each study have been previously described [18–20,29]. The histopathological appearance of the tumors (degree of retinal involvement and extension to other ocular structures, severity of necrosis, degree of tumor differentiation, number of mitotic figures, and calcium deposits) was scored by a masked reviewer. The extent and character of the inflammation was also graded [18,19].

Typically, one-way ANOVA was used to assess the effect of dose followed by paired t-tests when a significant effect was found. Also typically, the tumor areas were transformed to the log scale before analysis to obtain uniform variability. Please see specific manuscripts for exact methods [18–20,29].

C. Analysis of Tumor Cell Death

Histological methods of detecting DNA fragmentation were used to identify dying cells in tumors. Terminal transferase dUTP end labeling (TUNEL) was carried out as described previously [21–23] on paraffin sections of xenograft tumors harvested 5 weeks after treatment. Basically, the 3′ ends of nicked DNA were labeled by the addition of biotin-conjugated dUTP using terminal deoxynucleotide transferase (TdT). Labeled DNA was identified by reacting the sections with an avidin peroxidase ABC kit followed by staining with diaminobenzidine. Since TUNEL labels degraded nuclei in both apoptotic and necrotic nuclei, we also stained sections using the ligation method of Didenko and Hornsby [24]. This method specifically labels double-strand DNA strand breaks that have 3′ overhanging ends, typical of apoptotic but not necrotic cells. A 200-bp DNA fragment, corresponding to the multiple cloning site of the plasmid vector pBK-CMV, was generated by Taq DNA polymerase and PCR using Texas red-conjugated nucleotides. DNA fragments generated by Taq also contain 3′ overhanging ends, which can be ligated to DNA fragments in apoptotic nuclei. Labeled DNA was then layered over tissue sections and ligated to nicked DNA using T4 DNA ligase enzyme. After extensive washing, unligated DNA was removed and labeled nuclei were visualized using a fluorescent microscope. With each method, the tissues were viewed using Nomarski interference optics and were not counterstained.

D. Immunohistochemistry

Paraffin-embedded tissue sections were labeled with antibodies to human *p53*, human *p21*, human *bax*, and the Ki-67 antigen. All antibodies were used with essentially the same protocol described previously [23]. Sections were deparaffinized and subjected to antigen retrieval by incubating them in 100 mM TRIS buffer (pH 9.5) at 90°C for 10 min (*p21*, BAX, and MIB-1) or 30 min (*p53*), followed by 60 min in the same buffer at room temperature. After incubation with primary antibody, the sections were washed and incubated with appropriate biotinylated secondary antibody and stained with the avidin peroxidase ABC kit. Sections were viewed with Nomarski optics and not counterstained.

III. RESULTS OF VITAMIN D EXPERIMENTS

A. The Presence of Vitamin D Receptors in Y-79 RB Cells

In studies carried out in 1988 [14], Scatchard analysis of the receptor assay showed a concentration of 94 fmol of calcitriol receptors per million Y-79 RB cells, or 56,000 receptors per cell. These receptors have a dissocation constant of 1.18 nmol/L.

B. PCR Amplification of VDR cDNA from Human RB Samples

A total of 23 RB samples taken from the enucleated eyes of different patients were analyzed by PCR for the original presence of VDR mRNA. In every sample, examination of the PCR product by agarose gel electrophoresis revealed a predicted 103-bp band corresponding to a targeted portion of the human VDR coding sequence (representative sample shown in Fig. 2, lane 1). The PCR primer pairs used in both the human and mouse experiments span an intron in order to control for residual genomic DNA. Using the same oligonucleotide primers, an identical 103-bp

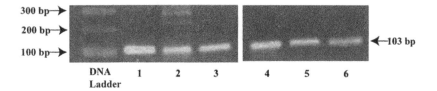

Figure 2 PCR amplification of vitamin D receptor (VDR) cDNA obtained from human and mouse tissue samples. Lane 1 contains VDR mRNA from a representative section of fresh human retinoblastoma. Lane 2 contains mRNA from human retinoblastoma cell line Y-79. Lane 3 contains mRNA from cultured HL60 human leukemia cells. Lane 4 contains a representative sample of murine intraocular retinoblastoma. Lane 5 shows a predicted 103 bp band for extraorbital metastasis in the mouse model. Lane 6 contains a representative sample of mouse kidney, which is known to express VDR mRNA.

band was amplified from Y-79 RB (Fig. 2, lane 2) and cultured HL60 human leukemia cells, a cell line known to express VDR [26,27] (Fig. 2, lane 3). DNA sequencing of the PCR product from one human RB sample confirmed that the 103˜-bp band encoded the expected VDR region. While all 23 samples were positive in this study, there remains a possibility that a future sample may not be positive. This potential variability is reflected a 95% confidence interval of (0.85,1) for the estimated probability of any RB sample being positive. This interval is calculated assuming binomially distributed outcomes.

C. PCR Amplification of VDR cDNA from a Mouse Model of Retinoblastoma

Retinoblastoma samples from five LHβ-Tag mice, along with one metastatic tumor sample and one whole kidney, were processed and analyzed essentially as described for the human RB samples. Mouse renal tissue is known to express VDR [27] and therefore serves as a positive control for these experiments. A predicted 103-bp band was visualized following agarose gel electrophoresis for all samples containing intraocular RB (representative sample shown in Fig. 2, lane 4), extraorbital metastasis (Fig. 2, lane 5), and whole kidney (Fig. 2, lane 6). Analogous to the human samples, the size of the band corresponds to a portion of the murine VDR coding sequence targeted by the murine-specific oligonucleotide primers used during PCR.

D. In Vitro Effects of Calcitriol

Concentrations of 10^{-9} and 10^{-6} mol/L of calcitriol were effective at inhibiting the growth of the RB cells in vitro (Fig. 3) [14]. This inhibition was statistically significant at 10^{-6} mol/L of calcitriol on day 6 and 10^{-9} mol/L of calcitriol on day 9 ($p < 0.05$). The 10^{-12} mol/L of calcitriol did not statistically significantly inhibit cell growth. The inhibition of cell growth was dose-dependent on days 3 and 6.

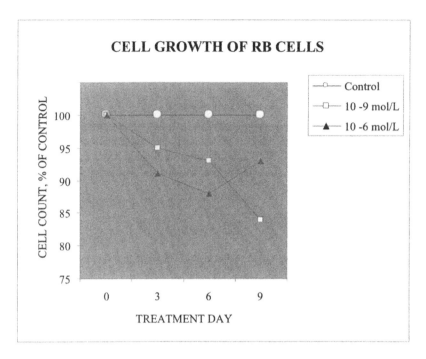

Figure 3 Relative counts of retinoblastoma cells expressed as percentage of control; 10^{-9} mol/L of calcitriol caused a 15% decrease in cell growth by day 9.

E. Effectiveness and Toxicity of Ergocalciferol in the Athymic Xenograft Model

Mice were treated with a high dose (7.8 mg/kg) of ergocalciferol and a low dose (2.8 mg/kg) of ergocalciferol. The geometric mean diameter (the cube root of length × width × height) was measured 33 days after treatment was initiated. The effect of ergocalciferol on tumor size is shown in Figure 4A. The survival data are summarized in Figure 4B. Histopathological examination showed a dose-dependent increase in tumor necrosis and calcification in the treated animals. A more detailed description of the results has been published [17].

F. Effectiveness and Toxicity of Calcitriol Treatment in the Athymic Xenograft Model

In this experiment, the treated group received 500 ng/kg of calcitriol. Tumor size was judged on the basis of geometric mean diameter (Fig. 5A). The results after 30 days of treatment are shown in Figure 5B. Histopathological examination showed no difference in calcification or necrosis between the control tumors and those in the treated animals. Further details regarding these results can be found in the original report [28].

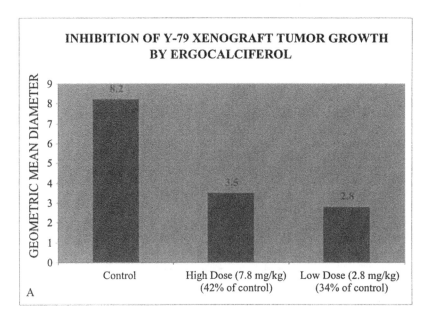

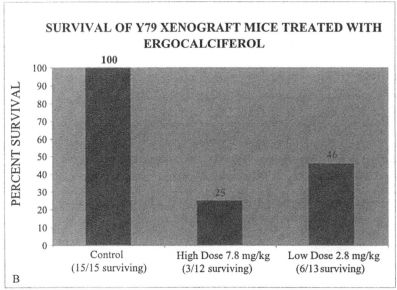

Figure 4 (A) Effect of ergocalciferol on growth of Y-79 retinoblastoma xenografts after 28 days of treatment. The low dose is most effective with $p < 0.05$ compared to calcitriol. Tumors were measured in terms of geometric mean diameter. (B) Survival of control and ergocalciferol-treated Y-79 retinoblastoma xenograft mice after 33 days of treatment.

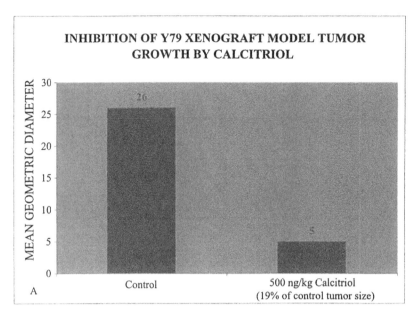

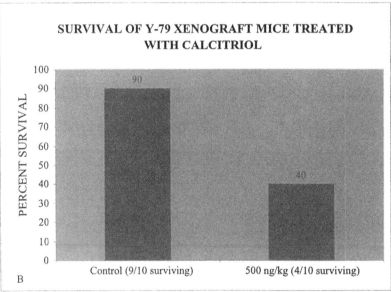

Figure 5 (A) Effect of calcitriol on growth of Y-79 retinoblastoma xenografts after 28 days of treatment. The low dose is most effective with $p < 0.05$ compared to controls. Tumors were measured in terms of geometric mean diameter. (B) Survival of control and calcitriol-treated Y-79 retinoblastoma xenograft mice after 33 days of treatment.

G. Effectiveness and Toxicity of Calcitriol in the LHβ-Tag Transgenic Model

In studying the antineoplastic effect of calcitriol in LHβ-Tag mice, toxicity studies were done using calcitriol doses of 0.05, 0.1, and 0.2 µg, which were compared to controls. In the dose-response studies, a high dose (0.05 µg) and a low dose (0.025 µg) were administered. Tumor size was measured by the mean largest cross-sectional area. The results after 5 weeks of treatment are shown in Figure 6A. The combined survival results for both the dose-response and toxicity studies following 5 weeks of treatment are summarized in Figure 6B.

Histopathological studies showed no increased calcification in the tumors of treated animals. There was, however, greater cell death in the tumors in the low-dose group ($p < 0.02$). More differentiation was noted in the low-dose group ($p < 0.003$), which was manifest by increased numbers of Homer-Wright rosettes and a smaller proportion of the tumor appearing undifferentiated. Additional information regarding these results is given in the original article [18].

H. Effectiveness and Toxicity of 16,23-D₃ in the Athymic Xenograft Model

Preliminary experiments determined the most efficacious dose of 16,23-D$_3$ to be 0.5 µg. The effectiveness and toxicity of this drug was evaluated using a negative control that received mineral oil alone and a positive control that received 0.5 µg of calcitriol. Results of tumor size (tumor volume) are given as of the 32nd day of treatment, because after that day there were insufficient calcitriol-treated mice surviving to permit analysis. The results after 5 weeks of treatment are compared in Figure 7A. Survival for the three groups following 5 weeks of treatment is shown in Figure 7B. On histopathological examination, no qualitative morphological difference was found among the three groups with regard to calcification, necrosis, or differentiation. A more detailed description of these results can be found in the original report [15].

I. Effectiveness and Toxicity of 16,23-D₃ in the LHβ-Tag Transgenic Model

In an initial study of the effectiveness of 16,23-D$_3$ [19], an extremely low dose of this vitamin D analogue was compared to a control (mineral oil). The results are shown in Figure 8A. All animals survived the 5-week treatment schedule.

Subsequent toxicity studies indicated that considerably larger doses of 16,23-D$_3$ were well tolerated by the transgenic mice [20]. Consequently, a second experiment was performed in which the treatment arms included 0.35-, 0.5-, and 0.75-µg doses. These treatment groups were compared to a control group receiving only mineral oil. Tumor size was measured as the average of the square root of the right and left eye tumor area. The results are presented in Figure 8B. Survival data are shown in Figure 8C. On histological examination of the tumors, no difference in appearance was found between the control and treated animals. Further details of results can be found in the original reports [19,20].

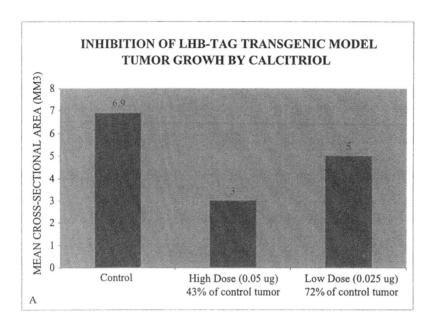

A

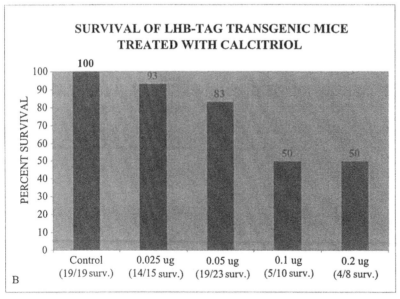

B

Figure 6 (A) Effect of calcitriol on growth of LHβ-Tag transgenic retinoblastomas after 5 weeks of treatment. The difference in tumor size was significant between the high dose and control ($p < 0.008$) and the low dose and control ($p < 0.014$). (B) Survival of control and calcitriol treated LHβ-Tag transgenic mice after 5 weeks of treatment.

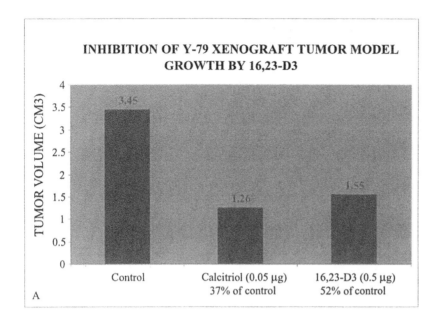

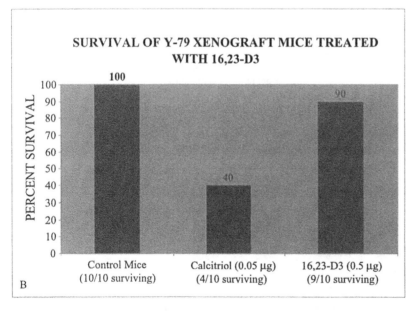

Figure 7 (A) Effect of 16,23-D_3 on growth of Y-79 retinoblastoma xenografts compared to control and calcitriol following 5 weeks of treatment. 16,23-D_3-treated mice had significantly smaller tumor size than controls ($p = 0.02$) but were not significantly different from the calcitriol-treated mice. (B) Survival of 16,23-D_3-treated Y-79 retinoblastoma xenograft mice compared to control and calcitriol-treated mice after 5 weeks of treatment.

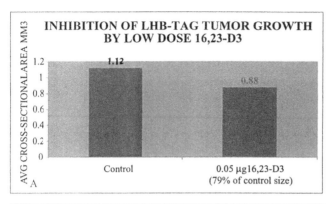

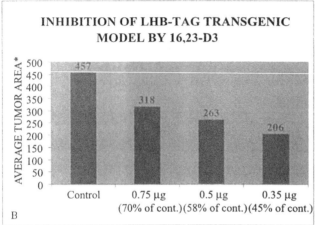

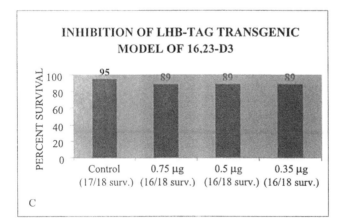

Figure 8 (A) Effect of an extremely low dose (0.05 mg) of 16,23-D$_3$ on growth of LHβ-Tag transgenic retinoblastoma after 5 weeks of treatment. The difference in tumor size was significant ($p = 0.02$). (B) Effect of 16,23-D$_3$ on growth of LHβ-Tag transgenic retinoblastoma after 5 weeks of treatment. The difference between the 0.35-μg-treated group and the controls was statistically significant ($p = 0.0056$). *Tumor size was calculated as the average of the square root of the right and left eye tumor area. (C) Survival of control and 16,23-D$_3$-treated LHβ-Tag transgenic mice after 5 weeks of treatment.

J. Effectiveness and Toxicity of 1α-OH-D$_2$ in the Athymic Xenograft Model

Following 5 weeks of treatment with 1α-OH-D$_2$, the size of tumors in animals receiving this analogue in 0.1-, 0.2-, 0.3-, and 0.6-μg doses were compared to controls that received coconut oil via oral gavage. The results are shown in Figure 9A. Survival data are summarized in Figure 9B [16].

K. Effectiveness and Toxicity of 1α-OH-D$_2$ in the LHβ-Tag Transgenic Model

Following 5 weeks of treatment with doses of 0.1, 0.3, 0.5, or 1.0 μg/day of 1α-OH-D$_2$, the size of tumors in animals was compared to controls that received coconut oil via oral gavage. The results are shown in Figure 10A [29]. Survival data are summarized in Figure 10B [29].

L. Characterization of the Mechanism of Arrest of Tumor Growth by Vitamin D Analogues

Specimens of Y-79 xenografts taken from athymic mice treated for 5 weeks with either 16,23-D$_3$ or calcitriol were compared with tumors from control animals at the same stage. Paraffin sections of tumors (two mice per treatment) were analyzed for cell death using terminal transferase dUTP-nick end labeling (TUNEL) and cell proliferation using the monoclonal antibody MIB-1. Figure 11 (sections A–C) shows that control tumors and tumors treated with calcitriol exhibit some TUNEL labeling (approximately 0.13 to 0.64% of the cells, respectively), but the level of cell death is more than six times greater in tumors treated with 16,23-D$_3$ (approximately 4.2% of the cells). In addition to an examination of the rate of cell death in these tumors, we also looked for evidence of the type of cell death (apoptosis or necrosis). The morphology of nuclear fragmentation was examined from sections of tumors stained with hematoxylin and eosin (Fig. 11, panel D). All tumors, but especially those treated with 16,23-D$_3$, contained highly pyknotic and fragmented nuclei, both morphologically consistent with apoptotic cell death [30,31]. Dying cells in these tumors also stained using the 3′ overhang ligation technique (Fig. 11, panel E). In addition to these results obtained with Y79 xenografts, similar features of apoptotic cell death were observed in dying cells found in spontaneous tumors of transgenic mice treated with vitamin D analogues (data not shown). Thus it is important to note that vitamin D–induced cell death in these tumors appears to be apoptotic and therefore controlled by genes being expressed in the dying cells.

    In a similar experiment, specimens of Y-79 xenografts taken from athymic mice treated for 5 weeks with 1α-OH-D$_2$ (2 μg per day) were compared with controls using TUNEL labeling. As with 16,23-D$_3$ and calcitriol, 1α-OH-D$_2$ caused an increase in cell death via apoptotic changes observed in the tumor sections (Fig. 12).

    Conversely, all four tumor specimens studied had relatively uniform labeling with the MIB-1 antibody (Fig. 13: 2.3%, 2.6%, and 3.3% for control, 16,23-D$_3$ and calcitriol, respectively; and Fig. 14 for 1α-OH-D$_2$) suggesting that the rate of cell proliferation is unaffected. The combined observations for tumors treated with calcitriol suggest that the mechanism of tumor growth arrest for this analogue is also

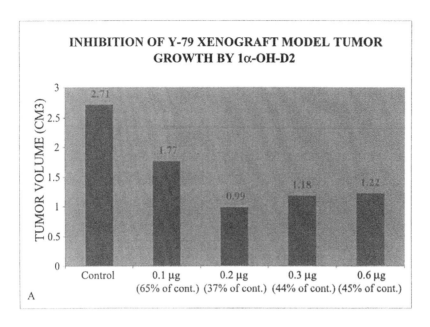

A

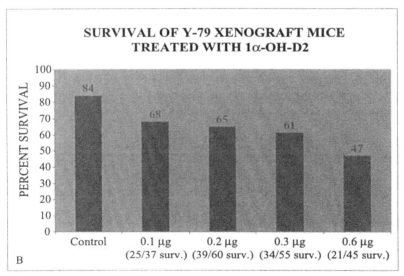

B

Figure 9 (A) Effect of 1a-OH-D$_2$ on growth of Y-79 retinoblastoma xenografts compared to controls following 5 weeks of treatment. The 0.3-μg and 0.2-μg groups were statistically significantly smaller than the control group ($p < 0.003$ and $p < 0.004$, respectively). (B) Survival of 1α-OH-D$_2$-treated xenograft mice compared to control mice after 5 weeks of treatment.

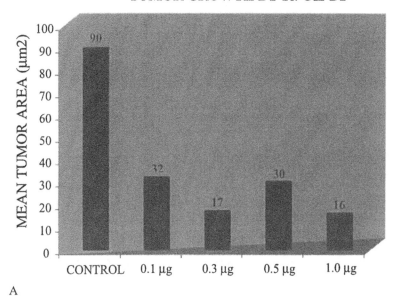

A

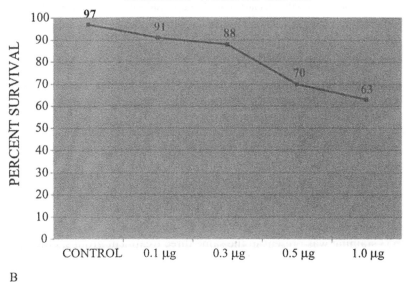

B

Figure 10 (A) Effect of 1a-OH-D$_2$ on growth of LHβ-Tag transgenic tumors as compared to controls following 5 weeks of treatment. All dose groups were statistically significantly smaller than the control group ($p < 0.0001$ for all dose groups). (B) Survival of 1α-OH-D$_2$-treated LHβ-Tag transgenic mice compared to control mice after 5 weeks of treatment.

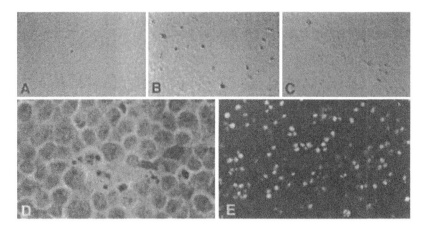

Figure 11 Cell death in Y79 xenograft tumors after 5 weeks of vitamin D treatment demonstrated by TUNEL staining in (A) untreated tumors, (B) tumors treated with 16,23-D$_3$, and (C) tumors treated with calcitriol. Panels A, B, and C exhibit signs of active cell death. 16,23-D$_3$ tumors had TUNEL staining that was six times greater than control or calcitriol tumors at this stage. D. Higher magnification of an H&E-stained section of a 16,23-D$_3$–treated tumor. Nuclear morphology of the cells is consistent with apoptotic cell death, including highly pyknotic nuclei and cells with extensive nuclear fragmentation. E. Fluorescence micrograph of dying cells in a tumor treated with 16,23-D$_3$ and labeled using the 3′ overhang ligation technique [24]. DNA fragments are apoptotic but not necrotic; nuclei containing a high proportion of similar 3′ overhanging nucleotides can be covalently linked to biotin-labeled DNA. Ligated DNA is visualized using streptavidin conjugated to Texas red. Morphological evidence combined with this labeling technique indicates that these tumor cells are dying by apoptosis.

mediated by an increase in cell death. It is possible, however, that the time point examined in this preliminary study was too late to observe the period of peak TUNEL activity for the calcitriol treatment.

Morphological and histochemical methods suggest that vitamin D analogues activate apoptotic cell death in retinoblastoma. Since this mechanism of cell death is genetically regulated, the expression patterns of three genes dissociated with cell death were investigated by immunohistochemistry in sections of 5-week-treated tumors treated with calcitriol, 16,23-D$_3$, and corresponding controls. The gene products examined included the tumor suppressor protein p53, and the gene products of two genes regulated by *p53* (*p21*$^{\text{waf-1/cip-1}}$ and *bax*).

Nuclear p53 staining was present in the same three treatment groups, although it was most abundant in tumors treated with 16,23-D$_3$. Similarly, both *p21* and *bax* immunoreactivity were strongest in the 16,23-D$_3$ groups. Since the expression of *p53*, and its downstream target genes, correlates with retinoblastoma cell death [23], it is not surprising to find elevated expression levels in the treatment group undergoing the greatest rate of cell death.

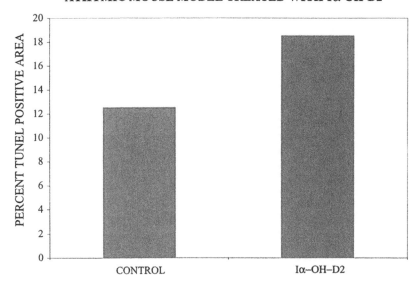

**TUNEL-STAINING OF Y-79 XENOGRAFTS IN THE
ATHYMIC MOUSE MODEL TREATED WITH 1α-OH-D2**

Figure 12   Percentage of TUNEL-positive areas compared to total surface area of tumor section. Specimens treated with 1α-OH-D$_2$ exhibit increased TUNEL staining when compared to controls ($N = 5$, $p < 0.05$, unpaired t-test).

IV. CONCLUSIONS

As we noted in the introduction to this chapter, alternatives to the current methods of RB therapies are needed [32]. Vitamin D analogues hold the promise of fulfilling this need. We initially studied ergocalciferol and calcitriol (Fig. 1) in the athymic Y-79 RB xenograft mouse model. Although these compounds showed impressive reductions in tumor growth as compared to controls, the doses required for this effect caused mortality with rates ranging from 25% to 46% [18,28]. It should be noted, however, that the immunocompromised athymic mouse model has an extremely high sensitivity to calcitriol, vitamin D$_2$, 16,23-D$_3$, and 1α-OH-D$_2$ and that immunocompetent mice, such as the transgenic strain, are a better indicator of actual drug toxicity. In an experiment in which calcitriol was administered to athymic mice in a dose required to reduce tumor growth to 36% of the control (i.e., 0.05 μg), there was still only a 40% survival rate of treated animals [15]. By withholding doses of ergocalciferol from sick animals, the survival rate could be improved to 75% [18]. In all of the experiments, the toxicity appeared to be related to the hypercalcemia induced by these compounds. Consequently, we concluded that ergocalciferol and calcitriol were excessively toxic, and were not suitable for treatment of children with RB.

We then turned our attention to a synthetic analogue of calcitriol, 16,23-D$_3$ (Fig. 1) which has an antineoplastic effect similar to that of calcitriol but with less hypercalcemic activity. In our initial experiments with this compound, animals treated with 0.05 μg of 16,23-D$_3$ were found to have a significantly smaller tumor

Control   1623-D$_3$ Calcitriol (D$_3$)

p53

p21

Bax

MIB-1

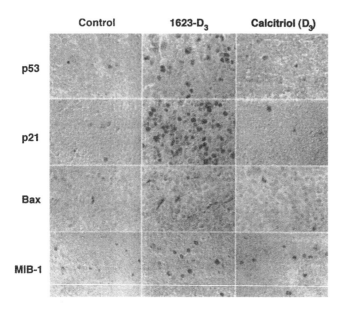

Figure 13 Immunohistochemical labeling of Y-79 tumors grown in athymic mice after 5 weeks of vitamin D treatment. Sections of untreated tumors, 16,23-D$_3$-treated tumors, and calcitriol-treated tumors were stained with the following proteins: p53 (monoclonal DO-1), p21 (monoclonal Ab-6), BAX (polyclonal Ab-1), and antibodies directed against the Ki-67 nuclear antigen (MIB-1). Each panel is a Normarski interference image taken near the center of the tumors because they exhibited uniform cell density. *p53* and *p53*-regulated genes (*p21* and *BAX*) are upregulated in tumors treated with 16,23-D$_3$. This change in gene expression mirrors the increased apoptotic activity seen in Fig. 10. MIB-1 staining is relatively equal among all the treatments, suggesting that cell proliferation is unaffected.

cross-sectional area when compared to corresponding controls ($p = 0.02$) [19]. All animals survived 5 weeks of treatment. In subsequent studies using higher doses (0.2–0.75 µg), the drug was effective in reducing tumor growth and the survival rate was approximately 90% [15,20]. This appears to be a promising drug for use in treatment of RB children. It was not approved by the Food and Drug Administration (FDA) until March 1999 for investigational use in human cancer patients. This led us to investigate an analogue of vitamin D$_2$, 1α-OH-D$_2$.

1α-OH-D$_2$ is a vitamin D analogue that was approved by the FDA in 1999 for oral use in the treatment of secondary hyperparathyroidism due to renal failure. This compound was approved earlier for investigational use in human tumor treatment in 1996 and is currently being used in phase 2 human clinical trials of prostate cancer (George Wilding, personal communication). Like 16,23-D$_3$, 1α-OH-D$_2$ is known to induce low levels of hypercalcemia while providing effective systemic serum drug levels for tumor treatment [33,34]. In a recent study [16], we found that 1α-OH-D$_2$ limited tumor growth of the human Y-79 RB cell line, which was subcutaneously injected in athymic "nude" mice. We reported a dose-response efficacy curve with minimal toxicity in both the athymic and transgenic mouse models of RB [16,29]. Our results indicate that 1α-OH-D$_2$, a compound not known to be a mutagen, can

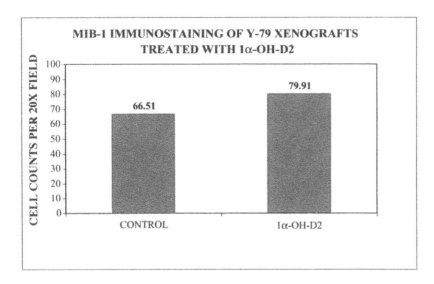

Figure 14 MIB-1 immunostaining of tumor sections to study cell proliferation. Labeled cells were counted using × 20 magnification; 10 fields per section were included in the analysis. No increase in MIB-1 immunostaining was seen after treatment of 1α-OH-D$_2$ ($N=5$, $p = 0.2495$, unpaired t-test).

limit tumor growth in a nontoxic dose range. In comparing our studies [16,29] to a similar study of 16,23-D$_3$ and calcitriol in same mouse models [15,19,20], 1α-OH-D$_2$ appears to be similar in tumor reduction capability at a 0.3-µg dose level when compared to 0.5 µg of 16,23-D$_3$ or 0.05 µg of calcitriol.

It is probable that tumor cells must contain VDR in order for vitamin D analogues to be effective in limiting their growth. Examination of 23 consecutively received RB samples with PCR amplification for the presence of VDR mRNA has been completed. Message encoding receptors were present in all specimens, providing convincing evidence that these tumor cells express receptor protein. The 95% confidence interval for the probability of any RB being positive is (0.85, 1), based on the binomial distribution.

Calcitriol and its analogues have been demonstrated to inhibit cellular proliferation in other malignant cell lines besides RB, including leukemic, breast, colon, renal, and lung carcinomas [35–38]. It is hypothesized that the antiprolifera- tive effect of these compounds is mediated by a vitamin D receptor–linked mechanism, although exceptions exist [39–42]. Considerable evidence exists that the antineoplastic and differentiating effects of vitamin D compounds affect funda- mental cellular processes of proliferation, differentiation, and apoptosis. The resulting key biochemical events are related to activation of cyclin-dependent kinase inhibitors, such as $p21^{waf-1/cip-1}$, and there are some reports that activated VDR can directly mediate the expression of this gene [43–47].

In this chapter, we present data showing that tumor growth attenuation of Y- 79 xenografts in athymic mice following treatment with 16,23-D$_3$ is due to apoptotic cell death. Calcitriol and vitamin D analogues can also induce apoptosis in leukemic (HL60) cells as well as human breast cancer and colon cancer cell lines [48–50].

Recent studies have shown that human RB and RB cell lines are extremely susceptible to p53-mediated apoptosis and elevated $p21^{waf-1/cip-1}$ expression [23,47]. These results indicate that the treatment of xenograft tumors elicits the increased expression of both *p53* and *p53*-regulated genes. These data are consistent with the role of bound VDR in stimulating the activation of apoptotic genes and may account for the decreased toxicity of these compounds without compromising efficacy. It is likely that 1α-OH-D_2 has a similar mechanism of action against RB tumors in the athymic mouse.

ACKNOWLEDGMENTS

This research was supported by the Research To Prevent Blindness (RPB) and NIH/ NEI RO1 grant EYO1917. 16,23-D_3 was graciously provided to us by Ilex Corporation. 1α-OH-D_2 and supplemental funds for animal care costs were graciously provided to us from BoneCare International, Inc. The authors also wish to thank the following physicians and their patients for donating human RB samples for vitamin D receptor analysis: David H. Abramson, Cornell Medical College; Thomas Lee, New York Presbyterian Hospital; J. William Harbour, Washington University Medical School; Jerry Shields, and Carol Shields, Wills Eye Hospital; Timothy Murray, Bascom Palmer Eye Institute; Ted Dryja, Massachusetts Eye & Ear Infirmary; Joan O'Brien, University of California, San Francisco; A. Linn Murphree, and Anita Fisher, PhD, Children's Hospital of Los Angeles; Monte Mills, Children's Hospital of Philadelphia; and Mansoor Movaghar, Davis Duehr Dean Eye Clinic.

The authors also wish to thank Drs. Robert Nickells and Cassandra Schlamp for their technical work associated with the mechanism of action of vitamin D analogues and Dr. David Gamm for expertise in the vitamin D receptor assays. The authors also wish to thank Drs. Steven M. Cohen, Amanda M. Saulenas, Ilona Slusker-Shternfeld, Sina Sabet, Craig Wilkerson, Paul J. Bryar, Richard Grostern, Boaz Lissauer, Daniel G. Dawson, Joel Gleiser, as well and Ms. Janice M. Lokken for their technical expertise on the vitamin D_2, calcitriol, 16,23-D_3, and 1α-OH-D_2 drug trials.

Portions of this chapter are reprinted with the permission of the editor and publishers from the article "Vitamin D analogs, a new treatment for retinoblastoma: The first Ellsworth Lecture," which appeared in *Ophthalmic Genetics*, Vol. 22, No. 3.

REFERENCES

1. Ferris FL, Chew EY. A new era for the treatment of RB. Arch Ophthalmol 1996;114:1412.
2. Eng C, Li FP, Abramson DH, Ellsworth RM, Wong FL, Goldman MB, Seddon J, Tarbell N, Boice JD Jr. Mortality from second tumors among the long-term survivors of RB. J Natl Cancer Inst 1993;85:1121–1128.
3. Roarty JD, McLean IW, Zimmerman LE. Incidence of second neoplasms in patients with bilateral RB. Ophthalmology 1988;95:1583–1587.
4. Abramson DH, Frank CM. Second nonocular tumors in survivors of bilateral RB. A possible age effect on radiation-related risk. Ophthalmology 1998;105:573–580.

5. Gallie BL, Budning A, DeBoer G, Thiessen JJ, Koren G, Verjee Z, Ling V, Chang H S-L. Chemotherapy with focal therapy can cure intraocular RB without radiotherapy. Arch Ophthalmol 1996;114:1321–1328.

6. Verhoeff R. RB undergoing spontaneous regression: Calcifying agents suggested in treatment of RB. Am J Ophthalmol 1966;62:573–574.

7. Reid TW, Albert DM, Rabson AS, Russell P, Craft J, Chu ES, Tralka TS, Wilcox J. Characteristics of an established cell line of RB. J Natl Cancer Inst 1974;53:347–360.

8. Gallie BL, Albert DM, Wong JJ, Buyukmihci N, Puliafito CA. Heterotransplantation of RB into the athymic "nude" mouse. Invest Ophthalmol Vis Sci 1977;16:256–299.

9. Windle JJ, Albert DM, O'Brien JM, Marcus DM, Disteche CM, Bernards R, Mellon PL. RB in transgenic mice. Nature 1990;343:665–669.

10. O'Brien JM, Marcus DM, Bernards R, Carpenter JL, Windle JJ, Mellon P, Albert DM. A transgenic mouse model for RB. Arch Ophthalmol 1990;108:1145–1151.

11. Koshy KT. Vitamin D: An update. J Pharm Sci 1982;71:137–152.

12. Jones G, Byrnes B, Palma F, Segev D, Mazur Y. Displacement potency of vitamin D_2 analogs in competitive protein-binding assays for 25-hydroyxvitamin D_3, 24.25-dihydroyvitamin D_3, and 1,25-idhydroxyvitamin D_3. J Clin Endocrinol Metab 1980;50(4):773–775.

13. Chomczynski P, Sacchi N. Single-step method of RNA isolation by acid guanidinium thiocyanate-phenol-chloroform extraction. Anal Biochem 1987;162:156–159.

14. Saulenas A, Cohen S, Key L, Winter C, Albert DM. Vitamin D and RB: The presence of receptors and inhibition of growth in vitro. Arch Ophthalmol 1988;106:533–535.

15. Sabet SJ, Darjatmoko SR, Lindstrom MJ, Albert DM. Antineoplastic effect and toxicity of 1,24-dihydroxy-16-cnc-23-ync-vitamin D_3 in athymic mice with Y-79 human RB tumors. Arch Ophthalmol 1999;117:365–370.

16. Grostern RJ, Bryar PJ, Zimbric ML, Darjatmoko SR, Lissauer BJ, Lindstrom MJ, Lokken JM, Strugnell SA, Albert DM. Toxicity and dose-response studies of 1α-hydroxyvitamin D_2 in a retinoblastoma xenograft model. Arch Ophthalmol 2002;120:607–612.

17. Albert DM, Saulenas AM, Cohen SM. Verhoeff's query: Is vitamin D effective against RB? Arch Ophthalmol 1988;106:536–540.

18. Albert DM, Marcus DM, Gallo JP, O'Brien JM. The antineoplastic effect of vitamin D in transgenic mice with RB. Invest Ophthalmol Vis Sci 1992;33(8):2354–2364.

19. Shternfeld IS, Lasudry JGH, Chappell RJ, Darjatmoko SR, Albert DM. Antineoplastic effect of 1,25-dihydroxy-16-ene-23-yne-Vitamin D_3 analogue in transgenic mice with RB. Arch Ophthalmol 1996;114:1396–1401.

20. Wilkerson CL, Darjatmoko SR, Lindstrom MJ, Albert DM. Toxicity and dose-response studies of 1,25-$(OH)_2$-16-ene-23-yne vitamin D_3 in transgenic mice. Clin Cancer Res 1998;4:2253–2256.

21. Gavrieli Y, Sherman Y, Ben-Sasson SA. Identification of programmed cell death in situ via specific labeling of nuclear DNA fragmentation. J Cell Biol 1992;119:493–501.

22. Quigley HA, Nickells RW, Kerrigan LA, Pease ME, Thibault DJ, Zack DJ. Retinal ganglion cell death in experimental glaucoma and after axotomy occurs by apoptosis. Invest Ophthalmol Vis Sci 1995;36:774–786.

23. Nork TM, Poulsen G, Millecchia LL, Jantz RG, Nickells RW. p53 regulates apoptosis in human RB. Arch Ophthalmol 1997;115:213–219.

24. Didenko VV, Hornsby PJ. Presence of double-strand breaks with single-ase 3′ overhangs in cells undergoing apoptosis but not necrosis. J Cell Biol 1996;135:1369–1376.

25. Reitsma PH, Rothberg PG, Astrin SM, Trial J, Bar-Shavit Z, Hall A, Teitelbaum SL, Kahn AJ. Regulation of myc gene expression in HL-60 leukaemia cells by a vitamin D metabolite. Nature 1983;306:492–494.

26. Mangelsdorf DJ, Koeffler HP, Donaldson CA, Pike JW, Haussler MR. 1,25-dihydroxyvitamin D_3-induced differentiation in a human promyelocytic leukemia cell line (HL-60): Receptor-mediated maturation to macrophage-like cells. J Cell Biol 1984;98:391–398.

27. Colston RW, Feldman D. Demonstration of a 1,25-dihydroxycholecalciferol cytoplasmic receptor-like binder in mouse kidney. J Clin Endocrinol Metab 1979;49:798–800.

28. Cohen SM, Saulenas AM, Sullivan CR, Albert DM. Further studies on the effect of vitamin D on RB. Arch Ophthalmol 1988; 106:541–543.

29. Dawson DG, Gleiser J, Zimbric ML, Darjatmoko SR, Frisbie JC, Lokken JM, Lindstrom MJ, Audo I, Strugnell SA, Albert DM. Toxcitiy and dose-response studies of 1α-hydroxyvitamin D2 in LHβ-Tag transgenic mice. Trans Am Ophthalmol Soc 2002; 100:125–130.

30. Kerr JFR, Wylli AH, Currie AR. Apoptosis: A basic biological phenomenon with wide-ranging implications in tissue kinetics. J Cell Biol 1972;26:239–257.

31. Nickells RW, Zack DJ. Apoptosis in ocular disease: A molecular overview. Ophthalm Genet 1996;17:145–165.

32. O'Brien JM. Alternative treatment in RB. Ophthalmology 1998;105:571–572.

33. Knutson JC, Hollis BW, LeVan LW, Valliere C, Gould KG, Bishop CW. Metabolism of 1α-hydroxyvitamin D_2 to activated dihydroxyvitamin D_2 metabolites decreases endogenous 1α-dihydroxyvitamin D_3 in rats and monkeys. Endocrinology 1995;136:4749–4753.

34. Strugnell S, Byford V, Makin HLJ, Moraiarty RM, Gilardi R, LeVan LW, Knutson JC, Bishop CW, Jones G. 1α,24S-dihydroxyvitamin D_2: A biologically active product of 1α-hydroxyvitamin D_2 made in the human hepatoma, HEP3B. Biochem J 1995;310:233–241.

35. Walters M. Newly identified actions of the vitamin D endocrine system. Endocr Rev 1992;13:719–764.

36. Brenner RV, Shabahang M, Schumacker LM, Nauta RJ, Uskokovic MR, Evans SR, Buras RR. The antiproliferative effect of vitamin D analogs on MCF-7 human breast cancer cells. Cancer Lett 1995;92:77–82.

37. Schwartz GG, Oeler TA, Uskokovic MR, Bahnson RR. Human prostate cancer cells: Inhibition of proliferation by vitamin D analogs. Anticancer Res 1994;14:1077–1082.

38. Pakkala S, deVos S, Elstner E, Rude RK, Uskokovic M, Binderup L, Koeffler HP. Vitamin D_3 analogs: Effect on leukemic clonal growth, differentiation, and serum calcium. Leuk Res 1995;19:65–72.

39. Inaba M, Okuno S, Koyama H, Nishizawa Y, Morii H. Dibutyryl cAMP enhances the effect of 1,25-dihydroxyvitamin D_3 on a human promyclocytic leukemia cell, HL-60, at both the receptor and the postreceptor steps. Arch Biochem Biophys 1992;29:181–186.

40. Kawa S, Yoshizawa K, Tokoo M, Imai H, Oguchi H, Kiyosawa K, Homma T, Nikaido T, Furihata K. Inhibitory effect of 22-oxa-1,25-dihydroxyvitamin D_3 on the proliferation of pancreatic cancer cell lines. Gastroenterology 1996;110:1605–1613.

41. Bhatia M, Kirkland JB, Meekling-Gill KA (1995). Monocytic differentiation of acute promyelocytic leukemia cells in response to 1,25-dihydroxyvitamin D_3 is independent of nuclear receptor binding. J Biol Chem 1995;270:15.962–15.965.

42. Brown AJ, Dusso A, Slatopolsky E. Selective vitamin D analogs and their therapeutic applications. Semin Nephrol 1974;14:156–174.

43. Frey MR, Zhao X, Evans SS, Black JD. Activation of protein kinase C (PKC) isozymes inhibits cell cycle progression, modulates phosphorylation of the RBs (Rb) protein, and induces expression of p21waf1/cip1 in intestinal epithelial cells. Proc Am Assoc Cancer Res 1996;37:51.

44. Wali R, Bissonnette M, Khare S, Aquino B, Niedziela S, Sitrin M, Brasitus T. Protein kinase C isoforms in the chemopreventive effects of a novel vitamin D_3 analogue in rat colonic tumorigenesis. Gastroenterology 1996;111:118–126.
45. Millard SS, Koff A. Cyclin-dependent kinase inhibitors in restriction point control, genomic stability, and tumorigenesis. J Cell Biochem 1998;30/31:37–42.
46. Brugarolas JCC, Gordon JI, Beach D, Jacks T, Hannon CJ. Radiation-induced cell cycle arrest compromised by p21 deficiency. Nature 1995;377:552–557.
47. Kondo Y, Kondo S, Liu JB, Haqqi T, Barnett GH, Barna BP. Involvement of p53 and waf1/cip1 in gamma-irradiation-induced apoptosis of retinoblastoma cells. Exp Cell Res 1997;251:51–56.
48. Elstner E, Linker-Israeli M, Umiel T, Le J, Grillier I, Said J, Shintau IP, Krajewski S, Reed JC, Binderup L, Koeffler HP. Combination of a potent 20-epi-vitamin D_3 analogue (KH 1060) with 9-cis-retinoic acid irreversibly inhibits clonal growth, decreases bcl-2 expression, and induces apoptosis in HL-60 leukemic cells. Cancer Res 1996;56:3570–3576.
49. Vandewalle B, Hornez L, Wattez N, Revillion F, Lefebvre J. Vitamin-D3 derivatives and breast-tumor cell growth: Effect on intracellular calcium and apoptosis. Int J Cancer 1995;61:806–811.
50. Skarosi S, Abraham C, Bissonnette M, Scaglione-Sewell B, Sitrin MD, Brastius TA. 1,25-dihydroxyvitamin D_3 stimulates apoptosis in CaCo-2 cells. Gastroenterology 1997;112:A608.

15

Therapy of Uveal Melanoma: Methods and Risk Factors Associated with Treatment

DAN S. GOMBOS

M. D. Anderson Hospital, Houston, Texas, U.S.A.

WILLIAM F. MIELER

Baylor College of Medicine, Houston, Texas, U.S.A.

I. INTRODUCTION

The past century has seen a dramatic shift in the management of uveal melanoma. A disease once universally treated by enucleation is now managed by a range of techniques that can often preserve the eye and varying degrees of vision. While some treatment approaches remain controversial, others are widely accepted. The primary goal of management is to prevent both local tumor growth and spread of tumor outside of the eye, thereby altering the natural course of the malignancy with its associated morbidity and mortality. Unlike the case in other ocular conditions, preservation of life is the most important factor here, with retention of the eye and vision a secondary goal.

Treatment for patients with uveal melanoma can be divided into five broad categories (Table 1): observation, photocoagulation therapy, radiotherapy, local excision, and organ resection (enucleation). The treatments represent a spectrum of approaches applicable for tumors of various size and intraocular location. The indications for certain techniques overlap with others. Some of the modalities discussed here have evolved over decades with proven efficacy, while others remain in their infancy with limited long-term data. The clinician is cautioned to assess each treatment option carefully and proceed with an individualized plan tailored to the

Table 1 Treatment Options for a
Patient with a Uveal Melanoma

Observation
Laser therapies
Photocoagulation therapy
Transpupillary thermotherapy (TTT)
Photodynamic therapy (PDT)
Radiotherapy
Brachytherapy
Charged-particle radiation
Gamma knife
External-beam radiation therapy
Tumor resection techniques
Enucleation

---

specific needs of each patient. Detailed explanations of the risks and benefits will allow the patient to make an informed decision regarding the management option that suits him or her best.

II. OBSERVATION

As with most cancers, it is generally best to diagnose and treat uveal melanomas early in their natural course. Distinguishing small active melanomas from suspicious choroidal nevi, however, is an important consideration for the clinician before proceeding with therapy.

Small indeterminate lesions can remain stable for many years and often require no intervention. Some small tumors may transform and declare themselves as melanomas. When such a lesion presents itself, it is best to assess its risk for growth and malignant transformation. Such characteristics include tumor thickness greater than 2 mm, proximity to the optic nerve and the presence of symptoms, orange pigment, or subretinal fluid (Fig. 1). Small lesions that have dormant features can be followed closely with serial observation. Retinal drawings, fundus photographs, and echography should serve as a baseline for repeat assessment in 3 to 4 months. If the lesion remains stable, periodic review can be performed at greater intervals. Patients should be instructed to return for evaluation sooner if they develop any visual symptoms in the affected eye. Proceeding with therapy is reasonable if growth is documented (photographically or echographically) or the lesion demonstrates numerous risk factors [1].

Most tumors with documented growth should be treated. However in special circumstances, observation may be considered. Elderly monocular patients with small melanomas, who are at risk for visual loss with therapy are one such group. These cases require careful patient selection, informed consent, and close serial assessment.

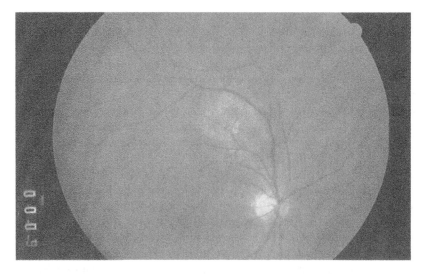

Figure 1 Photograph OD showing a juxtapapillary small uveal melanoma (2.2 mm thick) with orange pigmentation and subretinal fluid. The lesion grew within 6 months, eventually requiring ^{125}I brachytherapy treatment.

III. LASER THERAPIES: PHOTOCOAGULATION, THERMOTHERAPY, AND PHOTODYNAMIC THERAPY

While various types of lasers have been employed in the treatment of uveal melanomas, the therapeutic principle is similar for most modalities; energy directed to the lesion is absorbed and converted to heat, which destroys the malignancy. The majority of lasers cause immediate cell death through coagulation of proteins, while newer approaches heat tumor cells causing tissue necrosis—so called thermotherapy. Generally these methods are indicated for small melanomas with documented growth or those lesions at high risk for future growth.

Meyer-Schwickerath, a pioneer in photocoagulation, was the first to treat a uveal melanoma with this approach in 1957. Since then a number of studies have suggested that laser photocoagulation can be used to treat small melanomas [2–6]. Some clinicians have limited this modality to tumors less than 2 mm in height, while others have treated lesions up to 3.5–4.0 mm [7,8]. Limited tissue penetration restricts its use for thicker lesions. Local tumor control is successful in approximately 85% of cases; however, studies with increased follow-up have demonstrated a propensity for late recurrences [9]. Melanomas in close proximity to the optic nerve or macula were initially selected for laser photocoagulation as an alternative to brachytherapy, but these cases now often seem prone to failure. Lesions posterior to the equator, in eyes that dilate well with clear media, are most amenable to photocoagulation; however, with the advent of indirect ophthalmoscopic delivery of laser, virtually any tumor is amenable. On occasion, when brachytherapy is not successful and a local tumor recurrence develops, tumors are treated with photocoagulation [10].

A number of different lasers have been used to treat melanomas. While xenon arc photocoagulation was initially described, it has largely been replaced by argon and krypton lasers [7,9,11]. The general approach is to the treat the lesion with low-energy, long-exposure burns in multiple stages. The melanoma is first surrounded with two to three rows of laser spots. At follow up, heavy white burns are applied to the tumor surface. Treatments continue at 3- to 5-week intervals until the lesion flattens and develops into a flat atrophic scar (Fig. 2A–C). Some tumors require multiple treatments until an acceptable response is achieved. Late recurrences, years following therapy, have been described so careful serial follow-up is mandatory if this method is selected (Fig. 3A,B) [4,5,12–15].

With the introduction of the 810-nm diode laser, a number of centers have abandoned traditional photocoagulation for laser-induced hyperthermia [16–20]. While indications for this modality continue to evolve, small pigmented tumors, less than 2–3 mm in height, that are not contiguous with or overhang the optic nerve seem to have the best response [17,18]. Local control in some studies is reported as high as 95%; however, reports with longer follow-up demonstrate failure rates up to 22% at 3 years [19–21]. Treatments are usually administered via a slit-lamp delivery system under retrobulbar anesthesia. Using a 2 to 3-mm spot size, the laser is applied to the lesion with an exposure up to 60 sec. A slight blanching of the tumor surface is the desired endpoint. Most clinicians advocate two to four treatment sessions until a flat scar is achieved, but others have demonstrated treatment effects years after only one session [22–24]. In one report, tumors requiring more than three treatments for tumor control were more likely ultimately to recur [21]. Amelanotic lesions tend to be resistant to this modality, as there is very limited laser energy uptake. As a result,

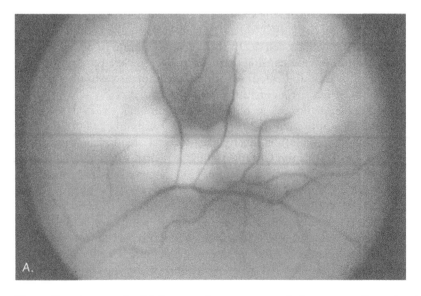

Figure 2 Photographs OS documenting xenon coagulation to a small uveal melanoma along the superotemporal arcade. (A) Initial treatment was placed around the margin of the tumor, followed by (B) treatment to the surface of the tumor, resulting in a (C) flat fibrotic scar.

some centers administer compounds such as indocyanine green (ICG) prior to therapy of amelanotic tumors to increase laser uptake.

Thermotherapy has been used as an adjunct to plaque brachytherapy. So-called sandwich therapy has been described in the management of large choroidal melanomas treated with ruthenium plaques. Application of thermotherapy is used to lower the applied dose of radiation [22,25–26]. While tumor regression and survival are favorable with the approach, some studies demonstrate a significant loss of central vision. Thermotherapy has also been used as a salvage technique for eyes failing primary brachytherapy and photocoagulation.

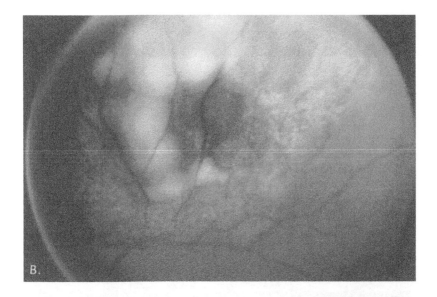

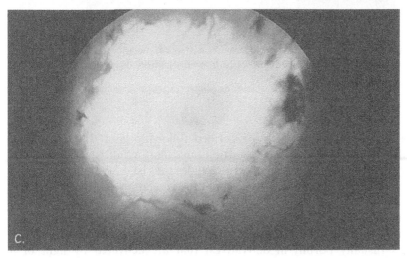

Figure 2   Continued.

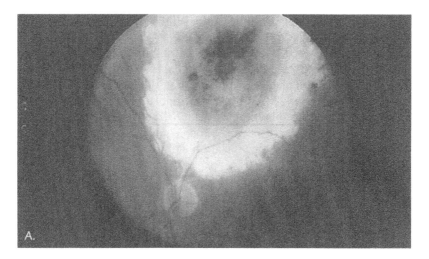

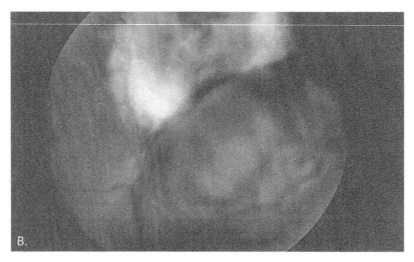

Figure 3 Photographs showing (A) a stable laser treated small melanoma, which eventually regrew (B) two years following treatment, necessitating enucleation surgery.

   Multiple complications have been described following laser therapies. They include vascular occlusions, neovascularization, macular wrinkling, edema, and exudation [13,15,17,18,20]. A serious concern includes the risk of extraocular tumor extension, a complication described with both photocoagulation and thermotherapy [12,21,27–33].
   Reports have described the treatment of melanomas with photodynamic (PDT) or photoradiation therapy [34,35]. These approaches involve the administration of systemic agents (usually porphyrin derivatives) that are activated by light of a specific wavelength. The mechanism of action seems to involve vascular closure but may include a direct cytotoxic effect on tumor cells [36]. Small human trials have

been published with short-term results [37]. While promising, this approach is not widely employed and requires further investigation.

IV. RADIOTHERAPY

Foster Moore is largely credited with the first use of local radiation to treat an intraocular tumor. His implantation of radon seeds into an ocular "sarcoma" is perhaps the first documented case of brachytherapy for a choroidal tumor [38]. Today ocular plaques are among the most widely used organ-sparing treatment options available for small and medium-sized uveal melanomas. Teletherapy in the form of charged particles is an alternate means of delivering targeted radiation and is available at selected centers in the United States and Europe.

A. Brachytherapy

Over the twentieth century, advances in the design and construction of plaques have led to their expanded use in treating uveal melanomas. Following Moore's initial work, Stallard experimented with brachytherapy by suturing radioactive seeds to the sclera overlying intraocular tumors [39]. Later, to ensure uniform dosimetry, he constructed metallic carriers that housed the seeds and could be directly sutured to the eye. Though melanomas were initially felt to be radioresistant, Stallard found that melanomas regressed if treated at doses greater than previously used. Plaques offer a means of delivering high-dose radiation directly to the tumor with reduced side effects to adjacent structures [40].

Cobalt 60 initially became the standard radiation source due to its availability, long half-life, and consistent dosimetry [41–43]. Plaques could be constructed and reused over a period of years (Fig. 4). The difficulty of shielding cobalt and the unintentional radiation of adjacent ocular structures led to experimentation with alternative radioactive sources. Gold, strontium, iridium, and palladium plaques have all been described in the literature [44–46]. Each source varies in its availability, complexity of dosimetry planning, type of radiation emitted, and ability to be shielded [47]. The past decade has seen a gradual trend toward the use of two major isotopes, iodine 125 (^{125}I) and ruthenium 106 (^{106}RU). 125I is primarily used in North America and was the source selected for the COMS study [48]. It is an emitter of low-energy gamma x-rays and can be used to treat tumors of various heights, generally up to 10.0 mm in thickness [49]. It is readily available and easily shielded with a thin rim of gold (Fig. 5A,B) [50–52]. By constructing plaques with standard inserts [53], the COMS study was able to ensure uniform dosimetry for tumors treated in this trial. Ruthenium was introduced by Lommatzsch in the 1960s, and it gradually replaced cobalt in most European oncology centers [54–57]. Unlike iodine, ruthenium is a beta emitter and is coated on a silver carrier. Worldwide, these two sources are used in the majority of plaques constructed for the treatment of uveal melanomas.

Clinically, plaques are best suited for the management of medium size and actively growing small uveal melanomas. Dosimetry plans are based on the apical measurements of the tumor, desired apex dose, and dose rate of the emitting source. Tumors of greater height require treatment plans that deliver larger doses to the

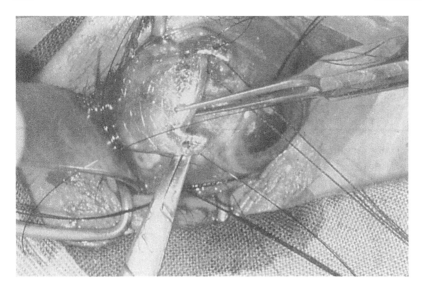

Figure 4 Photograph showing a ^{60}Co radioactive plaque being placed over the base of a uveal melanoma.

underlying sclera. Doses of 70–120 cGy to the tumor apex are described in the literature, but most centers treat melanomas at doses of 80–100 cGy [38,43,54,58–61]. The COMS study initially chose a dose of 100 cGy, but reassessment of the

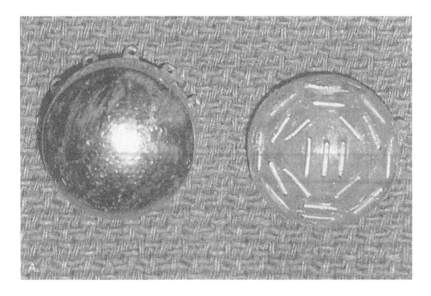

Figure 5 Photograph (A) depicting a gold-plated plaque with a Silastic insert designed for use with the radioactive isotope[125]I. This plaque was utilized in the Collaborative Ocular Melanoma Study (COMS). (B) Photograph showing plaque sutured in place over the base of the uveal melanoma.

initial dosimetry suggests that tumors actually received closer to 85 cGY [62]. Tumors with apex heights of 2.5 to 10 mm are well suited for this modality. Its use in larger tumors is limited by the increased radiation administered to the adjacent sclera. The reduced tissue penetration of beta rays often limits the use of ruthenium plaques to tumors ranging up to 5–6 mm in height [54–57,63,64]. However, some European centers have modified their treatment plans to include tumors of greater apical dimensions [65–67]. Recently there have been reports of ruthenium brachytherapy combined with adjuvant thermotherapy (sandwich therapy) in the management of larger melanomas [25,26,68,69] (see discussion of laser therapies in Sec. III, above).

Intraocular location and tumor basal dimensions are factors used to select a plaque of appropriate size and shape. While some clinicians have reported plaquing tumors with basal dimensions as large as 20 mm others feel the technique is best limited to lesions measuring 15–16 mm [59,70]. Initial plaque designs were circular and well suited for equatorial uveal melanomas. Such is the case for the COMS plaques. Modifications in design have expanded the applications of brachytherapy for most melanomas. Notched and curved plaques are commercially available or can be custom-made and have been used to treat iris, ciliary body, and peripapillary tumors [71–74].

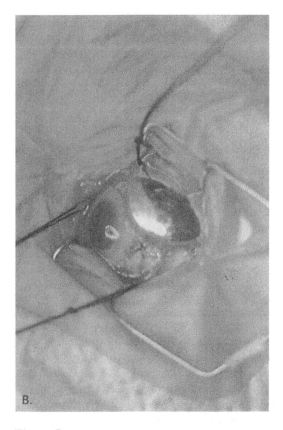

Figure 5 Continued.

The key to successful treatment of a tumor with an ocular plaque is its accurate placement. Surgically, the technique begins with a peritomy followed by surgical isolation of the extraocular muscles. The tumor is localized using transillumination or scleral indentation and a dummy plaque is sutured to the overlying sclera. Some centers use intraoperative ultrasonography to confirm the position of the plaque in relation to the tumor [75]. Once this has been done, the active plaque is sutured and left in place for a prescribed period of time (often 3–7 days), after which it is surgically removed. At a number of centers, radiotherapists and dosimetrists are present in the operating room to ensure proper orientation and placement of the plaque.

Tumor regression following radiotherapy can be delayed up to a year. Initial response may include resorption of subretinal fluid followed later by pigmentary changes and decreased tumor height (Fig. 6A,B). Over time, vascular changes can be appreciated on fluorescein angiography, and certain tumors demonstrate increased internal reflectivity on echography [90]. Some clinicians consider lack of tumor growth a successful response to radiotherapy. Partly because of the various definitions used by authors to assess tumor regression, studies vary in published response rate. Nonetheless most findings suggest a local control rate of 85–90% following plaque brachytherapy [40,43,63,84,91–94]. The majority of tumors stabilize in height or regress over the first 2–6 years after treatment.

Tumor recurrence has been described years after radiotherapy and thus obligates the ocular oncologist to long-term serial assessment of his or her patient. Generally, recurrence is seen within 3 years of therapy and can be managed with enucleation, additional plaque radiotherapy, or adjuvant laser treatment [95]. Margin failure may be more amenable to the last two approaches. Enucleation following failed plaque radiotherapy is most commonly due to tumor recurrence or neovascular glaucoma [55,89,96,97].

Complications to this technique vary. Initially patients may complain of diplopia or ocular irritation. Uveitis can be observed following radiation of an anterior segment lesion; rarely, there may be scleral melting (Fig. 7). Retinal detachment (exudative and rhegmatogenous), subretinal exudation, and vitreous hemorrhage may occur [76]. Radiation-related toxicities are often delayed for 2–3 years and include cataracts, radiation vasculopathy (Fig. 8A,B), papillopathy (Fig. 9A,B) and neovascular glaucoma [42,43,56,57,60,70,77–84]. Visual loss is more likely to occur when there is increased proximity to the fovea and optic nerve [72,84–88]. Complications tend to occur in those eyes with larger tumors treated at higher dose rates [77,89].

B. Charged-Particle Radiotherapy

The availability of charged particles at a number of research institutions and their use in treating other malignancies led to the development of protons and helium ions for the treatment of uveal melanomas [98]. This modality, in theory, offers advantages over traditional brachytherapy. The Bragg peak effect affords less radiation to adjacent structures and provides a uniform dose to the entire tumor. This differs from brachytherapy, where the tumor base receives a larger dose than the tumor apex. In addition, the use of charged particles avoids radiation exposure to the operative team.

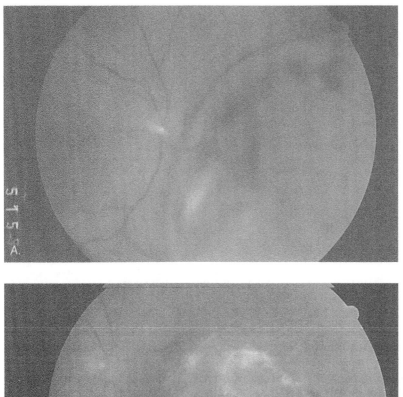

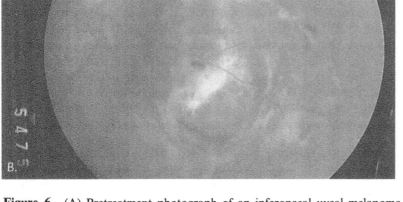

Figure 6 (A) Pretreatment photograph of an inferonasal uveal melanoma 7.4 mm thick. (B) Two years following ^{125}I brachytherapy treatment, the tumor has shrunk to a height of 2.4 mm and shows pigmentary mottling with secondary fibrotic scarring.

The surgical technique is similar to that used for brachytherapy. After the lesion is localized, a series of tantalum marker clips are sutured to the sclera in a circumferential pattern surrounding the tumor. Unlike plaque radiotherapy, only one surgical procedure is required. Once in place, the clips are used as localizing markers for physicists planning treatment. Patients are immobilized during therapy using a bite block and mask. Treatments are often fractionated over three to five sessions.

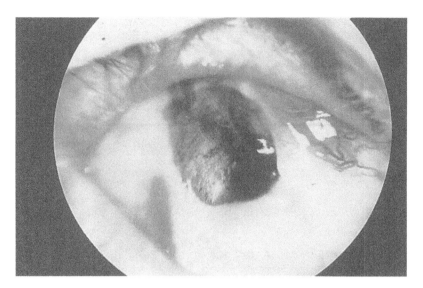

Figure 7 Photograph documenting a scleral melt following ^{125}I brachytherapy treatment. A scleral patch graft was required.

Tumor response following charged-particle radiotherapy is similar to that after brachytherapy [99]. Some reports suggest local control rates as high as 98% and an ocular retention rate of 90% [100]. However, charged-particle radiotherapy carries an increased risk of anterior segment complications, including dry eye and lash loss [98,101–104]. Neovascular glaucoma is more likely to develop when a significant portion of the anterior segment is irradiated [105,106]. Some authors advocate a two-field technique to decrease this complication. Poor visual outcomes following charged-particle radiotherapy correlate not only with tumor location (fovea, optic nerve) but also with tumor size greater than 8 mm [103,107–111].

Some centers use this form of radiation exclusively for all choroidal and ciliary body melanomas. Others limit its use to lesions less amenable to plaque radiotherapy, such as juxta- and circumpapillary tumors. A few centers have treated selected iris melanomas with reported success. The greatest limitation of charged-particle radiotherapy is the associated cost and requirement of a cyclotron. This has limited its use to two or three centers in the United States.

C. Gamma Knife and LINAC Stereotactic Radiotherapy

The increased use of stereotactic and gamma-knife radiotherapy to treat intracranial as well as head and neck lesions of various shapes has made it appealing in the management of intraocular tumors [112]. The Leksell gamma knife is a computer-controlled device that delivers radiotherapy precisely through a series of cobalt ports [113–115]. A similar modality, stereotactic LINAC radiotherapy, offers the advantage of external-beam radiation that can be fractionated and conformed to any tumor size and shape [116,117]. Plans can be constructed that allow radiation to enter the eye in such a fashion as to avoid critical anterior segment structures. Early studies with both modalities are encouraging, but long-term follow-up is still pending. Complications are similar to those of other forms of radiation and include neovascular glaucoma and optic neuropathy [90,112,118–123]. With the increased use of conformational techniques to treat other malignancies, stereotactic radiotherapy may become increasingly available for intraocular use.

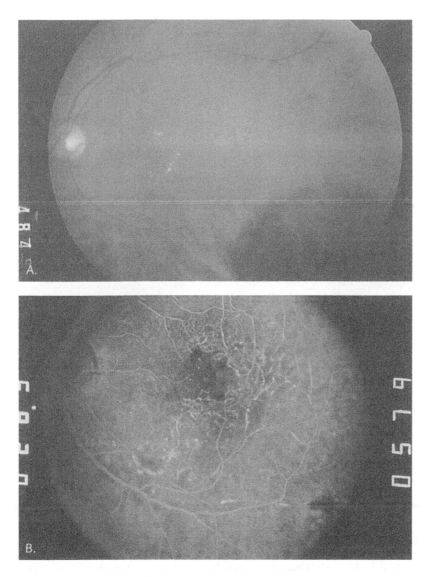

Figure 8 (A) Photograph OS showing a uveal melanoma along the inferotemporal arcade that had been treated with brachytherapy 5 years previously. Note the exudates in the macular region. (B) Fluorescein angiogram documents radiation-induced macular capillary nonperfusion, with loss of vision to the 20/200 level.

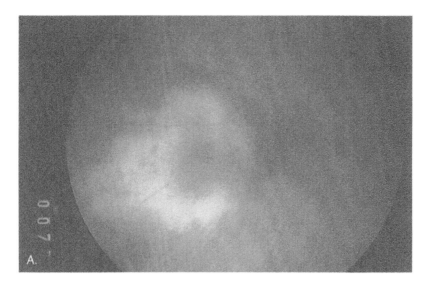

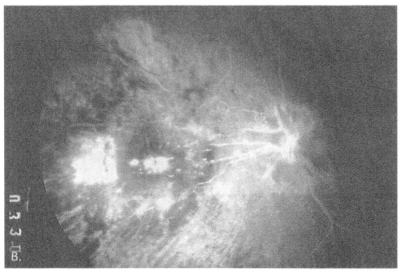

Figure 9   (A) Photograph OS taken 1 year following ^{125}I brachytherapy treatment of a uveal melanoma nasal to the optic disc. (B) Fluorescein angiogram documenting development of radiation-induced optic neuopathy with loss of vision to the hand motion level. The vision remained permanently reduced, though the tumor remained stable.

D.   External-Beam Radiotherapy

Traditional external-beam radiotherapy is used largely as an adjuvant modality for extraocular melanomas. Indications include gross orbital disease detected on presentation or after enucleation and microscopic extraocular extension appreciated on pathological review. Patients with painful bone and brain metastasis may also benefit from palliative radiation.

Pre-enucleation radiotherapy (PERT) was once administered as a means of decreasing the risk of hematogenous dissemination ascribed to surgical intervention. Numerous studies, including early results from the COMS trial, have failed to demonstrate a benefit from this approach; as a result it has largely been abandoned [124–130] (see discussion of enucleation, Sec. VII).

V. THERMORADIOTHERAPY

The response of uveal melanomas to hyperthermia and radiotherapy has led to techniques that incorporate both modalities. This approach is successful in managing other malignancies and often permits the use of lower doses of radiation.

Methods used to administer thermoradiotherapy include modified iodine plaques that deliver hyperthermia via microwave applicators or ferromagnetic thermoseeds [131–134]. Ultrasound-induced hyperthermia has also been combined with proton-bean radiotherapy [135]. Recent reports describe transpupillary thermotherapy (TTT) used in conjunction with brachytherapy. The "sandwich" technique involves the administration of diode laser hyperthermia in combination with traditional plaque radiation. The timing and frequency of laser treatments vary among different protocols. Some centers administer TTT prior to plaque surgery, while others do so months later. Early results suggest high rates of local tumor control; however, significant visual loss can occur [22,25,26,68,69]. At this time there is limited data to suggest the optimum method of combining these modalities.

VI. LOCAL TUMOR RESECTION

Local tumor excision is an approach used in the management of many other solid tumors, such as breast, lung, and gastrointestinal cancer. Resection of intraocular melanoma was first reported in the early twentieth century, Initially to treat anterior segment tumors. Later, ophthalmologists such as Peyman, Foulds, and Shields advanced methods to resect posterior uveal lesions. While the procedures vary in technique, they all represent means of surgically resecting the tumor while maintaining the structural and physiological integrity of the eye and surrounding structures. Unlike brachytherapy, they provide the patient with pathological confirmation of the diagnosis and avoid potential radiation-induced side effects. Selecting which method to use involves consideration of tumor size, location, and potential complications.

Surgical iridectomy is indicated for the excision of isolated iris tumors not involving the ciliary body or angle. Following a limbal incision, the tumor is resected using scissors. Depending on the size of the tumor, the pupil can be reapproximated with nonabsorbable suture. While this procedure is often successful in resecting the lesion, some patients are left with large iris defects that can cause polyopia and photophobia. Colored contact lenses and iris implants may be helpful in addressing these complaints.

Iridocyclectomy is a procedure used to resect tumors of the ciliary body and adjacent iris (Fig. 10 A,B). The technique begins with construction of a scleral flap hinged at the limbus. After application of diathermy to the scleral bed, the underlying tumor is excised with scissors. The sclera is then closed with interrupted

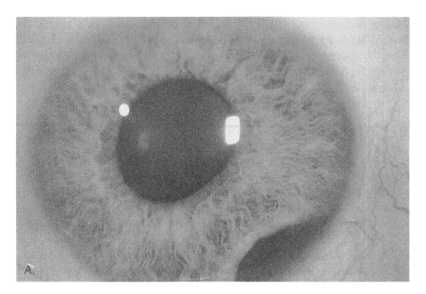

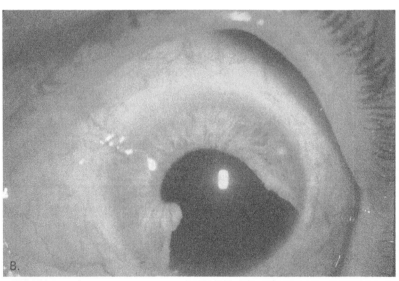

Figure 10 Photograph showing (A) the anterior extent of an iridociliary body melanoma and (B) postoperative appearance two years following an iridocyclectomy procedure. The patient remains free of tumor.

sutures. The technique works best when less than four clock hours of ciliary body are involved; excision of larger areas is technically feasible but associated with a higher rate of complications, such as hypotony [136].

Posterior lesions can be excised from both the ab interno and ab externo approaches. Eye wall resections involve a full-thickness excision of sclera, choroid, and overlying retina. Some clinicians advocate treating the tumor and its margins with cryotherapy or laser photocoagulation preoperatively to create retinal adhesions and reduce the risk of detachment. A ring stabilizer or eye-wall basket is used to maintain ocular integrity during the procedure. Following tumor localization, the sclera, choroid, and overlying retina are excised in toto. A vitrectomy is performed and the ocular defect is closed with a patch graft of donor sclera or dacron [137–139].

Modification of this approach includes dissection of a flap prior to the excision of the underlying tumor. Partial lamellar sclerouvectomy maintains the integrity of the outer wall by first dissecting a hinged 90% scleral flap (Fig. 11 A,B). Following diathermy to the scleral bed, the tumor is resected using scissors and is teased away from the retina using a blunt-tipped instrument. The sclera is then closed with interrupted suture. An encircling band is applied by some surgeons [140–142].

Resection of a posterior uveal tumor can be a technically difficult procedure. Some authors recommend that the surgery be performed under hypotensive conditions to minimize complications. For certain patients, this is an absolute contraindication to use of this modality [143]. A number of acute and long-term complications have been described with this technique, including retinal detachment, vitreous hemorrhage, macular edema, and hypotony. Among the more serious complications are expulsive choroidal hemorrhage and orbital seeding. Results suggest that tumors less than 10 mm in diameter located anterior to the equator have the best outcome, although lesions up to 18 mm have been removed successfully [140–142,144–147]. Intraocular and orbital recurrence is possible and has been described following what was felt to be complete surgical excision. Given these complications, some centers advocate adjuvant brachytherapy when proceeding with lamellar sclerouvectomy; following removal of the lesion, the sclera is reapproximated and a plaque is sutured to the overlying the area [148,149].

Tumors not accessible to external excision can be removed using an ab interno approach. Endoresection is best suited to posterior tumors, including those that are peripapillary in location. Lesions nasal to the disc afford the best postoperative visual potential [150,151]. Following pretreatment laser hyperthermia, a three-port vitrectomy is performed. A retinotomy is made and the tumor is removed in piecemeal fashion using the vitrector. Following excision, endodiathermy, gas-fluid exchange, and endolaser are used to prevent rebleeding, create retinal adhesions, and destroy residual tumor cells. Silicone oil is then injected and the sclerotomy ports are treated with cryotherapy [152,153]. The potential risk of incomplete resection, dispersion of tumor cells following a piecemeal excision, and extraocular extension through sclerotomy sites has led to controversy regarding the use of this technique. As a result, some clinicians limit its role to tumors within one disc diameter of the optic nerve and those less than 10 mm in basal diameter [151,154]. Attempts at pretreating larger tumors with gamma-knife radiotherapy have also been described [155].

VII. ENUCLEATION

As the number of therapeutic options available for uveal melanomas continues to expand, there remain fewer indications for primary enucleation. For much of the early twentieth century, most eyes thought to be harboring melanomas were removed. As a result, some patients underwent unnecessary surgery. The poor

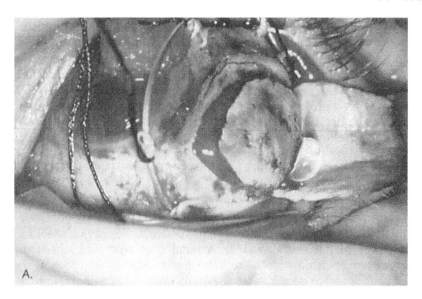

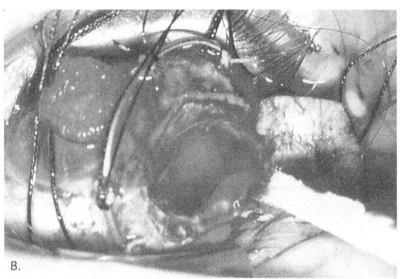

Figure 11 Intraoperative photographs of a lamellar sclerouvectomy procedure. (A) A partial thickness scleral flap has been raised over the base of the tumor, which was then followed by placement of diathermy around the base of the tumor. (B) Surgical removal of the tumor, leaving intact the underlying retina. The scleral flap was then closed and a pars plana vitrectomy procedure was performed.

prognosis associated with metastasis of this cancer was considered justification for this aggressive approach.

As plaque radiotherapy grew in acceptance and smaller lesions were observed with greater confidence, an increasing number of eyes that would have been enucleated were spared. Yet there remained concern that these modalities might worsen a patient's overall survival and risk for metastasis. In the late 1970s, some researchers presented data suggesting an increased risk of mortality following enucleation [156–159]. The Zimmerman hypothesis maintained that increased pressure associated with surgical intervention, such as an enucleation, disseminated tumor cells, resulting in an increased risk of hematogenous spread. Some clinicians advocated a "no-touch" technique, where gentle manipulation of the eye was combined with freezing of the tumor base [160,161]. However, there were only limited data to suggest that either the hypothesis or the technique was clinically applicable. A number of studies comparing patients treated with brachytherapy versus enucleation failed to show a difference in mortality [83,124,162–165]. The COMS trial addressed this question by randomizing patients with medium-sized tumors to brachytherapy or enucleation [166]; preliminary results have not demonstrated a difference in melanoma-associated mortality between the two groups. Most clinicians no longer advocate enucleation by "no touch" method, although some still adhere to an approach of minimal manipulation.

Today primary enucleations are reserved for eyes with massive tumor involvement (greater than 40–50% tumor volume), no useful vision, total retinal detachment, or neovascular glaucoma (Fig. 12). Ciliary body tumors that are too large for excision or brachytherapy, ring melanomas, and circumpapillary lesions are also treated with this approach. Secondary enucleations are indicated for eyes failing local therapies. Finally, patients with small and medium-sized tumors who, after informed consent, elect not to proceed with eye-sparing techniques may also be considered candidates for organ removal.

Enucleations are usually performed under general anesthesia. Re-examination of the affected eye is recommended intraoperatively prior to the start of the procedure. Following a peritomy, the muscles are disinserted from the globe. The

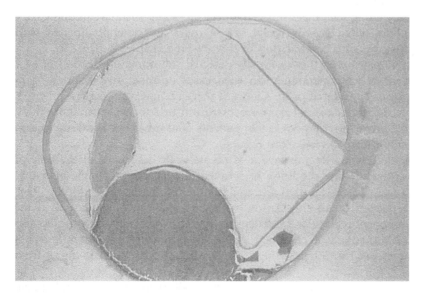

Figure 12 Histopathology of an enucleated globe containing a large ciliochoroidal melanoma, with a secondary retinal detachment.

optic nerve is transected with scissors using a nasal approach and gentle temporal traction. Following excision, the globe and orbit are carefully inspected for signs of extraocular involvement. If none is appreciated, an orbital implant is inserted. Many surgeons prefer a biointegrated material such as hydroxyapatite. If such a method is used, the implant is first wrapped (with donor tissue or Vicryl mesh) and the rectus muscles are attached in an anatomically correct fashion. Tenon's capsule is then meticulously closed prior to suturing of the conjunctiva. A pressure patch is applied and the patient is referred for fitting of an ocular prosthesis after postoperative edema has resolved. Cosmetic results are excellent, with good prosthetic motility. The pathology is later reviewed for diagnostic confirmation and complete surgical excision.

Given the concerns raised by the Zimmerman hypothesis, some clinicians have advocated the use of pre-enucleation radiotherapy (PERT). Similar techniques used for other systemic malignancies have been shown to decrease patient morbidity. Yet retrospective studies failed to demonstrate a benefit or improved survival with PERT. The large-tumor COMS group addressed this question in a prospective trial that randomized eyes prior to enucleation. Early results at 5-year follow-up have failed to demonstrate either benefit or harm with PERT [127,130]. As a result, this approach has largely been abandoned.

VIII. EXTRAOCULAR INVOLVEMENT

The management of extraocular melanoma depends largely on the nature and extent of extraocular disease. In this respect, periocular involvement must be distinguished from systemic metastatic disease. Large uveal melanomas, including those with increased basal diameters, are at risk for extrascleral involvement [167]. Tumor cells can spread locally along scleral emissary channels, including vortex veins and ciliary nerves, leaving the sclera grossly intact. These cases are generally treated with surgery, radiotherapy, or a combination of the two [168,169].

Microscopic metastasis is occasionally detected following enucleation of eyes that appeared intact intraoperatively. In such cases postoperative external-beam radiotherapy can be considered [170]. Adjuvant therapy, however, increases the risk of complications, including orbital exposure, extrusion, and socket contracture [171]. Some clinicians prefer to monitor such patients and treat with external-beam radiotherapy only if orbital recurrence occurs.

Unanticipated extrascleral extension is occasionally diagnosed at the time of surgical intervention. If this condition is detected at the time of plaque insertion, management varies based on the size and nature of extraocular disease. One approach is to convert to an enucleation, with local excision of the lesion. If the extraocular component is large and nodular, postoperative radiotherapy should also be considered. Alternatively, in cases with small, flat extrascleral extension (less than 2 mm), one can proceed with brachytherapy following dissection of the tumor from the scleral wall [172].

In proceeding with a planned enucleation, small areas of extrascleral spread can be removed en bloc with the globe and adjacent Tenon's capsule (tenonectomy) [172–174]. Some reports suggest these cases carry an 8–18% risk of orbital recurrence. Given these results, adjuvant radiotherapy should be considered in this setting [170,175].

In cases presenting with massive orbital involvement or those following prior enucleation, exenteration may be indicated (Fig. 13) [172,176,177]. There remains debate as to whether this radical procedure actually improves patient survival. Nonetheless, tumor debulking with this approach can be the most cosmetically acceptable option for the patient. Adjuvant external-beam radiotherapy is usually recommended and can be given preoperatively. Many of these patients have systemic disease; therefore a metastatic workup should be considered prior to surgical intervention.

Only a small percentage (approximately 1%) of patients present with both ocular and systemic uveal melanoma. Hepatic involvement is the most common area of organ metastasis, followed by the subcutaneous tissue and lungs. When systemic disease is detected, it is best to refer the patient to a medical oncologist with experience in treating melanomas. Patients with isolated hepatic metastasis have benefited from arterial chemoembolization and local resection [178–181]. A number of systemic chemotherapeutic protocols have been tested, with poor results [182–

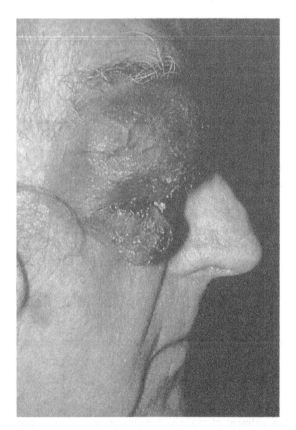

Figure 13 Photograph showing prominent orbital extension of melanoma from a ciliochoroidal lesion. The patient refused treatment and died of metastatic disease within 6 months.

185]. Adjuvant therapies with interleukins and interferon have failed to live up to their expectations [186,187]. The EORTC oncology task force recently reported data from a phase II trial of chemoimmunotherapy with bleomycin, vincristine, lomustine, dacarbazine (BOLD), and recombinant alpha 2b interferon. The results to date have demonstrated a limited response. Palliative radiotherapy can be effective for patients with painful metastasis to the brain and bones. Generally these patients carry a very poor prognosis [188]. Ocular therapy is therefore deferred for patients with a life expectancy of less that 1 year if the eye is intact, without neovascular changes, and pain free. Should neovascular glaucoma develop in this setting, options include enucleation versus ciliary body ablation.

Given the poor prognosis associated with metastatic disease, a number of centers have considered adjuvant therapies to prevent systemic spread. As discussed elsewhere, pre-enucleation external-beam radiotherapy was advocated by some in an attempt to prevent dissemination of tumor cells at the time of surgery. Preliminary results from the COMS study have not demonstrated any benefit from this approach. Some researchers have vaccinated patients with melanoma antigens [189–191]. There is a single case report of a choroidal melanoma responding to the administration of a melanoma vaccine [192]. Other studies have investigated the empirical use of systemic agents such as interferon after local therapy. To date, no single method has been shown to significantly alter the course of this disease, prevent metastasis, or lengthen long-term survival.

IX. CONCLUSIONS

Unlike that of many other cancers, diagnosis of the intraocular tumor is often associated with a unique motivation for organ preservation. Today there is a range of therapeutic options available in the management of uveal melanomas. While methods and indications vary, a trend toward eye-sparing techniques whenever possible has clearly emerged. Increasing numbers of patients can be cured and maintain their eyes and vision. Advances in photocoagulation therapies, radiation, and surgical techniques hold great promise for the future.

This optimism is tempered only by the limited progress in the management of systemic disease. Greater understanding is necessary regarding the biological events associated with extraocular and systemic metastasis. Only when these pathways are delineated will the ophthalmologist develop therapies that achieve all the goals of treatment, including (1) curing the intraocular tumor, (2) preventing extraocular disease, and (3) preserving the eye and vision.

REFERENCES

1. Manschot WA, van Peperzeel HA. Choroidal melanoma. Enucleation or observation? A new approach. Arch Ophthalmol 1980;98:71–77.
2. Meyer-Schwickerath G, Vogel M. Treatment of malignant melanomas of the choroid by photocoagulation. Trans Ophthalmol Soc UK 1977;97:416–420.
3. Tse DT. Laser photocoagulation of choroidal malignant melanoma. Biomed Pharmacother 1986;40:323–325.

4. Vogel M, Meyer-Schwickerath G. Results of photocoagulation treatment of malignant melanomas of the choroid. In: Jakobiec, F E, ed. Ocular and Adnexal Tumors. Birmingham, AL: Aesculapius, 1978, pp 70–75.

5. Vogel MH. Treatment of malignant choroidal melanomas with photocoagulation. Evaluation of 10-year follow-up data. Am J Ophthalmol 1972;74:1–10.

6. Meyer-Schwickerath G, Vogel MH. Malignant melanoma of the choroid treated with photocoagulation. A 10-year follow-up. Mod Prob Ophthalmol 1974;12:544–549.

7. Foulds WS, Damato BE. Low-energy long-exposure laser therapy in the management of choroidal melanoma. Graefes Arch Clin Exp Ophthalmol 1986;224:26–31.

8. Francois, J. Treatment of malignant melanoma of the choroid by light coagulation. Mod Prov Ophthalmol 1974;12:550–555.

9. Minckler D, Thompson FB Photocoagulation of malignant melanoma. Arch Ophthalmol 1979;97:120–123.

10. Augsberger, JJ, Mullen D, Kleinedidam, M. Indirect ophthalmoscope laser treatment as supplement to 125-I plaque therapy for choroidal melanoma. Trans Am Ophthalmol Soc 1992;90:303–316.

11. Jaffe GJ, Mieler WF, Burke JM, et al. Photoablation of ocular melanoma with high-powered argon endolaser. Arch Ophthalmol 1989;107:113–118.

12. Barr CC, Norton EW. Recurrence of choroidal melanoma after photocoagulation therapy. Arch Ophthalmol 1983;101:1737–1740.

13. Bornfield N Wessing A. Photocoagulation of choroidal melanoma. In: Ryan SJ ed. Retina. VolI. St. Louis: Mosby, pp. 815–823.

14. Francois J, Hanssens M, DeLaey JJ. Recurrence of malignant melanoma of the choroid seven and eight years after light coagulation. Ophthalmologica 1971;162:188–192.

15. Hepler RS, Allen RA, Straatsma BR. Photocoagulation of choroidal melanoma. Arch Ophthalmol 1968;79:177–181.

16. Brancato R, Pratesi R, Leoni G, et al. Semiconductor diode laser photocoagulation of human malignant melanoma. Am J Ophthalmol 1989;107:295.

17. Oosterhuis JA, Journee-de Korver HG, Keunen JEE. Transpupillary thermotherapy: Results in 50 patients with choroidal melanoma. Arch Ophthalmol 1998;116:157–161.

18. Oosterhuis JA, Journee de Korver HG, Kakebeeke Keeme HM, Bleeker JC. Transpupillary thermotherapy in choroidal melanomas. Arch Ophthalmol 1995;113:315–321.

19. Godfrey DG, Waldro RG, Capone A Jr. Transpupilary thermotherapy for small choroidal melanomas. Am J Ophthalmol 1999;128:88–93.

20. Shields CL, Shields JA Carter J, Lois N, Edelstein C, Gunduz K, Mercado G. Transpupillary thermotherapy for choroidal melanoma: Tumor control and visual results in 100 consecutive cases. Ophthalmology 1998;105:581–590.

21. Shields CL, Shields JA, Perez N, et al. Primary transpupillary thermotherapy for choroidal melanoma in 256 consecutive cases: Outcomes and limitations (abstr). Program of the Xth International Congress of Ocular Oncology Meeting, Amsterdam, the Netherlands, June 17–21, 2001, p 174.

22. Keunen JEE, Journee-de Korver JG, Oosterhuis JA. Transpupillary thermotherapy of choroidal melanoma with or without brachytherapy: A dilemma. Br J Ophthalmol 1999;83:987–988.

23. Robertson DM, Buettner H, Bennett SR. Transpupillary thermotherapy as primary treatment for small choroidal melanomas. Arch Ophthalmol 1999;117:1512–1519.

24. Robertson DM, Buettner H, Bennett SR. Transpupillary thermotherapy as primary treatment for small choroidal melanomas. Trans Am Ophthalmol Soc 1999;97:407–427.

25. Starzyeka M, Romanowska-Dixon B, Slomska J, et al. Transpupillary thermotherapy combined with 106Ru as a method of managing choroidal melanoma. Klin Oczna 2000;102(4):249–252.

26. Seregard S, Landau I. Transpupillary thermotherapy as an adjunct to ruthenium plaque radiotherapy for choroidal melanoma. Acta Ophthalmol Scand 2001;79(1):19–22.

27. Boniuk M, Choen JS. Combined use of radiation plaques and photocoagulation in the treatment of choroidal melanomas. In: Jakobiec FA, ed. Ocular and Adnexal Tumors. Birmingham, AL: Aesculapius, 1978, p 80.

28. Finger PT, Lipka AC, Lipowitz JL, et al. Failure of transpupillary thermotherapy(TTT) for choroidal melanoma: two cases with histopathological correlation. Br J Ophthalmol 2000;78(9):1075–1076.

29. Duvall J, Lucas DR. Argon laser and xenon arc coagulation of malignant choroidal melanoma: Histological findings in 6 cases. Br J Ophthalmol 1981;65:464–468.

30. Francois J. Treatment of malignant choroidal melanomas by xenon photocoagulation. In: Lommatzsch PK, Blodi, FC, eds. Intraocular Tumors. New York: Springer-Verlag, 1983, pp 277–285.

31. Lund OE. Changes in choroidal tumors after light coagulation (and diathermy coagulation). Arch Ophthalmol 1966;75:458–466.

32. Meyer-Schwickerath G, Bornfield N. Photocoagulation of choroidal melanomas— Thirty years experience. In: Lommatzsch PK, Blodi FC. eds. Intraocular Tumors. New York: Springer-Verlag, 1983, pp 269–276.

33. Vogel MH. Histopathological observations of photocoagulated malignant melanomas of the choroid. Am J Ophthalmol 1972;74:466–472.

34. Foster BS, Gragoudas ES, Young LH. Photodynamic therapy of choroidal melanoma. Int Ophthalmol Clin 1997;37:117–126.

35. Lewis RA, Tse DT, Phelps CD, Weingeist TA. Neovascular glaucoma after photoradiation therapy for uveal melanoma. Arch Ophthalmol 1984;102:839–842.

36. Fingar VH, Wieman TJ, McMahon KS, et al. Photodynamic therapy using a protoporphyrinogen oxidase inhibitor. Cancer Res 1997;57:4551–4556.

37. Bruce RA. Evaluation of hematoporphyrin photoradiation therapy to treat choroidal melanoma. Lasers Surg Med 1984;4:59–64.

38. Moore RF. Choroidal sarcoma treated by the intraocular insertion of radiation seeds. Br J Ophthalmol 1930;14:145–156.

39. Stallard HB. A case of malignant melanoma of the choroid successfully treated by radon seeds. Trans Ophthalmol Soc UK 1949;69:293–296.

40. Stallard HB. Radiotherapy for malignant melanoma of the choroid. Br J Ophthalmol 1966;50:147–155.

41. Beitler JJ, McCormick B, Ellsworth RM, et al. Ocular melanoma: Total dose and dose rate effects with Co-60 plaque therapy. Radiology 1990;176:275–278

42. Ellsworth RM. Cobalt plaques for melanoma of the choroid. In: Jakobieck FA, ed. Ocular and Adnexal Tumors, Birmingham, AL: Aesculapius, 1978, pp 76–79.

43. Shields JA, Augsburger JJ, Brady LW, et al. Cobalt plaque therapy for posterior uveal melanomas. Ophthalmology 1982;89:1202–1207.

44. Finger PT, Bernson A, Szechter A Palladium-103 plaque radiotherapy for choroidal melanoma. Ophthalmology 1999;106:606–613.

45. Luxton G, Astrahan MA, Liggett PE, et al. Dosimetric calculations and measurements of gold plaque ophthalmic irradiators using iridium-192 and iodine-125 seeds. Int J Radiat Oncol Biol Phys 1988;15:167–176.

46. Missotten L, Dirven W, Van der Schueren A, et al. Results of treatment of choroidal malignant melanoma with high-dose-rate strontium-90 brachytherapy. A retrospective study of 46 patients treated between 1983 and 1995. Graefes Arch Clin Exp Ophthalmol 1998;236:164–173.

47. Finger PT, Lu D, Buffa A, et al. Palladium-103 versus iodine-125 for ophthalmic plaque radiotherapy. Int J Radiat Oncol Biol Phys 1993;27:849–854.

48. Earle J, Kline RW, Robertson DM. Selection of Iodine-125 for the collaborative ocular melanoma study. Arch Ophthalmol 1987;105:763–764.

49. Ling CC, Chen GT, Boothby JW, et al. Computer assisted treatment planning for [125]L ophthalmic plaque radiotherapy. Int J Radiat Oncol Biol Phys 1989;17:405–410.

50. Alberti W, Pothmann B, Tabor P, et al. Dosimetry and physical treatment planning for iodine eye plaque therapy. Int J Radiat Oncol Biol Phys 1991;20:1087–1092.

51. Hartnett AN, Thomson EE, An iodine-125 plaque for radiotherapy of the eye: Manufacture and dosimetric considerations. Br J Radiol 1988;61:835–838.

52. Wu A, Krasin F. Film dosimetry analyses on the effect of gold shielding for iodine-125 eye plaque therapy for choroidal melanoma. Med Phys 1990;17:843–846.

53. Karolis C, Frost RB, Billson FA. A thin I-125 seed eye plaque to treat intraocular tumors using an acrylic insert to precisely position the sources. Int J Radiat Oncol Biol Phys 1990;18:1209–1213.

54. Lommatzsch P. Treatment of choroidal melanomas with 106Ru/106Rh beta-ray applicators. Surv Ophthalmol 1974;19:85–100.

55. Lommatzsch PK. Results after (-irradiation (106Ru/106Rh) of choroidal melanomas: 20 years' experience. Br J Ophthalmol 1986;70:844–851.

56. Lommatzsch PK. Treatment of choroidal melanomas with 106Ru/106Rh beta ray applications. In: Alberti WE, Sagerman RH, eds. Radiotherapy of Intraocular and Orbital Tumors. Berlin: Springer-Verlag, 1993, pp 23–30.

57. Lommatzsch PK, Werschnik C, Schuster E. Long-term follow-up of Ru-106/ Rh-106 brachytherapy for posterior uveal melanoma. Graefes Arch Clin Exp Ophthalmol 2000;238:129–137.

58. Packer S, Fairchild RG, Salanitro P. New techniques for iodine-125 radiotherapy of intraocular tumors. Ann Ophthalmol 1987;19:26–30.

59. Packer S, Rothman M. Radiotherapy of choroidal melanoma with Iodine-125. Ophthalmology 1980;87:582–590.

60. Rousseau A, Boudreault G, Packer S, et al. Radiation therapy of choroidal melanoma. Trans Ophthalmol Soc UK 1977;97:431–435.

61. Straatsma BR, Fine SL, Earle JD, et al. Enucleation versus plaque irradiation for choroidal melanoma. Ophthalmology 1988;95:1000–1004.

62. Ray SK, Bhatnagar R, Hartsell WF, Desai GR. Review of eye plaque dosimetry based on AAPM Task Group 43 recommendations. American Association of Physicists in Medicine. Int J Radiat Oncol Biol Phys 1998;41(3):701–706.

63. Seregard S, Trampe E, Lax I, et al. Results following episcleral ruthenium plaque radiotherapy for posterior uveal melanoma: The Swedish experience. Acta Opthalmol Scand 1997;75:11–16.

64. Wessing A, Foerster M, Bornfield N. Ruthenium plaque treatment of malignant choroidal melanomas. In: Oosterhuis JA ed. Ophthalmic Tumors. Dordrecht, The Netherlands: Junk Publishers 1985, pp 71–85.

65. Poier E, Langmann G, Leitner H, Vidic V. Optimierung der Zielvolumserfassung bei der Bestrahlung intraokularer melanome Mittels Rutheniumapplikatoren. Fortschr Ophthalmol 1991;88:158–160.

66. Potter R, Janssen K, Prott FJ, et al. Ruthenium-106 eye plaque brachytherapy in the conservative treatment of uveal melanoma: Evaluation of 175 patients treated with 150 Gy from 1981–1989. Front Radiat Ther Oncol 1997;30:143–149.

67. Hallerman D. Treatment of intraocular melanomas by ruthenium-106 beta irradiation. In: Oosterhuis JA, ed. Ophthalmic Tumors. Dordrecht, The Netherlands: Junk Publishers, 1985, pp 55–75.

68. Kreusel K-M, Bechrakis N, Riese J, et al. Regression of large choroidal melanoma after combined plaque therapy and transpupillary thermotherapy (abstr). Program of the

Xth International Congress of Ocular Oncology Meeting, Amsterdam, June 17–21, 2001, p 175.

69. Bartlema YM, Keunen JEE, Oosterhuis JG, et al. Five year follow-up of 50 patients with choroidal melanoma after combined treatment with brachytherapy and transpupillary thermotherapy (abstr). Program of the Xth International Congress of Ocular Oncology Meeting, Amsterdam, June 17–21, 2001, p 176.

70. Packer S, Rotman M, Salanitro PT. Iodine-125 irradiation of choroidal melanoma. Ophthalmology 1984;91:1700–1708.

71. Abdel-Dayem HK, Trese MT. A technique for suturing peripapillary radioactive plaques. Am J Ophthalmol 1999;127:224–226.

72. DePotter P, Shields JA, et al. Plaque radiotherapy for juxtapapillary choroidal melanoma. Arch Ophthalmol 1996;114:1357–1365.

73. Shields CL, Shields JA, De Potter P, Singh AD, Hernandez C, Brady LW. Treatment of non-resectable malignant iris tumours with custom designed plaque radiotherapy. Br J Ophthalmol 1995;79:306–312.

74. Vine AK, Tenhaken RK, Diaz RF, et al. A new inexpensive customized plaque for choroidal melanoma iodine-125 plaque therapy. Ophthalmology 1989;96:543–546.

75. Pavlin CJ, Japp B, Simpson ER, et al. Ultrasound determination of the relationship of radioactive plaques to the base of choroidal melanomas. Ophthalmology 1989;96:538–542.

76. Radtke ND, Augsburger JJ, Schmitt T. Management of exudative retinal detachment after plaque therapy for intraocular melanoma. Am J Ophthalmol 1991;112:92–94.

77. Char DH, Lonn LI, Margolis LW. Complications of cobalt plaque therapy of choroidal melanomas. Am J Ophthalmol 1977;84:536–541.

78. Foerster MH, Bornfeld N, Schulz U, et al. Complications of local beta radiation of uveal melanomas. Graefes Arch Clin Exp Ophthalmol 1986;336–340.

79. Summanen P, Immonen I, Kivela T, et al. Radiation related complications after ruthenium plaque radiotherapy of uveal melanoma. Br J Ophthalmol 1996;80:732–739.

80. Stallard HB. Malignant melanoblastoma of the choroid. Mod Prob Ophthalmol 1968;7:16–38.

81. MacFaul PA. Local radiotherapy in the treatment of malignant melanoma of the choroid. Trans Ophthalml Soc UK 1977;97:421–427.

82. Zografos L, Gailloud C. Cobalt plaque treatment of choroidal melanomas. In: Oosterhuis JA ed. Ophthalmic Tumors. Dordrecht, The Netherland Junk Publishers, 1985, pp 87–92.

83. Gass JD. Comparison of prognosis after enucleation vs. cobalt 60 irradiation of melanomas. Arch Ophthalmol 1985;103:916–923.

84. Garretson BR, Robertson DM, Earle JD. Choroidal melanoma treatment with iodine 125 brachytherapy. Arch Ophthalmol 1987;105:1394–1397.

85. Cruess AF, Augsburger JJ, Shields JA, et al. Visual results following cobalt plaque radiotherapy for posterior uveal melanomas. Ophthalmology 1984;91:131–136.

86. Gunduz K, Shields CL, Shields JA, et al. Radiation complications and tumor control after plaque radiotherapy of choroidal melanoma with macular involvement. Am J Ophthalmol 1999;127:579–589.

87. Kellner U, Bornfeld N, Forester MH. Radiation induced optic neuropathy following brachytherapy of uveal melanomas. Graefes Arch Clin Exp Ophthalmol 1993;231:267–270.

88. Summanen P, Immonen I, Kivela T, Tommila P, Heikkonen J, Tarkkanen A. Visual outcome of eyes with malignant melanoma of the uvea after ruthenium plaque radiotherapy. Ophthalm Surg 1995;26:449–460.

89. Char DH, Crawford JB, Kaleta-Michaels S, et al. Analysis of radiation failure after uveal melanoma brachytherapy. Am J Ophthalmol 1989;108:712–716.

90. Coleman DJ, Lizzi FL, Silverman RH, et al. Regression of uveal malignant melanomas following cobalt-60 plaque: Correlates between acoustic spectrum and tumor regression. Retina 1985;5:73–78.

91. Packer S, Stoller S, Lesser ML, Mandel FS, Finger PT. Long-term results of iodine 125 irradiation of uveal melanoma. Ophthalmology 1992;99:767–774.

92. Robertson DM, Earle J, Anderson JA. Preliminary observations regarding the use of iodine-125 in the management of choroidal melanoma. Trans Ophthalmol Soc UK 1983;103:155–160.

93. Tjho-Heslinga RE, Kakebeeke-Kemme HM, Davelaar J, et al. Results of ruthenium irradiation of uveal melanoma. Radiother Oncol 1993;29:33–38.

94. Tjho-Heslinga RE, Davelaar J, Kemme HM, et al. Results of ruthenium irradiation of uveal melanomas: the Dutch experience. Radiother Oncol 1999;53(2):133–137.

95. Duker JS, Augsburger JJ, Shields JA. Noncontiguous local recurrence of posterior uveal melanoma after cobalt 60 episcleral plaque therapy. Arch Ophthalmol 1989;107:1019–1022.

96. Shields CL, Shields JA, Karlsson U, et al. Reasons for enucleation after plaque radiotherapy for posterior uveal melanoma. Clinical findings. Ophthalmology 1989;96:919–924.

97. Lommatzsch PK, Kirsch IH. 106Ru/106Rh plaque radiotherapy for malignant melanomas of the choroid. With follow-up results more than 5 years. Doc Ophthalmol 1988;68:225–238.

98. Char DH, Castro JR, Kroll SM, Orvome AR, Quivey JM, Stone RD. Five-year follow-up of helium ion therapy for uveal melanoma. Ophthalmology 1990;108:209–214.

99. Wilson MW, Hungerford JL. Comparison of episcleral plaque and proton beam radiation therapy for the treatment of choroidal melanoma. Ophthalmology 1999;106:1579–1587.

100. Gragoudas ES, Egan KM, Seddon JM, et al. Intraocular recurrence of uveal melanoma after proton beam irradiation. Ophthalmology 1992;99:760–766.

101. Bercher L, Zografos L, Chamot L, Egger E, Perret C, Uffer S, Gailloud C. Functional results of 450 cases of uveal melanoma treated with proton beam. In: Bornfeld N, Gragoudas ES, Hopping W Lommatzsch PK, Wessing A, Zografos L, eds. Tumors of the Eye. Amsterdam: Kluger, 1991, pp 507–510.

102. Char DK, Kroll SM, Castro J. Ten-year follow-up of helium ion therapy for uveal melanoma. Am J Ophthalmol 1998;125:81–89.

103. Gragoudas ES, Egan KM, Walsh SM, et al. Lens changes after proton beam irradiation for uveal melanoma. Am J Ophthalmol 1995;119:157–164.

104. Meecham WJ, Char DH, Kroll SM, et al. Anterior segment complications after helium ion radiation therapy for uveal melanoma: Radiation cataract. Arch Ophthalmol 1994;112:197–203.

105. Kim MK, Char DH, Castro JL, Saunders WM, Chen GT, Stone RD. Neovascular glaucoma after helium ion irradiation for uveal melanoma. Ophthalmology 1986; 93:189–193.

106. Kincaid MC, Folberg R, Torczynski E, et al. Complications after proton beam therapy for uveal malignant melanoma. A clinical and histopathologic study of five cases. Ophthalmology 1988;95:982–991.

107. Goodman DF, Char DH, Crawford JV, et al. Uveal melanoma necrosis following helium ion therapy. Am J. Ophthalmol 1986;101:643–645.

108. Gragoudas ES, Li W, Ian AM, et al. Risk factors for radiation maculopathy and papillopathy after intraocular irradiation. Ophthalmology 1999;106:1571–15.

109. Guyer DR, Mukai S, Egan KM, Seddon JM, Walsh SM, Gragoudas ES. Radiation maculopathy after proton beam irradiation for choroidal melanoma. Ophthalmology 1992;99:1278–1285.

110. Seddon JM, Gragoudas ES, Polivogianis L, Hsieh CC, Egan KM, Goitein M, Verhey L, Munzenrider J, Austin-Seymour M, Urie M. et al. Visual outcome after proton beam irradiation of uveal melanoma. Ophthalmology 1986;93:666–674.

111. Seddon JM, Gragoudas ES, Egan KM, et al. Uveal melanomas near the optic disc or fovea: Visual results after proton beam irradiation. Ophthalmology 1987;94:354–361.

112. Chinela AB, Zambrano A, Bunge HJ, et al. Gamma knife radiosurgery in uveal melanomas. In: Steiner $$$ et al, eds. Radiosurgery: Baseline and Trends. New York: Raven Press; 1992, p 161–169.

113. Zehetmayer M, Menapace R, Kitz K, Ertl A, Strenn K, Ruhswurm I. Stereotactic irradiation of uveal melanoma with the Leksell gamma unit. In: Wiegel N, Bornfeld MH, Forester W, Hinkelbein W, eds. Radiotherapy of Ocular Disease. Vol. 30. Barel: Karger, 1997, pp 47–55.

114. Zehetmayer M, Menapace R, Kitz K, et al. Stereotactic irradiation of uveal melanoma with the Leksell gamma unit. Front Radiather Oncol 1997;30:47–55.

115. Logani S, Helenowski TK, Thakrar H, Pothiawala B. Gamma knife radiosurgery in the treatment of ocular melanoma. Stereotact Funct Neurosurg 1993;61 (Suppl 1):38–44.

116. Zehetmayer M, Dieckmann K, Kren G, et al. Fractionated stereotactic radiotherapy with linear accelerator for uveal melanoma—Preliminary Vienna results. Strahlenther Onkol 1999;175:74–75.

117. Dieckmann K, Bogner J, Zehtmayer M, et al. A LINAC-based stereotactic irradiation technique of uveal melanoma. Radiother Oncol 2001;61(1):49–56.

118. Girkin CA, Comey CH, Lunsford LV, et al. Radiation ophthalmolopathy after stereotactic radiosurgery. Ophthalmology 1997;104:1634–1643.

119. Marchini G, Babighian S, Tomazzoli L, Gerosa MQ, Nicolato A, Bricolo A, Piovan E, Zampieri PG, Allessandrini F, Benati A. et al. Stereotactic radiosurgery of uveal melanomas: Preliminary results with gamma knife treatment. Stereotact Funct Neurosurg 1995;64(Suppl 1):72–79.

120. Zehtmayer M, Kitz K, Menapace R, et al. Local tumor control and morbidity after one to three fractions of stereotactic external beam irradiation for uveal melanoma. J. Radiother Oncol 2000;55(2):135–144.

121. Langmann G, Pendl G, Klaus-Mullner, et al. Gamma knife radiosurgery for uveal melanomas: an 8-year experience. J Neurosurg 2000;93(Suppl 3): 184–188.

122. Langmann G, Pendl G, Papaefthymiou G, et al. High dose versus low(er) dose in radiosurgery for uveal melanomas with the Leksell gamma knife (abstr). Program of the Xth International Congress of Ocular Oncology Meeting, Amsterdam, the Netherlands, June 17–21, 2001, p 155.

123. Zehetmayer M, Georgopoulos M, Segur-Eltz N, et al. Fractionated stereotatic 6MV LINAC radiotherapy for uveal melanoma (abstr). Program of the Xth International Congress of Ocular Oncology Meeting, Amsterdam, the Netherlands, June 17–21, 2001, p 156.

124. Augsburger JJ, Lauritzen K, Gamel JK, et al. Matched group study of preenucleaton radiotherapy versus enucleation alone for primary malignant melanoma of the choroid and ciliary body. Am J Clin Oncol 1990;13:382–387.

125. Char DH, Phillips TL. Pre-enucleation irradiation of uveal melanoma. Br J Ophthalmol 1985;69:177–179.

126. Char DH, Phillips TL, Andejeski Y, et al. Failure of preenucleation radiation to decrease uveal melanoma mortality. Am J Ophthalmol 1988;106:21–26.

127. Collaborative Ocular Melanoma Study Group. The collaborative ocular melanoma study (COMS) randomized trial of pre-enucleation radiation of large choroidal melanoma II: COMS report no. 10. Initial mortality findings. Am J Ophthalmol 1998;125:779–796.

128. Gunlap I, Batioglu F. Effect of pre-enucleation irradiation on the survival of patients with uveal melanoma. Ophthalmologica 1998;212:231–235.

129. Luyten GP, Mooy CM, Eijkenboon WM, et al. No demonstrated effect of pre-enucleation irradiation on survival of patients with uveal melanoma. Am J Ophthalmol 1995;119:786–791.

130. Collaborative Ocular Melanoma Study (COMS). Randomized trial of pre-enucleation radiation of large choroidal melanoma III: local complications and observations following enucleation. COMS report no. 11. Am J Ophthalmol 1998;126:362–372.

131. Bollemiher JG, Lagendijk JJ, van Best JA, et al. Effects of microwave-induced hyperthermia on the anterior segment of healthy rabbit eyes. Graefes Arch Ophthalmol 1989;227:271–276.

132. Finger PT. Microwave thermoradiotherapy for uveal melanoma. Results of a 10-year study. Ophthalmology 1997;104:1794–1803.

133. Finger PT, Packer S, Svitra PP, et al. Thermoradiotherapy for intraocular tumors. Arch Ophthalmol 1985;103:1574–1578.

134. Finger PT, Packer S, Svitra PP, et al. Hyperthermic treatment of intraocular tumors. Arch Ophthalmol 1984;102:1477–1481.

135. Coleman DJ, Lizzi FL, Burgess SEP, et al. Ultrasonic hyperthermia and radiation in the management of intraocular malignant melanoma. Am J Ophthalmol 1986;101:635–642.

136. Naumann GOH, Rummelt, V. Block excision of tumors of the anterior uvea. Ophthalmology 1996;103:2017–2028.

137. Char DH, Crawford JB, Miller T. Eye wall resection of uveal tumors. Trans Am Ophthalmol Soc 2000;98:153–159.

138. Peyman GA, Gremillion CM. Eye wall resection in the management of uveal neoplasms. Jpn J Ophthalmol 1989;33:458–471.

139. Shields JA, Augsberger JJ, Stefanyszyn MA, et al. Sclerochorioretinal resection for choroidal melanoma. A clinicopathologic correlation of a post mortem eye. Ophthalmology 1984;91:1726–1730.

140. Shields JA. Local resection of posterior uveal melanoma. Br J Ophthalmol 1996;80:97–98.

141. Shields JA, Shields CL, Shah P, Sivalingam V, Partial lamellar sclerouvectomy for ciliary body and choroidal tumors. Ophthalmology 1991;98:971–983.

142. Shields JA, Shields CL. Surgical approach to lamellar sclerouvectomy for posterior uveal melanomas. The 1986 Schoenberg Lecture. Ophthalm Surg 1988;19:774–780.

143. Todd JG, Colvin JR. Ophthalmic surgery. In: MacRae WR, Wildsmith JAW, eds. Induced Hypotension. London: Elsevier Science, 1991; pp 257–269.

144. Damato B, Foulds WS. Indications for trans-scleral local resection of uveal melanoma. Br J Ophthalmol 1996;80:1029–1030.

145. Damato BE, Paul J, Foulds WS. Predictive factors of visual outcome after local resection of choroidal melanoma. Br J Ophthalmol 1993;77:616–623.

146. Peyman GA, Juarezs CP, Diamond JG, et al. Ten years experience with eye wall resection for uveal malignant melanomas. Ophthalmology 1984;91:1720–1725.

147. Kara GB. Excision of uveal melanomas: A 15-year experience. Trans Am Acad Ophthalmol Otol 1979;86:997–1023.

148. Damato BE. Adjunctive plaque radiotherapy after local resection of uveal melanoma. Front Radiat Ther Oncol 1997;30:123–132.

149. Damato BE, Paul J, Foulds WS. Risk factors for residual and recurrent uveal melanoma after trans-scleral local resection. Br J Ophthalmol 1996;80:102–108.

150. Damato BE, Groenewald C, McGalliard J, Wong D. Endoresection of choroidal melanoma. Br J Ophthalmol 1998;82:213–218.

151. Kertes PJ, Johnson JC, Peyman GA Internal resection of posterior uveal melanomas. Br J Ophthalmol 1998;82:1147–1153.

152. Peyman GA, Nelson NC Jr, Paris CL, et al. Internal choroidectomy of posterior uveal melanomas under a retinal flap. Int Ophthalmol 1992;16:439–444.

153. Peyman TGA, Charles H. Internal eye wall resection in the management of uveal melanoma. Can J Ophthalmol 1988;23:2190–2223.

154. Lee KJ, Peyman GA, Raichand S. Internal eye wall resection for posterior uveal melanoma. Jpn J Ophthalmol 1993;37:287–292.

155. Bornfield N, Talies S, Horstmann GA, Radiosurgical treatment of large uveal melanoma as a presurgical procedure (abstr). Program of the Xth International Congress of Ocular Oncology Meeting, Amsterdam, the Netherlands, June 17–21, 2001, p 154.

156. McLean IW, Foster WD, Zimmerman LE, Uveal melanoma: Location, size, cell type, and enucleation as risk factors in metastasis. Hum Pathol 1982;13:123–132.

157. Zimmerman LE, McLean IW. An evaluation of enucleation in the management of uveal melanomas. Am J Ophthalmol 1979;87:741–760.

158. Zimmerman LE, McLean IW, Foster WD Does enucleation of the eye containing a malignant melanoma prevent or accelerate the dissemination of tumour cells? Br J Ophthalmol 1978;62:420–425.

159. Zimmerman LE, McLean IW, Foster WD. Statistical analysis of follow-up data concerning uveal melanomas, and the influence of enucleation. Ophthalmology 1980;87:557–564.

160. Fraunfelder FT, Boozman FW, Wilson RA, et al. No-touch technique for intraocular malignant tumors. Arch Ophthalmol 1977;95:1616–1620.

161. Wilson RA, Fraunfelder FT. "No-touch" cryosurgical enucleation: A minimal trauma technique for eyes harboring intraocular malignancy. Ophthalmology 1978;85:1170–1175.

162. Seregard S. Long-term survival after ruthenium plaque radiotherapy for uveal melanoma. A meta-analysis of studies including 1,066 patients. Acta Ophthalmol Scand 1999;77:414–417.

163. Kiehl H, Kirsch I. Treatment of malignant choroidal melanomas: Comparison of survival after consecutive (106Ru/106Rh applicator) treatment and enucleation, first results of a GDR-wide study, 1960–1980. In: Lommatzsch PK, Blodi FC, eds. Intraocular Tumors. New York: Springer-Verlag 1983, pp 109–112.

164. Seddon JM, Gragoudas ES, Albert DM, et al. Comparison of survival rates for patients with uveal melanoma after treatment with proton beam irradiation or enucleation. Am J Ophthalmol 1985;99:282–290.

165. Augsburger JJ, Gamel JW, Sardi VF, et al. Enucleation vs cobalt plaque radiotherapy for malignant melanomas of the choroid and ciliary body. Arch Ophthalmol 1986;104:655–661.

166. Diener-West M, Earle JD, Fine SL, et al. The COMS randomized trial of iodine 125 brachytherapy for choroidal melanoma: III. Initial mortality findings. COMS Report No. 18. Arch Ophthalmol 2001 119(7):969–983.

167. Pach JM, Robertson DM, Taney BS, Martin JA, Campbell RJ, O'Brien PC. Prognostic factors in choroidal and ciliary body melanomas with extrascleral extension. Am J Ophthalmol 1986;101:321–331.

168. Shammas HF, Blodi FC. Orbital extension of choroidal and ciliary body melanomas. Arch Ophthalmol 1977;95:2002–2005.

169. Weissgold DJ, Gragoudas ES, Green JP, et al. Eye-sparing treatment of massive extrascleral extension of choroidal melanoma. Arch Ophthalmol 1998;116:531–533.

170. Hykin PG, McCartney ACE, Plowman PN, et al. Postenucleation orbital radiotherapy for the treatment of malignant melanoma of the choroid with extrascleral extension. Br J Ophthalmol 1990;74:36–39.

171. Sloan GH, McNab AA. Complications of hydroxyapatite implants. Ophthalmology 1997;104:1982.

172. Shields JA, Augsburger JJ, Corwin, S., et al. The management of uveal melanomas with extrascleral extension. Orbit 1986;6:31–37.

173. Wolter JR. Epibulbar extension of a choroidal melanoma treated with tenonectomy. Ophthalm Surg 1974;5:48–52.

174. Wolter JR. Tenonectomy. Treatment of epibulbar extension of choroidal melanomas. Arch Ophthalmol 1971;86:529–533.

175. Starr HJ, Zimmerman LE. Extrascleral extension and orbital recurrence of malignant melanomas of the choroid and ciliary body. Int Ophthalmol Clin 1962;2:369–384.

176. Kersten RC, Tse DT, Anderson RL, Blodi FC. The role of orbital exenteration in choroidal melanoma with extrascleral extension. Ophthalmology 1985;92:436–443.

177. Rini FJ, Jakobiec FA, Hornblass A, et al. The treatment of advanced choroidal melanoma with massive orbital extension. Am J Ophthalmol 1987;104:634–640.

178. Carrasco CH, Wallace S, Charnsangavej C, et al. Treatment of hepatic metastases in ocular melanoma. Embolization of the hepatic artery with polyvinyl sponge and cisplatin. JAMA 1986;255:3152–3154.

179. Fornier GA, Albert DM, Arrigg CA, et al. Resection of solitary metastasis: Approach to palliative treatment of hepatic involvement and choroidal melanoma. Arch Ophthalmol 1984;102:80–82.

180. Leyvraz S, Spataro V, Bauer J, Pampallona S, Salmon R, Dorval T, Meuli R, Gillet M, Lejeune F, Zografos L. Treatment of ocular melanoma metastatic to the liver by hepatic arterial chemotherapy. J Clin Oncol 1997;15:2589–2595.

181. Mavligit GM, Charnsangavej C, Carrasco H, et al. Regression of ocular melanoma metastatic to the liver after hepatic arterial chemoembolization with cisplatin and polyvinyl sponge. JAMA 1988;260:974–976.

182. Bedikian AY, Legha SS, Mavligit G, Carrasco CH, Khorana S, Plager C, Papadopoulos N, Benjamin RS. Treatment of uveal melanoma metastatic to the liver: a review of the MD Anderson Cancer Center experience and prognostic factors. Cancer 1995;76:1665–1670.

183. Creagan ET, Suman VJ, Dalton RJ, et al. Phase III clinical trial of the combination of cisplatin, dacarbazine, and carmustine with or without tamoxifen in patients with advanced malignant melanoma. J Clin Oncol 1999;17:1884–1890.

184. Sellami M, Weil M, Dhermy P, et al. Adjuvant chemotherapy in ocular malignant melanoma. Oncology 1986;43:221.

185. Young DW, Lever RS, English JS, MacKie RM. The use of BELD combination chemotherapy (bleomycin, vindesine CN, and DTIC) in advanced malignant melanoma. Cancer 1985;55:1879–1881.

186. Falkson CI, Ibrahim J, Kirkwood JM, et al. Phase III trial of dacarbazine versus dacarbazine with interferon alpha-2b versus dacarbazine with tamoxifen versus dacarbazine with interferon alpha-2b and tamoxifen in patients with metastatic malignant melanoma: An Eastern Cooperative Oncology Group Study. J Clin Oncol 1998;16:1743–1493.

187. Keilholz U, Goey SH, Punt CJA., et al. Interferon alfa-2a and interleukin-2 with or without cisplatin in metastatic melanoma: A randomized trial of the European Organization for Research and Treatment of Cancer Melanoma Cooperative Group. J Clin Oncol 1997;2:127–131.

188. Kath R, Hayungs J, Bornfeld N, Sauerwein W, Hoffken K, Seeber S. Prognosis and treatment of disseminated uveal melanoma. Cancer 1993;72:2219–2223.

189. Hoon DS, Okamoto T, Wang HJ, et al. Is the survival of melanoma patients receiving polyvalent melanoma cell vaccine linked to the human leukocyte antigen phenotype of patients? J Clin Oncol 1998;16:1430–1437.

190. McLean IW, Berd D, Mastrangelo MJ, et al. A randomized study of methanol-extraction residue of bacille Calmette-Guérin as postsurgical adjuvant therapy of uveal melanoma. Am J Ophthalmol 1990;110:522–526.

191. Spitler LE, del Rio, M., Khentigan, A., et al. Therapy of patients with malignant melanoma using a monoclonal antimelanoma antibody-ricin A chain immunotoxin. Cancer Res 1987;1717–1723.

192. Mitchell MS, Liggett PE, Green RL, et al. Sustained regression of a primary choroidal melanoma under the influence of a therapeutic melanoma vaccine. J Clin Oncol 1994;12:396–401.

16

The Treatment of Retinoblastoma

DAVID H. ABRAMSON and AMY C. SCHEFLER

New York Presbyterian Hospital, New York, New York, U.S.A.

I. INTRODUCTION

A. Historical Perspective and Present Survival

Retinoblastoma, first described by Pawius in 1657, virtually disappeared from the medical literature for 150 years [1]. Between 1767 and 1847, numerous cases were reported in Europe. In 1809, Wardrop published 35 cases of retinoblastoma treated successfully with enucleation, after which enucleations for retinoblastoma became widespread [2]. In the United States, the first case report appeared in 1818 in the register of The New York Hospital. The modern era of radiotherapy began with Reese and Martin at the Columbia Presbyterian Medical Center in New York in 1936 [1].

Survival rates for retinoblastoma patients in the developed world have increased dramatically over the past century. The mortality of retinoblastoma was reported as 87% in 1897 in children who were treated with enucleation and 41% in all children in 1931 [1]. Seventy-five years ago, retinoblastoma was rarely detected at an early stage, and the thought of retaining an affected eye with useful vision was inconceivable [3]. In contrast, recent cancer registry reports in Europe and the United States have demonstrated 5-year survival rates of 90 and 98% respectively [4,5]. The improved survival rate is due to earlier detection of the tumor and improved techniques for local tumor control rather than a change in the natural history of the disease [6]. In stark contrast to developed countries, developing nations report dramatically low survival rates, as patients in these countries typically present with widespread metastatic disease (Table 1) [7–13].

Table 1 Five-Year Survival Rates from Recent Retinoblastoma Series in the Developing
World

Author(s)	Year of report	Location	No. of patients in report	5-year survival rate
Saw et al. [7]	2000	Singapore	69	83%[a]
Wessels et al. [8]	1996	Tygerberg, South Africa	15	46%
Gunalp et al. [9]	1996	Ankara, Turkey	636	82%
Nandakumar et al. [10]	1996	Bangalore, India	24	73%
Ajaiyeoba et al. [11]	1993	Ibadan, Nigeria	44	43%
Erwenne et al. [13]	1989	Sao Paulo, Brazil	158	64%[a]
Sha [12]	1988	Zhengzhou, China	100	58%

[a] Three-year survival rate reported only.

B.   Goals of Treatment

The primary goal of retinoblastoma treatment is to ensure the survival of these
children. Secondary but also important goals include retention of the eye(s) and of
vision. A final goal is the avoidance of facial bony deformities or other physical
changes that can affect functional well-being [3].

C.   Unique Challenges in the Treatment of Retinoblastoma

Since 1949, clinicians involved in the treatment of retinoblastoma patients have
recognized that second nonocular cancers can develop years after successful
treatment of the primary disease [14]. It is important that young patients, as well
as their parents be counseled regarding their risk for additional malignancies and the
need for appropriate screening. The relationship between treatment type, genetics,
and the risk for additional nonocular tumors is complex and was elucidated
primarily at our center, where we have followed a large cohort of patients since 1916.
This extensive follow-up period has enabled us to assess specific risk factors
associated with the development of second cancers, as discussed in Sec. III.

D.   Diagnostic Considerations

1.   Extent of Disease Workup

Patients suspected to have retinoblastoma should undergo indirect ophthalmoscopy
and fundus photography as well as ophthalmic ultrasonography. Ultrasonography
can be useful for this disease, as it demonstrates masses with high reflectivity that
block sound, causing characteristic shadowing behind the tumor [6]. False-positive
results on ultrasound are not uncommon, however. Needle biopsies are rarely if ever
indicated in retinoblastoma, as puncturing of the eye can lead to tumor seeding and
orbital invasion [6].

Computed tomography (CT) scans may no longer be appropriate for
retinoblastoma patients, as a recent analysis has demonstrated an increased lifetime

risk of other cancers in pediatric patients subjected to this imaging modality [15]. Instead, as part of an extent of disease workup, magnetic resonance imaging (MRI) is routinely performed. In addition to its excellent resolution in the diagnosis of extraocular soft tissue disease, MRI can readily distinguish between retinoblastoma and Coats disease, as due to proteinaceous exudate, Coats disease appears brighter than retinoblastoma on T2-weighted images [6]. One disadvantage of MRI is that calcification, a key feature of retinoblastoma, is more easily demonstrated with CT than MRI.

2.   An Approach to the Treatment and Examination Schedule

In our center, 28 months is the oldest age at which a patient with a positive family history of retinoblastoma has developed his or her first tumor in a previously documented disease-free eye [16]. As a result, we have developed a predesigned examination schedule for newborns with a positive family history of retinoblastoma, in whom screening is initiated at birth. Infants are examined in the newborn nursery within 24–48 hr of birth and again at 3, 6, and 10 weeks of age. All of these initial examinations are performed without anesthesia. Serial examinations are typically performed at 16, 24, 34, 44, and 54 weeks of age under general anesthesia. Following the 54-week examination, patients are examined every 12 weeks until they are at least 28 months of age.

For all patients who are referred to our center with suspected retinoblastoma other than those described above, no predesigned examination schedule has been developed. The reason for this practice is that the rate of formation of new retinoblastoma foci, the rate of recurrence of previously treated tumors, and the rate of formation of tumors in the fellow eye vary widely from patient to patient. The examination and treatment schedule is highly individualized and catered toward the patient's specific risk factors.

Treatment approaches for retinoblastoma are based on whether the patient presents with extraocular or intraocular disease. The treatment of extraocular disease is reviewed in Chap. 23. A discussion of the treatment of intraocular disease follows.

II.   TREATMENT OF INTRAOCULAR DISEASE

A.   Enucleation

1.   History

The first surgical removal of an eye was an unsuccessful attempt performed by Hayes in 1767 [17]. James Wardrop was the first to propose early enucleation in a publication. He published 35 cases in 1809, after which time the clinical application of enucleation became widespread [2]. Currently, enucleation is the most commonly employed technique for treating retinoblastoma.

2. Indications

The patients considered for enucleation are those with unilateral or bilateral Reese-Ellsworth Group V eyes, patients with active tumor in a blind eye, and patients who develop glaucoma from tumor invasion. Patients are also considered for enucleation if they have failed all other forms of treatment or if they active tumor and cannot be followed [3].

3. Technique

In children, enucleation is performed under general anesthesia, though the patients do not require overnight hospitalization. A dilated fundoscopic exam is performed on both eyes prior to surgery. Critical elements of the surgery include avoiding any perforation of the globe and obtaining a long stump of optic nerve. To avoid perforation of the globe, the Brown-Addison forceps are preferred for aiding in traction. In the past, a suture was passed through the stump of the medial rectus muscle, resulting in several cases of inadvertent needle penetration into the eye and rupture of the globe [18]. To obtain a long stump of optic nerve, a gently curved enucleation scissors is used with a nasal approach and the nerve is cut in one motion. A silicone or plastic ball is inserted in place of the eye, and 3 weeks later a thin prosthesis similar to a contact lens is molded and painted by an ocularist to match the fellow eye.

4. Results

Greater than 99% of patients with unilateral retinoblastoma without microscopic or macroscopic extraocular disease are cured by enucleation [19]. The balls rarely need to be replaced, and the prosthesis is removed once a month to once a year for cleaning.

5. Complications

The main complications of enucleation are hemorrhage and infection. Hemorrhage is best controlled during surgery with direct digital pressure and, if necessary, thrombin-soaked patties, FloSeal, or Avitene (bovine collagen). Postoperative ecchymosis usually subsides with use of a pressure patch and ice compresses. Infection is rare in patients who are not receiving chemotherapy. Those patients who develop recurrent infections of the socket are managed effectively with topical antibiotic therapy. Giant papillary conjunctivitis (GPC) may develop years after successful prosthesis fitting and is treated with topical mast-cell stabilizers.

B. External-Beam Radiation

1. History

External-beam radiation therapy (EBR) has been successfully employed for retinoblastoma since Hilgartner experimented with x-ray treatments in Austin, Texas, in 1903 [20]. Early experience demonstrated the efficacy of tumor regression with radiation therapy. However, significant complications were frequently observed due to the techniques employed [14,21]. Complications included keratitis sicca, keratinization of conjunctiva and sclera, lacrimal gland atrophy/fibrosis, loss of lashes, corneal ulcers/perforation, hyphema, rubeosis iridis, glaucoma, iritis/uveitis, cataract, vitreous hemorrhage, retinal vascular damage, optic nerve infarction, fat atrophy in the orbit, and arrest of orbital growth [3]. Currently most of these complications have been eliminated or minimized by reducing the total radiation dose, by changing the source of radiation and positioning of the portals, and by utilizing fractionated doses.

2. Indications

EBR is one means of preserving vision in a child with retinoblastoma [18]. Unlike focal therapies—including photocoagulation, cryotherapy, and episcleral plaque therapy—fractionated external-beam radiation provides an excellent opportunity for useful vision in a macula undestroyed by tumor. EBR is considered as a primary treatment option in children with small tumors located within the macula, since treatment options other than systemic chemotherapy often destroy central vision. EBR is also considered for multifocal tumors for which focal therapy is ineffective. In cases of bilateral advanced intraocular disease in which clinical judgment cannot predict which eye is more likely to have useful vision, EBR can be used bilaterally. In these cases, one or both eyes may eventually require salvage enucleation. EBR is often the salvage treatment of choice after focal therapies have failed. Finally, for children with advanced extraocular or metastatic disease, radiation therapy also plays a role in palliation and even potential cure of these sites along with chemotherapy [18].

3. Technique

Radiation therapy for retinoblastoma in the unenucleated eye is designed to encompass the entire tumor-bearing portion of the globe and at least 1 cm of optic nerve. The fields are designed so that the radiosensitive lens receives a significantly lower dose than the tumor. For children with bilateral disease, parallel opposing lateral D-shaped fields are used to avoid subsequent radiation-induced cataracts, which are more common when anterior fields are used [22]. Fields are designed using a CT simulator or plain films taken in the conventional radiation therapy simulator unit. Information about globe size and lens position is derived from a head CT or MRI study. For children with bilateral disease who have had one eye enucleated, a similar field arrangement is employed that involves a single field or bilateral fields, with the empty orbit receiving some exit dose of radiation. For patients with unilateral disease, a pair of superior and anterior wedged oblique "D" fields are used, with more radiation supplied to the superior oblique field to avoid a significant exit dose to the frontal lobe [23].

The dose prescribed to the retinal target volume ranges from 4200 to 4600 cGy. Children under the age of 6 months typically receive lower doses, while children with advanced bilateral disease receive higher doses [6,18]. The dose is administered in 180 to 200 cGy daily fractions five times per week.

4.   Results

Survival of children who undergo external beam radiation in the United States is 85–100%, mirroring the excellent survival rates of children with this disease in general [18]. Local control in the radiated eye, defined as preservation of the eye, varies in different series from 58 to 88% [18,24–29]. In our series, preservation of the eye is 95% for Reese-Ellsworth stage I to III eyes that are treated with the lateral beam technique. Radiation therapy has only a 50% local control rate in Reese-Ellsworth stages IV and V [18]. Location of the tumor determines the likelihood that it will respond to EBR: tumors in the posterior pole tend to have the best results with this treatment.

Five regression patterns have been described following EBR for retinoblastoma [30]. Larger tumors are more likely to form a type I pattern. In this pattern, the tumor shrinks in size, loses vascularity, and forms an irregular, glistening white mass. This mass consists of DNA-calcium complexes that continue to change in shape and shrink over time [3,18]. Tumors as large as 15 disc diameters (dd) have been found to undergo this type of regression, although the median size of tumors that form a type I pattern is 5 dd. In the type II pattern, a gray, translucent color develops and there is less shrinkage and no calcification. These tumors may occasionally reactivate. The type III pattern is a combination of types I and II and is the type observed most frequently. The center of the tumor becomes calcified and is surrounded by a variable amount of amorphous translucent gray remnants. The type IV pattern is most often observed after the use of plaque radiotherapy and manifests itself as destruction of the overlying retina with a white appearance signifying visible sclera. In recent years, a fifth regression pattern has been observed, labeled type 0. This pattern describes a situation in which the posttreatment examination reveals no evidence of the previously existing retinoblastoma. It is uncommon except in the smallest tumors.

The pretreatment size of the tumor is the most important predictor of the regression pattern. In one study, the median size of 58 tumors that disappeared after radiation was 1 dd, and 95% of those that disappeared were 3 dd or less. The median size of 26 tumors that formed a type I regression pattern was 5 dd; 23% of these were 3 dd or less [31].

5.   Complications

All patients experience skin erythema within the area of the radiation portal, but the skin rarely becomes infected. For patients with lesions between the equator and the ora serrata, the anterior edge of the field is brought forward to include the lens, increasing the risk for a cataract [18].

Another potential side effect of EBR is damage to the vascular endothelium. Injury ranges from optic nerve damage to total retinal vascular occlusion and vitreous hemorrhage. At the doses currently employed, the incidence of vascular complications is approximately 5% [3].

Facial and temporal bone hypoplasia can occur following EBR in very young children. This deformity is most marked when both eyes are treated with parallel opposing fields and when children are treated under the age of 6 months [32]. With the use of the three field–modified lateral beam technique described above, hypoplasia is minimized because of the smaller entrance dose at each of the three fields.

The most serious complication of EBR is an increased risk of second nonocular tumors in children with the genetic form of retinoblastoma (see Sec. III). Because of this risk, there has been a renewed interest in focal treatments such as cryotherapy and photocoagulation for children with intraocular disease.

C. Brachytherapy

1. History

Episcleral brachytherapy was pioneered in 1933 by the British ophthalmologist Henry Stallard [33]. He utilized cobalt applicators that were curved to fit the child's eye with suture holes built in to attach the plaque to the sclerae. Plaques were left in place for 3–7 days and radiation was delivered at 4000 cGy to the tumor apex. The current technique is similar but refined.

2. Indications

Over the last few years, plaques have been used more commonly as primary therapy due to the increasing awareness among clinicians of the potential for secondary cancer development when EBR is given to certain patients. Relative indications for plaques include tumors that are classified as Reese-Ellsworth Stage IVa or less, tumors that are between 4 and 10 dd in size, and tumors that do not involve the macula. Brachytherapy can also be used as a salvage technique in eyes that have failed other types of therapy including EBR, photocoagulation, or cryotherapy. Relative contraindications to brachytherapy include tumors larger than 10 dd, tumors that involve the macula, and tumors that have produced total vitreous seeding [34].

3. Technique

^{125}I is currently the most commonly used isotope in brachytherapy for retinoblastoma. This isotope is advantageous because the radioactive seeds can be placed into a custom-built plaque designed to match the size of the lesion. The gold shields of ^{125}I plaques also minimize excess radiation exposure for the patient, the patient's family, and the medical staff [18]. Plaques composed of other isotopes have also been employed with success. These include beta sources such as ruthenium.

Plaque placement is performed in the operating room, typically under general anesthesia. First, the conjunctiva is dissected from the limbus in the quadrant harboring the tumor. If an extraocular muscle overlies the tumor, the muscle is disinserted. The tumor is carefully localized with the indirect ophthalmoscope, and diathermy or ink marks are placed to record the tumor's position. A dummy plaque of exactly the same size and with identical suture holes as the active plaque is attached to the sclera. The plaque placement is confirmed with the indirect ophthalmoscope and then the active plaque is inserted. The dose is 4000–4500 cGy to the apex of the tumor at a rate of approximately 1000 cGy per day. The plaque is removed in a second operation 3–5 days later, depending on the isotope used and the size of the tumor. The regression response most commonly seen after removal is a type 4 pattern.

4. Results

A tumor recurrence rate of 12% at 1 year posttreatment has been reported when plaques are used as primary treatment for retinoblastoma [35]. Figures 1 and 2 demonstrate a large retinoblastoma before and after brachytherapy was used as primary treatment. Plaques can even be successful when used as salvage therapy for eyes that have failed other treatment methods. Our group reported a overall success rate for salvage brachytherapy of 50% [36]. Shields et al. recently reported on 148 tumors treated after failure of other methods [35]. Tumor recurrence at 1 year was detected in 8% of tumors previously treated with chemoreduction, 25% of tumors previously treated with external-beam radiotherapy, 34% tumors previously treated with both chemoreduction and external-beam radiotherapy, and 8% of tumors previously treated with laser photocoagulation, thermotherapy, or cryotherapy. Risks for tumor recurrence included the presence of tumor seeds in the vitreous, the presence of subretinal tumor seeds, and increasing patient age. In all cases, visual results depend on the size and location of the tumor(s) initially.

5. Complications

Side effects from brachytherapy for retinoblastoma are rare. Low rates of optic neuropathy and radiation retinopathy arc reported [18]. Cataracts can occur when both cobalt and iodine plaques are placed on anteriorly located tumors. The cataracts can take years to become evident and often do not require surgery. Plaques have not been shown to increase the incidence of second tumors in patients who have also received external-beam radiation [18].

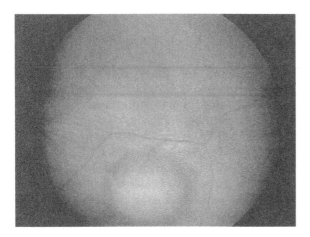

Figure 1 Retinoblastoma in a premature infant prior to placement of a radioactive ruthenium plaque.

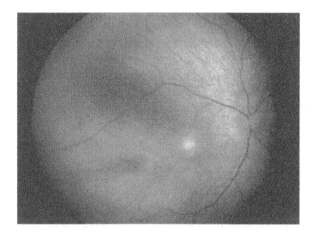

Figure 2   Appearance of the same lesion 2 months after treatment with the plaque.

D. Photocoagulation

1. History

Attempts to treat retinoblastoma without removing the eye were attempted as early as 1830, but it was not until the twentieth century that successful focal treatment became feasible. It is only during the past 50 years that retinoblastoma has been managed consistently without enucleation [37]. In 1953, Weve reported on the use of diathermy for the treatment of retinoblastoma tumor foci [38]. Light coagulation with the xenon arc photocoagulator was first described by Meyer-Schwickerath in 1957, initially for the purpose of closing macular holes and then for different diseases including the treatment of retinoblastoma.

2. Mechanism of Action

After passing through the anterior chamber, the laser burns the tiny blood vessels that supply the tumor and the tumor begins to involute within 1 week of treatment. Traditionally, xenon arc photocoagulation (wavelength 250–1500 nm) was used, but currently tumors can be treated with argon lasers in the visible range (wavelength 488–536 nm) or diode/infrared lasers in the invisible range (wavelength 810 nm) with success [6].

3. Indications

Photocoagulation is employed as primary treatment for selected small retinoblastomas. The following tumor features correlate with the success of photocoagulation: small size (less than 3 dd in diameter), anterior location, and low elevation (tumor equal to or less than half the base diameter) [37]. Photocoagulation is not used for tumors that involve the optic disc or fovea, as this technique would result in loss of central vision. In such cases, EBR was commonly employed in the past, and currently either EBR or chemoreduction are typically utilized.

4. Technique

Patients are treated while under general anesthesia with their pupils dilated. The light is aimed through the anterior chamber at the tumor's feeding vessels. One to three barriers of photocoagulation burns are applied without ever treating the tumor itself. With xenon arc photocoagulation, the light source is inhomogeneous, with a central hot spot that is heated more rapidly. The center of the burn becomes white while the edge becomes gray [37].

5. Results

Our group previously reported on the treatment of 278 retinoblastoma tumors at our center with photocoagulation, more than 70% of which were cured [37]. The mean number of photocoagulation sessions required for the tumors that were cured was 1.3. Of the tumors that failed photocoagulation, 44% went on to develop vitreous seeding and 55% required enucleation. Of eyes that were treated initially with photocoagulation, 50% went on to develop new local tumor foci. In all cases, new tumor foci appeared anterior to the equator. Patients who developed additional tumors in the eye were younger when photocoagulated (mean age, 5.5 months) than those who did not develop additional tumors (mean age, 47.8 months). We currently follow tumors that are treated with photocoagulation for at least 3 years before a cure is considered to be certain.

6. Complications

Potential complications of photocoagulation include cataracts, iris burns, vitreous hemorrhage, and traction effects.

E. Transpupillary Thermotherapy (TTT)

1. History

Transpupillary thermotherapy (TTT) was first used as treatment for retinoblastoma by Lagendijk, although other researchers in the Netherlands had previously studied its use as treatment for choroidal melanoma [39]. In 1982, Lagendijk designed a microwave applicator to deliver whole-eye hyperthermia and administered the treatment to two patients with recurrent retinoblastoma, both of whose disease regressed.

2. Mechanism of Action

The mechanism by which TTT causes tumor cell death is different from the mechanism by which classic laser photocoagulation destroys tumors. With TTT, the temperature is thought to be lower (45–60°C), and the thermal effect leads to apoptosis rather than burning. Because the effects of TTT rely on the direct killing of tumor cells, the laser beam is aimed directly at the tumor rather than at the feeding vessels as in photocoagulation.

3. Indications

Indications for TTT have not yet been established. In the largest series to date, patients with viable retinoblastoma within the retina or subretinal space with less than 1.0 mm of overlying subretinal fluid were included [40]. Larger tumors and vitreous seeding from the tumor to be treated with TTT were criteria for exclusion. Our group frequently treats only tumors that are 3 mm or less in base diameter that are not located in the periphery. Unlike the case with photocoagulation, peripapillary tumors can be treated effectively with TTT because the tumors, rather than their vascular beds, are treated directly. With photocoagulation, treatment in this area is often unsuccessful because it requires destruction of the feeding vessels, and the blood supply in the peripapillary area is extremely dense.

4. Technique

Thermal energy is delivered from an 810 mm infrared ophthalmic laser with modifications to the laser's hardware and software. Three different TTT techniques are utilized for the treatment of retinoblastoma. The first technique, described by Murphree et al. [41] and Murphree and Munier [42], utilizes a pediatric laser gonioscopy lens and an adaptor on the operating room microscope that delivers a transpupillary 3.0-mm spot of radiation. The power is set at 350–1500 mW and treatment typically lasts 1 min. Alternatively, the treatment can be delivered using an adaptor on the indirect ophthalmoscope and a 20 or 28D lens, which delivers a transpupillary 1.6-mm spot of radiation. For this technique, the power is also set at 350–1500 mW and treatment is performed for approximately 1 min. Finally, the radiation can be delivered transconjunctivally via Diopexy probe. For this technique, 1 min of treatment is performed using a handheld adaptor that delivers a 1-mm spot of radiation on a power setting of 500–1500 mW.

5. Results and Complications

In vitro and animal studies [43,44] demonstrating a synergistic effect of TTT and chemotherapy or EBR have prompted several studies exploring the use of TTT with single- or multiple-agent systemic chemotherapy in retinoblastoma patients [41–48]. Our unpublished experience has shown that the majority of retinoblastomas that are 3.0 mm or less in base diameter and not located in the periphery respond to TTT when it is combined with other therapies. Tumors typically regress to flat, pale scars that are less than 2 mm in size. Tumors that are close to the fovea can be treated successfully with no traction effects. Complications include cataracts, scarring/banding, and visual field defects.

Shields et al. have published the largest series of retinoblastomas treated with chemotherapy to date: 188 retinoblastomas in 80 eyes of 58 patients [40]. A total of 118 tumors were treated simultaneously with systemic chemotherapy and TTT; mean follow-up was 12 months. While 86% of the tumors demonstrated regression, complications were significant and included focal paraxial lens opacity (24%), sector optic disc atrophy (12%), retinal traction (5%), optic disc edema (5%), retinal vascular occlusion (2%), serous retinal detachment (2%), and corneal edema (1%). Focal iris atrophy, the most common complication (36%), was most strongly associated with an increasing number of treatment sessions ($p = 0.001$) and an increasing tumor base diameter ($p = 0.02$). Further studies with longer patient follow-up are needed to resolve questions related to tumor recurrence and ocular complications from TTT.

F. Cryotherapy

1. History

Cryotherapy was first introduced by Lincoff in 1967 in a report on one small peripheral retinoblastoma [49]. The use of cryotherapy for intraocular retinoblastoma quickly became widespread in many centers throughout the world. By 1969, Ellsworth noted that cryotherapy was as effective as photocoagulation for the treatment of small tumors [50].

2. Mechanism of Action

The tumor tissue is frozen rapidly ($-90°C/min$), resulting in intracellular ice crystal formation, protein denaturation, pH changes, and finally cell membrane rupture [51,52]. Cryotherapy also causes cell death by destroying circulation during the freeze via damage to the vascular endothelium and decreased blood flow. Platelet plugs are then formed that induce thrombosis, and the resulting ischemia leads to infarction within minutes or hours [53–55]. Cryotherapy may also influence tumor cell destruction by stimulating an immune reaction [56].

3. Indications

Cryotherapy may be used as the primary treatment for small peripheral retinoblastomas or as secondary treatment for recurrent tumors treated previously with EBR. Retinoblastomas that are successfully treated with cryotherapy include small tumors (less than 3–4 dd) not located at the vitreous base. Tumors with widespread vitreous seeding typically are not best treated with this method [57–59]. However, cryotherapy is uniquely useful for tumors with localized vitreous seeding overlying the tumor apex. In these cases, the freeze is extended in area to include the location of the seeds [58].

4. Technique

Patients are treated under general anesthesia and administered transrectal Tylenol. The tumor is localized via indentation with a cryoprobe and an indirect ophthalmoscope. Tumors anterior to the equator are treated transconjunctivally, while tumors posterior to the equator are treated through a small incision in the conjunctiva. The use of a curved cryotherapy probe aids in the treatment of posterior tumors. Freezing is applied in the center of the tumor until the entire tumor is transformed into a crystalline ball, freezing the overlying vitreous. Tumors are typically treated three times per session for as long as 3 to 4 min per freeze. If necessary, additional cryotherapy is applied until no viable or visible tumor remains, and the patient is left with a white chorioretinal scar.

5. Results

Cryotherapy is an effective method of focal therapy for retinoblastoma. In our center, 90% of tumors less than 3 mm in diameter are cured permanently [58].

6. Complications

The complications associated with cryotherapy for retinoblastoma are few and rarely serious. All patients demonstrate transient conjunctival edema and some experience transient lid edema. Vitreous hemorrhages can be observed in large or previously irradiated tumors [60]. Transient localized retinal detachments (ablation fugax) can occur but usually resolve within a few days to weeks after treatment.

G. Chemoreduction

1. History

Efforts to treat intraocular retinoblastoma with chemotherapy began with Kupfer in the 1950s. In 1953, Kupfer used intravenous nitrogen mustard as a primary treatment for retinoblastoma [61]. Then, in 1955, Reese et al. utilized intracarotid triethylenemelamine (TEM) in combination with EBR in order to decrease the required dose of EBR [62]. Currently chemoreduction is an area of active clinical and basic science research motivated by the desire to avoid enucleation and EBR [6].

2. Indications

The indications for chemoreduction are not yet well established. In general, however, chemoreduction is employed for three purposes. Most commonly, this treatment is used for patients who have visual potential in eyes containing tumors that are too large to treat with focal methods. Chemoreduction is used to shrink these tumors so that focal treatments such as photocoagulation, cryotherapy, thermotherapy, or radioactive plaques can then be administered. It is the focal treatment methods that cause permanent inactivation of the tumors. Chemoreduction is also used for patients below 1 year of age with advanced bilateral disease who require EBR to be cured. When administered to patients below 1 year of age, EBR increases the incidence of second nonocular cancers in these patients (see Sec. III.C). In these cases, chemotherapy is used just to control tumor growth until the patient is 1 year old and can safely undergo EBR. Finally, chemotherapy has also recently been utilized in some studies as a potential single-modality eye-preserving treatment. Permanent responses are rarely observed in these cases.

3. Technique

Most studies of chemoreduction for retinoblastoma have utilized vincristine, carboplatin, and an epipodophyllotoxin, either etoposide or teniposide (Table 2). The addition of cyclosporine as a P-glycoprotein inhibitor has been suggested to decrease the ability of tumor cells to transport antineoplastic drugs from the intracellular space, thereby allowing the cells to develop multidrug resistance [63,64]. Currently, the choice of agents as well as number and frequency of cycles varies at different institutions.

Table 2 Summary of Recent Reports on Chemoreduction for Retinoblastoma

Authors	No. of eyes	Agents	No. of cycles
Gallie, 1996 [63]	40	VRES	Various
Kingston, 1996 [66]	24	VRE	2 or 4, monthly
Murphree, 1996 [41]	35	VRE	3, monthly
Shields, 1996 [68][a]	31	VRE	2, monthly
Greenwald, 1996 [67]	11	RE	6–7, monthly
Chan, 1996 [64][b]	26	VRNS	Every 3 weeks for 3–12 months
Shields, 1997 [65][a]	52	VRE	2 or 6, monthly
Gunduz, 1998 [69]	27	VRE	2 or 6, monthly
Friedman, 2000 [70]	75	VRE	6, monthly
Beck, 2000 [72]	33	RE	Every 3–4 weeks for 2–5 cycles
Wilson, 2001 [71]	36	VR	Every 3 weeks for 6 months

Key: V, vincristine; R, carboplatin; E, etoposide; S, cyclosporine; N, teniposide.
[a] Twenty patients' results were published in both of these reports.
[b] This study is not included in Table 3 because the number of eyes in each Reese-Ellsworth group are not specified.

4. Results

The results of recent studies examining chemoreduction followed by focal therapies have been most promising for patients with Reese-Ellsworth stage I–III eyes. For these patients, several authors have demonstrated that enucleation can be successfully avoided almost 100% of the time [41,63–72]. Results for patients with Reese-Ellsworth stage IV and V eyes have been more discouraging. An analysis of all Reese-Ellsworth stage V eyes included in the eight published chemoreduction studies with applicable data is presented in Table 3. In patients treated with chemoreduction, only 30% of eyes avoided *both* EBR and enucleation. Forty-seven percent of eyes required EBR but avoided enucleation, and 35% of eyes required enucleation (with or without prior EBR). Thus, the goal of utilizing chemoreduction to avoid EBR and enucleation is achieved in only a minority of patients with Reese-Ellsworth stage V eyes.

Shields et al. recently suggested that chemoreduction may prevent trilateral retinoblastoma [73]. The authors retrospectively compared 142 patients treated with chemoreduction and 72 patients treated with nonchemoreduction methods from 1995 to 1999. One of 18 (5.5%) patients at risk for developing trilateral retinoblastoma in the nonchemoreduction group subsequently developed a pineoblastoma, a percentage consistent with a previously published series [74]. In contrast, none of the 99 patients at risk in the chemoreduction group developed trilateral retinoblastoma. The authors conclude that chemoreduction may play a role in preventing pineoblastoma. In this study, however, none of the patients in the chemoreduction group received EBR, which has been shown to be a risk factor for the development of pineoblastoma. The absence of EBR, rather than the addition of

Table 3 Metanalysis of Reese-Ellsworth Stage V Eyes Included in Recent Chemoreducation Studies

Authors	No. of R-E stage V eyes	Eyes not requiring EBR OR enucleation	Eyes requiring EBR	Eyes requiring enucleation (+/− prior EBR)	Median follow-up in months	Range of follow-up in months
Gallie, 1996 [63]	18	13 (72%)	4 (22%)	1 (8%)	3	1–57
Kingston, 1996 [66][a]	20[a]	0 (0%) [a]	20 (100%)[a]	6 (30%)	60	12–84
Murphree, 1996 [41]	21	0 (0%)	7 (33%)	17 (81%)	Unclear	Unclear
Shields, 1996 [68][b]	22	13 (59%)	9 (41%)	0 (0%)	6	2–13
Greenwald, 1996 [67]	6	1 (17%)	4 (67%)	2 (33%)	23	12–40
Shields, 1997 [65][b]	36	9 (25%)	19 (53%)	8 (22%)	17	13–27
Gunduz, 1998 [69]	27	5 (19%)	16 (59%)	10 (37%)	25	20–32
Friedman, 2000 [70]	30	14 (47%)	13 (43%)	9 (30%)	13	0–34
Beck, 2000 [72][c]	13	2 (15%)	7 (54%)	6 (46%)	31	4–41
Wilson, 2001 [71]	14	5 (36%)	8 (57%)	5 (36%)	19	3–42
Total	**165**	**49 (30%)**	**78 (47%)**	**58 (35%)**	—	—

[a] The protocol for this included EBRT for all patients, therefore the data is not included in the metanalysis.
[b] Twenty patients' results were published in both of these reports, thus only the data from the 1997 report are included in the analysis.
[c] One patient who lost to follow-up in this study was excluded in the analysis.

chemoreduction, may, in fact, explain the lack of pineoblastoma development in the chemoreduction arm of this study [75].

5. Complications

Short-term side effects of chemotherapy are common and include fever, nausea, vomiting, and diarrhea. Hematological problems such as leukopenia, thrombocytopenia, and anemia are also common. Serious but uncommon sequelae include neurological and cardiac disturbances. Less serious complications include alopecia and low-grade bacterial infections in an anopthalmic orbit [34].

Several ophthalmic complications have been reported in patients undergoing chemoreduction/local therapy for retinoblastoma. Anagoste et al. reported three cases of rhegmatogenous retinal detachments and active retinoblastoma, with retinal breaks adjacent to cryotherapy scars [76]. Gombos et al. published a case of cholesterosis in the anterior segment of an eye that underwent chemoreduction/local therapy for retinoblastoma [77].

In addition to noncancerous ophthalmic complications, there is evidence that new retinoblastomas can develop in patients while they are being treated with systemic chemotherapy. Scott et al. reported four such cases and theorize that the development of these new tumors could represent primary tumor resistance, selection of a resistant tumor cell line, or inadequate chemotherapeutic levels within small, minimally vascularized tumor cells [78]. Furthermore, our group recently reported on the development of new retinoblastomas in children who were treated with systemic carboplatin as their initial treatment. Children under 6 months of age had a 71% chance of developing new tumors, and children over the age of 6 months had a 25% chance [79].

Another potential complication of chemoreduction is the development of secondary nonocular cancers. Several agents utilized in current chemoreduction studies for retinoblastoma have been demonstrated to increase the risk for secondary cancers either in retinoblastoma patients or in patients treated with these drugs for other primary malignancies. The risk of secondary leukemias in survivors of ovarian cancer treated with platinum-based drugs is well documented [80,81]. One retinoblastoma survivor who received cisplatin developed acute myeloid leukemia (AML) [82]. AML has also been reported in two retinoblastoma patients who received vincristine [83,84]. Furthermore, teniposide has been reported to increase the risk of AML in survivors of childhood cancer, possibly in a pattern related to the schedule of drug delivery [85]. Although the drug is not presently being used in chemoreduction studies for retinoblastoma, cyclophosphamide has also been demonstrated to cause a significant increase in the incidence of second cancers in retinoblastoma patients [86]. The follow-up periods of chemoreduction studies with retinoblastoma patients to date are inadequate to assess the development of second cancers in these patients (Table 3).

6. Periocular Chemotherapy

Ideally, chemotherapy administered for intraocular retinoblastoma would be distributed exclusively to the intraocular space of the affected eye with no systemic exposure to the drug [87]. Based upon this goal, several groups have explored the local delivery of chemotherapeutic agents via intraocular injection. Murray et al. and

Harbour et al. demonstrated that transgenic mice with retinoblastoma experienced significant tumor control accompanied by little or no local toxicity using subconjunctivally injected carboplatin [88,89]. Our group reported that periocular carboplatin was well-tolerated in non-tumor-bearing primates and that higher levels of carboplatin were achieved in the vitreous after periocular administration than after intravenous administration [90]. These preclinical data prompted our group to study the efficacy and toxicity of subconjunctival carboplatin for intraocular retinoblastoma in a phase I/II trial with retinoblastoma patients. In the trial, a response was observed in some eyes with vitreous disease or retinal tumors but not in eyes with subretinal disease. In most patients, minor local toxicity and no systemic toxicities were observed. However, one patient did develop optic atrophy with decreased visual acuity. For patients who are treated with this modality for vitreous seeding, the source of the vitreous seeds must be treated with another method in order to achieve a cure. Further study and longer follow-up are needed to determine fully the safety and applicability of subconjunctival administration of carboplatin and other potential agents.

III. ADDITIONAL NONOCULAR CANCERS

A. Background

In 1949, it was first recognized that some retinoblastoma patients developed second nonocular neoplasms years after the successful treatment of the eye cancer [14]. Since then, the incidence of additional nonocular cancers in survivors of retinoblastoma who carry the RB1 mutation has been reviewed extensively [91]. Previous analyses have also shown that additional nonocular cancers are the leading cause of death in survivors of germinal retinoblastoma. These patients are not at an increased risk of dying of any other causes when compared to patients who have never had retinoblastoma [92].

B. Incidence and Timing of Additional Cancers

Nearly 95% of all children in the United States who develop retinoblastoma survive the disease. Of the survivors of germinal retinoblastoma, cumulative incidence reports of second cancers vary, but it is estimated that a rate of 1% per year of life approximates the rate [93]. Patients who develop a second cancer and then survive that cancer have an increased risk for the development of additional nonocular tumors of approximately 2% per year from the time of second tumor diagnosis [91]. The average latency period between subsequent tumor diagnoses becomes progressively shorter with each additional cancer that develops. Because females have a higher overall risk of dying of second tumors than males, more males are at risk for developing third tumors [91,92].

C. Risk Factors

A necessary risk factor for the development of additional nonocular tumors in retinoblastoma survivors is the presence of the germinal RB1 mutation. All patients with bilateral retinoblastoma are carriers of the germinal mutation and are at risk for additional nonocular cancers [91]. Identifying unilateral patients who carry the germinal mutation is less straightforward, but the following patients should be considered high risk for carrying the germinal mutation: most unilateral patients with a family history of retinoblastoma (including a family history of retinoma), unilateral patients who are diagnosed under the age of 6 months, and unilateral patients who present with multifocal tumors (not one tumor with seeding).

EBR is also a contributing factor to the development of additional cancers in retinoblastoma survivors. Children radiated during the first year of life are between two and eight times as likely to develop second cancers as those radiated after the age of 1 year [94,95]. Patients treated with higher doses and older methods of radiation delivery that lead to increased superficial skin and bone exposure are at higher risk for subsequent tumor development in the radiation field [91]. The radiation-induced risk for additional cancers applies only to patients with germinal retinoblastoma. Unilateral retinoblastoma patients who do not carry the constitutional mutation are at no increased risk for developing other cancers, even if they received EBR [6].

Additional nonocular cancers develop both within and outside the field of EBR. Our group has reported that in radiated patients who develop second malignancies, the tumors are within the radiation field two-thirds of the time and outside the field one-third of the time. In nonradiated patients who develop second tumors, the tumors are outside the hypothetical field two-thirds of the time and within the hypothetical field one-third of the time [94,96].

D. Types and Locations of Additional Malignancies

Second nonocular neoplasms observed in survivors of germinal retinoblastoma include, in order of most common to least, osteogenic sarcomas of the skull and long bones, soft tissue sarcomas, pineoblastomas, cutaneous melanomas, brain tumors, Hodgkin disease, lung cancer, and breast cancer [96,97]. Survivors of hereditary retinoblastoma are also at increased risk for the development of lipomas throughout the body. Patients who develop lipomas are at an even higher risk of developing second cancers [98].

Figure 3 demonstrates the timing of the development of each type of second cancer in retinoblastoma survivors. EBR treatment changes the age distribution of some of these cancers in two different patterns: one pattern if it was given before the age of 1 year and another if it was given afterward. In general, however, patients who have *not* received EBR are at highest risk for developing soft tissue sarcomas of the head and cutaneous melanomas beginning in their late twenties or early thirties. These patients are at highest risk for osteogenic sarcomas of the long bones and osteosarcomas of the skull during the mid-teenage years. Finally, retinoblastoma survivors at an equally elevated risk throughout their lives for developing brain tumors.

E. Third, Fourth, and Fifth Cancers

Our group recently published a report on the largest series of retinoblastoma survivors who developed a second cancer, survived, and went on to develop third, fourth, or fifth nonocular tumors [91]. Survivors of retinoblastoma who develop

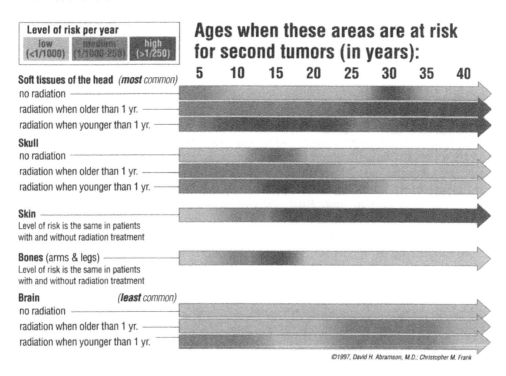

Level of risk per year		
low (<1/1000)	medium (1/1000-250)	high (>1/250)

Ages when these areas are at risk for second tumors (in years):

5   10   15   20   25   30   35   40

Soft tissues of the head *(most common)*
no radiation
radiation when older than 1 yr.
radiation when younger than 1 yr.

Skull
no radiation
radiation when older than 1 yr.
radiation when younger than 1 yr.

Skin
Level of risk is the same in patients with and without radiation treatment

Bones (arms & legs)
Level of risk is the same in patients with and without radiation treatment

Brain *(least common)*
no radiation
radiation when older than 1 yr.
radiation when younger than 1 yr.

©1997, David H. Abramson, M.D.; Christopher M. Frank

Figure 3 Patients who carry the germinal mutation for retinoblastoma are at risk for the development of additional nonocular cancers well into their adult lives.

second malignancies and survive are at an even higher risk for the development of additional cancers than they were for the development of a second tumor. The distribution of tumor sites in the second-tumor group suggests a nonrandom pattern of third, fourth, and fifth tumor development. Of patients with skin cancers as their second tumors, skin cancers also represent most of the third, fourth, and fifth tumors that develop in this group. Of patients treated for a second tumor in the skull in whom a third tumor develops, most are diagnosed with a soft tissue sarcoma in the head as the third tumor. The locations and expected ages at which soft tissue sarcomas of the head and osteogenic sarcomas of the long bones develop are consistent with the patterns observed in second tumors (see Fig. 3).

F. Recommendations to Patients to Minimize Subsequent Cancers

In order to minimize the role of subsequent cancers, retinoblastoma survivors at our center are advised to refrain from smoking, minimize their exposure to sunlight, and avoid unnecessary CT scans or x-rays. Although the relationship between degree of sunlight exposure and the development of cutaneous melanomas in the retinoblastoma survivor population is unclear, we continue to recommend limiting sunlight exposure because of the clear association with cutaneous melanomas in the general population. Regarding CT scans, our recommendation is based on a recent study that has demonstrated an increased risk for radiation-related cancers in children who undergo CT scans [15].

IV. CONCLUSION

The survival of retinoblastoma patients in the United States has improved significantly over the past century, while survival rates remain low in developing countries, where patients commonly present with metastatic disease. The implementation over the past 30 years of effective focal therapies such as photocoagulation, cryotherapy, and brachytherapy have helped prevent many patients from undergoing enucleation and EBR. Newer techniques such as transpupillary thermotherapy and chemoreduction hold additional promise for patients with intraocular disease. Unresolved issues in the treatment of retinoblastoma include effective screening protocols for additional nonocular malignancies, indications for chemoreduction, and appropriate therapies for widespread metastatic disease.

REFERENCES

1. Ellsworth R. Retinoblastoma: An overview. In: Blodi FC, ed. Retinoblastoma. New York: Churchill Livingstone, 1985.
2. Wardrop J. Observations on the Fungus Haematodes or Soft Cancer. Edinburgh: George Ramsay and Co, 1809.
3. Abramson DH. Treatment of retinoblastoma. In: Blodi FC, ed. Retinoblastoma. New York: Churchill Livingstone, 1985, pp 3–93.
4. Sant M, Capocaccia R, Badioni V. Survival for retinoblastoma in Europe. Eur J Cancer 2001; 37:730–735.
5. Novakovic B. U.S. childhood cancer survival, 1973–1987. Med Pediatr Oncol 1994; 23:480–486.
6. Abramson DH, Dunkel IJ, McCormick B. Neoplasms of the eye. Cancer Med 2000; 1:1083–1096.
7. Saw S, Tan N, Lee S, Au Eong K, Chia K. Incidence and survival characteristics of retinoblastoma in Singapore from 1968–1995. J Pediatr Ophthalmol Strabismus 2000; 37:87–93.
8. Wessels G, Hesseling P. Outcome of children treated for cancer in the Republic of Namibia. Med Pediatr Oncol 1996; 27:160–164.
9. Gunalp I, Gunduz K, Arslan Y. Retinoblastoma in Turkey—Treatment and prognosis. Jpn J Ophthalmol 1996; 40:95–102.
10. Nandakumar A, Anantha N, Appaji L, Swamy K, Mukherjee G, Venugopal T, Reddy S, Dhar M. Descriptive epidemiology of childhood cancers in Bangalore, India. Cancer Causes Control 1996; 7:405–410.
11. Ajaiyeoba IA, Akang EE, Campbell OB, Olurin IO, Aghadiuno PU. Retinoblastomas in Ibadan: treatment and prognosis. West Afr J Med 1993; 12:223–227.
12. Sha YH. Radiotherapy of retinoblastoma—Analysis of 100 patients. Zhonghua Zhong Liu Za Zhi 1988; 10:379–381.
13. Erwenne CM, Franco EL. Age and lateness of referral as determinants of extraocular retinoblastoma. Ophthalm Paediatr Genet 1989; 10:179–184.
14. Reese AB, Merriam GR, Martin HE. Treatment of bilateral retinoblastoma by irradiation and surgery. Report on 15-year results. Am J Ophthalmol 1949; 32:175–190.

15. Brenner D, Elliston C, Hall E, Berdon W. Estimated risks of radiation-induced fatal cancer from pediatric CT. Am J Roentgenol 2001; 176:289–296.
16. Abramson DH, Mendelsohn ME, Servodidio CA, Tretter T, Gombos DS. Familial retinoblastoma: where and when? Acta Ophthalmol Scand 1998; 76:334–338.
17. Hayes R. Medical Observations and Inquiries. Vol. 3. London: 1767, p 120.
18. McCormick B. Retinoblastoma. In: Leibel SA, Phillips TL, eds. Textbook of Radiation Oncology. Philadelphia: Saunders, 1988:1156–1164.
19. Abramson DH, Ellsworth RM. The surgical management of retinoblastoma. Ophthalmic Surg 1980; 11:596–598.
20. Hilgartner HL. Report of a case of a double glioma treated by x-ray. Tex Med 1903; 18:322.
21. Martin HE, Reese AB. Treatment of retinal gliomas by the fractionated or divided dose principal of roentgen radiation: Preliminary report. Arch Ophthalmol 1936; 16:733.
22. McCormick B, Ellsworth R, Abramson D, Haik B, Tome M, Grabowski E, LoSasso T. Radiation therapy for retinoblastoma: comparison of results with lenssparing versus lateral beam techniques. Int J Radiat Oncol Biol Phys 1988; 15:567–574.
23. McCormick B, Ellsworth R, Abramson D, LoSasso T, Grabowski E. Results of external beam radiation for children with retinoblastoma: A comparison of two techniques. J Pediatr Ophthalmol Strabismus 1989; 26:239–243.
24. Zelter M, Damel A, Gonzalez G, Schwartz L. A prospective study on the treatment of retinoblastoma in 72 patients. Cancer 1991; 68:1685–1690.
25. Shidnia H, Hornback NB, Helveston EM, Gettlefinger T, Biglan AW. Treatment results of retinoblastoma at Indiana University Hospitals. Cancer 1977; 40:2917–2922.
26. Amendola BE, Markoe AM, Augsburger JJ, Karlsson UL, Giblin M, Shields JA, Brady LW, Woodleigh R. Analysis of treatment results in 36 children with retinoblastoma treated by scleral plaque irradiation. Int J Radiat Oncol Biol Phys 1989; 17:63–70.
27. Foote RL, Garretson BR, Schomberg PJ, Buskirk SJ, Robertson DM, Earle JD. External beam irradiation for retinoblastoma: Patterns of failure and dose-response analysis. Int J Radiat Oncol Biol Phys 1989; 16:823–830.
28. Bedford MA, Bedotto C, Macfaul PA. Retinoblastoma. A study of 139 cases. Br J Ophthalmol 1971; 55:19–27.
29. Black L, McCormick B, Abramson DH. External beam radiation therapy and retinoblastoma: Long term results in the comparison of two techniques. Int J Radiat Oncol Biol Phys 1995; 35:45.
30. Reese AB. Tumors of the Eye. New York: Harper & Row, 1963.
31. Abramson DH, Jereb B, Ellsworth RM. External beam radiation for retinoblastoma. Bull N Y Acad Med 1981; 57:787–803.
32. Imhof SM, Mourits MP, Hofman P, Zonneveld FW, Schipper J, Moll AC, Tan KE. Quantification of orbital and mid-facial growth retardation after megavoltage external beam irradiation in children with retinoblastoma. Ophthalmology 1996; 103:263–268.
33. Stallard HB. The conservative treatment of retinoblastoma. Highlights Ophthalmol 1963; 6:129–130.
34. Shields JA, Shields CL. Intraocular Tumors: a Text and Atlas. Philadelphia: Saunders, 1992.
35. Shields CL, Shields JA, Cater J, Othmane I, Singh AD, Micaily B. Plaque radiotherapy for retinoblastoma: Long-term tumor control and treatment complications in 208 tumors. Ophthalmology 2001; 108:2116–2121.
36. Abramson DH, Ellsworth RM, Haik BG. Cobalt plaques in advanced retinoblastoma. Retina 1983; 3:12–15.
37. Abramson DH. The focal treatment of retinoblastoma with emphasis on xenon arc photocoagulation. Acta Ophthalmol Suppl 1989; 194:3–63.

38. Weve HJM. The Diathermy treatment of intraocular tumors. Trans Ophthalmol Soc Austr 1953; 13:47–58.
39. Lagendijk JJ. A microwave heating technique for the hyperthermic treatment of tumours in the eye, especially retinoblastoma. Phys Med Biol 1982; 27:1313–1324.
40. Shields CL, Santos MC, Diniz W, Gunduz K, Mercado G, Cater JR, Shields JA. Thermotherapy for retinoblastoma. Arch Ophthalmol 1999; 117:885–893.
41. Murphree AL, Villablanca JG, Deegan WF, 3rd, Sato JK, Malogolowkin M, Fisher A, Parker R, Reed E, Gomer CJ. Chemotherapy plus local treatment in the management of intraocular retinoblastoma. Arch Ophthalmol 1996; 114:1348–1356.
42. Murphree AL, Munier FL. Retinoblastoma. In: Ryan SJ, ed. Retina. St. Louis: Mosby-Year Book, 1994, pp 605–606.
43. Murray TG, O'Brien JM, Steeves RA, Smith BJ, Albert DM, Cicciarelli N, Markoe AM, Tompkins DT, Windle JJ. Radiation therapy and ferromagnetic hyperthermia in the treatment of murine transgenic retinoblastoma. Arch Ophthalmol 1996; 114:1376–1381.
44. Murray TG, Cicciarelli N, McCabe CM, Ksander B, Feuer W, Schiffman J, Mieler WF, O'Brien JM. In vitro efficacy of carboplatin and hyperthermia in a murine retinoblastoma cell line. Invest Ophthalmol Vis Sci 1997; 38:2516–2522.
45. Shields JA, Shields CL, De Potter P, Needle M. Bilateral macular retinoblastoma managed by chemoreduction and chemothermotherapy. Arch Ophthalmol 1996; 114:1426–1427.
46. Shields CL, Shields JA. Recent developments in the management of retinoblastoma. J Pediatr Ophthalmol Strabismus 1999; 36:8–18; quiz 35–16.
47. Lueder GT, Goyal R. Visual function after laser hyperthermia and chemotherapy for macular retinoblastoma. Am J Ophthalmol 1996; 121:582–584.
48. Levy C, Doz F, Quintana E, Pacquement H, Michon J, Schlienger P, Validire P, Asselain B, Desjardins L, Zucker JM. Role of chemotherapy alone or in combination with hyperthermia in the primary treatment of intraocular retinoblastoma: preliminary results. Br J Ophthalmol 1998; 82:1154–1158.
49. Lincoff H, McLean J, Long R. The cryosurgical treatment of intraocular tumors. Am J Ophthalmol 1967; 63:389.
50. Ellsworth RM. The practical management of retinoblastoma. Trans Am Ophthalmol Soc 1969; 67:462–534.
51. Neel HB, Ketcham AS, Hammond WG. Ischemia potentiating cryosurgery of primate liver. Ann Surg 1971; 174:309–318.
52. Amoils SP. Cryosurgery in Ophthalmology. Chicago: Year Book, 1975.
53. Bellman S, Adams RJ. Vascular reactions after experimental cold injury. Angiography 1956; 7:339–367.
54. Mundth AD. Studies on the pathogenesis of cold injury: microcirculatory changes in tissue induced by freezing. Proc Symp Aretic Biol Med 1964, p 4.
55. Rabb JM, Renaud ML, Brandt PA, Witt CW. Effect of freezing and thawing on the microcirculation and capillary endothelium of the hampster cheek pouch. Cryobiol 1974; 11:508–518.
56. Le Pivert PJ. Basic considerations of the cryolesion. In: Ablin RJ, ed. Handbook of Cryosurgery. Marcel Dekker, 1980.
57. Hopping W, Bunke-Schmidt A. Light coagulation and cryotherapy in retinoblastoma. In: Blodi FC, ed. Retinoblastoma. New York: Churchill Livingstone, 1985, pp 95–110.
58. Abramson DH, Ellsworth RM, Rozakis GW. Cryotherapy for retinoblastoma. Arch Ophthalmol 1982; 100:1253–1256.
59. Shields JA, Parsons H, Shields CL, Giblin ME. The role of cryotherapy in the management of retinoblastoma. Am J Ophthalmol 1989; 108:260–264.
60. Abramson DH. Cryotherapy in retinoblastoma. In: Jakobiec F, ed. Advanced Techniques in Ocular Surgery. Philadelphia: WB Saunders Co., 1984, pp 433–437.

61. Kupfer C. Retinoblastoma treated with intravenous nitrogen mustard. Am J Ophthalmol 1953; 36:1721.

62. Reese AB, Hyman GA, Merriam GR, Forrest AW. Treatment of retinoblastoma by radiation and triethylenemelamine. Arch Ophthalmol 1955; 53:505–513.

63. Gallie BL, Budning A, DeBoer G, Thiessen JJ, Koren G, Verjee Z, Ling V, Chan HS. Chemotherapy with focal therapy can cure intraocular retinoblastoma without radiotherapy. Arch Ophthalmol 1996; 114:1321–1328.

64. Chan HS, DeBoer G, Thiessen JJ, Budning A, Kingston JE, O'Brien JM, Koren G, Giesbrecht E, Haddad G, Verjee Z, Hungerford JL, Ling V, Gallie BL. Combining cyclosporin with chemotherapy controls intraocular retinoblastoma without requiring radiation. Clin Cancer Res 1996; 2:1499–1508.

65. Shields CL, Shields JA, Needle M, de Potter P, Kheterpal S, Hamada A, Meadows AT. Combined chemoreduction and adjuvant treatment for intraocular retinoblastoma. Ophthalmology 1997; 104:2101–2111.

66. Kingston JE, Hungerford JL, Madreperla SA, Plowman PN. Results of combined chemotherapy and radiotherapy for advanced intraocular retinoblastoma. Arch Ophthalmol 1996; 114:1339–1343.

67. Greenwald MJ, Strauss LC. Treatment of intraocular retinoblastoma with carboplatin and etoposide chemotherapy. Ophthalmology 1996; 103:1989–1997.

68. Shields CL, De Potter P, Himelstein BP, Shields JA, Meadows AT, Maris JM. Chemoreduction in the initial management of intraocular retinoblastoma. Arch Ophthalmol 1996; 114:1330–1338.

69. Gunduz K, Shields CL, Shields JA, Meadows AT, Gross N, Cater J, Needle M. The outcome of chemoreduction treatment in patients with Reese-Ellsworth group V retinoblastoma. Arch Ophthalmol 1998; 116:1613–1617.

70. Friedman DL, Himelstein B, Shields CL, Shields JA, Needle M, Miller D, Bunin GR, Meadows AT. Chemoreduction and local ophthalmic therapy for intraocular retinoblastoma. J Clin Oncol 2000; 18:12–17.

71. Wilson MW, Rodriguez-Galindo C, Haik BG, Moshfeghi DM, Merchant TE, Pratt CB. Multiagent chemotherapy as neoadjuvant treatment for multifocal intraocular retinoblastoma. Ophthalmology 2001; 108:2106–2114; discussion 2114–2105.

72. Beck MN, Balmer A, Dessing C, Pica A, Munier F. First-line chemotherapy with local treatment can prevent external-beam irradiation and enucleation in low-stage intraocular retinoblastoma. J Clin Oncol 2000; 18:2881–2887.

73. Shields CL, Meadows AT, Shields JA, Carvalho C, Smith AF. Chemoreduction for retinoblastoma may prevent intracranial neuroblastic malignancy (trilateral retinoblastoma). Arch Ophthalmol 2001; 119:1269–1272.

74. Blach LE, McCormick B, Abramson DH, Ellsworth RM. Trilateral retinoblastoma— incidence and outcome: a decade of experience. Int J Radiat Oncol Biol Phys 1994; 29:729–733.

75. Moll AC, Imhof SM, Schouten-Van Meeteren AY, Boers M. Screening for pineoblastoma in patients with retinoblastoma. Arch Ophthalmol 2002; 120:1774

76. Anagnoste SR, Scott IU, Murray TG, Kramer D, Toledano S. Rhegmatogenous retinal detachment in retinoblastoma patients undergoing chemoreduction and cryotherapy. Am J Ophthalmol 2000; 129:817–819.

77. Gombos DS, Howes E, O'Brien JM. Cholesterosis following chemoreduction for advanced retinoblastoma. Arch Ophthalmol 2000; 118:440–441.

78. Scott IU, Murray TG, Toledano S, O'Brien JM. New retinoblastoma tumors in children undergoing systemic chemotherapy. Arch Ophthalmol 1998; 116:1685–1686.

79. Lee TC, Hayashi N, Dunkel IJ, Novetski D, Beaverson KL, Abramson DH. New tumor formation in children with retinoblastoma treated with single agent carboplatin. American Academy of Ophthalmology, New Orleans, 2001.

80. Travis LB, Curtis RE, Stovall M, Holowaty EJ, van Leeuwen FE, Glimelius B, Lynch CF, Hagenbeek A, Li CY, Banks PM, et al. Risk of leukemia following treatment for non-Hodgkin's lymphoma. J Natl Cancer Inst 1994; 86:1450–1457.

81. Hawkins MM, Wilson LM, Stovall MA, Marsden HB, Potok MH, Kingston JE, Chessells JM. Epipodophyllotoxins, alkylating agents, and radiation and risk of secondary leukaemia after childhood cancer. BMJ 1992; 304:951–958.

82. Turner AR, Melynk A, Clark G. MDS and acute monocytic leukaemia after retinoblastoma. Br J Haematol 1996; 92:249.

83. Felice MS, Zubizarreta PA, Chantada GL, Alfaro E, Cygler AM, Gallego M, Rossi J, Sackmann-Muriel F. Acute myeloid leukemia as a second malignancy: Report of 9 pediatric patients in a single institution in Argentina. Med Pediatr Oncol 1998; 30:160–164.

84. White L, Ortega JA, Ying KL. Acute non-lymphocytic leukemia following multimodality therapy for retinoblastoma. Cancer 1985; 55:496–498.

85. Rivera GK, Pui CH, Santana VM, Pratt CB, Crist WM. Epipodophyllotoxins in the treatment of childhood cancer. Cancer Chemother Pharmacol 1994; 34:S89–95.

86. Draper GJ, Sanders BM, Kingston JE. Second primary neoplasms in patients with retinoblastoma. Br J Cancer 1986; 53:661–671.

87. Finger PT. Chemotherapy for retinoblastoma. Drugs 1999; 58:983–996.

88. Harbour JW, Murray TG, Hamasaki D, Cicciarelli N, Hernandez E, Smith B, Windle J, O'Brien JM. Local carboplatin therapy in transgenic murine retinoblastoma. Invest Ophthalmol Vis Sci 1996; 37:1892–1898.

89. Murray TG, Cicciarelli N, O'Brien JM, Hernandez E, Mueller RL, Smith BJ, Feuer W. Subconjunctival carboplatin therapy and cryotherapy in the treatment of transgenic murine retinoblastoma. Arch Ophthalmol 1997; 115:1286–1290.

90. Mendelsohn ME, Abramson DH, Madden T, Tong W, Tran HT, Dunkel IJ. Intraocular concentrations of chemotherapeutic agents after systemic or local administration. Arch Ophthalmol 1998; 116:1209–1212.

91. Abramson DH, Melson MR, Dunkel IJ, Frank CM. Third (fourth and fifth) nonocular tumors in survivors of retinoblastoma. Ophthalmology 2001; 108:1868–1876.

92. Eng C, Li FP, Abramson DH, Ellsworth RM, Wong FL, Goldman MB, Seddon J, Tarbell N, Boice JD Jr. Mortality from second tumors among long-term survivors of retinoblastoma. J Natl Cancer Inst 1993; 85:1121–1128.

93. Abramson DH. Second nonocular cancers in retinoblastoma: A unified hypothesis. The Franceschetti Lecture. Ophthalm Genet 1999; 20:193–204.

94. Abramson DH, Frank CM. Second nonocular tumors in survivors of bilateral retinoblastoma: A possible age effect on radiation-related risk. Ophthalmology 1998; 105:573–579; discussion 579–580.

95. Moll AC, Imhof SM, Schouten-Van Meeteren AY, Kuik DJ, Hofman P, Boers M. Second primary tumors in hereditary retinoblastoma: A register-based study, 1945–1997: Is there an age effect on radiation-related risk? Ophthalmology 2001; 108:1109–1114.

96. Wong FL, Boice JD, Jr., Abramson DH, Tarone RE, Kleinerman RA, Stovall M, Goldman MB, Seddon JM, Tarbell N, Fraumeni JF Jr, Li FP. Cancer incidence after retinoblastoma. Radiation does and sarcoma risk. JAMA 1997; 278:1262–1267.

97. Kleinerman RA, Tarone RE, Abramson DH, Seddon JM, Li FP, Tucker MA. Hereditary retinoblastoma and risk of lung cancer. J Natl Cancer Inst 2000; 92:2037–2039.

98. Li FP, Abramson DH, Tarone RE, Kleinerman RA, Fraumeni JF Jr, Boice JD Jr. Hereditary retinoblastoma, lipoma, and second primary cancers. J Natl Cancer Inst 1997; 89:83–84.

17

Clinical Trials in Uveal Melanoma: Patient Characteristics and the Treatment of Intraocular Tumors

TIMOTHY G. MURRAY and BRANDY C. HAYDEN

Bascom Palmer Eye Institute/University of Miami School of Medicine, Miami, Florida, U.S.A.

H. CULVER BOLDT

University of Iowa, Iowa City, Iowa, U.S.A.

CLAUDIA SCALA MOY

National Institutes of Health/National Institute of Neurological Disorders and Stroke, Bethesda, Maryland, U.S.A.

Clinical trials have established a framework to evaluate patient outcomes in the setting of standardized criteria for entry, treatment, and data analysis. The emphasis on clinical trials utilizing a prospective, randomized, multicentered design has centered, in its beginnings, on ophthalmic disease. The National Eye Institute's focus on clinical trials evaluation of ophthalmic disease has set a standard for clinical trials throughout the National Institutes of Health and worldwide.

The application of clinical trial methodology in the evaluation of uveal melanoma management highlights the unique problems associated with the study of relatively rare diseases, particularly those that require long-term outcome analysis, such as delayed mortality. Clinical trials may be also be limited by disparities in treatment (enucleation versus globe-conserving radiotherapy), evolving therapies (shift from cobalt 60 to iodine 125 for brachytherapy), and inability to achieve widespread investigator participation, including inability to comfortably randomize patients between study treatment arms. Prior to the implementation of a clinical trial, several factors must be considered, including (1) the clinical relevance of the study outcomes; (2) the ethical rationale to treatment randomization; (3) the existence of pilot data establishing a framework for accuracy of diagnosis, perceived efficacy of each treatment, and acceptable treatment associated complications; (4) the absence of definitive existing clinical data documenting a clear treatment benefit; (5) and the willingness of the medical community (and at risk patients) to participate in the proposed clinical trial. For the Collaborative Ocular Melanoma Study (COMS), the existing literature describing outcomes for uveal melanoma was investigated utilizing metanalysis techniques to determine a range of expected mortality for patients with small, medium, and large choroidal melanoma as defined by a standardized grading criteria focused on both tumor basal dimension and apical height. This information was combined with clinical parameters to establish an expected clinically relevant difference between each of two different treatments for the Medium Choroidal and Large Choroidal Melanoma Treatment Trials [1]. Preliminary safety and efficacy data for pre-enucleation external-beam radiotherapy, enucleation, and 125-iodine brachytherapy were also reviewed and standardized for the proposed clinical trials.

This information was integrated into the (COMS) planning phase beginning in 1984 and aimed at establishing the framework for submission of a series of three clinical studies to evaluate small, medium, and large posterior uveal (choroidal/ciliary body) melanoma treatment [2]. The overall design of the COMS incorporated six centralized units consisting of the chairman's office, a coordinating center, radiological physics center, echography center, photographic reading center, pathology center, and 41 individual clinical centers targeted toward patient screening for eligibility, randomization, treatment, and follow-up. The Small Tumor Trial was constituted to observe the outcome, in a nonrandomized fashion, for patients meeting the eligibility criteria with small choroidal melanoma. The second two arms of the COMS were constituted as prospective, randomized, multicentered clinical trials to evaluate the outcomes for patients with medium and large choroidal melanoma. Standardized inclusion criteria for these clinical trials included a primary, unilateral, unifocal choroidal tumor in an individual over the age of 18 years and competent to provide informed consent. The tumor was required to meet size eligibility criteria and to be evaluable by echography to accurately delineate the tumor height [3,4].

Patients were excluded from the COMS if 50% or more of the tumor volume involved the ciliary body; if extrascleral extension of 2 mm or more was present; if previous biopsy or treatment had been performed; if coexisting disease was expected to compromise survival; if other primary or metastatic malignancy was known; or if the patient had contraindications to surgery, radiation therapy, or general anesthesia. Specific to the medium tumor trial were exclusions that precluded plaque radiotherapy for tumors within 2 mm of the optic disc, media opacity that precluded indirect ophthalmoscopic visualization of the tumor, visual loss in the fellow eye of 20/200 or worse and involvement of the iris/angle by the tumor, or secondary/neovascular glaucoma.

The COMS utilized a manual of procedures, aimed at assuring uniformity throughout each individual study center that standardized all aspects of the two randomized trials [3,5]. This manual incorporated standard certification for each clinical center and individual center participants, including the treating surgeon, following ophthalmologist, radiation oncologist and physicist, clinic coordinator, echographer, photographer, visual acuity examiner, and reviewing pathologist. Standardized forms were developed for patient demographics, initial patient evaluation, treatment documentation, echography, photography, and patient follow-up [6]. Patient mortality, including pathological review for metastatic disease, was standardized and National Death Index review was included within the trial design to maximize data collection for the primary study outcome of mortality [7]. All data were collated at the centralized coordinating center and reviewed by the external Data and Safety Monitoring Committee.

The COMS was structured to ensure standardization of patient entry, treatment, follow-up, and outcome assessment [2]. This study employed centralized units to coordinate studywide activities and included the Chairman's Office, Coordinating Center, Echography Center, Pathology Center, Radiologic Physics Center, and Photograph Reading Center, along with the independent Data and Safety Monitoring Committee. Each study center maintained responsibility for oversight of patient eligibility, treatment, and study compliance. Individual patient data—including demographics, tumor characteristics, individual treatment parameters, and follow-up visits—were collated by the Coordinating Center. Baseline echograms and follow-up studies were evaluated for eligibility and tumor response by the Echography Center [3]. Enucleated globes and all biopsy tissues were reviewed within the Pathology Center. Treatment planning for eyes undergoing either fractionated external beam radiotherapy or iodine-125 brachytherapy was reviewed for compliance with standardized study treatment parameters at the Radiologic Physics Center [8]. Fundus photographs and fluorescein angiography were collated within the Photograph Reading Center. Overall study integration remained the responsibility of the Chairman's Office, while individual study centers were directed by an on-site principal investigator. This study design is a classic example of a large, multicentered, randomized clinical trial and played a significant role in assuring excellent standardization and compliance. This study design was also associated with the significant study costs incurred by the COMS throughout its trial period.

The COMS trial arms were first funded in 1985 by the National Eye Institute and then jointly funded in 1991 by the National Eye Institute and the National Cancer Institute. The Small Tumor Observational Study accrued 204 patients between December 1986 and August 1989 [9,10]. Small choroidal melanomas were eligible for this study if the tumor was between 1.0 and 3.0 mm in apical height and 5.0–16.0 mm in largest basal dimension. Patients were evaluated for all-cause mortality, melanoma-related mortality, and factors predictive of tumor growth and/or tumor treatment. The medium tumor trial accrued 1317 patients between February 1987 and July 1998. Medium choroidal melanomas were eligible for this study if the tumor was between 2.5 to 10.0 mm in apical height (3.0–8.0 mm until November 1990) and 5.0–16.0 mm in largest basal dimension. Patients were evaluated for the primary outcome of all-cause mortality and secondary outcomes including melanoma-related mortality, local tumor control, treatment-related complications, visual acuity, and quality of life. The large tumor trial accrued 1003 patients between November 1986 and December 1994. Large choroidal melanomas were eligible for this study if the tumor was greater than 10 mm in apical height (greater than 8.0 mm until November 1990) or greater than 16.0 mm in largest basal dimension. Patients were evaluated for the primary outcome of all-cause mortality and secondary outcomes including melanoma-related mortality, local tumor recurrence, orbital complications, or treatment-related complications.

The Small Tumor Observational Study focused on the outcome of study-eligible patients to determine the feasibility of a future randomized clinical trial [11]. A total of 204 patients with a median age of 62 years were followed for a median of 92 months. Of the 188 patients not treated immediately within the study, 46 exhibited local tumor growth within the follow-up window. Kaplan-Meier analysis of tumor growth documented a 21% 2-year and 31% 5-year incidence of tumor growth requiring definitive tumor treatment. Clinical factors predictive of tumor growth included greater initial tumor thickness and diameter, presence of orange pigment, absence of drusen and/or retinal pigment epithelial change, and presence of tumor pinpoint hyperfluorescence on angiography.

The Small Tumor Observational Study evaluated survival outcomes including all-cause mortality and melanoma-related mortality for all study participants. Kaplan-Meier analysis of 5-year all-cause mortality was 6%, and 8-year all-cause mortality was 14.9%. Kaplan-Meier analysis of melanoma-specific mortality was 1 and 3.7%, respectively, for 5 and 8 years. This study, though, suffers from the limitations of all nonrandomized reviews, including potentials for treatment bias, nonstandardized treatment, variability in follow-up, and absence of prospective data collection. Nonetheless, the Small Tumor Observational Study did establish data documenting the low mortality in patients participating within the framework of this observational study [11].

The Medium Choroidal Melanoma Trial evaluated 8712 patients during the study accrual window and noted 2882 patients who were eligible for study participation [12–15]. A total of 1317 patients with a mean age of 60 years participated in this clinical trial. Randomization between standardized enucleation and iodine-125 brachytherapy established overlapping treatment groups without evidence of clinically significant selection bias. Evaluation of eligible patients documented no clinically significant differences between patients enrolling and those not enrolling within the clinical trial, allowing for generalization of the study findings to patients eligible for the clinical trial [14].

Local treatment failure and enucleation were evaluated among the 657 patients assigned to iodine-125 brachytherapy [15]. Kaplan-Meier analysis of local tumor failure documented an incidence of 10.3% at 5 years posttreatment. Local treatment failure was the primary cause of enucleation within 3 years of treatment; while ocular pain without evidence of treatment failure was the most common cause of enucleation occurring more than 3 years from brachytherapy. Kaplan-Meier analysis of risk of enucleation by 5 years was 12.5%. Risk factors for treatment failure were older age at time of initial treatment, posterior tumor location, and greater tumor thickness; while risk factors for enucleation included greater tumor thickness, posterior tumor location, and poorer baseline visual acuity. Local tumor failure was weakly associated with reduced survival, with an adjusted risk ratio of 1.5 (Table 1).

Visual acuity was evaluated for patients undergoing standardized iodine-125 brachytherapy within the Medium Choroidal Melanoma Trial. Kaplan-Meier life-table analysis evaluated two clinically significant outcomes at a 36-month window: (1) decline of best-corrected visual acuity to 20/200 or worse and (2) loss of six lines

Table 1 Patient Demographics and Tumor Characteristics: Medium Choroidal Melanoma Treatment Trial

Variable	Risk ratio	95% Confidence interval	Chi Square	P value
Age at baseline				
<50 (ref.)	1.0		8.3	0.02
50–69	2.8	(1.3–6.5)		
≥69	2.9	(1.1–7.1)		
Gender				
Female (ref.)	1.0		3.5	0.06
Male	1.6	(1.0–2.7)		
Apical height, mm				
2.5–5.0 (ref.)	1.0		20.3	0.00004
5.1–7.5	3.1	(1.7–5.6)		
7.6–10.0	5.0	(2.4–10.5)		
Visual acuity, tumor eye				
≥20/20 (ref.)	1.0		16.3	0.001
20/25–20/40	2.0	(1.0–4.0)		
20/50–20/160	1.6	(0.7–3.6)		
≤20/200	1.4	(0.5–3.7)		
Distance tumor border to FAZ[a] center, mm				
0.0 (ref.)	1.0		12.6	0.006
0.1–2.0	0.6	(0.3–1.3)		
2.1–8.0	0.4	(0.2–0.9)		
≥8.0	0.5	(0.2–1.4)		

[a] Foveal avascular zone.
Source: Ref. 15.

or more of visual acuity from baseline (a quadrupling of the visual angle) [12]. All enucleated patients were counted as having poor vision for the purpose of this analysis. Life-table analysis of the rate of decrease in visual acuity equal to or worse than 20/200 noted an incidence of 17% of patients by 1 year and increased to 43% of patients by 3 years. Loss of six or more lines of visual acuity occurred in 18% of patients by 1 year, 34% by 2 years, and in 49% by 3 years postbrachytherapy. Recovery of visual acuity was rare, occurring in less than 5% of patients. Overall, on average, patients experienced a decline in visual acuity of two lines per year after brachytherapy (Tables 2 and 3). Risk factors associated with loss of visual acuity included greater tumor thickness, posterior tumor location [including the foreal avascular zone (FAZ)], poorer baseline visual acuity, non-dome-shaped tumors, greater radiation treatment dose to the fovea/optic nerve/opposite eye wall, and systemic diabetes mellitus.

Table 2 Visual Acuity in Treated Eye at Time Since Enrollment for Eyes Undergoing 125-Iodine Brachytherapy: Medium Choroidal Melanoma Treatment Trial

	Months since enrollment							
	0		12		24		36	
Visual acuity	*n*	%	*n*	%	*n*	%	*n*	%
≥20/20	208	33.4	152	24.4	97	16.8	62	12.4
20/25–20/40	230	36.9	203	32.6	136	23.6	93	18.6
20/50–20/80	80	12.8	70	11.2	75	13.0	53	10.6
20/100–20/160	38	6.1	35	5.6	34	5.9	43	8.6
20/200–20/320	25	4.0	37	5.9	39	6.8	32	6.4
20/400–20/640	13	2.1	27	4.3	27	4.7	24	4.8
≤20/800	23	3.7	73	11.7	98	17.0	116	23.2
Enucleated	0	0.0	9	1.4	23	4.0	31	6.2
Not available	6	1.0	17	2.7	48	8.3	47	9.4
Total patients	623	100	623	100	577	100	501	100
Median visual acuity	20/32		20/40		20/50		20/125	

Source: Ref. 12.

Table 3 Visual Acuity Assessment for Development of Visual Acuity of 20/200 or Less or Loss of Six or More Lines of Standardized Visual Acuity in Eyes Undergoing 125-Iodine Brachytherapy: Medium Choroidal Melanoma Treatment Trial

Visual acuity outcome	Midpoint of interval (months)	No. at risk at start of interval	No. of events during interval	No. censored during interval	Cumulative percentage with event	95% confidence interval
Loss of six or	6	589	60	27	10	(8–13)
more lines, with	12	502	40	29	18	(15–21)
confirmation at	18	433	35	29	25	(21–28)
the next visit	24	369	45	21	34	(30–38)
	30	303	33	19	42	(37–46)
	36	251	31	16	49	(44–53)
Visual acuity 20/	6	556	56	25	10	(8–13)
200 or less, with	12	475	33	26	17	(14–20)
confirmation at	18	416	37	27	24	(21–28)
the next visit	24	352	38	21	33	(29–37)
	30	293	17	24	37	(33–41)
	36	252	24	15	43	(38–48)

Source: Ref. 12.

The primary study outcome within the COMS was all-cause mortality and secondarily histopathologically confirmed melanoma metastasis with death [13]. Of the 1317 enrolled patients, 660 were assigned to enucleation and 657 to iodine-125 brachytherapy. Central review of all enucleated specimens documented misdiagnosis in only 2 patients (2 of 660 patients, 0.003%) undergoing randomization to enucleation. Sample size analysis was selected with a power to detect a 25% difference in mortality based on selected treatment and determined a minimal sample size of 1250 randomized patients. Kaplan-Meier analysis was utilized to determine time-to-death estimates, while survival rates by treatment arm were analyzed using the log-rank test. At the time of data analysis for publication, 1072 patients (81%) had been followed for 5 years, while 416 patients (32%) had been followed for at least 10 years from study entry. Kaplan-Meier analysis of cumulative all-cause mortality at 5 years was 18% for iodine-125 brachytherapy and 19% for enucleation. Kaplan-Meier analysis of mortality with histopathologically confirmed metastases at 5 years were 9% after iodine-125 brachytherapy and 11% after enucleation (Figs. 1 and 2). No statistically significant difference was noted for either treatment outcome based on the selected treatment of iodine-125 brachytherapy or enucleation. Risk factors associated with mortality included greater apical tumor height, increased longest tumor basal diameter, posterior tumor location, and older patient age.

The Large Choroidal Melanoma Trial evaluated 1302 eligible patients and accrued 1003 patients between November 1986 and December 1994 into the multicentered clinical trial [13,16–19]. Patients were randomized to primary enucleation or to fractionated pre-enucleation external-beam radiotherapy, followed by standardized enucleation. Pre-enucleation fractionated external-beam radiotherapy was delivered in five daily 4.0-Gy fractions for a total delivered dose of 20 Gy. Standardized enucleation was performed within 4 weeks of study entry and within 80 hr of completion of radiotherapy.

Of the 1003 study patients (mean age of 60 years), 506 patients were randomized to standard enucleation and 497 to pre-enucleation radiotherapy followed by enucleation [18]. The two treatment arms were, again, well balanced, and tumors were noted to have a mean apical height of 9.5 mm and a mean longest basal diameter of 17.3 mm. Local treatment complications were evaluated in all patients undergoing enucleation surgery. Orbital tumor recurrence (biopsy-confirmed) occurred in no patients with pre-enucleation radiotherapy followed by enucleation compared with 5 patients with orbital tumor recurrence undergoing standardized enucleation alone ($p = 0.03$, Fisher exact test). Additionally, severe ptosis had a statistically significant lower incidence for patients undergoing pre-enucleation radiotherapy followed by enucleation compared with the randomized group undergoing enucleation alone ($p = 0.007$, log-rank test). At 5 years follow-up, the most common complication was poor prosthetic motility occurring in 18% of patients (not statistically significant). Pre-enucleation radiotherapy was not associated with increased postsurgical orbital or lid complications [18].

Histopathological review of eyes enucleated within the COMS Large and Medium Choroidal Melanoma trials was significant for the large standardized sample size (1527 globes) and centralized independent ocular pathological grading [8,20]. The accuracy of diagnosis confirmed by this review was high (99.7%), with five misdiagnosis, of which four globes contained metastatic adenocarcinoma and one contained a choroidal hemangioma. Mixed cell type was noted in 86% of eyes, with

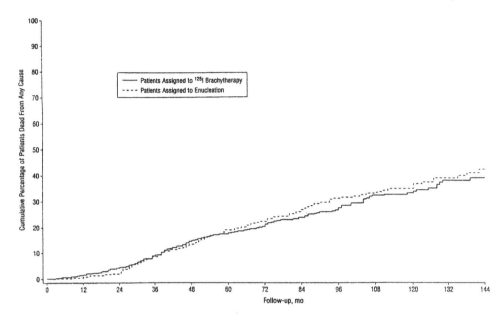

Figure 1 COMS randomized trial of iodine-125 brachytherapy or enucleation for medium-size choroidal melanoma: all-cause mortality outcomes. Cumulative proportion of patients who died from any cause by time from study enrollment. Patients are reported by treatment assignment to iodine-125 brachytherapy or primary enucleation.

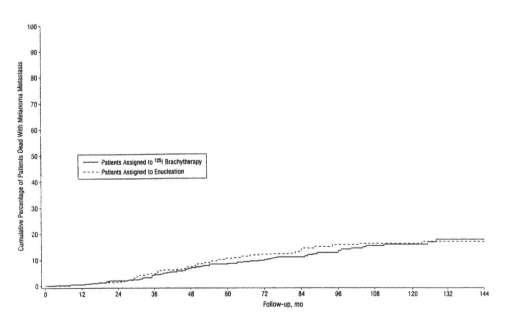

Figure 2 COMS randomized trial of iodine-125 brachytherapy or enucleation for medium-size choroidal melanoma: histopathologically confirmed metastatic melanoma related mortality outcomes. Cumulative proportion of patients who died with histopathological confirmation of melanoma metastasis. Patients are reported by treatment assignment to iodine-125 brachytherapy or primary enucleation.

only 5% of eyes containing primarily epithelioid cells. Local tumor invasion was significant, occurring in 81% of all study eyes. Extrascleral extension was present in 8% of eyes, while scleral invasion was noted in 56%. Retinal invasion and vitreous extension were present in 49 and 25% respectively. Mitotic activity was present in 9% of high-power fields in large choroidal tumors undergoing enucleation alone, in 5% of high-power fields in medium choroidal tumors undergoing enucleation, and in only 3% of high-power fields in eyes undergoing pre-enucleation radiotherapy followed by enucleation ($p = 0.001$). Increased intratumoral macrophage number was significantly associated with increased tumor pigmentation and increased tumor necrosis ($p = 0.001$ and $p = 0.01$ respectively).

The primary study outcome within the COMS was all-cause mortality and, secondarily, histopathologically confirmed melanoma metastasis with death [17]. In the Large Choroidal Melanoma Trial, the sample-size analysis was selected with a 90% power to detect a 20% difference in mortality based on selected treatment; it determined an effective sample size of 1003 randomized patients. Kaplan-Meier analysis was utilized to determine time-to-death estimates while survival rates by treatment arm were analyzed using the log-rank test. At the time of data analysis for publication, 734 patients (73%) had been followed for 5 years, while vital status at 10 years was available for 589 patients (59%) from study entry. Kaplan-Meier analysis of cumulative all-cause mortality at 5 years was 38% for pre-enucleation radiotherapy followed by enucleation and 42% for patients undergoing enucleation alone ($p = 0.32$, log-rank test) (Figs. 3 and 4). Cox proportional hazards analysis notes an overall risk ratio of 0.91 for pre-enucleation radiation therapy followed by enucleation when compared with enucleation alone. Kaplan-Meier analyses of mortality with histopathologically confirmed metastases at 5 years were 26% after pre-enucleation radiotherapy followed by enucleation and 28% after enucleation alone. No statistically significant difference was noted for either treatment outcome based on the selected treatment of pre-enucleation radiotherapy followed by enucleation or enucleation alone. Metastatic involvement was again most commonly noted to involve the liver (93%). Risk factors associated with mortality included increased longest tumor basal diameter and older patient age at study entry (Tables 4 and 5).

Evaluation of patient demographics to determine differences between evaluated patients with choroidal melanoma who are eligible versus those patients with choroidal melanoma who are ineligible, along with the correlate evaluation of eligible patients who elected to participate in the COMS and those who elected to be treated outside of the COMS, is key in determining both internal and external study validity [21]. This evaluation allows the clinician to determine study bias external to the randomization process and is paramount in determining the overall ability to generalize study data to patients outside of the study. Patient characteristics were reported for the Medium and Large Choroidal Melanoma trials and excellent internal and presumptive external validity was documented. These demographic data represent the single largest series of patients reported within a standardized environment, incorporating data generated from all 43 centers in North America.

The COMS evaluated 8712 patients with choroidal melanoma during the Medium Choroidal Melanoma Trial accrual study window [12–15]. A total of 5046 patients had tumors of eligible size, while 2882 met all study criteria for entry; 1317

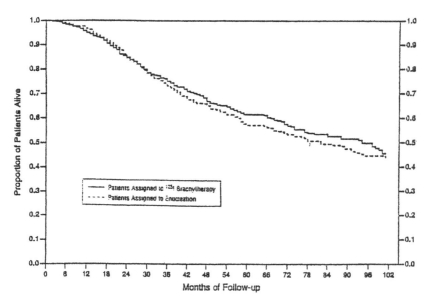

Figure 3 COMS randomized trial of pre-enucleation radiotherapy followed by enucleation or enucleation alone for large choroidal melanoma: all-cause mortality outcomes. Cumulative proportion of patients who survived to specified times since enrollment. Patients are reported by treatment assignment to pre-enucleation radiotherapy followed by enucleation or primary enucleation alone.

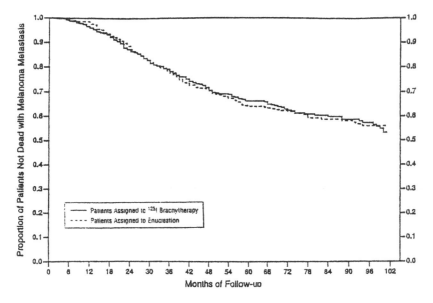

Figure 4 COMS randomized trial of pre-enucleation radiotherapy followed by enucleation or enucleation alone for large choroidal melanoma: Histopathologically confirmed metastatic melanoma–related mortality outcomes. Cumulative proportion of patients who survived without evidence of histopathologically confirmed melanoma metastases to specified times since enrollment. Patients are reported by treatment assignment to pre-enucleation radiotherapy followed by enucleation or primary enucleation alone.

patients elected to participate (46% of all eligible patients, 26% of all-size eligible tumors). Eligible patients had a mean age of 59 years, an equal number of men and women were eligible and participated, and 98% of patients were non-Hispanic whites. Patients were evaluated at the COMS clinical center at a median of 9 days from initial diagnosis. Visual acuity was 20/20 in 35% of the eligible patients' tumor-containing eye (Table 6) [12]. Tumor characteristics noted a mean apical height of 4.8 mm and longest basal diameter of 11.4 mm. The posterior border of the tumor was noted to be a mean distance of 4.0 mm from the optic disc and 3.0 mm from the center of the FAZ. Echographic characteristics documented a dome-shaped configuration in 77% of eyes, collar button in 16%, and lobulated in 5%, while internal reflectivity was low to low-medium in 79% of tumors (Table 7). Eligible patients who enrolled within the COMS Medium Tumor Trial were slightly older and had larger tumors than those patients who did not enroll [14]. These data suggest excellent internal reliability with no concerns for bias and suggest that enrolled patients were likely at higher risk for all-cause mortality than the cohort of patients who elected not to participate. This supports reasonable cause for external validity and allows the treating clinician to reasonably extrapolate these data to other patients with medium choroidal melanoma meeting the criteria for study eligibility.

The COMS evaluated 6078 patients with choroidal melanoma during the Large Choroidal Melanoma study accrual window [16–18]. A total of 1860 patients had tumors of eligible size; of these, 1302 were eligible for the clinical trial and 1003 enrolled in the randomized study (30% of all tumor patients and 77% of all-size eligible patients) (Table 8). The two principal reasons for the ineligibility of patients with large tumors were other independent primary cancers and greater than 50% of the tumor located within the ciliary body. Eligible patients had a mean age of 60 years, 56% were male, and 97% were non-Hispanic whites. Tumor characteristics at baseline included a mean apical tumor height of 9.5 mm and a longest mean basal diameter of 17.2 mm (Table 9). Echography noted collar-button configuration in 43%, dome shape in 38%, and lobulated in 15%; internal reflectivity was low to low-medium in 74% of tumors (Table 10). Only 26% of enrolling patients had a visual acuity of 20/40 or better at the time of enrollment (Table 11). Eligible patients who enrolled within the COMS Large Choroidal Melanoma Trial were similar to noneligible patients and to eligible patients who elected not to enroll in the trial with the exceptions that those who enrolled had larger tumor basal diameters, better visual acuity in the fellow eye, and less often had education beyond the high school level. These data, again, confirm high internal validity for the randomized treatment assignments and high external validity, allowing for application of these findings to patients with large choroidal melanoma meeting COMS criteria for study eligibility.

Quality-of-life analysis was included within the COMS study infrastructure to evaluate longitudinal and cross-sectional outcomes for patients treated within the Medium Choroidal Tumor trial [22,23]. In the absence of a survival outcome difference between treatments, along with the known decrease in visual function associated with iodine-125 brachytherapy, patient perceptions of quality of life become increasingly more pivotal to selection of treatment for the individual patient. Quality-of-life data are pending from the COMS and remain the major outcome variable yet to be reported.

The COMS utilized a classic study infrastructure incorporating a multi-centered, randomized, prospective evaluation of treatment for medium and large

Table 4 Baseline Tumor Characteristics: Large Choroidal Melanoma Treatment Trial

Tumor characteristic	Standard enucleation ($N = 506$)	Pre-enucleation radiation ($N = 497$)
Time since diagnosis (days)		
$\leqslant 30$	415 (82)	407 (82)
31–180	79 (16)	70 (14)
>180	12 (2)	20 (4)
Apical height (mm)		
<5.0	38 (8)	44 (9)
5.0–6.9	51 (10)	56 (11)
7.0–8.9	113 (22)	101 (20)
9.0–10.9	149 (30)	134 (27)
11.0–12.9	95 (19)	103 (21)
$\geqslant 13.0$	59 (12)	59 (12)
Not reported	1	0
Longest basal diameter (mm)		
<13.0	36 (7)	42 (8)
13.0–14.9	38 (8)	44 (9)
Proximity to optic disc (mm)		
$\geqslant 2.0$	331 (69)	345 (71)
<2.0	151 (31)	139 (29)
Not reported	24	13
Visible dilated feeder vessel to tumor		
Absent	383 (76)	393 (79)
Present	123 (24)	104 (21)
Associated RD		
None noted	82 (16)	90 (18)
Present, nonrhegmatogenous	411 (81)	396 (80)
Indeterminate or unknown	13 (3)	11 (2)
Shape/configuration		
Collar button	216 (43)	210 (42)
Dome	197 (39)	186 (37)
Lobulated or irregular	72 (14)	81 (16)
15.0–16.9	105 (21)	110 (22)
17.0–18.9	167 (33)	167 (34)
19.0–20.9	94 (19)	89 (18)
$\geqslant 21.0$	60 (12)	43 (9)
Indeterminate, not reported	6	2
Anterior border		
AC angle	28 (6)	29 (6)
Pars plicata	116 (23)	114 (24)
Pars plana	115 (23)	96 (20)
Between ora serrata and equator	181 (36)	176 (37)

Table 4 Continued

Tumor characteristic	Standard enucleation (N = 506)	Pre-enucleation radiation (N = 497)
Post to equator	60 (12)	65 (14)
Indeterminate, not reported	6	17
Peaked	12 (2)	10 (2)
Flat	4 (1)	5 (1)
Other	2 (<1)	2 (<1)
Indeterminate	3 (1)	3 (1)
Internal reflectivity		
Very low	22 (4)	17 (3)
Low	193 (38)	189 (38)
Low–medium	172 (34)	167 (34)
Medium	55 (11)	55 (11)
Medium–high	10 (2)	18 (4)
High or very high	3 (1)	2 (<1)
Irregular	34 (7)	36 (7)
Indeterminate	17 (3)	13 (3)

Source: Ref. 17.

choroidal melanoma to determine best treatment practices [2]. Utilizing this study infrastructure, overall study compliance was excellent, with compliance rates in excess of 90% in each of the study arms including patient eligibility, treatment application including external-beam radiotherapy, iodine-125 brachytherapy and enucleation, confirmation of tumor pathology, standardization of echography and photography, documentation of follow-up, and confirmation of vital status (Tables 12 and 13). This quality assurance, over a 17-year study interval, is a testament to the study design and the focus of the study participants.

Table 5 Histopathological Assessment of Metastatic Status: Large Choroidal Melanoma Treatment Trial

Status at death	Standard enucleation (N = 238)	Pre-enucleation radiation (N = 219)
Melanoma metastasis	130 (57)	139 (67)
Malignant tumor present, primary uncertain	51 (22)	41 (20)
Malignant tumor present, not metastatic melanoma	18 (8)	4 (2)
No evidence of malignancy	21 (9)	17 (8)
Insufficient evidence to establish presence of malignancy	8 (4)	6 (3)
Not yet assessed	10	12

Source: Ref. 17.

Table 6 Baseline Visual Acuity: Large Choroidal Melanoma Treatment Trial

	No. (%) of patients			
	Eligible patients			Ineligible patients
Visual acuity	Enrolled ($n = 1317$)	Not enrolled ($n = 2882$)	Total eligible ($n = 2882$)	patients ($n = 2164$)
Eye with choroidal melanoma				
20/20 or better	413 (32)	592 (38)	1005 (35)	368 (17)
20/25 to 20/32	343 (26)	409 (26)	752 (26)	487 (23)
20/40 to 20/50	236 (18)	228 (15)	464 (16)	360 (17)
20/63 to 20/80	92 (7)	130 (8)	222 (8)	254 (12)
20/100 to 20/125	62 (5)	44 (3)	106 (4)	104 (5)
20/160 to 20/200	50 (4)	61 (4)	111 (4)	161 (8)
Worse than 20/200	110 (8)	85 (6)	195 (7)	376 (18)
Not reported	11	16	27	54
Median	20/32	20/25	20/32	20/50
Fellow eye	917 (70)	1000 (64)	1917 (67)	999 (47)
20/20 or better	294 (22)	403 (26)	697 (24)	645 (30)
20/25 to 20/32	77 (6)	104 (7)	181 (6)	233 (11)
20/40 to 20/50	14 (1)	32 (2)	46 (2)	83 (4)
20/63 to 20/80	6 (<1)	7 (<1)	13 (<1)	13 (1)
20/100 to 20/125	3 (<1)	5 (<1)	8 (<1)	41 (2)
20/160 to 20/200	...a	...	...	110 (5)
Worse than 20/200	6	14	20	40
Not reported	≥20/20	≥20/20	≥20/20	20/25
Median				

a Ellipses indicate "not applicable."
Source: Ref. 14.

Single-institution clinical trials also play a role in our understanding of treatment benefits for patients with choroidal melanoma. Char and colleagues evaluated, in a prospective, randomized clinical trial, the application of helium ion charged-particle radiotherapy compared with iodine-125 brachytherapy [24]. This trial enrolled patients with medium choroidal/ciliary body melanoma and evaluated melanoma-specific mortality, local tumor recurrence, rates of enucleation, and treatment-related complications. Eighty-six patients were treated with helium ion charged-particle radiotherapy applied to a target 70 GyE to the tumor apex, with a 2-mm treatment margin, while 98 patients received iodine-125 brachytherapy applied to a target dose of 85 Gy to the tumor apex, with an initial treatment margin of 1 mm (later expanded to 2 mm after documentation of high local tumor failure rates). Char and colleagues reported high local tumor failure rates for iodine-125 brachytherapy with an event rate of 13.3% and an enucleation rate of 17.3% (mean follow-up 48 months) compared with helium ion charged particle radiotherapy with a local tumor failure rate of 0% and an enucleation rate of 9.3%. Metastatic ocular melanoma was noted in 8.2% of iodine-125 brachytherapy treated patients and in 9.3% of helium

Table 7 Echographic Baseline Characteristics: Medium Choroidal Melanoma Treatment Trial

	No. (%) of eligible patients	
Characteristic	Enrolled ($n = 1317$)	Not enrolled ($n = 1565$)
Tumor shape/configuration		
Dome	1014 (77)	327 (77)
Collar button	207 (16)	55 (13)
Lobulated or irregular	61 (5)	29 (7)
Peaked	31 (2)	9 (2)
Flat	3 (<1)	2 (<1)
Other	1 (<1)	0
Not available[a]	...[b]	1143
Internal reflectivity		
Very low	75 (6)	8 (10)
Low	503 (39)	49 (59)
Low–medium	523 (40)	17 (2)
Medium	85 (7)	7 (8)
Medium–high, high, or very high	37 (3)	2 (<1)
Irregular	75 (6)	0
Indeterminate	19	...
Not available	...	1482

[a] Not assessed after November 1989 for patients who did not enroll.
[b] Ellipses indicate "not applicable."
Source: Ref. 14.

ion treated patients. Melanoma related mortality was 8% in both treatment arms. Helium ion charged-particle radiotherapy was associated with lower tumor recurrence rates and lower enucleation rates than iodine-125 brachytherapy. Rates of local tumor recurrence and enucleation were significantly higher than reported within the COMS Medium Choroidal Melanoma Trial.

Gragoudas and colleagues evaluated, in a prospective randomized clinical trial, the application of proton-beam charged-particle radiotherapy at two different radiation doses to determine the effect on melanoma-specific mortality, local tumor control, visual acuity and visual field conservation, and treatment related complications [25]. A total of 188 patients were randomized to receive proton-beam radiotherapy at a targeted treatment dose of either 70 or 50 GyE to the tumor apex, with a treatment margin of 2 mm or greater. No difference in outcomes was noted for either treatment group with the exception of less loss of visual field noted for the lower-dose treatment arm. Melanoma metastatic disease was noted in 8% of treated patients, tumor recurrence was noted in 3% of treated eyes, while 55% of patients retained visual acuity of at least, 20/200. This single-institution clinical trial documented minimal benefit (and no significant risk) to a reduction in treatment dose to 50 GyE to the tumor apex for charged-particle radiotherapy for posterior uveal melanoma.

Table 8 Demographics of Ineligible, Eligible, Enrolled Eligible, and Not Enrolled but Eligible Patients (Evaluation of Internal and External Study Validity): Large Choroidal Melanoma Treatment Trial

	No. (%) of patients			
	Eligible patients			Ineligible patients ($n = 558$)
Characteristic	Enrolled ($n = 1003$)	Not enrolled ($n = 299$)	Total eligible ($n = 1302$)	
Age (years)				
<40	90 (9)	31 (11)	121 (9)	30 (5)
40–49	135 (13)	46 (16)	181 (14)	46 (8)
50–59	210 (21)	54 (18)	264 (20)	75 (13)
60–69	286 (29)	63 (21)	349 (27)	147 (26)
70–79	228 (23)	68 (23)	296 (23)	161 (29)
⩾80	54 (5)	33 (11)	87 (7)	99 (18)
Not reported	0	4	4	0
Mean age (years)	60.1	60.5	60.2	66.1
Sex				
Male	576 (57)	155 (53)	731 (56)	275 (49)
Female	427 (43)	140 (47)	567 (44)	283 (51)
Not reported	0	4	4	0
Race/ethnicity				
White, not Hispanic	970 (97)	288 (98)	1258 (97)	540 (97)
Hispanic	24 (2)	2 (1)	26 (2)	8 (1)
Black, not Hispanic	5 (<1)	4 (1)	9 (1)	8 (1)
Asian or Pacific Islander	2 (<1)	1 (<1)	3 (<1)	2 (<1)
American Indian or Eskimo	2 (<1)	0	2 (<1)	0
Not reported	0	4	4	0

Source: Ref. 16.

Clinical trials data approximate the "gold standard" for determination of treatment benefits particularly when the study design incorporates a clinically important question, standardizes inclusion and exclusion criteria, and maintains excellent study compliance, allowing for extrapolation of the study data to patients outside of the study. Clinical trials using this classic design tend to be expensive endeavors and require widespread participation of the medical community and eligible patients [26,27]. The Collaborative Ocular Melanoma Study has definitively answered the question of pre-enucleation radiotherapy as an unnecessary adjunctive treatment to primary enucleation alone in the management of large choroidal melanoma, has definitively answered the question of safety and efficacy of iodine-125 brachytherapy in the treatment of medium choroidal melanoma, and has noted no difference in mortality between this globe-conserving therapy and primary enucleation. Of significant import is the development of a national infrastructure that established standards of excellence within participating clinical centers of the

COMS for patients with choroidal melanoma, further broadening access of care for patients with this life-threatening ocular malignancy [28]. Further application of clinical trials methodology would play a significant role in evaluating evolving technologies in the management of posterior uveal melanoma, particularly treatment advances focused at enhanced globe conservation coupled with improved functional preservation of vision. Additionally, the COMS has defined a framework for a future clinical trial to evaluate the timing and treatment outcomes for patients with small choroidal melanoma.

Table 9 Tumor Characteristics for Ineligible, Eligible, Enrolled Eligible, and Not Enrolled but Eligible Patients: Large Choroidal Melanoma Treatment Trial

	No. (%) of patients			
	Eligible patients			Ineligible patients ($n = 558$)
Characteristic	Enrolled ($n = 1003$)	Not enrolled ($n = 299$)	Total eligible ($n = 1302$)	
Time since initial diagnosis (days)				
⩽30	864 (86)	244 (82)	1108 (85)	431 (77)
31–180	106 (11)	40 (13)	146 (11)	63 (11)
181–365	8 (1)	4 (1)	12 (1)	16 (3)
>365	25 (2)	9 (3)	34 (3)	48 (9)
Not reported	0	2	2	0
Median days	7	7	7	7
Laterality				
Right eye	507 (51)	148 (49)	655 (50)	275 (49)
Left eye	496 (49)	151 (51)	647 (50)	283 (51)
Apical height (mm)				
⩽5.0	90 (9)	22 (7)	112 (9)	48 (9)
5.1–7.0	109 (11)	26 (9)	135 (10)	46 (8)
7.1–9.0	230 (23)	64 (21)	294 (23)	103 (19)
9.1–11.0	281 (28)	100 (33)	381 (29)	153 (28)
11.1–13.0	191 (19)	65 (22)	256 (20)	115 (21)
13.1–15.0	73 (7)	18 (6)	91 (7)	61 (11)
>15.0	28 (3)	4 (1)	32 (2)	30 (5)
Not reported	1	0	1	2
Mean (mm)	9.5	9.6	9.5	10.1
Longest basal diameter (mm)				
<13.0	78 (8)	34 (12)	112 (9)	49 (9)
13.0–14.9	82 (8)	37 (13)	119 (9)	38 (7)
15.0–16.9	215 (22)	66 (23)	281 (22)	89 (17)
17.0–18.9	334 (34)	84 (29)	418 (32)	166 (31)
19.0–20.9	183 (18)	52 (18)	235 (18)	119 (22)
21.0–22.9	73 (7)	14 (5)	87 (7)	41 (8)
⩾23.0	30 (3)	6 (2)	36 (3)	29 (5)
Indeterminate, not reported	8	6	14	27
Mean (mm)	17.3	16.7	17.2	17.6
Location of posterior tumor border				
Posterior to equator	885 (89)	281 (95)	1166 (90)	389 (79)
Between ora serrata and equator	31 (3)	8 (3)	39 (3)	64 (13)
Ciliary body	0	0	0	8 (2)

Table 9 Continued

Characteristic	No. (%) of patients			
	Eligible patients			Ineligible patients ($n = 558$)
	Enrolled ($n = 1003$)	Not enrolled ($n = 299$)	Total eligible ($n = 1302$)	
Indeterminate	79 (8)	7 (2)	86 (7)	32 (6)
Not reported, not requested	8	3	11	65[a]
Location of anterior tumor border				
Posterior to equator	125 (12)	30 (10)	155 (12)	41 (8)
Between ora serrata and equator	357 (36)	121 (41)	478 (37)	129 (26)
Pars plana	211 (21)	70 (23)	281 (22)	60 (12)
Pars plicata	230 (23)	64 (21)	294 (23)	128 (26)
Anterior chamber angle	57 (6)	8 (3)	65 (5)	42 (9)
Iris	0	0	0	70 (14)
Indeterminate	21 (2)	5 (2)	26 (2)	22 (4)
Not reported, not requested	2	1	3	66[a]

[a]Data requested for patients in this category only until March 1994.
Source: Ref. 16.

Table 10 Baseline Echographic Characteristics: Large Choroidal Melanoma Treatment Trial

Characteristic	No. (%) of eligible patients	
	Enrolled ($n = 1003$)	Not enrolled ($n = 299$)
Tumor shape/configuration		
Collar button	426 (43)	61 (47)
Dome	383 (38)	47 (36)
Lobulated or irregular	153 (15)	20 (15)
Peaked	22 (2)	2 (2)
Flat	9 (1)	0
Other	4 (<1)	0
Indeterminate, not reported	6	169[a]
Internal reflectivity		
Very low	39 (4)	20[b]
Low	382 (39)	
Low–medium	339 (35)	
Medium	110 (11)	
Medium–high	28 (3)	4[c]
High	4 (<1)	
Very high	1 (<1)	
Irregular	70 (7)	
Indeterminate, not assessed	30	275

[a] Not classified after November 1989 for patients not enrolled.
[b] Total of very low, low, low–medium, and medium.
[c] Total of medium-high, high, very high, and irregular.
Source: Ref. 16.

Table 11 Baseline Visual Acuity: Large Choroidal Melanoma Treatment Trial

	No. (%) of patients			
	Eligible patients			Ineligible patients (n = 558)
Visual Acuity	Enrolled (n = 1003)	Not enrolled (n = 299)	Total eligible (n = 1302)	
Eye with choroidal melanoma				
20/20 or better	123 (12)	39 (16)	162 (13)	30 (6)
20/25–20/32	136 (14)	49 (20)	185 (15)	74 (16)
20/40–20/50	149 (15)	31 (12)	180 (14)	55 (12)
20/63–20/80	116 (12)	27 (11)	143 (12)	55 (12)
20/100–20/125	86 (9)	18 (7)	104 (8)	20 (4)
20/160–20/200	58 (6)	15 (6)	73 (6)	31 (7)
Worse than 20/200	324 (33)	71 (28)	395 (32)	204 (43)
Not reported	11	49	60	89
Median visual acuity	20/80	20/63	20/80	20/160
Fellow Eye				
20/20 or better	690 (69)	146 (49)	836 (66)	218 (44)
20/25–20/32	229 (23)	71 (29)	300 (23)	148 (30)
20/40–20/50	47 (5)	17 (6)	64 (5)	62 (13)
20/63–20/80	15 (1)	10 (3)	25 (2)	34 (7)
20/100–20/125	5 (<1)	4 (1)	9 (1)	4 (1)
20/160–20/200	4 (<1)	1 (<1)	5 (<1)	11 (2)
Worse than 20/200	8 (1)	3 (1)	11 (1)	17 (3)
Not reported	5	47	52	64
Median visual acuity	⩾20/20	⩾20/20	⩾20/20	20/25

Source: Ref. 16.

Table 12 Patient Baseline Demographics Medium Choroidal Melanoma Treatment Trial

| Characteristic | No. % of patients | | | |
| | Eligible patients | | | Ineligible patients (n = 2164) |
	Enrolled (n = 1317)	Not enrolled (n = 1565)	Total eligible (n = 2882)	
Age (year)				
<40	125 (9)	176 (11)	301 (10)	162 (7)
40–49	178 (14)	262 (17)	440 (15)	236 (11)
50–59	268 (20)	328 (21)	596 (21)	346 (16)
60–69	408 (31)	382 (24)	790 (27)	526 (24)
70–79	282 (21)	320 (20)	602 (21)	622 (29)
⩾80	56 (4)	91 (6)	147 (5)	271 (13)
Not reported	0	6	6	1
Mean age (years)	60	59	59	64
Sex				
Men	665 (50)	813 (52)	1478 (51)	1056 (49)
Women	652 (50)	746 (48)	1398 (49)	1107 (51)
Not reported	0	6	6	1
Race/ethnicity				
White, not Hispanic	1289 (98)	1534 (98)	2823 (98)	2117 (98)
Hispanic	14 (1)	14 (1)	28 (1)	29 (1)
Black, not Hispanic	8 (1)	7 (<1)	15 (1)	13 (1)
Asian or Pacific Islander	5 (<1)	4 (<1)	9 (<1)	3 (<1)
Native American	1 (<1)	0	1 (<1)	1 (<1)
Not reported	0	6	6	1

Source: Ref. 14.

Table 13 Tumor Baseline Characteristics: Medium Choroidal Melanoma Treatment Trial

	No. (%) of patients			
	Eligible patients			Ineligible patients ($n = 2164$)
Characteristic	Enrolled ($n = 1317$)	Not enrolled ($n = 1565$)	Total eligible ($n = 2882$)	
Time since initial diagnosis, days				
≤ 30	944 (72)	1190 (76)	2134 (74)	1572 (73)
31–180	188 (14)	170 (11)	358 (12)	254 (12)
181–365	67 (5)	56 (4)	123 (4)	78 (4)
> 365	117 (9)	148 (9)	265 (9)	246 (11)
Not reported	1	1	2	13
Median time, days	9	8	8	7
Laterality				
Right eye	663 (50)	821 (52)	1484 (51)	1075 (50)
Left eye	654 (50)	744 (48)	1398 (49)	1084 (50)
Both eyes	. . . [a]	. . .	. . .	5 (<1)
Apical height, mm				
2.5–3.0	162 (12)	297 (19)	459 (16)	294 (14)
3.1–4.0	430 (33)	472 (30)	902 (31)	613 (28)
4.1–5.0	243 (18)	268 (17)	511 (18)	372 (17)
5.1–6.0	154 (12)	199 (13)	353 (12)	288 (13)
6.1–7.0	139 (11)	138 (9)	277 (10)	233 (11)
7.1–8.0	114 (9)	104 (7)	218 (8)	192 (9)
8.1–10.0	75 (6)	87 (6)	162 (6)	171 (8)
Not reported	. . .	. . .	. . .	1
Mean height, mm	4.8	4.7	4.7	5.0
Longest basal diameter, mm				
≤ 8.0	185 (14)	252 (16)	437 (15)	378 (18)
8.1–10.0	275 (21)	378 (24)	653 (23)	797 (23)
10.1–12.0	371 (28)	426 (27)	797 (28)	539 (25)
12.1–14.0	276 (21)	302 (19)	578 (20)	378 (18)
14.1–16.0	210 (16)	207 (13)	417 (15)	348 (16)
Indeterminate	. . .	. . .	. . .	24
Mean diameter, mm	11.4	11.1	11.2	11.2
Location of posterior tumor border				
Posterior to equator	1279 (97)	1487 (97)	2766 (97)	1108 (85)
Between equator and ora serrata	38 (3)	46 (3)	84 (3)	145 (11)
Ciliary body	. . .	. . .	. . .	36 (3)
Anterior chamber angle	. . .	. . .	. . .	2 (<1)
Indeterminate	. . .	2	2	11
Not available	. . .	30	30	862

Table 13 Continued

Characteristic	No. (%) of patients			
	Eligible patients			Ineligible patients ($n = 2164$)
	Enrolled ($n = 1317$)	Not enrolled ($n = 1565$)	Total eligible ($n = 2882$)	
Location of anterior tumor border				
Posterior to equator	728 (55)	757 (49)	1485 (51)	725 (57)
Between equator and ora serrata	446 (34)	604 (39)	1050 (37)	270 (21)
Ciliary body	143 (11)	172 (11)	315 (11)	167 (13)
Anterior chamber angle	...	...	...	55 (4)
Iris	...	...	...	67 (5)
Indeterminate	...	2	2	18
Not available	...	30	30	862
Location of tumor apex relative to fovea				
Centered over fovea	9 (1)	4 (<1)	13 (<1)	32 (2)
Temporal	632 (48)	328 (40)	960 (45)	379 (29)
Superior	262 (20)	202 (25)	464 (22)	301 (23)
Inferior	255 (19)	167 (20)	422 (20)	285 (22)
Nasal	159 (12)	116 (14)	275 (13)	298 (23)
Not available†	...	748	748	869
Distance from closest tumor border to edge of optic disc, mm				
≤2.0	216 (16)	27 (17)	...	...
2.1–4.0	423 (32)	41 (26)	...	...
4.1–6.0	311 (24)	33 (21)	...	...
6.1–8.0	156 (12)	23 (14)	...	...
>8.0	207 (16)	35 (22)	...	...
Not available[b]	4	1406	...	...
Median, mm	4.0	4.5		
Closest distance between tumor and FAZ center, mm				
0	190 (15)	17 (11)	...	...
0.1–2.0	345 (26)	33 (21)	...	...
2.1–5.0	342 (26)	41 (26)	...	...
5.1–8.0	226 (17)	33 (21)	...	...
>8.0	201 (15)	35 (22)	...	...
Not available[6]	13	1406	...	...
Median, mm	3.0	4.5		

[a] Ellipses indicate "not applicable" or "inappropriate calculation"; FAZ, foveal avascular zone.
[b] Requested only during early years for patients not enrolled. Missing data for enrolled patients.
Source: Ref. 14.

REFERENCES

1. Collaborative Ocular Melanoma Study Group. Complications of enucleation surgery. COMS report no. 2. In: Franklin RM, ed. Proceedings of the New Orleans Academy of Ophthalmology Symposium on Retina and Vitreous. New York: Kugler, 1993, pp 181–190.
2. Collaborative Ocular Melanoma Study Group. Design and methods of a clinical trial for a rare condition: The Collaborative Ocular Melanoma Study. COMS report no. 3. Control Clin Trials 1993; 14:362–391.
3. Collaborative Ocular Melanoma Study Group. Echography (ultrasound) procedures for the Collaborative Ocular Melanoma Study. COMS report no. 12, part II. J Ophthalm Nurs Technol 1999; 18:219–232.
4. Byrne SF, Marsh MJ, Boldt HC, Green RL, Johnson RN, Wilson DJ. Consistency of observations from echograms made centrally in the Collaborative Ocular Melanoma Study. COMS report no. 13. Ophthalm Epidemiol 2002; 9:11–27.
5. Collaborative Ocular Melanoma Study Group. COMS Manual of Procedures. Accession no. PB95–179693. Springfield, VA: National Technical Information Service, 1995.
6. Collaborative Ocular Melanoma Study Group. COMS Forms Book. Accession no. PB91–217315. Springfield, VA: National Technical Information Service, 1991.
7. Moy CS, Albert DM, Diener-West M, et al. Cause-specific mortality coding. methods in the collaborative ocular melanoma study. COMS report no. 14. Control Clin Trials 2001; 22:248–262.
8. Collaborative Ocular Melanoma Study Group. Histopathologic characteristics of uveal melanomas in eyes enucleated from the Collaborative Ocular Melanoma Study. COMS report no. 6. Am J Ophthalmol 1998; 125:745–766.
9. Collaborative Ocular Melanoma Study Group. Factors predictive of growth and treatment of small choroidal melanoma. COMS report no. 5. Arch Ophthalmol 1997; 115:1537–1544.
10. Murray TG. Small choroidal melanoma. Arch Ophthalmol 1997; 115:1577–1578.
11. Collaborative Ocular Melanoma Study Group. Mortality in patients with small choroidal melanoma. COMS report no. 4. Arch Ophthalmol 1997; 115:886–893.
12. Melia BM, Abramson DH, Albert DM, et al. Collaborative ocular melanoma study (COMS) randomized trial of I-125 brachytherapy for medium choroidal melanoma: I. Visual acuity after 3 years. COMS report no. 16. Ophthalmology 2001; 108:348–366.
13. Diener-West M, Earle JD, Fine SL, et al. The COMS randomized trial of iodine 125 brachytherapy for choroidal melanoma: III. Initial mortality findings. COMS report no. 18. Arch Ophthalmol 2001; 119:969–982.
14. Diener-West M, Earle JD, Fine SL, et al. The COMS randomized trial of iodine 125 brachytherapy for choroidal melanoma: II. Characteristics of patients enrolled and not enrolled. COMS report no. 17. Arch Ophthalmol 2001; 119:951–965.
15. Collaborative Ocular Melanoma Study Group. The COMS randomized trial of iodine 125 brachytherapy for choroidal melanoma: IV. Local treatment failure and enucleation in the first five years following brachytherapy. COMS report no. 19. Arch Ophthalmology 2002. In press.
16. Collaborative Ocular Melanoma Study Group. The Collaborative Ocular Melanoma Study (COMS) randomized trial of pre-enucleation radiation of large choroidal melanoma I: Characteristics of patients enrolled and not enrolled. COMS report no. 9. Am J Ophthalmol 1998; 125:767–778.
17. Collaborative Ocular Melanoma Study Group. The Collaborative Ocular Melanoma Study (COMS) randomized trial of pre-enucleation radiation of large choroidal melanoma: II. Initial mortality findings. COMS report no. 10. Am J Ophthalmol 1998; 125:779–796.

18. Collaborative Ocular Melanoma Study Group. The Collaborative Ocular Melanoma Study (COMS) randomized trial of pre-enucleation radiation of large choroidal melanoma: III. Local complications and observations following enucleation. COMS report no. 11. Am J Ophthalmol 1998; 126:362–372.

19. Collaborative Ocular Melanoma Study Group. Assessment of metastatic disease status at death in 435 patients with large choroidal melanoma in the Collaborative Ocular Melanoma Study (COMS). COMS report no. 15. Arch Ophthalmol 2001; 119:670–676.

20. Grossniklaus HE, Albert DM, Green WR, Conway BP, Hovland KR. Clear cell differentiation in choroidal melanoma. COMS report no. 8. Collaborative Ocular Melanoma Study Group. Arch Ophthalmol 1997; 115:894–898.

21. Collaborative Ocular Melanoma Study Group. Sociodemographic and clinical predictors of participation in two randomized trials: findings from the Collaborative Ocular Melanoma Study. COMS report no. 7. Control Clin Trials 2001; 22:526–537.

22. Melia BM, Moy CS, McCaffrey L. Quality of life in patients with choroidal melanoma: A pilot study. Ophthalm Epidemiol 1999; 6:19–28.

23. COMS Quality of Life Study Group. Quality of life assessment in the collaborative ocular melanoma study: Design and methods. COMS-QOLS report no. 1. Ophthalm Epidemiol 1999; 6:5–17.

24. Char DH, Quivey JM, Castro JR, Kroll S, Phillips T. Helium ions versus iodine 125 brachytherapy in the management of uveal melanoma. A prospective, randomized, dynamically balanced trial. Ophthalmology 1993; 100:1547–1554.

25. Gragoudas ES, Lane AM, Regan S et al. A randomized controlled trial of varying radiation doses in the treatment of choroidal melanoma. Arch Ophthalmol 2000; 118:773–778.

26. Benson WE. The COMS: Why was it not stopped sooner? (letter). Arch Ophthalmol 2002; 120:672–673.

27. Fine S. The COMS: Why was it not stopped sooner? (reply to letter). Arch Ophthalmol 2002; 120:673.

28. Sieving PA. Fifteen years of work: The COMS outcomes for medium-sized choroidal melanoma. Arch Ophthalmol 2001; 119:1067–1068.

18

Clinical Trials in Retinoblastoma

EMILY Y. CHEW

National Eye Institute/National Institutes of Health, Bethesda, Maryland, U.S.A.

I. INTRODUCTION

Retinoblastoma is a rare tumor of both scientific and public health importance. Scientifically, this ocular condition provides unique opportunities for the evaluation of specific genetic abnormalities associated with tumorigenesis [1]. These data help elucidate the processes whereby both ocular and systemic tumors may develop [2,3]. From a public health perspective, the importance of retinoblastoma transcends even the tragedy associated with the death of a child. Although current treatments have resulted in survival better than 90%, these children and society have the burden of coping with long-term visual and systemic morbidity. More recently, systemic chemotherapy coupled with local intraocular therapy have become accepted treatment to avoid the use of external-beam radiation, which has been associated with disfigurement of the face, poor visual results, and a 35% risk of secondary cancers during a 30-year period [4–9]. Treatment of large tumors, especially those with vitreous seeding, remains difficult, as they have responded poorly to both the chemotherapy and the traditional treatment of radiation. Such eyes have often required enucleation. Once the tumor extends outside the eye, the prognosis is dismal.

The need for improved treatment in retinoblastoma remains a priority for all clinicians taking care of these young children and their devastated families. This can be achieved only with the collaborative effort of enthusiastic investigators, as this is a rare disorder. An initial meeting held on the campus of the National Institutes of Health in February 1995 resulted in the establishment of a core group of interested investigators, the Retinoblastoma Study Group, who collaborated on the development of a protocol for a standardized chemotherapy using carboplatin, etoposide, and vincristine. Since this meeting, clinicians from a number of countries have embraced this protocol, which uses chemotherapy and local intraocular therapy as the standard of care for a number of patients with retinoblastoma. This treatment protocol needs to be continuously refined to achieve improved visual and systemic results. The treatment for childhood cancers, such as leukemia, has evolved, with high success rates for survival through the process of collaborative research conducted over decades by dedicated investigators in the Children's Cancer Study Group and the Pediatric Oncology Group, both multicentered clinical research groups using common treatment protocols and evaluating common outcome variables. Networks of clinicians such as the Retinoblastoma Study Group need to be supported and maintained to conduct epidemiological studies and clinical trials in the therapy of retinoblastoma.

II. EPIDEMIOLOGICAL STUDIES AND CLINICAL TRIALS

Retinoblastoma is a rare ocular disorder with a limited number of patients treated in major clinical centers. For epidemiological studies such as the assessment of associated risk factors and clinical trials to evaluate treatment modalities, multicentered studies are necessary in order to provide sufficient numbers to make meaningful comparisons. Clinical trials may not be necessary to answer all research questions. However, treatment modalities that have small to moderate beneficial effects must be assessed, usually with a controlled clinical trial. Rarely are treatment effects so large that only a small number of patients will be required to be enrolled in a study to achieve statistical and clinical meaningful significance.

By sharing the data, the network of clinician may be able to identify future research questions more readily. It is important to identify future research questions regarding retinoblastoma.

A. Design Issues

1. Interdisciplinary Approach

Treatment strategies in the retinoblastoma require interdisciplinary collaboration among medical oncologists, pediatric ophthalmologist/retinal specialists, and ophthalmic oncologists. The design and conduct of clinical trials require additional team members—statisticians, clinical trialists, and epidemiologists [10]. It is imperative that all such participants of the clinical trial be involved with the process from the conception of the study to the interpretation of the data and drafting of the final manuscript of the study results. Additional expertise in regulatory issues dealing with the Food and Drug Administration (FDA) may be necessary for the conduct of such trials.

Because the number of patients with this rare ocular disorder seen in each major clinical center or major ophthalmic center throughout the United States, Canada, and Europe is limited, a clinical trial is feasible only if the collaborative efforts of a number of investigators in different geographic localities are combined. This requires also the efforts of a coordinating center that is adept in dealing with the issues of clinical trials to provide the necessary support for a large number of clinical centers providing limited number of participants for trials of a rare condition. In addition, a successful trial requires the direction of a chair and/or an advisory group willing to facilitate such collaborative efforts. Adequate funding to establish the essential infrastructure—i.e., clinical coordinator, data management, data analyses, and others—will also be crucial to the success of a randomized, controlled clinical trial. Clinical trials are unfortunately expensive, but they do provide the "gold standards" for guidance of treatment. It is important for the ophthalmic community to support such efforts of controlled clinical trials by referring patients and contributing in the design and conduct of trials.

2. Standardized Common Protocol

The protocol to be followed by all investigators, who may reside in different parts of the world, must be standardized to ensure that similar patients are receiving the same types of treatment. This requires standardized methods of evaluating eligibility and exclusion criteria and primary as well as secondary outcome measures of interest. Certification of the treating investigators and the technicians may also help with the standardization of the protocol. Monitoring of the trial is needed to determine compliance with the manual of operations of the study. Clinical trials should have an independent data and safety monitoring committee, which will evaluate the data periodically during the course of the study so as to provide protection for the study subjects. If the data indicate a clear beneficial effect of treatment on the primary outcome or if harmful effects are seen with treatment, an early termination of the study should be considered.

3. Eligibility Criteria

Once a clinical research issue has been identified, the study population must be defined, with reproducible methods of classifying the severity, location, and other characteristics of the tumors found in the eye, as well as other patient characteristics. The previously published classification, known as the Reese-Ellsworth classification, is no longer an adequate classification, as it was based on prognosis for mortality. Obviously, the prognostic characteristics for survival of the patient remain important factors to consider in treatment. However, a more refined classification of the status of retinoblastoma in the eye is required. A more recent ocular classification of retinoblastoma involvement, established by Murphree and other investigators, may be a clinically relevant and reproducible system. This classification is currently available at the following website: *https://www.unhres.utoronto.ca/abc/*. Within the context of a clinical trial, such a classification of ocular lesions of retinoblastoma can be further validated and refined. The classification for diabetic retinopathy as it is used today has its roots in the Airlie House Classification, which predated the beginning of the Diabetic Retinopathy Study (DRS) [11,12]. During the course of the randomized clinical trials of diabetic retinopathy, the DRS, and the Early Treatment Diabetic Retinopathy, the validity and reproducibility of the classification of diabetic retinopathy were further evaluated. This classification has provided the gold standard for all trials of diabetic retinopathy throughout the world.

An example of a possible clinical trial may include subjects with eyes manifesting the most severe form of retinoblastoma, in which there is vitreous seeding and tumors of large volume, resulting in exudative retinal detachment. The eligibility criteria for a trial of such eyes may require specific tests—i.e., ultrasonography, fundus photography, optical coherence tomography (OCT), and others. Standardization of the protocol that establishes both eligibility criteria is essential. When possible, the grading of some of these tests should be done at a centralized reading center that has no prior knowledge of the patients' characteristics or the assigned treatment.

4. Outcome Measurements

The main measurements of outcome would include the assessment of visual function in a standardized fashion. In order to obtain best-corrected visual acuities, the pediatric patients other methods of visual acuity measurement in addition to the traditional best-corrected visual acuity measured on the logarithmic visual acuity charts (Early Treatment Diabetic Retinopathy Study (ETDRS) visual acuity charts) may be required [13–15]. Secondary outcome measurements include ultrasonography, which will measure both the tumor height and volume as well as the presence of exudative retinal detachment in these cases. All of these assessments should be done with masked examiners who have no knowledge of the treatment modalities to be used.

B. Adverse Effects

Immediate adverse side effects associated with treatment of retinoblastoma will be collected as part of the clinical trial, with adverse report forms that must be submitted to central agencies such as the FDA if the drug/device is an investigative new drug or an approved drug with a new indication for use in this ocular disease.

An important adverse side effects associated with chemotherapy is the potential to develop secondary tumors. Patients with retinoblastoma already have this propensity, which is accelerated by radiation. It is important to gather such data during the course of the clinical trial and many years following the completion of the trial. This propensity may result in increased mortality decades following the administration of the chemotherapy. It may not be feasible to provide decades of follow-up in a clinical trial. Creative design of simple trials may be able to gather data on these long-term adverse effects. Alternative methods of obtaining such information may include periodic assessment of potential deaths of this cohort of individuals through agencies such as the National Death Index from the National Health Statistics. This means that essential information required for such surveys must be gathered at baseline. It is also important to obtain informed consents from all subjects and their families for the future collection of this information. With increasing scrutiny of the Institutional Review Boards (IRBs), these procedures may not be possible. It is important, however, for these studies of children, that the devastating effects of such adverse events be collected.

C. Masking of Treatment

Depending on the research question to be addressed, it may be difficult to mask the patient, his or her parents, and the treating ophthalmologists and oncologists as to the randomly assigned treatment. The placebo effect is real and, whenever possible, both the treating physician and the patient and his or her family should be masked. The technicians who are evaluating the major outcome measures, however, can and should definitely be masked to assigned treatment to prevent a biased assessment of the treatment effects. If possible, the patient care chart should not be available to the technicians who measure outcomes such as visual acuity, tumor regression measured by ultrasonography or optical coherence tomography, etc.

D. Natural History Data

Like all controlled clinical trials, studies in retinoblastoma will be valuable in providing important longitudinal clinical data. It is unexpected that trials in retinoblastoma will provided a pure placebo treatment group because no investigators would be willing to participate in such a trial. However, the natural history of the "standard of care" provides important information for the care of patients with retinoblastoma. In addition, risk-factor analyses of baseline characteristics as predictors of treatment outcome may also be valuable.

III. CONCLUSION

To further our knowledge of treatment for retinoblastoma, well-designed, controlled clinical trials are needed to provide data on both the beneficial effects as well as the long-term adverse effects of treatment. Such efforts deserve the support of the ophthalmic community because, in the case of such a rare ocular condition, it is imperative to evaluate treatment modalities within the context of a multicentered study. Establishing a retinoblastoma network will also enhance the chance of sharing precious tissues, which may lead to further tests at the basic science level to elucidate tumor formation as well as possible leads for new treatment techniques.

REFERENCES

1. Knudson AG. Antioncogenes and human cancer. Proc Natl Acad Sci USA 1993; 90:10914–10921.
2. Hamel PA, Phillips RA, Muncaster M, et al. Speculations on the roles of RB1 in tissue-specific differentiation, tumor initiation, and tumor progression. FASEB J 1993; 7:846–54.
3. Weinberg RA. The retinoblastoma protein and cell cycle control. Cell 1995; 81:323–330.
4. Eng C, Li FP, Abramson DH, et al. Mortality from second tumors among the long-term survivors of retinoblastoma. J Natl Cancer Inst 1993; 85:1121–1128.
5. Gallie BL, Budning A, DeBoer G, et al. Chemotherapy with focal therapy can cure intraocular retinoblastoma without radiotherapy. Arch Ophthalmol 1996; 114:1321–1328.
6. Kingston JE, Hungerford JL, Madreperla SA, et al. Results of combined chemotherapy and radiotherapy for advanced intraocular retinoblastoma. Arch Ophthalmol 1996; 114:1321–1328.
7. Murphree AL, Villablanca JG, Deegan WF III, et al. Chemotherapy plus local therapy in the treatment of intraocular retinoblastoma. Arch Ophthalmol 1996; 114:1348–1356.

8. Shields CL, De Potter P, Himelstein BP, et al. Chemoreduction in the initial management of intraocular retinoblastoma. Arch Ophthalmol 1996; 114:1330–1338.
9. Shields CL, Shields JA, Needle M, et al. Combined chemoreduction and adjuvant treatment for intraocular retinoblastoma. Ophthalmology 1997; 104:2101–2111.
10. Meinert CL. Clinical Trials: Design, Conduct, and Analyses. New York: Oxford University Press, 1986.
11. The Diabetic Retinopathy Study Research Group. DRS report #6: Design, methods, and baseline results. Invest Ophthalmol 1981; 21(1):149–209.
12. The Diabetic Retinopathy Study Research Group. DRS Report No. 7: A modification of the Airlie House classification of diabetic retinopathy. Invest-Ophthalmol Vis Sci 1981; 21:210–226.
13. Ferris FL, Kassoff A, Bresnick GH, et al. New visual acuity charts for clinical research. Am J Ophthalmol 1982; 94(1):91–96.
14. Holmes JM, Beck RW, Repka MX, et al. The Amblyopia Treatment Study visual acuity testing protocol. Arch Ophthalmol 2001; 119:1345–1353.
15. Cryotherapy for Retinopathy of Prematurity Cooperative Group. Multicenter trial of cryotherapy for retinopathy of prematurity: preliminary results. Arch Ophthalmol 1988; 106:471–479.

19

Pathology of Uveal Melanoma: Histological Parameters and Patient Prognosis

ROBERT FOLBERG

University of Illinois at Chicago, Chicago, Illinois, U.S.A.

JACOB PE'ER

Hadassah-Hebrew University Hospital, Jerusalem, Israel

I. INTRODUCTION

Dermatologists and dermatopathologists employ a dazzling array of terms to describe pigmented cutaneous lesions. There are melanomas of the lentigo maligna type, superficial spreading type, acral lentiginous type, and nodular melanoma. The criteria to describe regression in cutaneous melanoma were delineated nearly 25 years ago. Borderline pigmented cutaneous lesions (between melanomas and nevi) are described. Aside from acquired nevi, there are congenital nevi of the small and garment type, dysplastic nevi, Spitz nevi, blue and cellular blue nevi, and many others.

Ophthalmic pathologists, on the other hand, are handicapped by an impoverished lexicon for describing melanocytic uveal lesions: *nevus* and *melanoma*. Among nevi, ophthalmic pathologists recognize only two variants: congenital melanosis oculi and melanocytoma. There is no vocabulary to describe precursor lesions of uveal melanoma [1].

Are there no dysplastic nevi, Spitz tumors, or cellular blue nevi of the choroid or ciliary body? Is it possible that there are biologically indolent lesions mislabeled clinically and histologically as melanoma? The relative inaccessibility of uveal melanocytic lesions to biopsy without compromise of vision has been the most formidable obstacle to progress in their descriptive pathology. By contrast, dermatologists and dermatopathologists collaborated to develop precise clinico-pathological correlations, and long-term follow-up studies provided information on the biological behavior of many of types of pigmented cutaneous lesions.

When precise clinicopathological correlations are possible, as in iris melanomas, which are easily visible during slit-lamp examination and accessible to excision, a robust pathological classification is possible. The classification of iris melanomas proposed by Jakobiec and Silbert [2] is remarkable because it addresses not only the issue of prognosis for life but also the prognosis for retention of vision. Melanomas confined to the iris are seldom life-threatening unless there is invasion into the filtration angle or involvement of the ciliary body. One of the principal contributions of the Jakobiec and Silbert [2] classification is the recognition of a surface plaque—a thin layer of melanoma cells that may extend from a stromal thickening along the surface of the iris—as a risk factor for recurrence (Fig. 1). Clinical effacement or flattening of iris crypts and folds on slit-lamp examination by an "invisible" membrane may be the only clinical clue to the existence of the surface plaque histologically. When present, excision of the easily visible nodule may leave the thin membrane of tumor behind: there may be no clinically visible recurrence in the form of a nodule or tumefaction. However, a recurrence may appear many years after resection, or the flat membrane may grow over the trabecular meshwork and contribute to peripheral anterior synechiae and extensive spread of tumor, reminiscent of the diffuse spreading of the membranes of epithelial downgrowth.

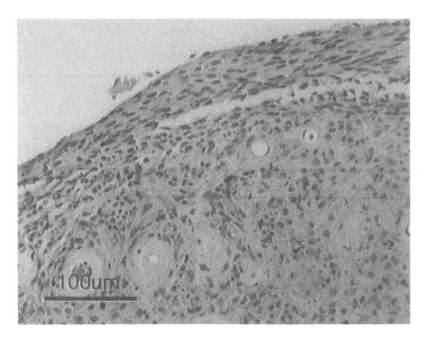

Figure 1   Iris nevus with surface plaque. The iris stroma is distended by nevus cells. A plaque of bland spindle cells lines the anterior surface of the iris. (H&E.)

Few prognostic risk factors are identified for melanomas confined to the iris aside from cell type and markers of proliferation.

Considerably more attention is focused on the pathology of ciliary body and choroidal melanomas because they are relatively more common than tumors confined to the iris and because of a significantly greater tendency for these tumors to follow an aggressive course. Most information about the prognostically relevant features of choroidal and ciliary body melanomas stems from intensive correlative studies that were done when most of these lesions were treated by enucleation. In the past, some experts, convinced of the inevitable progression of even the smallest pigmented lesions to life-threatening melanoma, advised enucleation to prevent any future risk to the patient's health [3]. Subsequently, careful clinical observations documented the relative "safety" of observing such small lesions because many of them did not grow and did not prove to be life-threatening [4]. Thus, only a short window of time was available for ophthalmic pathologists to accumulate histological material from small uveal melanocytic lesions. Tissue from these small lesions is now seldom available except from large archival collections and in rare instances when eyes are removed and the presence of the small pigmented lesion is incidental to the event that precipitates enucleation.

Ophthalmic pathologists are likely to encounter fewer tumors for examination because of the emergence of nonsurgical, vision-sparing treatments. The innate fear of losing vision together with the instinctive fear of loss of life pose terrible dilemmas for patients with choroidal or ciliary body melanomas and their physicians. Two polls conducted by the Gallup Organization posed the following question to Americans: what disease do you fear most? The most feared disease before public awareness of AIDS and Alzheimer disease was cancer. The second most feared disease was blindness. (The Gallup Organization, Inc.: "Public Knowledge and Attitudes Concerning Blindness"—a survey sponsored by Research to Prevent Blindness, Inc., New York, October 1965, April 1976, unpublished data.) If an ophthalmic oncologist can preserve vision while eradicating the risk to the patient's life, then many patients will opt for a treatment that does not require removal of the eye. Indeed, a comparison between surgical enucleation and primary radiation therapy by the Collaborative Ocular Melanoma Study (COMS) showed no substantial difference in survival between enucleation and vision-sparing radiation therapy [5]. Thus, pathologists are now likely to encounter only large, advanced tumors or tumors situated within the eye in anatomical locations that preclude nonsurgical treatment without loss of vision.

Even when tissue is available, one may ask why it is necessary to classify patients into prognostic categories if there is no adjuvant treatment to prevent or delay the onset of metastases or to treat metastatic melanoma. Except for the rare case in which the tumor erodes through the anterior coats of the eye and gains access to conjunctival lymphatics—after which spread to regional lymph nodes may occur [6]—uveal melanoma spreads hematogenously (there are no lymphatics within the uvea or the uveal melanoma [7]) and preferentially to the liver [8,9]. By the time sufficient quantities of hepatic parenchyma are compromised to permit detection of metastases either biochemically (through elevated liver enzymes) or by imaging studies [10], the tumor burden is frequently quite high, adding to the challenge of the medical oncologist. Of course, one can argue that it is worthwhile to develop tissue-based prognostic indicators for metastasis in the hope that effective adjuvant therapies will emerge from a better understanding of the molecular pathogenesis of uveal melanoma, but the pathologist must recognize that even if these prognostic indicators are validated, a substantial number of patients will still elect to be treated by modalities that do not provide any source of tissue for analysis.

Thus, the motivation for studying tissue-based prognostic markers in uveal melanoma is in part for the sake of historical interest and in part to classify into emerging treatment protocols those patients for whom tissue is available. There are, however, at least two compelling reasons why tissue based prognostic indicators should still be studied and new indicators developed: (1) tissue-based studies frequently identify tumor characteristics that can be the basis of novel investigations into the mechanisms of metastasis and (2) observations from mechanistically driven in vitro cell biological observations and animal models must be validated in human tissue for clinical relevance.

The remainder of this discussion therefore focuses on melanomas that involve the ciliary body or choroid and is divided into three parts: (1) a description of tissue-based prognostic features developed largely during the era when enucleation was the dominant form of treatment, (2) a discussion of the application of tissue-based prognostic features in the contemporary era of vision-sparing therapies, and (3) the development of new tissue-based prognostic features to identify important biological pathways for tumor progression and metastasis that can be investigated by in vitro manipulations and in animal models and, conversely, the issue of validating in vitro experiments and animal models through the study of human tissue.

II. CHOROIDAL AND CILIARY BODY MELANOMAS

A. Prognostic Histological Features in the Era of Enucleation as the Primary Treatment Modality

Larger melanomas tend to have a worse outcome than smaller tumors [11–16]. For purposes of prognostication, tumor size is measured as the largest basal dimension (LBD) in contact with the sclera (LTD for largest tumor dimension). This would seem at first to be at odds with the technique for measuring cutaneous melanomas: measuring the depth of invasion from the top of the granular cell layer of the epidermis to the deepest point of invasion (in ciliary body melanomas, the tumor height does not carry significant prognostic significance). In some studies, pathologists have measured both the major and minor axes in contact with the sclera as well as the height and have attempted to calculate tumor volume. Because of the irregular growth contours of these tumors, precise calculation of tumor volume is difficult; most pathologists, therefore, record only the LBD.

The technique by which LBD is recorded has been the subject of some controversy. Transmission of light through the eye during gross examination of the enucleation specimen typically reveals a shadow. Some pathologists choose to measure LBD from the shadow [17]. Others claim that blood or turbid fluid in a retinal detachment adjacent to the tumor might also block transmission of light and thereby lead to exaggeration of the LBD: these pathologists tend to measure LBD directly from the cut surface of the tumor [18]. If the pathologist measures LBD from the cut surface and the eye has been opened conventionally (through the pupil, optic nerve, and tumor shadow), there is no guarantee that the cut surface of the tumor actually captures the LBD. It is altogether possible that the LBD does not lie on an axis that intersects the optic nerve. The technique by which LBD is measured would seem to be trivial were it not for the fact that the major criterion for separating patients into risk categories for treatment protocols is LBD, and it is not clear that ophthalmic oncologists restrict their measurements of LBD to an axis that intersects the optic nerve. Although differences between clinical measurements of LBD and the pathologist's record of LBD have been attributed to the effects of fixation, it is more likely that ophthalmic oncologists and pathologists may be recording different measurements of tumor size.

To more precisely correlate clinical and pathological measurements, it has been recommended that pathologists open an eye containing a ciliary body or choroidal melanoma by first removing the cap of sclera *parallel* to the apex of the tumor, thereby permitting the pathologist to view the tumor from a panoramic perspective more closely resembling that viewed by the clinician; in the case of a melanoma of the posterior pole, the anterior segment is removed en bloc. The tumor can then be sectioned by direct visualization and measurement of LBD may be taken through the same axis used by the oncologist for clinical measurements [19].

For the purposes of entering prognostic data on pathology reports or for retrospective studies, either the direct measurement of LBD from the cut surface of the tumor or a measurement of LBD from the glass slides is acceptable [20].

It is widely suspected that tumor location is also associated with outcome: melanomas with a component in the ciliary body tend to have a worse outcome than tumors confined to the choroid [3,12,15,16,21]. In at least one study in which multivariate analyses were used, tumor location was not found to have an independent effect on outcome [22] (see below), but differences in chromosomal karyotyping between melanomas of the ciliary body and melanomas confined to the choroid [23–25] lend some support to the suspicion that more anteriorly situated tumors involving the ciliary body are more aggressive than more posteriorly situated tumors confined to the choroid.

Although not cited in many lists of prognostic factors, the melanoma *growth pattern* is associated with outcome. Diffuse melanomas [26], typically flat and encompassing large areas of the choroid and ciliary body, have an adverse outcome, as do melanomas that grow circumferentially around the major arterial circle of the iris (ring melanomas) [27]. In comparison with these two growth patterns, circumscribed melanomas have a more favorable outcome.

Melanomas that have extended through the sclera have a worse outcome than melanomas confined within the eye [28]. It was suspected for many years that invasion into vortex veins might be related to aggressive tumor behavior, and many pathologists were trained to take separate sections of vortex veins and study each for evidence of invasion. It is not clear, however, if extension of the tumor along vortex veins to reach an extraocular location is more or less ominous than direct extension of the tumor through the sclera or extension along emissary nerves. As mentioned above, uveal melanomas may invade through the sclera near the limbus, gain access to lymphatics, and thereby undergo spread to regional lymph nodes—an exceptionally rare event [6].

The morphology of the melanoma cell is undoubtedly a histologic marker of aggressive uveal melanoma behavior. The Callender classification [29] and its modification are used widely. In its contemporary usage, tumors composed of spindle A and spindle B melanoma cells are classified as melanomas of the spindle-cell type [30,31]. Tumors composed of either type of spindle cells and epithelioid cells are classified as being of the mixed-cell type (Fig. 2) and tumors composed predominantly of epithelioid cells as being of the epithelioid-cell type. In general, the more epithelioid cells in a tumor, the worse the prognosis [12,32]. Tumors that are largely or entirely necrotic carry the same prognosis as tumors of the mixed-cell type [31].

Despite repeated studies documenting the association between the presence of epithelioid cells histologically and adverse outcome, the classification is of limited usefulness because of difficulty in achieving intraobserver reproducibility in classification. Cross sections of spindle cells may look histologically like small epithelioid cells. Also, it is not clear how many epithelioid cells need to be present for a tumor to shift from being classified as a spindle-cell melanoma to a melanoma of the mixed-cell type or from a melanoma of the mixed-cell type to an epithelioid melanoma. To circumvent difficulties with the reproducibility of cell-type classifications, some have advocated a quantitative approach to describing pleomorphism (differences in cell shapes and sizes), especially measurements of nucleolar area or largest nucleolar diameter [33–37]. Measurements obtained from silver-stained preparations have yielded significantly improved reproducibility [38].

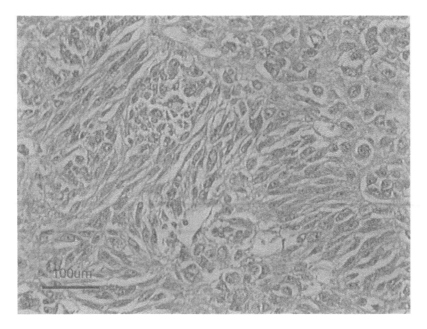

Figure 2 Malignant melanoma, choroid, mixed cell type. Spindle melanoma cells predominate in the lower two-thirds of the illustration. Note the open nuclei and the presence of prominent nucleoli. Epithelioid melanoma cells are featured in the upper right portion of the photomicrograph. Note the large cells with indistinct cell borders and large, round nuclei with very prominent nucleoli that vary in size and shape. (H&E.)

In many studies, the presence of mitotic figures in choroidal and ciliary body melanomas is related to adverse outcome: the greater the number of mitoses, the worse the prognosis [16,39,40]. In many areas of tumor pathology, counts of mitotic figures are now being replaced by the calculation of proliferation indices, determined by staining histological sections for markers of proliferation (e.g., PCNA, MIB-1, Ki-67). In recent studies of the histology of uveal melanoma, proliferation indices have been related to adverse outcome [41–43].

The presence of tumor-infiltrating lymphocytes (Fig. 3) has been associated with an adverse outcome (100 tumor infiltrating lymphocytes per 20 high-power fields) in multiple studies [16,44]. By contrast, the presence of tumor-infiltrating lymphocytes in cutaneous melanomas is associated with a favorable outcome [45].

B. Prognostic Histological Features in the Era of Vision-Sparing Therapies

Recognizing that many patients may be treated without any examination of tissue, some ophthalmic oncologists advocate what is termed in the ophthalmic literature as *fine-needle aspiration biopsy* (FNAB) to obtain tumor tissue for the purposes of assigning patients to prognostic categories [46]. This technique has been used in some institutions to distinguish between lesions that simulate melanoma (such as metastases to the eye) and primary melanomas [47,48]; for this purpose, the

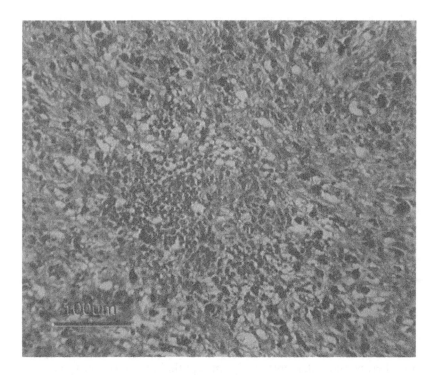

Figure 3 A cluster of tumor infiltrating lymphocytes is present between spindle melanoma cells. (H&E.)

technique has a high measure of accuracy. The indications for using FNAB to discriminate between uveal melanomas and simulating lesions may have diminished somewhat because of vastly improved accuracy in correctly diagnosing melanomas on the basis of noninvasive clinical criteria [49].

The use of FNAB to extract tumor tissue for prognostic studies is problematic because uveal melanomas, like most malignant neoplasms [50,51], tend to be heterogeneous, and the technique that ophthalmic oncologists use to extract tissue does not ensure representative sampling of the entire lesion. An ophthalmic intraocular FNAB involves only a single pass into the tumor, utilizing insertion of the needle and aspiration to secure a sample [47,48]. Although a single pass with a thin needle may provide tissue that is sufficient to distinguish melanoma from simulating lesions, it is unlikely that a restricted sample would yield information that is representative of the most malignant components of the lesion unless the feature of interest were distributed uniformly throughout the neoplasm.

It is important that ophthalmologists and pathologists understand that the technique of ophthalmic intraocular FNAB is not the same FNAB technique used in diagnostic cytology for most tumors. In conventional FNAB procedures, the pathologist, radiologist, or surgeon who performs the biopsy uses the needle to *cut* a thin tissue sample by inserting the needle into the tumor and withdrawing the needle. To ensure representative sampling of the tumor, the individual performing the biopsy typically reinserts the needle several times at different angles and approaches into the tumor so as to ensure representative sampling within the lesion [52].

In one histological study of an eye removed for uveal melanoma after an ophthalmic FNAB, the needle track was traced by serial sections, and it was shown that the needle track terminated in a zone of tumor populated by spindle melanoma cells, just missing a population of epithelioid melanoma cells [53]. In another study, cytomorphometry of the nucleolus was performed on both cells retrieved by ophthalmic FNAB and on histological sections of the same eye removed subsequently: significant differences existed in the cytomorphometric measurements between FNAB sample and the entire histological section [54]. Given the heterogeneity of tumors in general and uveal melanomas in specific, investigators who advocate using an ophthalmic onepass FNAB to obtain tumor tissue that is prognostically relevant must show that the prognostic marker of interest (antigenic, enzymatic, chromosomal, or otherwise) is distributed so uniformly that a random penetration of a thin needle will likely capture tumor cells that express the prognostic marker of interest.

Two other issues are relevant to a discussion of the application of ophthalmic FNAB to the prognostication of uveal melanoma. First, some investigators are concerned that tumor cells may be seeded along the aspiration track: extraocular extension by tumor, as mentioned above, is an ominous prognostic finding. Although tumor cells have been identified within the needle track [55,56], ophthalmic intraocular FNAB has been used for many years and there are no reports that would attribute dissemination of tumor to the application of this technique. Second, some uveal pigmented lesions are observed clinically for evidence of growth or change in behavior before therapeutic intervention. If an ophthalmic oncologist were to perform a one-pass FNAB and the results of the examination of tumor tissue were to indicate a relatively indolent process, would the oncologist and the patient be prepared for repeated FNAB procedures at varying time intervals in order to follow the lesion for tissue evidence of change in behavior?

To address the two concerns about FNAB—sampling error and the need to repeat examinations periodically—ophthalmic pathologists and oncologists have collaborated to develop histological criteria that reflect the tumor's biological behavior and can be detected by means of noninvasive imaging. The ultimate goal of this type of collaboration is the development of a noninvasive surrogate for biopsy.

Current imaging techniques do not permit the detection of cell type [57]. Even if it were possible to image individual cell sizes and shapes, it would be necessary to overcome the challenge of poor reproducibility of assignment of cell type.

Looping patterns of extracellular matrix deposition have been associated with death from metastatic melanoma [16,58–60]. Specifically, closed loops that are positive with the periodic acid–Schiff (PAS) stain and networks (at least three back-to-back loops) have been shown in repeated independent studies to be a strong prognostic marker (Fig. 4). Unlike cell type, the detection of these patterns is highly reproducible [16,60], especially if hematoxylin counterstaining is omitted and the sections viewed either with a green filter or by digital imaging and selection of the green channel. These patterns appear in metastases from uveal melanoma [61], regardless of the location of the metastatic deposit. The looping PAS-positive patterns can be reconstituted in vitro by aggressive uveal and cutaneous melanoma cells but not by nonaggressive cells, thus reinforcing a relationship between the appearance of these patterns in vitro and death from metastatic melanoma [1,62].

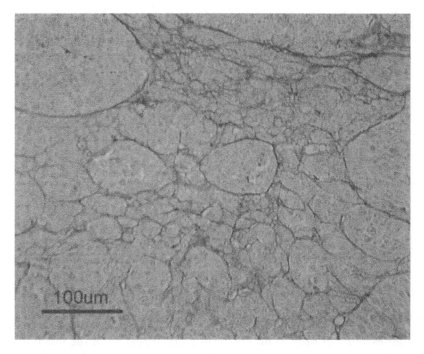

Figure 4   Back-to-back loops in melanoma of the choroid. (Periodic acid–Schiff without hematoxylin counterstaining.)

The diameter of spheroidal packets of melanoma cells encircled by these looping matrix patterns ranges from approximately 15 to 150 μm [63]. The shape and size of these packets is remarkable, because Coleman et al. [57] documented the prognostic association between acoustic scatterers detected by ultrasonography and outcome, and the size of the ultrasonographic scatterers detected by power-spectrum analysis of raw ultrasound radiofrequency data was nearly identical to packets of cells delimited by PAS-positive looping matrix patterns. A correspondence between the histological presence of PAS-positive looping patterns and acoustic scatterers of prognostic significance has been reported [64]; preliminary data from a prospective study relating the effectiveness of noninvasive ultrasonographic imaging to the detection of histological PAS-positive looping patterns suggest that it may be possible to use this noninvasive specialized ultrasound technique to detect a histological feature associated with outcome [65], thus achieving one type of noninvasive substitute for biopsy.

In vitro, matrix-rich (PAS-positive) patterns are capable of containing and conducting dye [1,62]. It has been suggested that these tumor-cell generated patterns, which are not blood vessels, contribute to the microcirculation of uveal melanomas, but this assertion has been challenged [66,67]. Despite these criticisms, it has been shown in an animal model that tracer material injected into the systemic circulation colocalizes to PAS-positive looping patterns that are devoid of endothelium [68,69]. Moreover, plasma and red blood cells have been demonstrated within these patterns in human tissue samples [70]. Finally, a correspondence between the detection of looping structures in tissue and detected in patients by means of laser scanning confocal ophthalmoscopy after injection of indocyanine green (ICG) has been reported [71,72]. In a prospective study of patients with indeterminate small melanocytic lesions of the choroid studied by confocal ophthalmoscopy and ICG, the presence of angiographically detectable loops (which are quite different angiographically from angiogenic vessels) was the strongest predictor of lesion growth [73].

Both ultrasound and angiographic approaches to detecting histological features of prognostic relevance are noninvasive and can be repeated as often as desired without any visual morbidity. Moreover, these techniques may be used to sample wide areas of the tumor to ensure a representative study. Although these noninvasive imaging studies detect attributes of tumors generated by aggressive genetically deregulated tumor cells [74,75], imaging studies only indirectly reflect the molecular or genetic profiles of the tumor cells. The issue assumes circular dimensions because, in order to extract cells from the tumor for the detection of these more specific markers, the ophthalmic oncologist must use a biopsy technique that does not disrupt vision: the one-pass ophthalmic intraocular FNAB, which may not yield a sample that is representative of the most malignant components of the tumor.

C. Developing New Prognostic Histological Characteristics

New tissue-based markers of prognostic significance are appearing in the literature with regularity [76]. Any listing or discussion of these markers here is therefore likely to be incomplete or outdated quickly.

It is important that new tissue markers of prognostic interest be evaluated very critically. Most investigators attempt to relate the presence or absence of a marker or a quantitative assessment of a marker (how much of it is present?) to outcome— death from metastatic melanoma. In studying reports of new markers, the critical reader should look for sufficient follow-up in the study set under analysis: although most uveal melanoma metastasize within 2.5 years after enucleation, the emergence of late metastases is far from uncommon [12,77]. Therefore databases used for analysis should include cases with long follow-up intervals.

Univariate analyses may be helpful in testing for possible associations between the presence of the marker under investigation and outcome; Kaplan-Meier [78] survival curves may be helpful in illustrating differences in survival between patients whose tumor contained and did not contain the marker of interest. Many investigators select a statistical sample that is large enough to permit a multivariate analysis, allowing for an examination of the prognostic marker under investigation and other well-established markers. The Cox proportional hazards model [79] is commonly used for these purposes.

Clinicians and researchers who follow descriptions of new histological markers in choroidal and ciliary body melanoma may become confused by conflicting claims for and against the usefulness of markers. There are a number of reasons for discrepancies between claims for and against the usefulness of new histological markers. First, the data sets used by different groups to study the same marker may vary. For example, one group studying the microcirculation of uveal melanoma "enriched" their study set with patients who had died from metastatic melanoma [80], while other investigators, studying the same phenomenon, did not and arrived at different conclusions about the utility of the marker under consideration [81]. Second, techniques for detecting the same marker may vary subtly between groups, but the differences may account for different assessments of marker validity. For example, Foss et al. [80] reported a relationship between vascularity in choroidal and ciliary body melanomas and adverse outcome, while Lane et al. [82] and Schaling et al. [83] did not. Foss et al. [80] not only used different reagents to count foci of endothelial marker staining in these tumors from those used by Lane et al. [82] and Schaling et al. [83] but also followed a convention established previously of obtaining their counts in "hot spots" [84], a technique not used by groups that did not find an association between vascularity and outcome. On the other hand, Foss et al. [85] found a relationship between PAS-positive matrix patterns and outcome by univariate analysis, but these patterns did not appear in a Cox model in multivariate analysis after microvascular counts were permitted to enter the model. Makitie et al. [81] validated the observation by Foss et al. [80] concerning microvascular counts and outcome, but they also validated numerous independent observations relating PAS-positive matrix patterns to outcome (both patterns and microvascular density appeared in the Cox model published by Makitie et al. [81]). Finally, Makitie et al. [81] pointed out that the frequency distribution of PAS-positive patterns in the study published by Foss et al. [85] was markedly different from that published by groups [16,58–60,81,86] that found an independent relationship between these patterns and outcome. This therefore raised the question of whether Foss et al. [85] had identified the PAS-positive patterns using the same criteria as other investigators.

One must also be cautious in examining conflicting claims between research groups in which a marker found to be valid by one group appears to "disappear" when entered into a Cox model prepared by a different group. If the marker in question is found by both groups to relate to outcome in univariate analyses, it is altogether possible that the marker does not appear in Cox models because of a relationship between the marker of interest and other tumor characteristics already in the model. For example, let us assume that the expression of molecule X, when demonstrated in tissue sections, is related to adverse outcome: there is a statistically valid separation in survival in Kaplan-Meier survival curves between patients whose tumor expresses molecule X and those whose tumor lacks expression of this marker. Let us further assume that the presence of molecule X appears in Cox models from a number of groups. A new tissue marker is described—a quantification of Y—by an independent research group. Quantification of Y appears in the Cox model, but the presence of molecule X drops out of the model. This does not at all mean that the presence of molecule X is irrelevant to the pathogenesis of metastasis in choroidal and ciliary body melanomas. Rather, there may be a relationship biologically between "quantification of Y" and the "presence of molecule X" such that prognostic information contained within "presence of molecule X" is accounted for by the "quantification of attribute Y." In fact, rather than dismiss the "presence of molecule X," one should now begin to search for the new biological relationship between these two markers.

Statistical associations developed from the study of tissue sections may *suggest* pathogenetic mechanisms and new forms of therapy, but these associations require examination of mechanisms by in vitro or animal model studies. For example, using the example of vascularity cited above, two groups [80,81] have now established that tumors containing "hot spots" of high microvascular density tend to have an adverse outcome. In these two studies, microvascular density entered Cox models along with many conventional tumor characteristics, such as cell type and LBD. One might be tempted to extrapolate from these studies and conclude that the tumor characteristic measured by these investigators—microvascular density—equates with angiogenesis. Equating angiogenesis with microvascular density may indeed be valid; if so, it could be argued that antiangiogenic therapies might play an important role in the treatment of patients with high-risk uveal melanoma. If uveal melanomas at high risk for metastasis are also highly angiogenic, it might be argued that antiangiogenic therapies may play an important and effective role in the treatment of uveal melanomas. By identifying a prognostic marker in tissue studies, ophthalmic pathologists would have contributed to a new rational basis for therapy.

However, one must be exceptionally cautious in extending tissue-based prognostic associations to pathogenic mechanisms. Microarray studies and studies of gene expression in uveal melanoma now suggest that highly aggressive tumor cells may express markers typically associated with endothelial cells, including CD31 and VE cadherin [1,62,74,75,87]. It is argued that as tumor cells become genetically deregulated, they express inappropriate markers. Aggressive melanoma cells, for example, express fetal keratins 8 and 18 in vitro [88,89], a marker inappropriate for melanocytes. The masquerading of tumor cells as endothelial cells may be striking: the cell line ECV-304—which was originally reported to be an immortalized endothelial (HUVEC) cell line by virtue of expression of factor VIII, ultrastructural features such as Weibel-Palade bodies, and the formation of tubules in vitro on Matrigel [90,91]—was discovered to be a derivative of the human bladder tumor cell line T14 [92]. Thus, in equating the tumor characteristic of microvascular density with angiogenesis, one must assume that the endothelial cell markers used in the studies were specific for endothelium and were not expressed on tumor cells. It has been shown recently that endothelial cell markers are indeed expressed in uveal melanoma cells in tissue section and that the parameter called "microvascular density" measures both the number of blood vessels and genetically deregulated tumor cells [92a]. In fact, even students of angiogenesis [93] concede that, at the time of this writing, there are no markers, either ultrastructural or immunohistochemical, specific for endothelium. Perhaps, then, the attribute described as microvascular density includes not only counts of blood vessels but also highly aggressive, genetically deregulated tumor cells. In a tumor that lacks lymphatics [7], both new blood vessels and aggressive tumor cells might contribute to metastasis.

When observations originate from in vitro experiments, it is necessary to confirm the observations in human tissue samples. For example, although it has been validated repeatedly that the expression of keratins 8 and 18 by melanoma cells is associated with aggressive behavior in vitro [88,89,94,95]; studies of the labeling of melanoma cells in histological sections of eyes removed for uveal melanoma with this marker suggest an association with invasive behavior [96] but have failed to establish any association between keratin labeling and adverse outcome [97].

Likewise, animal models may mirror the behavior of human disease for some attributes and not others [98]. For example, there are elegant animal models of human uveal melanoma in which tumor cells disseminate to the liver [99], mimicking the behavior of most choroidal and ciliary body melanomas. Nevertheless, many animal models of uveal melanoma established by the xenotransplantation of human or animal melanoma cell lines to the eyes of immunosuppressed mice show evidence of extensive necrosis in the tumor (accompanied by robust angiogenesis) [62]. Extensive necrosis is not a feature typical of most human melanomas, and it becomes challenging to determine if the angiogenesis in these models is in response to necrosis or an intrinsic property of the tumor in the model. Thus, one of the most important reasons for maintaining large data sets of human uveal melanoma tissues is to test the validity of observations made in vitro and from animal models on robust human tissue sample repositories for which long-term outcome is known.

New markers identified from tissue studies of larger series of melanoma have now associated the expression of insulin growth factor receptor [100], integrins [101,102], ezrin [103], markers of cell cycling and apoptosis [41–43,104,104–109], HLA expression [110], and tissue macrophages [111] with adverse outcome. Cytogenetic studies, once restricted to analyses on fresh tissue samples, may now be applied to tissue sections by fluorescent in situ hybridization (FISH) techniques [112]. From these studies, one may then design experiments to delineate mechanisms associated with metastasis and thus develop new therapeutic strategies. Thus, the importance of the pathologist's identification of new prognostic markers extends far beyond the goal of stratifying patients into risk categories and places the ophthalmic pathologist who studies tissue markers of prognosis on the front lines of cancer research.

ACKNOWLEDGMENTS

Supported by NIH grant E410457.

REFERENCES

1. Maniotis AJ, Folberg R, Hess A, Seftor EA, Gardner LMG, Pe'er J, Trent JM, Meltzer PS, Hendrix MJC. Vascular channel formation by human melanoma cells in vivo and in vitro: vasculogenic mimicry. Am J Pathol 1999; 155:739–752.
2. Jakobiec FA, Silbert G. Are most iris "melanomas" really nevi? Arch Ophthalmol 1981; 99:2117–2132.
3. Shammas HF, Blodi FC. Prognostic factors in choroidal and ciliary body melanomas. Arch Ophthalmol 1977; 95:63–69.
4. Gass JDM. Observations of suspected choroidal and ciliary body melanomas for evidence of growth prior to enucleation. Ophthalmology 1980; 87:523–528.
5. Diener-West M, Earle JD, Fine SL, Hawkins BS, Moy CS, Reynolds SM, Schachat AP, Straatsma BR. The COMS randomized trial of iodine 125 brachytherapy for choroidal melanoma: III. Initial mortality findings. Arch Ophthalmol 2001; 119:969–982.
6. Dithmar S, Diaz CE, Grossniklaus HE. Intraocular melanoma spread to regional lymph nodes—Report of two cases. Retina 2000; 20:76–79.
7. Clarijs R, Schalkwijk L, Ruiter DJ, de Waal RMW. Lack of lymphangiogenesis despite coexpression of VEGF-C and its receptor Flt-4 in uveal melanoma. Invest Ophthalmol Vis Sci 2001; 42:1422–1428.
8. McLean IW. The biology of haematogenous metastasis in human uveal malignant melanoma. Virchows Arch A Pathol Anat 1993; 422:433–437.
9. Willson JKV, Albert DM, Diener-West M, McCaffrey L, Moy CS, Scully RE. Assessment of metastatic disease status at death in 435 patients with large choroidal melanoma in the Collaborative Ocular Melanoma Study (COMS). Arch Ophthalmol 2001; 119:670–676.
10. Donoso LA, Shields JA, Augsburger JA, Orth DH, Johnson P. Metastatic uveal melanoma: diffuse hepatic metastasis in a patient with concurrent normal serum enzyme levels and liver scan. Arch Ophthalmol 1985; 103:758–758.
11. McLean IW, Foster WD, Zimmerman LE. Uveal melanoma: Location, size, cell type, and enucleation as risk factors in metastasis. Hum Pathol 1982; 13:123–132.
12. Seddon JM, Albert DM, Lavin PT, Robinson N. A prognostic factor study of disease-free interval and survival following enucleation for uveal melanoma. Arch Ophthalmol 1983; 101:1894–1899.
13. Miller MV, Herdson PB, Hitchcock GC. Malignant melanoma of the uveal tract—A review of the Auckland experience. Pathology 1985; 17:281–284.
14. Gamel JW, McLean IW, McCurdy JB. Biologic distinctions between cure and time to death in 2892 patients with intraocular melanoma. Cancer 1993; 71:2299–2305.
15. Seregard S, Kock E. Prognostic indicators following enucleation for posterior uveal melanoma—A multivariate analysis of long-term survival with minimized loss to follow-up. Acta Ophthalmol Scand 1995; 73:340–344.
16. Folberg R, Rummelt V, Parys-Van Ginderdeuren R, Hwang T, Woolson RF, Pe'er J, Gruman LM. The prognostic value of tumor blood vessel morphology in primary uveal melanoma. Ophthalmology 1993; 100:1389–1398.
17. Umlas J, Dienerwest M, Robinson NL, Green WR, Grossniklaus HE, Albert DM. Comparison of transillumination and histologic slide measurements of choroidal melanoma. Arch Ophthalmol 1997; 115:474–477.
18. Folberg R, Verdick RE, Weingeist TA, Montague PR. Gross examination of eyes removed for ciliary body or choroidal melanoma. Ophthalmology 1986; 93:1643–1647.
19. Montague PR, Meyer M, Folberg R. Technique for the digital imaging of histopathologic preparations of eyes for research and publication. Ophthalmology 1995; 102:1248–1251.

20. Folberg R, Gamel JW, Greenberg RA, Donoso LA, Naids RM. Comparison of direct and microslide pathology measurements of uveal melanomas. Invest Ophthalmol Vis Sci 1985; 26:1788–1791.

21. Augsburger JJ, Gamel JW. Clinical prognostic factors in patients with posterior uveal malignant melanoma. Cancer 1990; 66:1596–1600.

22. Rummelt V, Folberg R, Woolson RF, Hwang T, Pe'er J. Relation between the microcirculation architecture and the aggressive behavior of ciliary body melanomas. Ophthalmology 1995; 102:844–851.

23. Prescher G, Bornfeld N, Becher R. Nonrandom chromosomal abnormalities in primary uveal melanoma. J Natl Cancer Inst 1990; 82:1765–1769.

24. Sisley K, Rennie IG, Parsons MA, Jacques R, Hammond DW, Bell SM, Potter AM, Rees RC. Abnormalities of chromosomes 3 and 8 in posterior uveal melanoma correlate with prognosis. Genes Chromosomes Cancer 1997; 19:22–28.

25. Sisley K, Parsons MA, Garnham J, Potter AM, Curtis D, Rees RC, Rennie IG. Association of specific chromosome alterations with tumour phenotype in posterior uveal melanoma. Br J Cancer 2000; 82:330–338.

26. Braun UC, Rummelt VC, Naumann GO. Diffuse malignant melanomas of the uvea. A clinico-pathologic study of 39 patients. Klin Monatsbl Augenheilkd 1998; 213:331–340.

27. Demirci H, Shields CL, Shields JA, Eagle RC, Honavar S. Ring melanoma of the anterior chamber angle: A report of fourteen cases. Am J Ophthalmol 2001; 132:336–342.

28. Shammas HF, Blodi FC. Orbital extension of choroidal and ciliary body melanomas. Arch Ophthalmol 1977; 95:2002–2005.

29. Callender GR. Malignant melanotic tumors of the eye: A study of histologic types in 111 cases. Trans Am Acad Ophthalmol Otolaryngol 1931; 36:131–142.

30. McLean IW, Zimmerman LE, Evans RM. Reappraisal of Callender's spindle A type of malignant melanoma of choroid and ciliary body. Am J Ophthalmol 1978; 86:557–564.

31. McLean IW, Foster WD, Zimmerman LE, Gamel JW. Modifications of Callender's classification of uveal melanoma at the Armed Forces Institute of Pathology. Am J Ophthalmol 1983; 96:502–509.

32. Albert DM. The ocular melanoma story: LIII. Edward Jackson Memorial Lecture: Part II. Am J Ophthalmol 1997; 123:729–741.

33. Gamel JW, McLean IW, Greenberg RA, Zimmerman LE, Lichtenstein SJ. Computerized histologic assessment of malignant potential: a method for determining the prognosis of uveal melanomas. Hum Pathol 1982; 13:893–897.

34. Gamel JW, McLean IW. Computerized histopathologic assessment of malignant potential: II. A practical method for predicting survival following enucleation for uveal melanoma. Cancer 1983; 52:1032–1038.

35. Gamel JW, McLean IW. Computerized histopathologic assessment of malignant potential. III. Refinements of measurement and data analysis. Anal Quant Cytol 1984; 6:37–44.

36. McLean IW, Gamel JW. Prediction of metastasis of uveal melanoma: Comparison of morphometric determination of nucleolar size and spectrophotometric determination of DNA. Invest Ophthalmol Vis Sci 1988; 29:507–511.

37. McCurdy J, Gamel J, McLean I. A simple, efficient, and reproducible method for estimating the malignant potential of uveal melanoma from routine H&E slides. Pathol Res Pract 1991; 187:1025–1027.

38. McLean IW, Sibug ME, Becker RL, McCurdy JB. Uveal melanoma—The importance of large nucleoli in predicting patient outcome. An automated image analysis study. Cancer 1997; 79:982–988.

39. McLean IW, Foster WD, Zimmerman LE. Prognostic factors in small malignant melanomas of choroid and ciliary body. Arch Ophthalmol 1977; 95:48–58.

40. Seddon JM, Gragoudas ES, Albert DM. Ciliary body and choroidal melanomas treated by proton beam irradiation: Histopathologic study of eyes. Arch Ophthalmol 1983; 101:1402–1408.
41. Pe'er J, Gnessin H, Shargal Y, Livni N. PC-10 immunostaining of proliferating cell nuclear antigen (PCNA) in posterior uveal melanoma. Ophthalmology 1994; 101:56–62.
42. Karlsson M, Boeryd B, Carstensen J, Franlund B, Gustafsson B, Kagedal B, Sun XF, Wingren S. Correlations of Ki-67 and PCNA to DNA ploidy, S-phase fraction and survival in uveal melanoma. Eur J Cancer 1996; 32A:357–362.
43. Seregard S, Oskarsson M, Spangberg B. PC-10 as a predictor of prognosis after antigen retrieval in posterior uveal melanoma. Invest Ophthalmol Vis Sci 1996; 37:1451–1458.
44. de la Cruz POJ, Specht CS, McLean IW. Lymphocytic infiltration in uveal malignant melanoma. Cancer 1990; 65:112–115.
45. Clemente CG, Mihm MC Jr, Bufalino R, Zurrida S, Collini P, Cascinelli N. Prognostic value of tumor infiltrating lymphocytes in the vertical growth phase of primary cutaneous melanoma. Cancer 1996; 77:1303–1310.
46. Sisley K, Nichols C, Parsons MA, Farr R, Rees RC, Rennie IG. Clinical applications of chromosome analysis, from fine needle aspiration biopsies, of posterior uveal melanomas. Eye 1998; 12:203–207.
47. Augsburger JJ, Shields JA, Folberg R, Lang WR, O'Hara BJ, Claricci, JD. Fine needle aspiration biopsy in the diagnosis of intraocular cancer cytologic-histologic correlations. Ophthalmology 1985; 92:39–49.
48. Shields JA, Shields CL, Ehya H, Eagle RC Jr, De Potter P. Fine-needle aspiration biopsy of suspected intraocular tumors. The 1992 Urwick Lecture. Ophthalmology 1993; 100:1677–1684.
49. Accuracy of diagnosis of choroidal melanomas in the Collaborative Ocular Melanoma Study COMS report no 1. Arch Ophthalmol 1990; 108:1268–1273.
50. Hart IR, Fidler IJ. The implications of tumor heterogeneity for studies on the biology and therapy of cancer metastasis. Biochim Biophys Acta 1981; 651:37–50.
51. Yoon SS, Fidler IJ, Beltran PJ, Bucana CD, Wang YF, Fan D. Intratumoral heterogeneity for epigenetic modulation of MDR-1 expression in murine melanoma. Melanoma Res 1997; 7:275–287.
52. DeMay RM. The art and science of cytopathology. 1996; 1:463–492.
53. Folberg R, Augsburger JJ, Gamel JW, Shields JA, Lang WR. Fine-needle aspirates of uveal melanomas and prognosis. Am J Ophthalmol 1985; 100:654–657.
54. Char DH, Kroll SM, Stoloff A, Kaleta-Michaels S, Crawford JB, Miller TR, Howes EL, Jr, Ljung B-M. Cytomorphometry of uveal melanoma: Comparison of fine needle aspiration biopsy samples with histologic sections. Anal Quant Cytol Histol 1991; 13:293–299.
55. Karciolgu ZA, Gordon RA, Karciolglu GL. Tumor seeding in ocular fine needle aspiration biopsy. Ophthalmology 1985; 92:1763–1767.
56. Glasgow BJ, Brown HH, Zargoza, AM, Foos RY. Quantitation of tumor seeding from fine needle aspiration of ocular melanomas. Am J Ophthalmol 1988; 105:538–546.
57. Coleman DJ, Silverman RH, Rondeau, MJ, Lizzi FL, McLean IW, Jakobiec FA. Correlations of acoustic tissue typing of malignant melanoma and histopathologic features as a predictor of death. Am J Ophthalmol 1990; 110:380–388.
58. Sakamoto T, Sakamoto M, Yoshikawa H, Hata Y, Ishibashi T, Ohnishi Y, Inomata H. Histologic findings and prognosis of uveal malignant melanoma in Japanese patients. Am J Ophthalmol 1996; 121:276–283.
59. Seregard S, Spangberg B, Juul C, Oskarsson M. Prognostic accuracy of the mean of the largest nucleoli, vascular patterns, and PC-10 in posterior uveal melanoma. Ophthalmology 1998; 105:485–491.

60. Makitie T, Summanen P, Tarkannen A, Kivela T. Microvascular loops and networks as prognostic indicators in choroidal and ciliary body melanomas. J Natl Cancer Inst 1999; 91:359–367.
61. Rummelt V, Mehaffey MG, Campbell RJ, Peer J, Bentler SE, Woolson RF, Naumann GOH, Folberg R. Microcirculation architecture of metastases from primary ciliary body and choroidal melanomas. Am J Ophthalmol 1998; 126:303–305.
62. Folberg R, Hendrix MJ, Maniotis AJ. Vasculogenic mimicry and tumor angiogenesis. Am J Pathol 2000; 156:361–381.
63. Folberg R, Pe'er J, Gruman LM, Woolson RF, Jeng G, Montague PR, Moninger TO Yi H, Moore KC. The morphologic characteristics of tumor blood vessels as a marker of tumor progression in primary human uveal melanoma: A matched case-control study. Hum Pathol 1992; 23:1298–1305.
64. Coleman DJ, Rondeau MJ, Silverman RH, Folberg R, Rummelt V, Woods SM, Lizzi FL. Correlation of microcirculation architecture with ultrasound parameters of uveal melanoma. Eur J Ophthalmol 1995; 5:96–106.
65. Silverman RH, Folberg R, Boldt HC, Rondeau MJ, Lloyd HO, Mehaffey MG, Lizzi FL, Coleman DJ. Correlation of ultrasound parameter imaging with microcirculatory patterns in uveal melanomas. Ultrasound Med Biol 1997; 23:573–581.
66. McDonald DM, Munn L, Jain RK. Vasculogenic mimicry: How convincing, how novel, and how significant? Am J Pathol 2000; 156:383–388.
67. McDonald DM, Foss AJE. Endothelial cells of tumor vessels: Abnormal but not absent. Cancer Metastasis Rev 2000; 19:109–120.
68. Potgens AJG, Lubsen NH, Vanaltena MC, Schoenmakers JGG, Ruiter DJ, Dewaal RMW. Vascular permeability factor expression influences tumor angiogenesis in human melanoma lines xenografted to nude mice. Am J Pathol 1995; 146:197–209.
69. Potgens AJG, van Altena MC, Lubsen NH, Ruiter DJ, de Waal RMW. Analysis of the tumor vasculature and metastatic behavior of xenografts of human melanoma cell lines transfected with vascular permeability factor. Am J Pathol 1996; 148:1203–1217.
70. Chen X, Maniotis A, Folberg R. Composition of solid PAS-positive patterns in primary human uveal melanoma: an explanation for the paradoxical appearance of vascular mimicry in tissue sections. Invest Ophthalmol Vis Sci (Suppl) 2001; 42:S110–S110.
71. Mueller AJ, Bartsch DU, Folberg R, Mehaffey MG, Boldt HC, Meyer M, Gardner LM, Goldbaum MH, Peer J, Freeman WR. Imaging the microvasculature of choroidal melanomas with confocal indocyanine green scanning laser ophthalmoscopy. Arch Ophthalmol 1998; 116:31–39.
72. Mueller AJ, Freeman WR, Folberg R, Bartsch DU, Scheider A, Schaller U, Kampik A. Evaluation of microvascularization pattern visibility in human choroidal melanomas: Comparison of confocal fluorescein with indocyanine green angiography. Graefes Arch Clin Exp Ophthalmol 1999; 237:448–456.
73. Mueller AJ, Schaller U, Freeman W, Folberg R, Kampik A. Complex microcirculation patterns detected by confocal indocyanine green angiography predict time to growth of small choroidal melanocytic tumors. MuSIC-Report II. Ophthalmology 2002; 12:2207–2214.
74. Bittner M, Meltzer P, Chen Y, Jiang Y, Seftor E, Hendrix M, Radmacher M, Simon R, Yakhini Z, Ben-Dor A, Dougherty E, Wang E, Marincola F, Gooden C, Leuders J, Glatfelter A, Pollock P, Carpten J, Gillanders E, Leja D, Dietrich K, Beaudry C, Berens M, Alberts D, Sondak V, Hayward N, Trent J. Molecular classification of cutaneous melanoma by gene expression profiling. Nature 2000; 406:536–540.
75. Seftor EA, Meltzer PS, Kirschmann DA, Pe'er J, Maniotis AJ, Trent JM, Folberg R, Hendrix MJC. Molecular determinants of uveal melanoma invasion and metastasis. Clin Exp Metastasis 2002; 19:233–246.

76. Mooy CM, De Jong PTVM. Prognostic parameters in uveal melanoma: A review. Surv Ophthalmol 1996; 41:215–228.

77. McLean IW, Foster WD, Zimmerman LE, Martin DG. Inferred natural history of uveal melanoma. Invest Ophthalmol Vis Sci 1980; 19:760–770.

78. Kalbfleisch J, Prentice RL. The Statistical Analysis of Failure Time Data. New York: John Wiley & Sons, 1980, pp 70–118.

79. Cox DR. Regression models and life tables. J R Stat Soc Series B 1972; 34:187–220.

80. Foss AJE, Alexander RA, Jefferies LW, Hungerford JL, Harris AL, Lightman S. Microvessel count predicts survival in uveal melanoma. Cancer Res 1996; 56:2900–2903.

81. Makitie T, Summanen P, Tarkkanen A, Kivela T. Microvascular density in predicting survival of patients with choroidal and ciliary body melanoma. Invest Ophthalmol Vis Sci 1999; 40:2471–2480.

82. Lane AM, Egan KM, Gragoudas ES, Yang J, Saornil MA, Alroy J, Albert D. An evaluation of tumour vascularity as a prognostic indicator in uveal melanoma. Melanoma Res 1997; 7:237–242.

83. Schaling DF, van der Pol JP, Schlingemann RO, Parys-Van Ginderdeuren R, Jager MJ. Vascular density and vascular patterns in the prognosis of choroidal melanoma. 1996; 43–54.

84. Weidner N, Semple JP, Welch WR, Folkman J. Tumor angiogenesis and metastasis — correlation in invasive breast carcinoma. N Engl J Med 1991; 324:1–8.

85. Foss AJE, Alexander RA, Hungerford JL, Harris AL, Cree IA, Lightman S. Reassessment of the PAS patterns in uveal melanoma. Br J Ophthalmol 1997; 81:240–246.

86. McLean IW, Keefe KS, Burnier MN. Uveal melanoma: Comparison of the prognostic value of fibrovascular loops, mean of the ten largest nucleoli, cell type and tumor size. Ophthalmology 1997; 104:777–780.

87. Hendrix MJC, Seftor EA, Meltzer PS, Gardner LMG, Hess AR, Kirschmann DA, Schatteman GC, Seftor REB. Expression and functional significance of VE-cadherin in aggressive melanoma cells: Role in vasculogenic mimicry. Proc Nat Acad Sci USA 2001; 98:8018–8023.

88. Hendrix MJC, Seftor EA, Chu Y-W, Seftor REB, Nagle RB, McDaniel KM, Leong SPL, Yohem KH, Liebovitz AM, Meyskens FL Jr, Conaway DH, Welch DR, Liotta La, Stetler-Stevenson WG. Coexpression of vimentin and keratins by human melanoma tumor cells: Correlation with invasive and metastatic potential. J Natl Cancer Inst 1992; 84:165–174.

89. Hendrix MJC, Seftor EA, Seftor RB, Gardner LM, Boldt HC, Meyer M, Peer J, Folberg R. Biologic determinants of uveal melanoma metastatic phenotype—Role of intermediate filaments as predictive markers. Lab Invest 1998; 78:153–163.

90. Takahashi K, Sawasaki Y, Hata J, Mukai K, Goto T. Spontaneous transformation and immortalization of human endothelial cells. In Vitro Cell Dev Biol 1990; 26:265–274.

91. Hughes SE. Functional characterization of the spontaneously transformed human umbilical vein endothelial cell line ECV304: Use in an *in vitro* model of angiogenesis. Exp Cell Res 1996; 225:171–185.

92. Lucas M, Rose PE, Morris AG. Contrasting effects of HSP72 expression on apoptosis in human umbilical vein endothelial cells and an angiogenic cell line, ECV304. Br J Haematol 2000; 110:957–964.

92a. Chen X, Maniotis AJ, Majundar D, Pe'er J, Folberg R. Uveal melanoma cell staining and assessment of tumor vascularity. Invest Opthalmol Vis Sci 2002; 43:2533–2539.

93. Chang YS, di Tomaso E, McDonald DM, Jones R, Jain RK, Munn LL. Mosaic blood vessels in tumor: Frequency of cancer cells in contact with flowing blood. Proc Natl Acad Sci USA 2000; 97:14608–14613.

94. Chu YW, Seftor EA, Romer LH, Hendrix MJC. Experimental coexpression of vimentin and keratin intermediate filaments in human melanoma cells augments motility. Am J Pathol 1996; 148:63–69.

95. Hendrix MJC, Seftor EA, Chu YW, Trevor KT, Seftor REB. Role of intermediate filaments in migration, invasion and metastasis. Cancer Met Rev 1996; 15:507–525.

96. Kivela T, Summanen, P. Retinoinvasive malignant melanoma of the uvea. Br J Ophthalmol 1997; 81:691–697.

97. Fuchs U, Kivela T, Summanen P, Immonen I, Tarkkanen A. An immunohistochemical and prognostic analysis of cytokeratin expression in malignant uveal melanoma. Am J Pathol 1992; 141:169–181.

98. Grossniklaus HE, Dithmar S, Albert DM. Animal models of uveal melanoma (review). Mel Res 2000; 10:195–211.

99. Grossniklaus HE. Tumor vascularity and hematogenous metastasis in experimental murine intraocular melanoma. Trans Am Ophthalmol Soc 1998; 96:721–752.

100. All-Ericsson C, Girnita L, Seregard S, Bartolazzi A, Jager MJ, Larsson O. Insulin-like growth factor-1 receptor in uveal melanoma: a predictor for metastatic disease and a potential therapeutic target. Invest Ophthalmol Vis Sci 2002; 43:1–8.

101. Anastassiou G, Schilling H, Djakovic S, Bornfeld N. Expression of VLA-2, VLA-3, and alpha(v) integrin receptors in uveal melanoma: Association with microvascular architecture of the tumour and prognostic value. Br J Ophthalmol 2000; 84:899–902.

102. Elshaw SR, Sisley K, Cross N, Murray AK, MacNeil SM, Wagner M, Nichols CE, Rennie IG. A comparison of ocular melanocyte and uveal melanoma cell invasion and the implication of alpha 1 beta 1, alpha 4 beta 1, and alpha 6 beta 1 integrins. Br J Ophthalmol 2001; 85:732–738.

103. Makitie T, Carpen O, Vaheri A, Kivela T. Ezrin as a prognostic indicator and its relationship to tumor characteristics in uveal malignant melanoma. Invest Ophthalmol Vis Sci 2001; 42:2442–2449.

104. Mooy CM, Luyten GPM, Dejong PTVM, Luider TM, Stijnen T, van de Ham F, van Vroonhoven CCJ, Bosman FT. Immunohistochemical and prognostic analysis of apoptosis and proliferation in uveal melanoma. Am J Pathol 1995; 147:1098–1104.

105. Ghazvini S, Kroll S, Char DH, Frigillana H. Comparative analysis of proliferating cell nuclear antigen, bromodeoxyuridine, and mitotic index in uveal melanoma. Invest Ophthalmol Vis Sci 1995; 36:2762–2767.

106. Pe'er J, Stefani FH, Seregard S, Kivela T, Lommatzsch P, Prause JU, Sobottka B, Damato B, Chowers I. Cell proliferation activity in posterior uveal melanoma after Ru-106 brachytherapy: An EORTC ocular oncology group study. Br J Ophthalmol 2001; 85:1208–1212.

107. Baldi G, Baldi F, Maguire M, Massaro-Giordan M. Prognostic factors for survival after enucleation for choroidal melanoma. Int J Oncol 1998; 13:1185–1189.

108. Coupland SE, Anastassiou G, Stang A, Schilling H, Anagnostopoulos I, Bornfeld N, Stein H. The prognostic value of cyclin D1, p53, and MDM2 protein expression in uveal melanoma. J Pathol 2000; 191:120–126.

109. Mooy CM, De Jong PTVM, Van der Kwast TH, Mulder PGH, Jager MJ, Ruiter DJ. Ki-67 immunostaining in uveal melanoma: The effect of pre-eunucleation radiotherapy. Ophthalmology 1990; 97:1275–1280.

110. Hurks HMH, Valter MM, Wilson L, Hilgert I, van den Elsen PJ, Jager MJ. Uveal melanoma: No expression of HLA-G. Invest Ophthalmol Vis Sci 2001; 42:3081–3084.

111. Makitie T, Summanen P, Tarkkanen A, Kivela T. Tumor-infiltrating macrophages (CD68(+) cells) and prognosis in malignant uveal melanoma. Invest Ophthalmol Vis Sci 2001; 42:1414–1421.

112. Parrella P, Caballero OL, Sidransky D, Merbs SL. Detection of c-myc amplification in uveal melanoma by fluorescent in situ hybridization. Invest Ophthalmol Vis Sci 2001; 42:1679–1684.

20

Retinoblastoma: Pathology and Prognosis

IAN W. McLEAN

Armed Forces Institute of Pathology, Washington, D.C., U.S.A.

Retinoblastoma is the most common intraocular tumor of childhood and the most common tumor of the retina. In the United States, uveal malignant melanoma occurs more frequently in adults than retinoblastoma occurs in children. In a series based on pathological specimens received by the Armed Forces Institute of Pathology, 188 of 235 retinal tumors and pseudotumors (80%) were retinoblastomas [1]. Because uveal melanoma is unusual in blacks, retinoblastoma is far more common than any other intraocular tumor in African countries with predominately black populations [2].

Retinocytoma is the very rare benign counterpart to retinoblastoma. The incidence of retinocytoma is less than 1% that of retinoblastoma. Flexner-Wintersteiner rosettes were considered the highest degree of differentiation prior to 1969, when Tso et al. [3] described cytologically benign cells in retinoblastomas. These cells individually or in small bouquet-like clusters ("fleurettes") exhibited photoreceptor differentiation [4,5] (Fig. 1). In most instances, such areas of benign-appearing tumor cells represented only a small component within an otherwise typical retinoblastoma, but rare tumors were composed entirely of cells with benign cytological features [4]. In 1983, Margo et al. [6] introduced into the English literature the term *retinocytoma* for these benign tumors.

Based on long-term clinical observations, Gallie and coworkers [7] introduced a different name, *retinoma*, for small, often partially calcified retinal tumors exhibiting no growth. Although they studied 36 eyes with such lesions clinically, none was examined histologically. It seems clear, however, that the tumors they

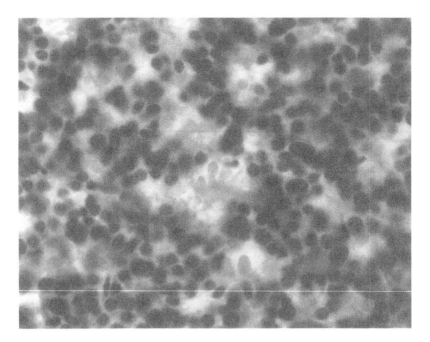

Figure 1 Retinocytoma. Bland retinocytes with small nuclei and no mitotic activity have formed fleurettes.

studied clinically are identical to the retinocytomas of Margo and coworkers [6]. These benign tumors have a very similar appearance to retinoblastomas that have undergone regression after radiation therapy [8], and for this reason some investigators consider them to be spontaneously regressed retinoblastomas. Eagle et al. [9] described an interesting case in which a benign retinocytoma or retinoma, after remaining stable in this patient from age 4 until age 7, suddenly began to grow rapidly. Histology indicated that there were two distinct components to the tumor. The inner component was a typical endophytic retinoblastoma and the outer component was a typical retinocytoma. The delayed rapid growth of this tumor would be very unusual behavior if this were a spontaneously regressed tumor.

The pseudoretinoblastomas are nonneoplastic conditions that mimic retinoblastoma clinically. They include a variety of lesions, but the most common are Coats disease, which probably represents a vascular malformation of the retina; persistent hyperplastic primary vitreous, a congenital anomaly; and *Toxocara* endophthalmitis, a nematode infection. In series based on clinical experience, the frequency of pseudotumors (approximately 50%) is higher than in series based on pathological specimens, because when these entities are correctly diagnosed, they are usually managed without generating a pathological specimen [10].

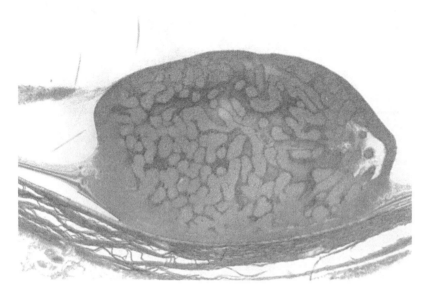

Figure 2 Endophytic retinoblastoma. Tumor grows from inner surface of retina into the vitreous. Well-defined sleeve pattern with cuffs of retinoblasts surrounding blood vessels.

I. PATHOLOGICAL FEATURES

The gross features of intraocular retinoblastoma are dependent on the growth pattern of the tumor. Five growth patterns are recognized in retinoblastomas, which explain certain variations in clinical presentation as well as differences in intraocular and extraocular spread:

A. Endophytic Retinoblastomas

Endophytic retinoblastomas (Figs. 2 and 3) grow from the inner surface of the retina into the vitreous. Thus, on ophthalmoscopic examination, the tumor is viewed directly. Retinal vessels are typically lost from view as they enter the tumor (Fig. 4). As endophytic tumors grow large and become friable, tumor cells tend to be shed from the tumor into the vitreous, where they grow into separate tiny spheroidal masses that appear as fluff balls or cotton balls. These spheroidal masses of tumor can mimic inflammatory conditions such as mycotic or nematodal endophthalmitis. Tumor cells in the vitreous may seed onto the inner surface of the retina (Fig. 3), where they may invade the retina, making it very difficult to distinguish histologically between seeding and multicentricity.

It is important to distinguish multicentric retinoblastoma (Fig. 4) from retinal seeding (Fig. 3), because the presence of multiple tumors indicates a germinal mutation and the heritable form of retinoblastoma. This distinction is impossible once there is extensive vitreous seeding. Tumors that lie mainly on the inner surface

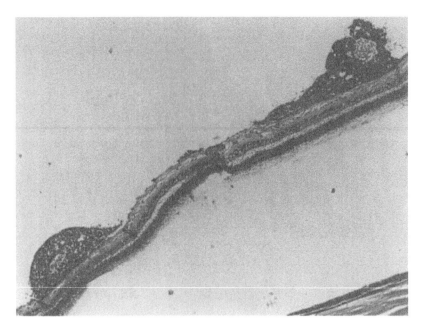

Figure 3   Endophytic retinoblastoma. Seeding of retinoblasts on the inner surface of the retina.

of the retina rather than within it or consist of clusters of tumor cell within the vitreous are tumors in which retinal seeding is more likely than multifocality.

Tumor cells in the vitreous may invade posteriorly into the optic nerve and spread to the brain. They may spread anteriorly into the posterior chamber and then into the anterior chamber by aqueous flow. Secondary deposits on the lens, zonular fibers, ciliary epithelium, iris, corneal endothelium, and trabecular meshwork may be observed, and tumor cells may clog the aqueous outflow pathways, causing glaucoma. In such cases, the anterior segment changes may be misinterpreted clinically as those of granulomatous iridocyclitis.

B.   Exophytic Retinoblastomas

Exophytic retinoblastomas (Figs. 4 and 5) grow from the outer retinal surface toward the choroid, producing a retinal detachment. On ophthalmoscopic examination, the tumor is viewed through the retina and the retinal vessels course over the tumor. As the tumor grows larger, causing subretinal exudation, tumor cells may escape into the subretinal exudate. Secondary implants may then develop on the outer retinal surface, where they can invade the retina or the inner surface of the retinal pigment epithelium. These implants may replace the pigment epithelium and eventually infiltrate through Bruch's membrane into the choroid. From the choroid, tumor cells may escape along ciliary vessels and nerves into the orbit and conjunctiva. From the orbit and conjunctiva, they can gain access to blood vessels and lymphatics and metastasize.

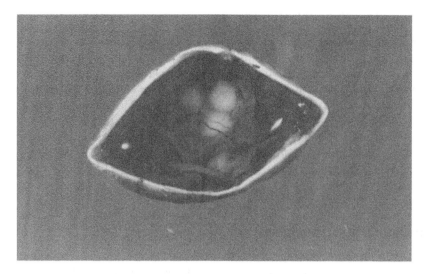

Figure 4 Multicentric retinoblastoma. Cluster of three small tumors. The upper two are endophytic. The lower one is exophytic with retinal blood vessels passing over the tumor.

C. Mixed Endophytic-Exophytic Tumors

Mixed endophytic-exophytic tumors are probably more common than either purely endophytic or exophytic retinoblastomas, especially among the larger tumors. The combined features of both endophytic and exophytic growth characterize these tumors.

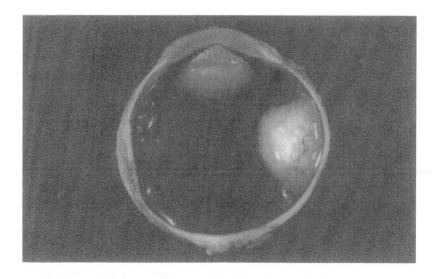

Figure 5 Exophytic retinoblastoma. Retinal blood vessel passes over the tumor.

D. Diffuse Infiltrating Retinoblastomas

Diffuse infiltrating retinoblastomas (Figs. 6 and 7) are the least common and often give rise to the greatest difficulty in clinical diagnosis [11–13]. It occurs later in life than other forms of retinoblastoma, with a mean age of 6 years, compared to 1.5 years for other forms of retinoblastoma. These tumors grow diffusely within the peripheral retina without greatly thickening it. Tumor cells are discharged into the vitreous, often with seeding of the anterior chamber producing a pseudohypopion. Because of the absence of a retinal mass, this type of retinoblastoma masquerades as a vitritis or *Toxocara* endophthalmitis. With anterior chamber involvement, hyperacute iritis with hypopyon, juvenile xanthogranuloma, or tuberculosis may be suspected [13].

E. Complete Spontaneous Regression

Complete spontaneous regression (Figs. 8 and 9) is believed to occur more frequently in retinoblastoma than in any other malignant neoplasm [7]. Typically, there is a severe inflammatory reaction followed by phthisis bulbi [14]. The mechanism or mechanisms by which regression occurs are unknown. In several cases of bilateral retinoblastoma from the American Registry of Ophthalmic Pathology there was total necrosis and phthisis bulbi on one side, while, on the other, a viable tumor massively filled the eye and invaded the orbit [14]. Such cases would seem to exclude the possibility of a systemic mechanism for tumor necrosis. The cells of a retinoblastoma have not only a high growth fraction but also a high death rate. If

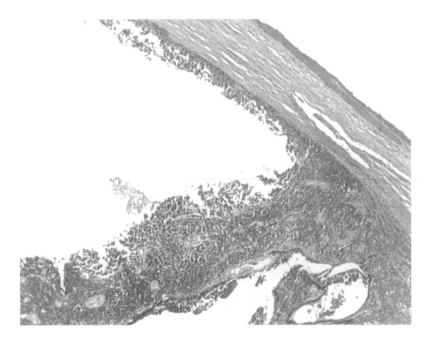

Figure 6   Diffuse infiltrating retinoblastoma. Retinoblasts have infiltrated the iris and ciliary body, occluded the chamber angle, and seeded the corneal endothelium.

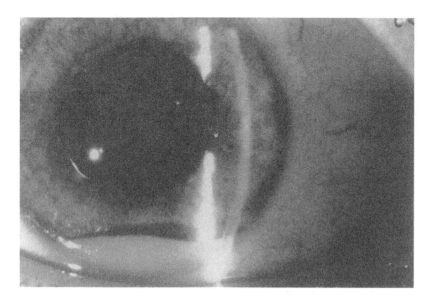

Figure 7 Diffuse infiltrating retinoblastoma. There are small nodules of tumor on the surface of the iris and a pseudohypopion.

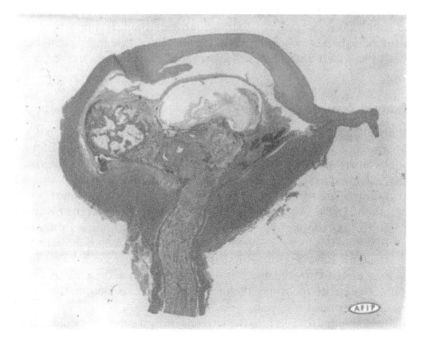

Figure 8 Spontaneously regressed retinoblastoma. The eye is phthisic. There is disorganization and bone formation.

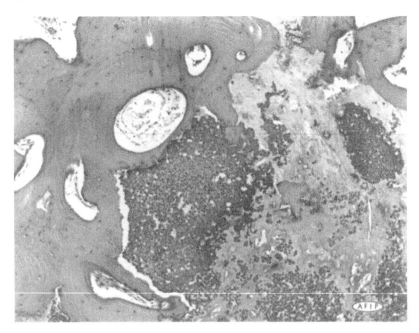

Figure 9 Spontaneously regressed retinoblastoma. There is bone formation and clumps of necrotic ossified retinoblasts.

for some reason the growth rate is slowed down, then the high death rate gets the upper hand and total necrosis occurs. Extraocular extension is important in determining this outcome, because once the tumor reaches the vascular supply to the orbit, the retinoblastoma, if left untreated, will grow rapidly until it kills the patient.

F. Histopathology

Retinoblastomas are malignant neuroblastic tumors. The predominant cell has a large basophilic nucleus of variable size and shape and scanty cytoplasm. Mitotic figures are typically numerous. The tumor cells have a striking tendency to outgrow their blood supply. Characteristically, especially in large tumors, sleeves of viable cells are present, cuffing dilated blood vessels (Figs. 2 and 10). As the tumor cells become displaced more than 90–110 μm away from the vessel, they undergo ischemic coagulative necrosis [15,16]. Although this is a relatively constant finding from one tumor to the next, the thickness of the sleeves is dependent on the metabolic activity of the cells within the cuff. Burnier et al. [16] demonstrated an inverse relationship between the thickness of the cuff and the mitotic activity within the cuff. A cuff thickness of 100 μm represents the approximate distance that oxygen can diffuse before it is completely consumed in rapidly growing neoplasms.

When viable tumor cells are shed into the vitreous or into subretinal fluid, they may grow into spheroidal aggregates with diameters that rarely exceed 1 mm [15]. Within the spheroids, the more peripherally situated cells derive their nutrition from the vitreous or subretinal fluid and the more central cells undergo necrosis. This represents the opposite situation from the cuffs of viable tumor cells that surround the vessels in retinoblastomas. If viable cells in the vitreous or subretinal space become attached to the retina, they may gain oxygen from the retinal vasculature and secrete angiogenic molecules that stimulate the proliferation of capillaries from the retina into the tumor. Similarly, tumor cells in the subretinal exudate may seed onto the outer surface of the retina. Tumor cells can seed on the inner surface of the retinal pigment epithelium or invade beneath the retinal pigment epithelium, remaining viable by deriving nutrition from the choriocapillaris.

As the retinoblastoma grows to fill the vitreous cavity, almost without exception, the tumor's intrinsic blood vessels cannot keep pace with the proliferation of the neoplastic cells. This implies that at this stage, the growth rate of the tumor is limited by the ability of the tumor to induce new vessel formation. This results in extensive areas of coagulative necrosis. Foci of dystrophic calcification occur frequently within the areas of necrosis (Fig. 10). In most instances, the necrotic portions of retinoblastomas do not seem to provoke much of an inflammatory response. With marked necrosis, the DNA liberated from the tumor's nuclei may become absorbed preferentially in the walls of blood vessels (Fig. 11) and by the internal limiting membrane of the retina, giving a deep blue (hematoxylinophilic) or Feulgen-positive staining to these tissues [17]. Similar basophilic staining of the lens capsule, vessels in the iris, or tissues adjacent to Schlemm's canal may occur when some of the fragmented DNA escapes into the aqueous.

The formation of Flexner-Wintersteiner rosettes (Fig. 12) is highly character-istic of retinoblastomas. Pineoblastoma and medulloepithelioma are the only other

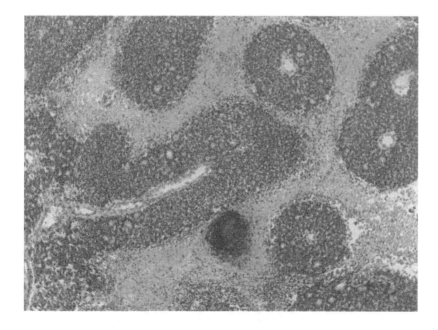

Figure 10   Retinoblastoma sleeve pattern. The sleeves of viable retinoblasts surrounding blood vessels are remarkably uniform in thickness. They all contain Flexner-Wintersteiner rosettes. Within the necrotic tissue is a calcified nodule.

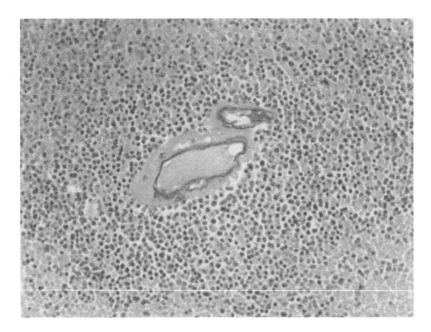

Figure 11 Blood vessels in necrotic area of retinoblastoma. There is dark staining of the wall of the blood vessel due to DNA deposition from the necrotic retinoblasts.

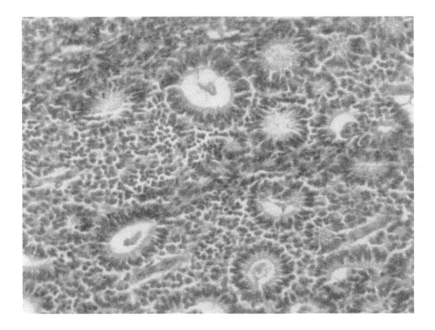

Figure 12 Flexner-Wintersteiner rosettes. Columnar cells with basal nuclei surround an apical lumen. Many cells have a small projection from the apical surface into the lumen.

neoplasms in which Flexner-Wintersteiner rosettes have been observed. The Flexner-Wintersteiner rosette represents photoreceptor differentiation by the tumor, but the cells of the rosettes are not benign. Characteristically Flexner-Wintersteiner rosettes are found within areas of undifferentiated malignant cells exhibiting mitotic activity, and the cells that form the rosettes may also contain mitotic figures. Some rosettes are incompletely formed and the cells blend with the surrounding undifferentiated cells.

The typical Flexner-Wintersteiner rosette (Fig. 12) is lined by columnar cells that circumscribe an apical lumen. The basal ends of the cells that form the rosettes contain the nuclei. The apical ends of the columnar cells are held together by terminal bars and the cells may have apical cytoplasmic projections into the lumen of the rosette. Electron microscopy has demonstrated that these projections represent primitive inner and outer segments. In the lumens of the rosettes, Alcian blue and colloidal iron stains reveal a coating of hyaluronidase-resistant acid mucopolysaccharide that has similar staining characteristics to the glycosaminogycan matrix that surrounds the rod and cones of the retina [18]. Tso and coworkers [19] described several additional ultrastructural features that the cells forming Flexner-Wintersteiner rosettes share with retinal photoreceptors: zonula occludens that form a luminal limiting membrane analogous to the cellular junctions that form the outer limiting membrane of the retina, cytoplasmic microtubules, cilia with the $9+0$ pattern of microtubules, and lamellated membranous structures resembling the discs of rod outer segments. Immunohistochemical and lectin histochemical studies have also supported the concept that retinoblastomas are composed of neuroblastic cells that may differentiate into photoreceptor-like cells [20–22].

Homer Wright rosettes (Fig. 13) are much less commonly seen in retinoblastomas than Flexner-Wintersteiner rosettes. Because they are found in a variety of neuroblastic tumors, they are less specific for retinoblastoma. These rosettes do not contain photoreceptor elements, and Wright first described this rosette in a neuroblastoma of the adrenal gland. They are also highly characteristic of cerebellar medulloblastomas [23]. The cells in these rosettes are not arranged about a lumen but, instead, send out neurofibrillary processes that form a tangle within the center of the rosette. Therefore, Homer White rosettes represent differentiation toward neurons similar to the retinal bipolar cells.

In 1970, Tso and coworkers [4] reported that in 18 of 300 retinoblastomas (6%) treated by enucleation, there were foci of cytologically benign cells that had features of photoreceptors (Figs. 1, 14, and 15). In most of these 18 tumors, the areas exhibiting photoreceptor differentiation could easily be spotted at low magnification as discrete, comparatively eosinophilic islands standing out in contrast to the much more intensely basophilic portions of the tumor. The tumor cells that exhibited photoreceptor differentiation had more abundant cytoplasm and smaller, less basophilic nuclei. In these areas, mitotic figures were uncommon and necrosis was absent, but scattered deposits of calcium were occasionally present. This calcification differed from that in the undifferentiated areas because it was not associated with necrosis. Scattered among the differentiated cells were individual cells and clusters of cells with long cytoplasmic processes that stained brightly with eosin. The cytoplasmic processes project through a fenestrated membrane and, when present in a cluster, tended to fan out like a bouquet of flowers (hence the name *fleurette*) (Figs. 1 and 14). Electron microscopy has revealed that the cells of the fleurettes

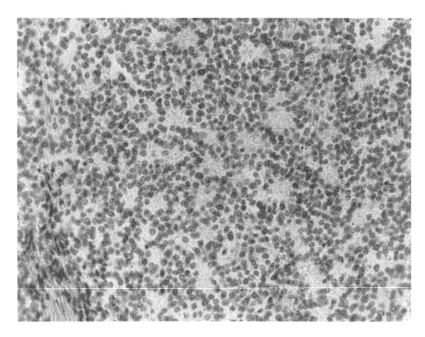

Figure 13   Homer Wright rosettes. Retinoblasts surround a central tangle of neurofilaments. Homer Wright rosettes are not as sharply delimited as Flexner-Wintersteiner rosettes.

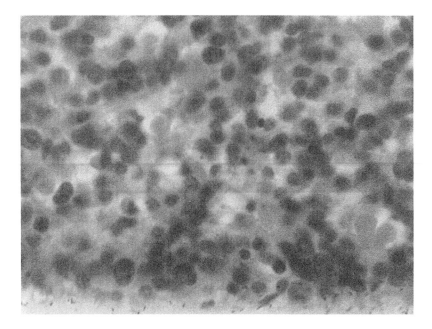

Figure 14   Fleurettes. Retinocytes surround little pockets of extracellular space. Projecting into some of these spaces are the bulbous processes of fleurettes.

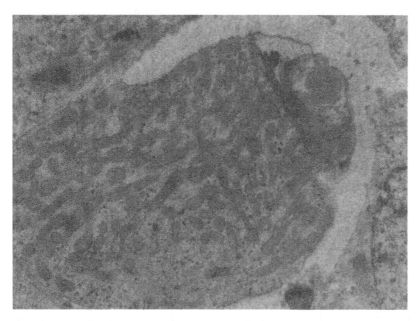

Figure 15 Fleurette. Electron micrographic evidence of photoreceptor differentiation. The bulbous process is composed of two components. The inner part has numerous mitochondria-like the inner segment of retinal cones and the outer part has a stack of lamella like the outer segments of cones.

contain structures that resemble retinal cones [5]. The bulbous eosinophilic processes contained numerous mitochondria (Fig. 15) and resembled cone inner segments.

In a subsequent study, Tso et al. [24] examined retinoblastomas in 54 eyes enucleated after having been irradiated. Of these, 42 eyes contained viable tumor cells and 17 of these tumors (40%) exhibited photoreceptor differentiation. In seven cases, the residual tumor was composed entirely of cells showing photoreceptor differentiation. Consequently, these investigators suggested that tumors containing such benign components might be incompletely radioresponsive because, as a general rule, benign and highly differentiated tumors are more radioresistant. Follow-up information was obtained in 13 of the 17 cases; there was only one tumor death. Despite uncontrolled tumor growth, the parents of this child refused to permit enucleation. The patient died of intracranial extension of the retinoblastoma. Histological study revealed this tumor to be composed of areas of undifferentiated retinoblastoma and areas of benign-appearing cells that exhibited photoreceptor differentiation.

Tumors composed entirely of benign-appearing cells are now diagnosed as retinocytomas. In addition to the cells exhibiting photoreceptor differentiation, there are cells that resemble bipolar neurons, astrocytes, and Müller cells [6]. The presence of glia has been demonstrated using glial fibrillary acid protein immunohistochemistry and electron microscopy and probably represents reactive gliosis in these benign variants of retinoblastoma [6].

In phthisic eyes with totally necrotic "regressed" retinoblastomas, it may be difficult to diagnose the retinoblastoma. Histological examination reveals dense calcification in a tumor that exhibits complete coagulative necrosis (Figures 8 and 9). Under high magnification, one can usually make out the ghostly outlines of fossilized tumor cells. Further confusion may be created by exuberant reactive proliferation of retinal pigment epithelial cells, ciliary epithelial cells, and glial cells and by ossification [25].

II. EXTRAOCULAR EXTENSION, SPREAD, AND METASTASIS

Most retinoblastomas exhibit relentlessly progressive, rapidly invasive growth. If left untreated, they usually fill the eye and completely destroy the internal architecture of the globe (Fig. 16). The most common method of spread is by invasion through the optic disc into the optic nerve (Figs. 17 and 18). Once into the nerve, the tumor may spread directly along the nerve fiber bundles back toward the optic chiasm, or it may infiltrate through the pia into the subarachnoid space. From the subarachnoid space, tumor cells may be carried via the circulating cerebrospinal fluid to the brain and spinal cord. Once the tumor has invaded the choroid (Fig. 19), it may then spread into the orbit via the scleral canals or by massively replacing the sclera (Fig. 16). It has been estimated that an average of approximately 6 months is required from when the retinoblastoma produces its first symptoms to when it invades beyond the eye [26]. Extraocular invasion dramatically increases the chances of hematogenous

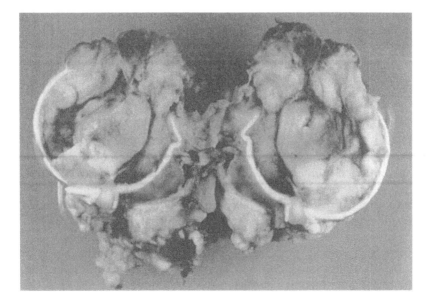

Figure 16   Advanced retinoblastoma. The bisected eye shows that the tumor has destroyed the intraocular structures and cornea. It has invaded outside the eye to form extraocular masses anteriorly and posteriorly.

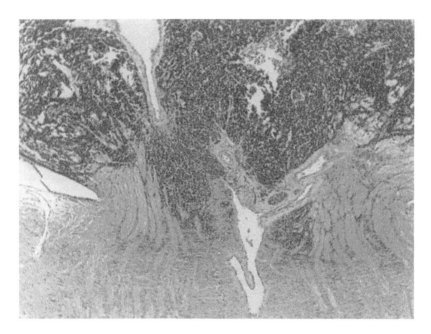

Figure 17 Retinoblastoma. Minimal optic nerve invasion. Centrally there are a few retinoblasts posterior to the lamina cribrosa.

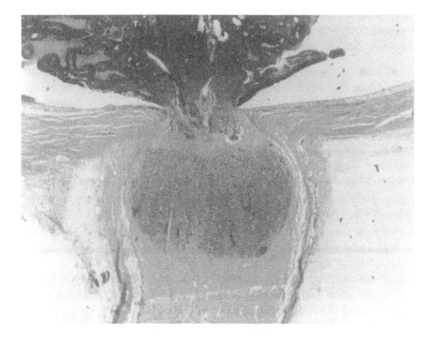

Figure 18 Retinoblastoma. Optic nerve invasion has not reached the resection margin. Tumor cells have come very close to the subarachnoid space.

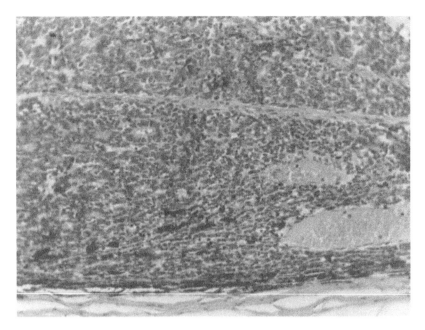

Figure 19   Exophytic retinoblastoma. Retinoblasts have completely infiltrated the choroid. An unusual feature in this tumor is the presence of Flexner-Wintersteiner rosettes within the choroidal infiltrate.

dissemination and permits access to conjunctival lymphatics and metastasis to regional lymph nodes.

Retinoblastomas exhibit metastatic potential in four ways:

1.   Direct infiltrative spread may occur along the optic nerve from the eye to the brain. Once the orbital soft tissues have been invaded, the tumor may spread directly into the orbital bones, through the sinuses into the nasopharynx, or via the various foramina into the cranium.
2.   Dispersion of tumor cells may occur after cells in the optic nerve have invaded the leptomeninges and gained access to the circulating subarachnoid fluid. This may occur without involvement of cut end of the optic nerve. Flow of cerebrospinal fluid can carry tumor cells from the eye to the brain and spinal cord; in monocular cases, spread to the optic nerve on the opposite side has been observed.
3.   Hematogenous dissemination leads to widespread metastasis to the lungs, bones, brain, and other viscera. Extraocular invasion and to a lesser degree choroidal invasion increase the risk for hematogenous spread.
4.   Lymphatic spread occurs in those cases in which there has been anteriorly located or massive extraocular extension. There are no intraocular or posterior orbital lymphatic channels, but the lacrimal gland, bulbar conjunctiva, and eyelids are richly supplied with lymphatic vessels.

When metastasis occurs, it is generally becomes symptomatic and kills within the first year or two following treatment. Kopelman et al. [27] found that the median time to death with fatal retinoblastoma was 6.4 months in unilateral cases and 14.2 months in bilateral cases. In contrast, Gamel et al. [28] estimated the median time to death for patients dying of metastatic uveal melanoma to be 7.2 years. Late death from metastasis, which occurs so frequently following enucleation for uveal melanomas, is rare after treatment for retinoblastoma—so much so that when late metastasis is suspected, the question of an independent new primary tumor must be considered. Hematogenous metastasis from retinoblastoma is characteristically widespread, but—unlike uveal melanoma—is frequently preceded by spread to regional lymph nodes. The brain may be selectively affected when spread has occurred via the optic nerve. Invasion of leptomeninges of the optic nerve typically gives rise to a thick accumulation of tumor cells in the meninges along the basilar surface of the brain and in the ventricles, which can be detected by computed tomography [29].

In metastatic lesions, retinoblastoma typically appears much less differentiated than in the intraocular primary tumor. Rosettes, which may be numerous and highly organized in the primary tumors, are typically very difficult to find and poorly formed in metastatic lesions. Fleurettes are never observed in metastatic lesions. In a study of 17 autopsies [30] on children who died of metastatic retinoblastoma, 9 had distant bone involvement, 8 had visceral involvement, and 8 had lymph node involvement. The metastases of retinoblastoma, unlike those of uveal melanoma, do not home to the liver.

The primary retinoblastoma-like tumors observed in the pineal and in parasellar sites [27,31] and primitive neuroectodermal tumors that have been encountered as second primary neoplasms in patients with heritable retinoblastoma have been confused with metastatic retinoblastoma. In distinction from metastatic retinoblastoma, these second primary tumors are initially solitary and frequently not located in sites of predilection for metastatic retinoblastoma. They often appear several years after the successful treatment of intraocular retinoblastomas that do not have a high risk of metastasis. The intracranial primary tumors may exhibit photoreceptor differentiation, with numerous rosettes and fleurettes, which one would not expect in a metastatic retinoblastoma.

Recurrence of retinoblastoma in the orbit following enucleation is usually the result of tumor cells that were left untreated in the orbit. In some instances this may be the result of subclinical orbital involvement that also may have escaped histopathological recognition. More frequently, it has been a consequence of incomplete initial treatment of known invasion of the orbit or optic nerve beyond the margin of surgical transection. Very rarely, orbital recurrence may be the result of lymphatic or hematogenous spread to the bony walls and soft tissues of the orbit or the lids.

III. PROGNOSIS

There are many risk factors affecting prognosis, but most important is the extent of invasion by the retinoblastoma outside of the eye. Kopelman et al. [27], in an analysis of cases from the Registry of Ophthalmic Pathology, found that the extent of invasion into the optic nerve and through the ocular coats were the two most important predictors of patient outcome. Extraocular invasion as the most important predictor of death is supported by a number of studies [32–36]. When the data were evaluated by multivariate analysis, bilaterality was the only variable that proved to be more significantly associated with a fatal outcome than in univariate analysis, suggesting that bilaterality is related to death for reasons unrelated to the primary tumor. In some of these cases the cause of death was attributed to spread of retinoblastoma to the brain, yet there was no optic nerve invasion. One must consider the possibility that new intracranial primary tumors (trilateral retinoblastomas) were responsible for the deaths in these cases.

A problem with the study by Kopelman et al. [27] was that it was based on cases of retinoblastoma that were treated prior to 1962, and the possibility existed that more modern treatment could affect the results. A more recent study was performed in Germany [37], but in this study there were few deaths, making statistically significant inferences about prognostic factors difficult. Mclean et al. [38] compared 514 cases of retinoblastoma from the Registry of Ophthalmic Pathology obtained between 1917 and 1962 (mean, 1945) with 460 cases from Germany obtained between 1963 to 1986 (mean, 1976). The cause-specific survival rate, in which only deaths attributed to spread or metastasis of the retinoblastoma are considered, was lower in the older sample from the United States (66% at 5 years) than that in the German sample (93% at 5 years). Because of the rapid growth rate of retinoblastoma, 5-year survival rates essentially represent cure rates. Invasion of the ocular coats and invasion into the optic nerve were the most significant prognostic factors in both samples. A multivariate logistic model using seven variables (post-1962 German versus pre-1963 American case, unilateral versus bilateral, invasion of choroid, invasion of sclera, invasion of orbit, invasion of retrolaminar optic nerve, and invasion of the resected margin of the optic nerve) described well the observed mortality patterns (Table 1). In the absence of these prognostic factors, there were no deaths in the German series and eight deaths in the series from the Registry of Ophthalmic Pathology. Because metastasis of retinoblastoma is very unlikely in the absence of extraocular invasion, many oncologists no longer recommend lumbar punctures and bone marrow aspirates when retinoblastoma does not invade outside the eye [39].

Table 1 Prognostic Factors Determined by Logistic Regression of 514 American Cases Obtained Prior to 1963 and 460 German Cases Obtained After 1962

Variable	Odds ratio	p Value
Invasion of ocular coats		
Into choroid	2.9	<0.0001
Into sclera	9.1	<0.0001
Into orbit	37.6	<0.0001
Invasion of optic nerve		
Resected	4.4	<0.0001
Unresected	13.3	<0.0001
Bilaterality	2.9	0.0001
Pre-1963 American case	4.1	<0.0001

Source: Ref. 38.

McLean et al. [1] have reviewed 12 cases of fatal unilateral retinoblastoma from the Registry of Ophthalmic Pathology in which the tumors were believed to be confined to the eye without invasion into the optic nerve or sclera. In 6 of the 12 cases, there was choroidal invasion. In 8 cases, 4 with choroidal invasion and 4 without choroidal invasion, there was an orbital recurrence, which preceded the development of distant metastasis. These histories suggest that there was probably microscopic extraocular spread that was not detected by histological examination. This emphasizes the importance of extraocular invasion as the pathway leading to metastasis of retinoblastoma and the great need for careful histological examination aimed at the detection of microscopic extraocular extension for accurate staging. A problem arises when globes are opened to get fresh tissue for genetic and molecular biology studies. This often spreads tumor cells to suprachoroidal and episcleral locations, making it very difficult to tell if there was extraocular invasion by the tumor.

IV. UNSUSPECTED RETINOBLASTOMA

Stafford and coworkers [40], in their analysis of 618 histologically proven cases of retinoblastoma for which adequate clinical data were available, found that almost 15% had been misdiagnosed initially. In 6.6% of the 618 cases, the incorrect initial diagnosis had led to a delay in enucleation while treatment was given for panophthalmitis, endophthalmitis, tuberculosis, or other forms of uveitis. In the other 8.3%, a variety of noninflammatory, nonneoplastic conditions had been diagnosed. Shields et al. [41] described five patients with retinoblastoma who presented with orbital cellulitis without extraocular extension of the tumor. In all five cases, the retinoblastoma was large and had undergone extensive necrosis. Delays in enucleation were associated with a greater mortality than in the cases where a correct initial diagnosis had been followed promptly by enucleation. Kopelman et al. [27] found that the odds of death were 2.5 times greater with clinically undiagnosed retinoblastoma.

REFERENCES

1. McLean IW, Burnier MN, Zimmerman LE, Jakobiec FA. Tumors of the eye and ocular adnexa. In: Atlas of Tumor Pathology, 3rd Series, Fascicle 12. Washington, DC: Armed Forces Institute of Pathology, 1994; pp 101–127.
2. Klauss V, Chana HS. Ocular tumors in Africa. Soc Sci Med 1983; 17:1743–1750.
3. Tso MOM, Fine BS, Zimmerman LE, et al. Photoreceptor elements in retinoblastoma. A preliminary report. Arch Ophthalmol 1969; 82:57–59.
4. Tso MOM, Zimmerman LE, Fine BS. The nature of retinoblastoma: I. Photoreceptor differentiation: A clinical and histologic study. Am J Ophthalmol 1970; 69:339–649.
5. Tso MOM, Fine BS, Zimmerman LE. The nature of retinoblastoma: II. Photoreceptor differentiation: An electron microscopic study. Am J Ophthalmol 1970; 69:350–359.
6. Margo C, Hidayat A, Kopelman J, Zimmerman LE. Retinocytoma: A benign variant of retinoblastoma. Arch Ophthalmol 1983; 101:1519–1531.
7. Gallie BL, Phillips RA, Ellsworth RM, et al. Significance of retinoma and phthisis bulbi for retinoblastoma. Ophthalmology 1982; 89:1393–1399.

8. Abramson DH, McCormick B, Fass D, et al. Retinoblastoma. The long-term appearance of radiated intraocular tumors. Cancer 1991; 67:2753–2755.

9. Eagle RC Jr, Shields JA, Donoso L, Milner RS. Malignant transformation of spontaneously regressed retinoblastoma, retinoma/retinocytoma variant. Ophthalmology 1989; 96:1389–1395.

10. Shields JA, Shields CL. Intraocular Tumors: A Text and Atlas. Philadelphia: Saunders, 1992.

11. Mansour AM, Greenwald MJ, O'Grady R. Diffuse infiltrating retinoblastoma. J Pediatr Ophthalmol Strabismus 1989; 26:152–154.

12. Nicholson DH, Norton EW. Diffuse infiltrating retinoblastoma. Trans Am Ophthalmol Soc 1980; 78:265–289.

13. Shields JA, Shields CL, Eagle RC, Blair CJ. Spontaneous pseudohypopyon secondary to diffuse infiltrating retinoblastoma. Arch Ophthalmol 1988; 106:1301–1302.

14. Boniuk M, Zimmerman LE. Spontaneous regression of retinoblastoma. Int Ophthalmol Clin 1962; 2:525–542.

15. Schipper J. Retinoblastoma: A medical and Experimental Study (thesis). Utrecht: University of Utrecht, 1980, p 144.

16. Burnier MN, McLean IW, Zimmerman LE, Rosenberg SH. Retinoblastoma. The relationship of proliferating cells to blood vessels. Invest Ophthalmol Vis Sci 1990; 31:2037–2040.

17. Bunt AH, Tso MO. Feulgen-positive deposits in retinoblastoma. Incidence, composition, and ultrastructure. Arch Ophthalmol 1981; 99:144–150.

18. Zimmerman LE. Retinoblastoma and retinocytoma. In: Spencer WH, ed. Ophthalmic Pathology: An Atlas and Textbook. Philadelphia: Saunders, 1985, pp 1292–1351.

19. Tso MOM, Fine BS, Zimmerman LE. The Flexner-Wintersteiner rosettes in retinoblastoma. Arch Pathol 1969; 88:665–671.

20. Donoso LA, Shields CL, Lee EY. Immunohistochemistry of retinoblastoma. A review. Ophthalm Paediatr Genet 1989; 10:3–32.

21. Kivela T. Glycoconjugates in retinoblastoma. A lectin histochemical study of ten formalin-fixed and paraffin-embedded tumours. Virchows Arch [A] 1987; 410:471–479.

22. Vrabec T, Arbizo V, Adamus G, McDowell JH, Hargrave PA, Donoso LA. Rod cell-specific antigens in retinoblastoma. Arch Ophthalmol 1989; 107:1061–1063.

23. Rubinstein LJ. Tumors of the central nervous system. In: Atlas of Tumor Pathology, Suppl to Fascicle 6, 2nd Series. Washington, DC: Armed Forces Institute of Pathology, 1982, pp 15–20.

24. Tso MOM, Zimmerman LE, Fine BS, et al. A cause of radioresistance in retinoblastoma: Photoreceptor differentiation. Trans Am Acad Ophthalmol Otolaryngol 1970; 74:959–969.

25. Smith JLS. Histology and spontaneous regression of retinoblastoma. Trans Ophthalmol Soc UK 1974; 94:953–967.

26. Erwenne CM, Franco EL. Age and lateness of referral as determinants of extra-ocular retinoblastoma. Ophthalm Paediatr Genet 1989; 10:179–184.

27. Kopelman JE, McLean IW, Rosenberg SH. Multivariate analysis of risk factors for metastasis in retinoblastoma treated by enucleation. Ophthalmology 1987; 94:371–377.

28. Gamel JW, McLean IW, Rosenberg SH. Proportion cured and mean log survival time as functions of tumor size. Statist Med 1990; 9:999–1006.

29. Meli FJ, Boccaleri CA, Manzitti J, Lylyk P. Meningeal dissemination of retinoblastoma: CT findings in eight patients. AJNR 1990; 11:983–986.

30. Merriam GR. Retinoblastoma: Analysis of 17 autopsies. Arch Ophthalmol 1950; 44:71–108.

31. Bader JL, Meadows AT, Zimmerman LE, et al. Bilateral retinoblastoma with ectopic intracranial retinoblastoma: Trilateral retinoblastoma. Cancer Genet Cytogenet 1982; 5:203–213.
32. The Committee for the National Registry of Retinoblastoma. Survival rate and risk factors for patients with retinoblastoma in Japan. Jpn J Ophthalmol 1992; 36:121–131.
33. Hungerford J, Kingston J, Plowman N. Orbital recurrence of retinoblastoma. Ophthalm Paediatr Genet 1987; 8:63–68.
34. Magramm I, Abramson DH, Ellsworth RM. Optic nerve involvement in retinoblastoma. Ophthalmology 1989; 96:217–222.
35. Messmer EP, Heinrich T, Höpping W, de Sutter E, Havers W, Sauerwein W. Risk factors for metastases in patients with retinoblastoma. Ophthalmology 1991; 98:136–141.
36. Stannard C, Lipper S, Sealy R, Sevel D. Retinoblastoma: Correlation of invasion of the optic nerve and choroid with prognosis and metastases. Br J Ophthalmol 1979; 63:560–570.
37. Messmer EP, Heinrich T, Höpping W, de Sutter E, Havers W, Sauerwein W. Risk factors for metastases in patients with retinoblastoma. Ophthalmology 1991; 98:136–141.
38. McLean IW, Rosenberg SH, Messmer EP, Heinrich T, Hopping W, Havers W. Prognostic factors in cases of retinoblastoma: Analysis of 974 patients from Germany and the United States treated by enucleation. In: Bornfeld N, Gragoudas ES, Lommatzsch PK., eds. Tumors of the Eye. Proceedings of the International Symposium on Tumors of the Eye. Amsterdam: Kugler Publications, 1991, pp 69–72.
39. Pratt CB, Meyer D, Chenaille P, Crom DB. The use of bone marrow aspirations and lumbar punctures at the time of diagnosis of retinoblastoma. J Clin Oncol 1989; 7:140–143.
40. Stafford WR, Yanoff M, Parnell B. Retinoblastoma initially misdiagnosed as primary ocular inflammation. Arch Ophthalmol 1969; 82:771–773.
41. Shields JA, Shields CL, Suvarnamani C, Schroeder RP, DePotter P. Retinoblastoma manifesting as orbital cellulitis. Am J Ophthalmol 1991; 112:442–449.

21

Molecular Genetics of Retinoblastoma

ISABELLE AUDO and JOSÉ SAHEL

Hôpital Saint Antoine, Paris, France

I. INTRODUCTION

Retinoblastoma (RNB) is the most frequent primary ocular tumor of early childhood. It affects 1 in 14,000 to 1 in 20,000 births [1], with both sporadic and hereditary forms. This tumor originates from a retinal precursor cell, and the underlying defect is the successive inactivation of both alleles of the same retinoblastoma susceptibility gene, *RB1* (OMIM 180200), following a two-hit model described by Knudson [2]. The *RB1* gene has been identified after genetic analysis of hereditary RNB in the long arm of chromosome 13 [3–6], and studying its mutations allows a better understanding of the disease and accurate genetic counseling helpful for treatment. *RB1* was also the first tumor suppressor gene to be identified, and the discovery of its central role in cell cycle control opened the field to a better understanding of normal cell proliferation and the malignant development of other cancers [7,8] that goes beyond the gene's involvement in retinoblastoma.

II. KNUDSON'S TWO-HIT HYPOTHESIS AND DISCOVERY OF *RB1* THE RETINOBLASTOMA SUSCEPTIBILITY GENE

After ophthalmoscopes came into general use for the early diagnosis of RNB and subsequent enucleation, hereditary forms of RNB, mostly bilateral, and their autosomal dominant transmission were recognized, allowing earlier diagnosis, treatment and improved survival [9].

In 1971, Alfred Knudson presented a two-hit hypothesis model explaining the development of RNB and predicting the existence of recessive cancer genes or tumor suppressor genes [2]. He reported a statistical analysis of 48 cases of RNB. From his results, based on unilaterality or bilaterality, sex, age at diagnosis (bilateral average at 15 months and unilateral average at 24 months), family history, and published reports [10], the author suggested that two genetic mutations are required for the development of a retinoblastoma (two-mutation or two-hit hypothesis). Each of those alterations was calculated to occur at a rate of approximately 2×10^{-7} per year. Since a great deal of cell divisions take place in the developing retina, the chance of one mutation occurring is very good. In the dominantly hereditary forms, a first mutation occurring in the germline (either transmitted by one of the parents or occurring de novo) represents the first hit; it will be carried in all developing cells and can be transmitted to descendants. RNB arises from a retinoblast hit by a second somatic mutation. Because this second mutation is likely to occur in more than one embryonic retinal cell that already bears a mutation, most individuals carrying a germline mutation will develop "early" multifocal and/or bilateral disease (in his publication, Knudson took an average of $m = 3$ for the number of tumors), although 12% develop a unilateral, unifocal lesion [11]. If no second somatic mutation occurs in the developing retina, no tumor will develop. In patients with nonhereditary RNB, the tumor develops from on single retinoblast hit by two successive somatic mutations. Because the occurrence of two consecutive somatic mutations in more than one retinal cell is very unlikely, these patients develop one "late" unifocal unilateral tumor. This two-hit hypothesis does not imply that those two mutations are sufficient for the development of RNB; it remains controversial whether mutations of other genes are also needed, representing the rate-limiting step in tumorigenesis.

Comings, in 1973, subsequently suggested that in an autosomal dominantly inherited tumor such as RNB, the two successive mutations inactivate both alleles of a specific regulatory gene and a tumor suppressor gene and that each mutation is recessive at the cellular level [12]. Benedict et al. later proposed a similar model [13].

In 1983, Benedict et al. and Cavanee at al. obtained the evidence that the two mutations required for tumor formation affected two alleles of the same gene [14]. Thus homozygous loss of function of the *RB1* gene initiates retinoblastoma tumor formation. Because the wild-type allele prevents tumor formation, the *RB1* gene was called a tumor suppressor gene. The *RB1* locus was then mapped to the long arm of chromosome 13 [13q14] by linkage and deletion analysis of the RNB family, in a region close to the gene coding for the esterase D (*ESD*) [3–6]. The *RB1* gene was subsequently cloned in 1986 and characterized [15–18].

III. *RB1* GENE STRUCTURE AND PROTEIN STRUCTURE AND FUNCTION

RB1 was the first gene described as a tumor suppressor, and this opened the way to a better understanding of cancer genesis. The structure and function of this gene in the cell cycle and in differentiation are coming to be more understood and are the subjects of extensive reviews [19–26].

A. The *RB1* Gene

The *RB1* gene is located on chromosome 13 at band q14. It is a large gene that spreads over 180 kb, contains 27 exons that range in size from 31–1873 bp and

26 introns ranging from 80–70,500 bp [27]. The promoter region of *RB1* is located at 186–206 bp upstream from the initiation codon; it contains binding sites for different transcription factors (RBF-1, Sp1, ATF, and E2F) [28]. Mutations at those sites, which have been described in hereditary RNB, inhibit binding of transcription factors, thus reducing promoter activity [29]. At this 5′ end, CpG islands are present that actually encompass the promoter region and are normally not methylated. Hypermethylation of these regions plays a role in tumorigenesis and promoter inactivation [30]. Transcription of *RB1* produces a 4.8-kb mRNA [31]. A 2.7-kb open reading frame results from this mRNA and encodes for a 110-kDa ubiquitously expressed nuclear phosphoprotein, pRB, containing 928 amino acid residues.

B. The Retinoblastoma Protein, pRb (Fig. 1)

1. The Function of pRb in Cell Proliferation and Differentiation

pRb plays a major role in cell proliferation and differentiation. It belongs to a small family of nuclear proteins comprising two other members, p107 and p130 (for review, see Ref. 32). Those three proteins share sequence homology in two separate domains that interact to form a pocket in the tertiary structure, the A/B pocket—hence the name *pocket proteins* given to this family. They are involved in distinct functions in the cell cycle and differentiation, but they also have overlapping roles and a partial ability to compensate for each other.

pRb fulfils its tumor suppressor role by controlling the cell cycle at the G1/S phase restriction point and thus the entry into S phase [33]. If pRb is functionally inactivated by a mutation, its control upon the restriction point is lost, potentially resulting in a constant activation of the cell cycle.

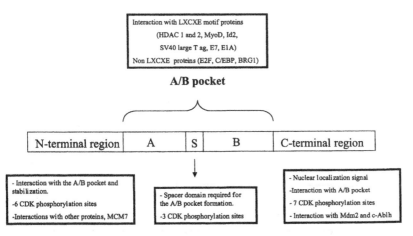

Figure 1   pRb structure and function. pRb is composed of different structural domains that are important for its function: two central domains, A and B which form the A/B central pocket, a C-terminal and a N-terminal region. Specific protein-protein interactions and phosphorylation sites have been described for each of these domains and are essential for pRb function.

pRB lacks DNA binding domains. Thus it will interact with gene promoters through its binding with other transcription factors. One of pRB's key targets is the E2F family of transcription factors (six known members differentially involved in cell proliferation, differentiation, and apoptosis), which heterodimerize with their obligate partner DP (three members). E2F/DP activate transcription of genes essential for DNA synthesis and for further cell cycle progression, including dihydrofolate reductase (*DHFR*) thymidine kinase, DNA polymerase alpha, *cdc2*, cyclin A and E, c-*myc*, b-*myb*, *pRB, p107*, and *E2F1* itself.

The ability to bind E2F and other transcription factors depends on pRB phosphorylation status, which changes throughout the cell cycle by sequential action of specific G1 cyclin-dependent kinases (CDK) bound to specific cyclins (Fig. 2): pRb is hypophosphorylated in G0/G1, which is its active status. It is then able to bind to and repress transcription factor E2F. pRb also actively represses transcription by physically recruiting transcriptional repression complexes to promoters containing E2F sites. In addition, pRb can inhibit E2F transactivation through the recruitment of chromatin remodeling factors, such as histone deacetylases (HDAC) and SWI/SNF complexes, DNA methyltransferase I (DNMT1), and histone H3 methyltransferase. This remodels chromatin to a more condensed state, physically blocking access to the promoter regions [34,35].

pRB becomes hyperphosphorylated during the transition phase between G1 and S phase, which leads to its inactivation and the release of E2F, driving S phase progression. The RB/E2F regulation pathway is thus critical for the control of cell proliferation and is disrupted in virtually every cancer.

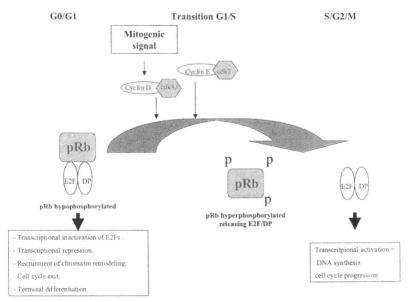

Figure 2 pRb function in cell proliferation and differentiation. pRb function is mediated through interactions with E2F and other transcription factors. Its ability to interact with other proteins depends on its phosphorylation status which changes throughout the cell cycle by sequential action of specific G1 cyclin-dependent kinases (CDK). During G0/G1 phase, pRb is hypophosphorylated and represses transcriptional activation. It becomes hyperphosphory-lated during the G1/S transition which releases E2F and initiates cell cycle progression.

Hypophosphorylated pRB binds to and regulates the function of other proteins involved in cell proliferation, including BRG-1, c-Abl, Mdm2, and MCM7. It also plays a unique role in differentiation pathways by leading the precursor cell to exit the cell cycle and start terminal differentiation (for review, see Refs. 25 and 26). Its role in myogenesis, hematopoiesis, and neurogenesis has been described, and different transcription factors seem to be regulated by pRb: CAAAT/enhancer binding proteins C-EBP, the HMG family member HBP1, and the basic helix-loop-helix (bHLH) transcription factors MyoD and Id-2.

2. Structure of pRb (Fig. 1)

pRB is composed of different structural domains that are important for its function. A better knowledge of the relation between structure and function helps us to understand the consequences of mutations and to build strategies for better screening.

Two central domains, the *A and B boxes*, highly conserved among species and separated by a less conserved spacer region, are required to form the *central pocket*. This A/B pocket is fundamental for pRB function through its ability to interact with different types of proteins. Two types of bindings have been described: interaction involving an *LXCXE motif* (Lys-X-Cys-X-Glu), such as interaction with endogenous proteins like HDAC 1 and 2 or viral oncoproteins (simian virus 40 large T antigen, human papillomavirus E7, and adenovirus E1A), and interaction with a *non-LXCXE motif*, such as interaction with the E2F family of transcription factors, C/EBP and BRG1. In 1998, Lee et al. elucidated the crystal structure of the LXCXE binding site in the pocket and discovered that it consists of five highly conserved amino acid residues separated in the linear peptide sequence [36]. The LXCXE binding site is located inside the B box in a well-conserved sequence, but the A box is essential for proper folding and the formation of an active pocket. Phosphorylation of this site disrupts the interface of the A/B boxes and could be a possible mechanism of reversible inactivation of pRB during the cell cycle.

Although no single "hot spot" for a preferential mutation site has been identified in the *RB1* gene, most of the mutations giving rise to a stable mutant pRB affect the protein-binding function of this pocket, pointing out its fundamental role in cell cycle control [37]. Functional assays for the pocket binding activity have even been proposed as a screening method for *RB1* mutation [38].

The carboxy-terminal region also plays an important role for tumor suppression, but it is less structured than the A/B pocket. It contains several functional sites, including a nuclear localizing signal, cyclin binding motifs, and seven consensus cyclin-dependent kinase (CDK) phosphorylation sites, and a second E2F binding site. The C-terminal region can also bind the oncoproteins Mdm2 and c-Abl. It can interact with the A/B pocket and regulate its activity. This interaction is strengthened by phosphorylation of the C-terminal residues, which disrupt the interaction A/B pocket/LXCXE proteins.

The N-terminal region is the least-characterized portion. It is also able to interact with the A/B pocket and regulates its activity, probably in promoting a stable active pRB conformational state. It also contains six consensus CDK phosphorylation sites, which may play a role in regulating pRB in the cell cycle and binding sites for different proteins such as MCM7.

IV. RETINOBLASTOMA TUMOR AND MUTATIONS OF *RB1*

Some 55–65% of patients affected by retinoblastoma are sporadic cases with unilateral lesions, and the first hit involves a somatic mutation. Those sporadic cases are at no risk for transmitting the disease to their offspring. At the opposite extreme are the other 35–45% of hereditary cases of RNB either by transmission of a germline mutation from an affected parent (10% of the patients present a family history) or by a new germline mutation that can be transmitted to offspring. The paternal allele is most often the carrier of the de novo mutation [39,40]. Indeed, 85% of new germline mutations affect the father's allele [41], but no paternal age effect has been found [40]. This paternal preference is very helpful in predicting the copy of the gene that will be the carrier of the first mutation. Its explanation could be found in the greater number of cell divisions occurring during spermatogenesis than during oogenesis, since mutations usually arise during DNA replication. On the other hand, a somatic mutation does not disclose any maternal or paternal preference for the first inactivated allele.

The hereditary condition is segregated as a Mendelian autosomal dominant trait with 90% penetrance. Among those genetic cases, patients typically develop multifocal and bilateral lesions, although 10–12% develop unilateral tumor [11]. Patients carrying a germline mutation will also be more susceptible to the development of secondary malignancies, especially sarcomas, and 5–7% present midline intracranial primitive neuroectodermal tumor (trilateral retinoblastoma) [42]. Thus, identification of a germline mutation is essential for better follow-up and improved vision and survival prognosis (see Fig. 3 to report the actual risk data for genetic counseling).

A. Mutation Detection

Whenever possible, analysis of tumor cells will give the best information, since the mutation is always present there and homozygous in 70% of cases [14]. If tumor samples are not available for DNA analysis (no fresh tissue harvested from an enucleated eye or local treatment chosen), constitutional cells, most often leukocytes from peripheral blood, will be studied for mutation analysis in clinical laboratories.

Different tests that vary in applicability and cost have been used to study mutations in RNB. Genetic linkage analysis has been developed but it can be applied only to RNB families, necessitating the availability of multiple informative family members (representing only 10% of RNB cases) and are not suitable for de novo mutations, which represent most of the hereditary cases [43,44]. Cytogenetic testing looking for chromosomal anomalies in 13q14 detects only very large chromosomal anomalies, and its low resolution allows the detection of only 7–8% of the patients with bilateral retinoblastoma and 1–4.9% in sporadic unilateral retinoblastoma [45]. Patients carrying a large cytogenetic deletion may be affected by a 13q deletion syndrome, which is associated with developmental delay, mental retardation, and facial dysmorphism. With the isolation and sequencing of *RB1*, it became possible to analyze the coding region of the gene directly. More sophisticated techniques have thus been developed to allow a greater resolution for the identification of small deletions, insertions, or point mutations, which constitute most of the germline mutations: DNA fragment analysis techniques using Southern blot hybridization

→ The index patient has a **family history of retinobastoma:**

. Index patient with RNB:
90%x50% = **45%** risk to have an affected child.
. Index patient without RNB:
10% risk to be a carrier and not developing a tumor:
10%x50%x90% = **4.5%** to have an affected child.

→ The index patient has **no family history of retinoblastoma:**

. Proband has **bilateral and/or multifocal tumor**: carrier of a germ line mutation:
- 90%x50%= **45%** risk to have an affected child.
. Proband has **unilateral, unifocal tumor**: 12% risk carrier of a germ line mutation:
- 50%x12%= **6%** risk to transmit to the offspring.
- 45%x12%= **5.4%** risk to have an affected child.
If the first child doesn't develop the disease then the risk for the second child is smaller. If at the opposite one child develops a RNB, then the proband is carrier for a germ line mutation and the transmission risk is the same as for every parent carrying a germ line mutation.

Figure 3 Evaluation of the genetic risk of retinoblastoma (RNB).

with cDNA and genomic clones, which allow only about 15% of mutations in hereditary retinoblastoma to be identified [46,47]; ribonuclease protection assay and the polymerase chain reaction (PCR) [48]; direct genomic sequencing [49,50]; high-resolution gel electrophoresis and multiplex PCR [51]; single-strand conformation polymorphism (SSCP) analysis [52]; and exon-by-exon PCR-SSCP analysis [53,54].

These techniques can be costly and time-consuming in routine clinical testing. To assess this question, Noorani et al. have compared the cost of molecular screening to conventional repeated ophthalmological examinations for a proto-typical family of a proband and seven at-risk relatives and demonstrated the value of genetic screening [55]. They found that genetic testing (using fragment analysis by quantitative multiplex PCR and if negative, sequencing of the promoter region and the 27 exons until a mutation was found) was four times less expensive than conventional screening [56]. They suggest complete retinal examination without anesthesia at birth and every 6 weeks until 3 months of age, thus three exams, then examination under general anesthesia at 5, 7, 9, 12, and 16 months and thereafter every 6 or 12 months up to at least 6 years of age, depending of the actual risk of developing a new tumor. The molecular approach is also valuable, since it spares stressful ophthalmological examinations to unaffected siblings and increases vigilance for an appropriate treatment and follow-up for the tested carriers. It also provides more information for a better understanding of the pathogenesis of retinoblastoma.

B. Mosaiscism—To Be Taken into Account in Genetic Analysis

According to Lohmann et al., however, genetic testing fails to detect about 17–20%
of the mutations [57]. In those cases, it is possible that the mutation was missed, but
they could also reflect a mosaicism that would not be detected in the peripheral
blood.

   The mosaic could be either the first affected patient in a family or one of the
parents. Mosaicism occurs when a mutation in *RB1* arises at some point during
embryogenesis, and the time point at which the mutation occurs determines the
number and type of cells that will carry the defect. The possibility of this mosaicism
should be taken into account during genetic counseling, because it could cause
significant errors in predicting the actual risk: a patient with retinoblastoma could be
a mosaic, bearing the mutation in leukocytes but not in the germline, and thus could
be improperly considered to be at risk of transmitting the trait to descendants. At the
opposite extreme, the mutation could be present in the germline and in some somatic
cells without being detectable in the leukocytes. This could then give false
reassurance about the genetic risk for the offspring and also about the occurrence
of multifocal and/or bilateral disease for the patient [58]. Sippel et al. studied 156
documented RBN families to evaluate the incidence of mosaicism among them [59].
The investigators were able to determine a mosaicism in 10% of those families, either
in the proband or in one of his or her parents. This percentage might be higher since,
for some cases, the authors could not gather all the elements characterizing a
mosaicism. Thus mosaicism should be taken into account in providing genetic
counseling based on DNA analysis, and Sippel et al. propose that genetic tests of
germline DNA be performed when feasible for an accurate evaluation of the actual
risk.

C. Nature of the First Hit

RNB results from inactivation of both copies of the *RB1* tumor suppressor gene. The
first allele is usually inactivated by an intragenic mutation (either in the germline or
in a somatic cell). The inactivation of the second copy can occur by any mechanisms
involved in the first mutation but most commonly (65–70% of cases) is lost by
mechanisms involving chromosomal interaction leading to loss of heterozygosity
(LOH) at the *RB1* locus [14].

   Oncogenic mutations leading to at least the inactivation of one of the *RB1*
alleles have been well documented in the literature. The majority of initial mutations
found are predicted to create premature stop codons as a result of nonsense or
frameshift mutations due to points mutations, deletions, and/or insertions or to
affect the A/B pocket structure. Lohmann et al. studied 119 patients with hereditary
RNB; among 83% causal mutations identified in peripheral blood, the authors found
15% of large deletions, 26% of short-length mutations, and 42% of single-base
substitutions [57]. No "hot spot" was found on the *RB1* gene for a preferential
location for single base-pair substitution, but mutations were unequally distributed
along the gene. Blanquet et al. found that exons 3, 8, 18, and 19 were preferential
targets for mutations among 232 patients affected by hereditary and sporadic RNB
[60]. Nevertheless, no mutation was identified in the last three exons, 25, 26, and 27.

This observation led the authors to suggest that mutations in the 3' end might not be oncogenic.

Harbour performed a metanalysis from 19 international reports published from January 1987 to June 1997, comprising 192 patients [61]. The author studied the distribution of reported germline mutations on the *RB1* gene for retinoblastoma patients and found that 43% of reported mutations were nonsense mutations and 35% frameshift mutations. These two types of mutations are the most deleterious for protein function, since they usually induce premature stop codons and thus give rise to a truncated protein. Of these mutations, 12% were found in a conserved 5' or 3' splice site of an intron and probably led to aberrant splicing and deletion of one or more exons and thus to a truncated protein. At the opposite extreme, 6% were missense mutations and 3% small in-frame deletions. Those mutations do not result in a truncated protein but rather affect amino acids that are critical for pRb function (amino acid substitution that will disrupt the A/B pocket interaction). Some 2% of the mutations were located in the promoter region and were all associated with low-penetrance RNB, which represents 4% of the cases included in this metanalysis. In 59%, the mutation was a base substitution. These are mostly recurrent C-to-T transitions located at CGA arginine codons within the open reading frame, which gives rise to a stop codon. This reflects the high mutability of 5'-methylated cytosines CpG in CpG dinucleotides through deamination [62]. Local quasirepeat sequences creating a misalignment can also associate to CpG deamination to originate a point mutation [63]. Some 32% of mutations were due to small deletions and 9% to small insertions. The deleted or inserted sequence usually ranges from -39 to $+55$ bp [64]. Only minimal variability was found among publications from different countries. Lohmann, in 1999, reported similar results [64]. The author also created a useful database on a website listing all the oncogenic mutations reported on the *RB1* gene (http://www.dlohmann.de/Rb/).

D. Second Hit and Loss of Heterozygosity

Loss of the homologous normal allele is the most common somatic event that leads to the inactivation of the second wild-type allele of the *RB1* gene (second hit) in a cell that is already heterozygous after inactivation by a first mutation in the other allele. This results in homozygosity or hemizygosity for the abnormal allele. Loss of heterozygosity (LOH) was first described in retinoblatoma by Cavenee et al. in 1983 in cultured RNB cells [14] and confirmed by Dryja et al. on RNB family studies [65]. This mechanism plays an important role in the expression of recessive mutations and inactivation of other tumor suppressor genes [66].

LOH represents 50–70% of all retinoblastomas and can occur by different chromosomal mechanisms: (Fig. 4): mitotic nondisjunction with loss of the wild-type chromosome or duplication of the mutant chromosome, mitotic recombination between the retinoblastoma locus and the centromere, or gene conversion and deletion [14]. To establish the relative frequencies of those different events, Hagstrom et al. studied 158 cases of matched RNB and leukocyte DNA samples using polymorphic markers and found 64% of LOH [67]. Among those LOH cases, 7% were hemizygous after a deletion or nondisjunction without duplication and 93% homozygous (equal to about 55% chromosomal nondisjunction with duplication and 45% mitotic recombination). The authors also found no difference in the occurrence

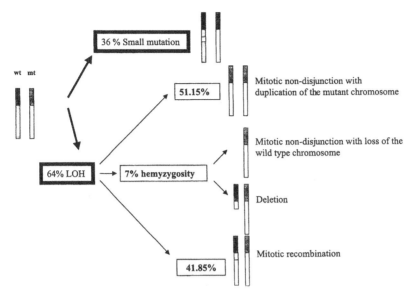

Figure 4   Mechanisms leading to loss of the second *RB1* allele [67]. The loss of the second *RB1* allele can occur either after a small mutation or more frequently by the loss of the homologous normal allele (loss of heterozygosity, LOH). This event can occur by different chromosomal mechanisms (mitotic nondisjunction, deletion, and mitotic recombination). Hagstrom et al. have studied the frequencies of each event and their results are reported in this figure [67].

of LOH whether the patient was a man or a woman, whether the initial mutation was located in the germline or in a somatic cell, or whether the initial mutation arose from the paternal or maternal allele.

E.   Low-Penetrance Retinoblastoma

About 10% of RNB families exhibit reduced penetrance (with unaffected obligate carriers) and variable expressivity of the disease (occurrence of RNB at an older age than usually expected in familial cases, with a high number of unilateral cases or benign retinocytomas) [68]. Some of those cases may be classified by mistake as unilateral sporadic cases. Characterization of those families and the underlying molecular mechanisms is relevant for accurate genetic counseling but also to further our understanding of the physiopathology of retinoblastoma and other cancers. To identify quantitatively low-penetrance retinoblastoma families, Lohmann et al. propose to calculate a disease:eye ratio (DER) that takes into account both penetrance and expressivity [69]. The DER is the number of eyes affected by RNB divided by the number of mutation carriers in the family. It is expected that families with complete penetrance and expressivity will typically have a ratio of 1.5 or higher, whereas most low-penetrance RNB families will have a DER inferior to 1.5.

It has been suggested that "weak" *RB1* alleles could account for the low penetrance of retinoblastoma: the presence of those two alleles would be sufficient for tumor suppression, whereas the presence of only one (after loss of heterozygosity, leading to nondisjunction without reduplication or small intragenic mutation) would lead to retinoblastoma.

The underlying nature of those weak alleles causing low penetrance retinoblastoma involves a mutational process that either induce a reduction in the amount of pRB synthesized or the production of a partially nonfunctional pRB [70]. Otterson et al. proposed the classification of those two kinds of mutational mechanisms into two classes [71]: class 1 comprising mutations leading to a reduction of pRB expression and class 2 including mutations leading to the production of a partially inactivated pRB. Harbour reviewed all the mutations described in low-penetrance retinoblastoma, classified them according to these two groups, and provided an insight into their consequences for tumorigenesis [72]. Class 1 mutations are less common and either affect the promoter region, disturbing binding with transcription factors required for an efficient pRB expression (e.g., SP1 or ATF), or involve splice-site sequences. Class 2 mutations affect the coding region of *RB1*. They consist mainly of small in-frame deletions or point mutations affecting amino acid residues critical for pRB structure and function (localization in the LXCXE or non-LXCXE binding site, E2F binding in particular). Thus, the identification of these mutations provides further information on pRB.

F. Genetic Anomalies Associated to pRB Inactivation and Concept of a Third Hit

RNB often displays other genetic changes in association with *RB1* inactivation [73]. This observation has led to the concept of a third hit, which would be involved in tumorigenesis, tumor progression, and resistance to treatment [74]. A third additional mutation could disrupt signals that would normally lead to apoptosis in the absence of a functional pRB, giving rise to a tumor. This could be the case if the chormosome imbalance resulted in an additional copy of a portion of a chromosome at an oncogene location or a monosomy at a tumor suppressor gene locus, thus providing a growth advantage. The most frequently described genetic anomaly is the gain of one or two extra copies of the short arm of chomosome 6, often as an isochromosome i6p, which is unique to RNB. This anomaly is found in 60% of the tumors [75] and has been shown to be associated with a worse prognosis and undifferentiated histological forms [76]. The other most common chromosomal imbalances found in RNB are a partial or complete trisomy of 1q (50% of RNB), monosomy 16 (46%), and extra copies of 2p (37.5%) [77]. Interestingly, Herzog et al. found more common and complex chromosomal imbalances on older patients at the age of surgery, which suggests that mutational abnormalities leading to the progression of RNB might be different in younger versus older patients [78]. Different authors are focusing on identifying potential candidates—oncogene or tumor suppressor gene—localized in those portions of chromosomal imbalance. Among the candidates are *Notch*, a receptor involved in neuronal development [74]; the oncogene *MYCN*, located in 2p [77]; glioblastoma amplification on chromosome 1; the *GAC1* gene and the renin gene, *REN*, located in 1q32 [78]; and the kinesin-like gene, *RBKIN*, in 6p22 [79]. The identification of these potential candidates will give us a better understanding of the genesis of retinoblastoma.

V. CONCLUSION

Since the two-hit hypothesis was announced by Knudson, our understanding of the molecular genetics underlying the development of retinoblastoma has increased dramatically. This has led to a better evaluation of patient risks, enabling a more informed choice of appropriate treatment and follow-up. Our increased knowledge of the structure and function of pRB and its implication in the development of retinoblastoma also gives us a better understanding of its involvement in cell proliferation and of tumorigenesis in other tissues.

REFERENCES

1. Tamboli A, Podgor MJ, Horm JW. The incidence of RNB in the United States: 1974 through 1985. Arch Ophthalmol 1990; 108:128–132.
2. Knudson AG Jr. Mutation and cancer: Statistical study of retinoblastoma. Proc Nat Acad Sci USA 1971; 68:820–823.
3. Yunis JJ, Ramsy N. Retinoblastoma and subband deletion of chromosome 13. Am J Dis Child 1978; 132:161–163.
4. Sparkes RS, Sparkes MC, Wilson MG, Towner JW, Benedict W, Murphree AL, Yunis JJ. Regional assignment of genes for human esterase D and retinoblastoma to chromosome band 13q14. Science 1980; 208:1042–1044.
5. Sparkes RS, Murphree AL, Lingua RW, Sparkes MC, Field LL, Funderburk SJ, Benedict WF. Gene for hereditary retinoblastoma assigned to human chromosome 13 by linkage to esterase D. Science 1983; 219(4587):971–973.
6. Connolly MJ, Payne RH, Johnson G, Gallie BL, Alderdice PW, Marshall WH, Lawton RD. Familial, EsD-linked, retinoblastoma with reduced penetranceand variable expressivity. Hum Genet 1983; 65:122–124.
7. Harbour JW, Lai SL, Whang-Peng J, Gazdar AF, Minna JD, Kaye FJ. Abnormalities in structure and expression of the human retinoblastoma gene in SCLC. Science 1988; 241:353–357.
8. Lee EY, To H, Shew JY, Bookstein R, Scully P, Lee WH. Inactivation of the retinoblastoma susceptibility gene in human breast cancers. Science 1988; 241:218–221.
9. Smith SM, Sorsby A. Retinoblastoma: some genetic aspects. Ann Hum Genet 1958; 23:50–58
10. Ashley DJ. The two "hit" and multiple "hit" theories of carcinogenesis. Br J Cancer 1969; 23(2):313–328.
11. Vogel F. Genetics of retinoblastoma. Hum Genet 1979; 52:1–54.
12. Commings DE. A general theory of carcinogenesis. Proc Natl Acad Sci USA 1973; 70:3324–3328.
13. Benedict WF, Murphree AL, Banerjee A, Spina CA, Sparkes MC, Sparkes RS. Patient with 13 chromosome deletion: Evidence that retinoblastoma gene is a recessive cancer genes. Science 1983; 219:973–975.
14. Cavenee WK, Dryja TP, Phillips RA, Benedict WF, Godbout R, Gallie BL, Murphree AL, Strong LC, White RL. Expression of recessive alleles by chromosomal mechanisms in retinoblastoma. Nature 1983; 305:779–784.
15. Friend SH, Bernards R, Rogelj S, Weinberg RA, Rapaport JM, Albert DM, Dryja TP. A human DNA segment with properties of the gene that predisposes to retinoblastoma and osteosarcoma. Nature 1986; 323:643–646.
16. Lee WH, Bookstein R, Hong F, Young LJ, Shew JY, Lee EY. Human retinoblastoma susceptibility gene: Cloning, identification, and sequence. Science 1987; 235:1394–1399.

17. Fung Y-KT, Murphree AL, T'Ang A, Qian J, Hinrichs SH, Benedict WF. Structural evidence for the authenticity of the human retinoblastoma gene. Science 1987; 236:1657–1661.
18. Goodrich DW, Lee W-H. Molecular characterization of the retinoblastoma susceptibility gene. Biochem Biophys Acta 1993; 1155:43–61.
19. Kaelin WG, Jr. Functions of the retinoblastoma protein. Bioessays 1999; 21:950–958.
20. DiCiommo D, Gallie BL, Bremner R. Retinoblastoma: The disease, gene and protein provide critical leads to understand cancer. Cancer Biol 2000; 10:255–269.
21. Nevins JR. The Rb/E2F pathway and cancer. Hum Mol Genet 2001; 10:699–703.
22. Harbour JW, Dean DC. The RB/E2F pathway: Expanding roles and emerging paradigms. Genes Dev 2000; 14:2393–2409.
23. Zheng L, Lee W-H. The retinoblastoma gene: A prototypic and multifunctional tumor suppressor. Exp Cell Res 2001; 264:2–18.
24. Sears RC, Nevins JR. Signaling networks that link cell proliferation and cell fate. J Biol Chem 2002; 277:11617–11620.
25. Lipinski MM, Jacks T. The retinoblastoma gene family in differentiation and development. Oncogene 1999; 18:7873–7882.
26. Ferguson KL, Slack RS. The Rb pathway in neurogenesis. Neuroreport 2001; 12:55–62.
27. Toguchida J, McGee TL, Paterson JC, Eagle JR, Tucker S, Yandell DW, Dryja TP. Complete genomic sequence of human retinoblastoma susceptibility gene. Genomics 1993; 17:535–543.
28. Ohtani-Fujita N, Fujita T, Aoike A, Ofsifchin NE, Robbins PD, Sakai T. CpG methylation inactivates the promoter activity of the human retinoblastoma tumor suppressor gene. Oncogene 1993; 8:1063–1067.
29. Sakai T, Othani N, McGee TL, Robbins PD, Dryja TP. Oncogenic germ-line mutations in Sp1 and ATF sites in the human retinoblastoma gene. Nature 1991; 353:83–86.
30. Sakai T, Toguchida J, Ohtani N, Yandell DW, Rapaport JM, Dryja T. Allelic-specific hypermethylation of the retinoblastoma tumor-suppressor gene. Am J Hum Genet 1991; 48:880–888.
31. T'Ang A, Varley JM, Chakraborty S, Murphee AL, Fung YKT. Structural rearrangement of the retinoblastoma gene in human breast carcinoma. Science 1988; 241:263–266.
32. Classon M, Dyson N. p107 and p130: versatile proteins with interesting pockets. Exp Cell Res 2001; 264:135–147.
33. DeCaprio JA, Ludlow JW, Lynch D, Furukawa Y, Griffin J, Piwnica-Worms H, Huang CM, Livingston DM. The product of the retinoblastoma susceptibility gene has properties of a cell cycle regulatory element. Cell 1989; 58:1085–1095.
34. Harbour JW, Dean DC. Chromatin remodeling and Rb activity. Curr Opin Cell Biol 2000; 12:685–689.
35. Ferreira R, Naguibneva I, Pritchard LL, Ait-Si-Ali S, Harel-Bellan A. The Rb/chromatin connection and epigenetic control: Opinion. Oncogene 2001; 20:3128–3133.
36. Lee JO, Russo AA, Pavlvetich NP. Structure of the retinoblastoma tumour-suppressor pocket domain bound to a peptide form HPV E7. Nature 1998; 391:859–865.
37. Kaye FJ, Kratze RA, Gerster JL, Horowitz JM. A single amino acid substitution results in a retinoblastoma protein defective in phosphorylation and oncoprotein binding. Proc Natl Acad Sci USA 1990; 87:6922–6926.
38. Paggi MG, Martelli F, Fanciulli M, et al. Defective human retinoblastoma protein identified by lack of interaction with E1A oncoprotein. Cancer Res 1994; 54:1098–2104.
39. Zhu XP, Dunn JM, Phillips RA, Goddard AD, Paton KE, Becker A, Gallie BL. Preferential germline mutation of the paternal allele in retinoblastoma. Nature 1989; 340:312–313.
40. Dryja TP, Mukai S, Petersen R, Rapaport JM, Walton D, Yandell DW. Parental origin of mutations of the retinoblastoma gene. Nature 1989; 339:556–558.

41. Dryja TP, Morrow JF, Rapaport JM. Quantification of the paternal allele bias for new germline mutations in the retinoblastoma gene. Hum Genet 1997; 100:446–449.

42. Bader JL, Meadows AT, Zimmerman LE, Rorke LB, Voute PA, Champion LA, Miller RW. Bilateral retinoblastoma with ectopic intracranial retinoblastoma: Trilateral retinoblastoma. Cancer Genet Cytogenet 1982; 5:203–213.

43. Wiggs JL, Dryja TP. Predicting the risk of hereditary retinoblastoma. Am J Opthalmol 1988; 106:346–351.

44. Mukai S. Molecular genetic diagnosis of retinoblastoma. Semin Ophthalmol 1993; 8:292–299.

45. Bunin GR, Emanuel BS, Meadows AT, Buckley JD, Woods WG, Hammond GD. Frequency of 13q abnormalities among 203 patients with retinoblastoma. J Natl Cancer Inst 1989; 81:370–374.

46. Kloss K, Währisch P, Greger V, Messmer E, Fritze H, Höpping W, Passarge E, Horsthemke B. Characterization of deletions at the retinoblastoma locus in patients with bilateral retinoblastoma. Am J Med Genet 1991; 39:196–200.

47. Blanquet V, Creau-Goldberg N, de Grouchy J, Turleau C. Molecular detection of constitutional deletions in patients with retinoblastoma. Am J Med Genet 1991; 39:355–361.

48. Dunn JM, Phillips RA, Zhu X, Becker A, Gallie BL. Mutations in the RB1 gene and their effects on transcription. Mol Cell Biol 1989; 9:4596–604.

49. Yandell DW, Campbell TA, Dayton SH, Petersen R, Walton D, Little JB, McConkie-Rosell A, Buckley EG, Dryja TP. Oncogenic point mutations in the human retinoblastoma gene: Their application to genetic counseling. N Engl J Med 1989; 321:1689–1695.

50. Yandell DW, Dryja TP. Detection of DNA sequence polymorphisms by enzymatic amplification and direct genomic sequencing. Am J Hum Genet 1989; 45:547–555.

51. Lohmann D, Horsthemke B, Gillessen-Kaesbach G, Stefani FH, Hofler H. Detection of small RB1 gene deletions in retinoblastoma by multiplex PCR and high-resolution gel electrophoresis. Hum Genet 1992; 89:49–53.

52. Hogg A, Onadim Z, Baird PN, Cowell JK. Detection of heterozygous mutations in the RB1 gene in retinoblastoma patients using single-strand conformation polymorphism analysis and polymerase chain reaction sequencing. Oncogene 1992; 7:1445–1451.

53. Shimizu T, Toguchida J, Kato MV, Kaneko A, Ishizaki K, Sasaki MS. Detection of mutation of the *RB1* gene in retinoblastoma patients by using exon-by-exon PCR-SSCP analysis. Am J Hum Genet 1994; 54:793–800.

54. Mastrangelo D, Squitieri N, Bruni S, Hadjistilianou T, Frezzotti R. The polymerase chain reaction (PCR) in the routine genetic characterization of retinoblastoma: A tool for the clinical laboratory. Surv Ophthalmol 1997; 41:331–340.

55. Noorani HZ, Khan HZ, Gallie BL, Destky AS. Cost comparison of molecular versus conventional screening of relatives at risk for retinoblastoma. Am J Hum Genet 1996; 59:301–307.

56. Musarella MA, Gallie BL. A simplified scheme for genetic counseling in retinoblastoma. J Pediatr Ophthalmol Strabismus 1987; 24:124–125.

57. Lohmann DR, Brandt B, Höpping W, Passarge E, Horsthemke B. The spectrum of the *RB1* germ line mutations in hereditary retinoblastoma. Am J Human Genet 1996; 58:940–949.

58. Greger V, Passarge E, Horsthemke B. Somatic mosaicism in patient with bilateral retinoblastoma. Am J Hum Genet 1990; 46:1187–1193.

59. Sippel KC, Fraioli RE, Smith GD, Schalkoff ME, Sutherland J, Gallie BL, Dryja TP. Frequency of somatic and germ-line mosaicism in retinobalstoma: Implications for genetic counseling. Am J Hum Genet 1998; 62:610–619.

60. Blanquet V, Turleau C, Gross-Morand MS, Senamaud-Beaufort C, Doz F, Besmond C. Spectrum of germline mutations in the RB1 gene: A study of 232 patients with hereditary and non hereditary retinoblastoma. Hum Mol Genet 1995; 4:383–388.
61. Harbour JW. Overview of RB gene mutations in patients with retinoblastoma. Implications for clinical genetic screening. Ophthalmology 1998; 105:1442–1447.
62. Mancini D, Singh S, Ainsworth P, Rodenhiser D. Constitutively methylated CpG dinucleotides as mutation hot spots in the retinoblastoma gene (RB1). Am J Hum Genet 1997; 61:80–87.
63. Hogg A, Bia B, Onadim Z, Cowell JK. Molecular mechanisms of oncogenic mutations in tumors from patients with bilateral and unilateral retinoblastoma. Proc Natl Acad Sci USA 1993; 90:7351–7355.
64. Lohmann DR. RB1 gene mutations in retinoblastoma. Hum Mutat 1999; 14:283–288.
65. Dryja TP, Cavenee W, White R, Rapaport JM, Petersen R, Albert DM, Bruns GAP. Homozygosity of chromosome 13 in retinoblastoma. N Engl J Med 1984; 310:550–553.
66. Knudson AG. Antioncogenes and human cancer. Proc Natl Acad Sci USA 1993; 90:10914–10921.
67. Hagstrom SA, Dryja TP. Mitotic recombination map of 13cen-13q14 derived from a an investigation of loss of heterozygosity in retinoblastomas. Proc Natl Acad Sci USA 1999; 96:2952–2957.
68. Matsunaga E. Hereditary retinoblastoma: penetrance, expressivity and age of onset. Hum Genet 1976; 33:1–15.
69. Lohmann DR, Brandt B, Hopping W, Passarge E, Horsthemke B. Distinct *RB1* gene mutations in patients with low penetrance in hereditary retinoblastoma. Hum Genet 1994; 94:349–354.
70. Sakai T, Othani N, McGee TL, Robbins PD, Dryja TP. Oncogenic germ-line mutations in Sp1 and ATF sites in the human retinoblastoma gene. Nature 1991; 353:83–86.
71. Otterson GA, Chen WD, Coxon AB, Khleif SN, Kaye FJ. Incomplete penetrance of familial retinoblastoma linked to germ-line mutation that result in partial loss of RB function. Proc Natl Acad Sci USA 1997; 94:12036–12040.
72. William Harbour JW. Molecular basis of low-penetrance retinoblastoma. Arch Ophthalmol 2001; 119:1699–1704.
73. Squire J, Gallie BL, Phillips RA. A detailed analysis of chromosomal changes in heritable and non-heritable retinoblastoma. Hum Genet 1985; 70:291–301.
74. Gallie BL, Campbell C, Devlin H, Duckett A, Squire JA. Developmental basis of retinal-specific induction of cancer by RB mutation. Cancer Res 1999; 59:1731s–1735s.
75. Squire J, Phillips RA, Boyce S, Godbout R, Rogers B, Gallie BL. Isochromosome 6p, a unique chromosomal abnormality in retinoblastoma: Verification by standard staining techniques, new densitometric methods, and somatic hybridization. Hum Genet 1984; 66:46–53.
76. Cano J, Oliveros O, Yunis E. Phenotype variants, malignacy, and additional copies of 6p in retinoblastoma. Cancer Genet Cytogenet 1994; 76:112–115.
77. Mairal A, Pinglier E, Gilbert E, Peter M, Validire P, Desjardins L, Doz F, Aurias A, Couturier J. Detection of chormosome imbalances in retinoblastoma by parallel karyotype and CGH analyses. Genes Chromosomes Cancer 2000; 28:370–379.
78. Herzog S, Lohmann DR, Buitingt K, Schüler A, Horsthemke B, Rehder H, Rieder H. Marked differences in unilateral isolated retinoblastomas from young and older children studied by comparative genomic hybridization. Hum Genet 2001; 108:98–104.
79. Chen D, Pajovic S, Duckett A, Brown VD, Squire JA, Gallie BL. Genomic amplification in retinoblastoma narrowed to 0.6 megabase on chromosome 6p containing a kinesin-like gene, *RBKIN*. Cancer Res 2002; 62:967–971.

22

Genetically Engineered Mouse Models of Retinoblastoma

JOLENE J. WINDLE

Virginia Commonwealth University, Richmond, Virginia, U.S.A.

DANIEL M. ALBERT

University of Wisconsin, Madison, Wisconsin, U.S.A.

I. INTRODUCTION

Retinoblastoma is a uniquely human form of cancer. Nonexperimental hereditary retinoblastoma has never been observed in a nonhuman species, and sporadic retinal tumors in animals are extremely rare [1]. Thus, a variety of strategies have been employed to create animal models for retinoblastoma, to be used both for furthering our basic understanding of the pathophysiology and molecular genetics of this disease and to serve as tools in the development of new therapeutic approaches. The most widely used strategy for creating animal models of retinoblastoma has involved the xenograft of human retinoblastoma tumor cell lines into immune-compromised mice (or rats), either subcutaneously [2] or into the eye [3–5]. While human tumor xenografts in mice have been an invaluable tool in cancer research, there are a number of significant limitations to this approach. Most notably, xenograft models do not allow for the study of the natural course of development and progression of cancer, and they largely fail to model the complex interactions between cancer cells and the host [6]. An additional strategy that has been employed for creating animal models of retinoblastoma involves the injection of adenovirus into the eyes of newborn rats or baboons [7,8]. Although tumors arising in these models closely resemble human retinoblastoma histologically, the models are technically cumbersome to create and tumors arise with a relatively low incidence.

The development of technologies for introducing specific mutations into the germline of mice has led to the creation of several new models of retinoblastoma, which have been employed both for studying the molecular genetics of retinoblastoma and for evaluating novel therapeutic strategies. The basic methods for creating these mice are briefly described below, followed by a description of various mouse models and their application to the study of retinoblastoma.

II. METHODS FOR THE CREATION OF GENETICALLY ENGINEERED MICE

In the past two decades, several related methods have been developed for introducing specific genetic modifications into the mouse genome [9,10], allowing for the creation of a wide range of mouse models of human disease, including cancer. The most straightforward of these methods involves the introduction of new genes into the mouse genome to create "transgenic mice." In cancer research, this approach is well suited for creating models involving expression of dominantly acting oncogenes. Alternatively, targeted mutations that specifically inactivate genes normally present in the mouse genome can be introduced to create "knockout" mice. This approach allows one to model loss-of-function mutations, such as the heterozygous or homozygous inactivation of tumor suppressor genes. More recently, a variety of refinements of these strategies have been developed that allow for conditional transgene expression or gene inactivation, greatly amplifying the power of these technologies for modeling human disease [11,12].

A. Production of Transgenic Mice

Although the term *transgenic* can strictly be applied to any mouse carrying experimentally introduced DNA, including knockout mice, the term is generally used to refer to mice in which a new gene or segment of DNA is experimentally introduced into the germline by nonhomologous recombination. Most often, this involves microinjection of a solution containing experimentally modified DNA into one of the two pronuclei of fertilized mouse eggs and reimplantation of the microinjected eggs into the oviducts of recipient females for subsequent development (Fig. 1). The resulting pups are screened for the presence of the "transgene" in their genome by biopsying a small piece of tail or other tissue at the time of weaning and preparing genomic DNA for polymerase chain reaction (PCR) or Southern blot analysis. In order for the transgene to be retained in the cells of the fully developed mouse, it must physically integrate into one of the chromosomes of the microinjected pronucleus, an event that occurs in approximately 10–20% of injected eggs on average. When the transgene does integrate into a chromosome, it becomes part of the genetic makeup of the resulting "founder" mouse and is subsequently transmitted to offspring in a Mendelian fashion. It should be noted that the site of chromosomal integration is random and can profoundly influence expression of the transgene. In addition, transgenes can integrate in single or multiple copies (usually in a tandem head-to-tail array at a single locus); copy number also influences transgene expression level. Thus, there can be considerable variability in transgene expression levels and resulting phenotype among lines of mice established

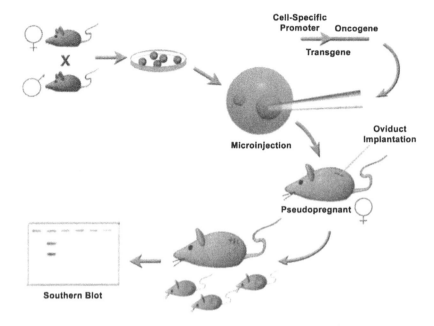

Figure 1 Production of transgenic mice by pronuclear injection.

from different founders carrying the same transgene. However, within any given line of mice, the patterns of transgene expression and phenotype are generally relatively consistent and stable over multiple generations.

A major consideration in the creation of transgenic mice is the design of the transgene to be introduced. Although full-length unmodified genes or even larger segments of chromosomes can be introduced, more often the transgene consists of an experimentally created gene containing two critical elements, a protein-coding region and a regulatory region. The protein-coding region (often derived from a cDNA) dictates the gene product to be produced by the transgene, while the promoter or regulatory region of the transgene determines the cell-type specificity, developmental timing, and level of transgene expression. For the creation of transgenic mouse models of cancer, the protein-coding region often encodes a known dominantly acting oncogene or gene whose expression can contribute to the development of cancer.

B. Production of Knockout Mice

In contrast to the genetic modification in transgenic mice, which involves the random integration of the transgene DNA into the genome, the genetic modification in knockout mice involves the introduction of a defined mutation into a specific gene in the mouse genome by a much less frequent homologous recombination event (Fig. 2). Thus, it becomes necessary to screen a large number of cells to identify those in which the desired homologous recombination event has occurred among a much larger number of cells in which the foreign DNA has randomly integrated into the genome. This is accomplished by introducing the "targeting

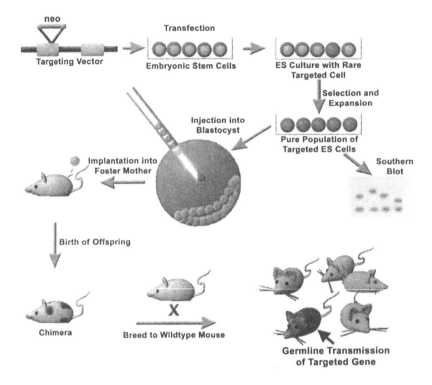

Figure 2   Production of knockout mice by gene targeting in ES cells.

vector" by electroporation into cultured embryonic stem (ES) cells, which are totipotent cells derived from the inner cell mass of day E3.5 mouse blastocysts [13]. The targeting vector usually contains several kilobases of DNA homologous to the gene being targeted for mutation as well as a gene encoding a drug-resistance enzyme (e.g., a bacterial neomycin resistance gene), which serves both to disrupt the coding region of the targeted gene, and to allow for the selection of cells that have incorporated the foreign DNA. Individual surviving clones of ES cells are then molecularly screened to identify the homologous recombinants. Once clones of correctly targeted ES cells are identified, these are microinjected into recipient blastocysts, where they commingle with cells of the endogenous inner cell mass. The blastocysts are then reimplanted into the uterus of foster females and allowed to develop to birth. The resulting mice are referred to as chimeras, since many or all of their tissues are derived from a mix of both normal and genetically modified ES cells. If any of the germline cells (e.g., sperm) of the chimeric mice are derived from the genetically modified ES cells, their offspring can inherit the mutation, which will subsequently be transmitted to future generations in a Mendelian fashion. The first generation offspring from the founding chimeras are heterozygous for the mutated gene and are usually either phenotypically normal or display only modest phenotypes. To observe the phenotype resulting from complete absence of expression of the targeted gene, heterozygotes must be interbred to generate homozygous offspring.

C. Production of Conditional (Cell Type–Specific) Knockout Mice

One enhancement of knockout technology developed in recent years is the ability to restrict gene inactivation to specific tissues or cell types [11,12]. This is particularly useful when inactivation of the gene in all cells results in embryonic lethality or a marked phenotype at one stage of development that precludes assessing the role of the inactivated gene at a later stage. The most commonly used approach for creating cell type-specific knockout mice takes advantage of the P1 bacteriophage *Cre/loxP* recombination system [14] (Fig. 3). Cre is a phage-encoded recombinase that mediates homologous recombination between repeats of 34-bp DNA elements called *loxP* sites. To utilize this system for creating cell type–specific knockouts, two separate lines of mice are generated and then interbred. In one line of mice, the gene to be inactivated is subtly modified by the introduction of two small repeats (*loxP* sites), generally into introns flanking essential exons, by homologous recombination in ES cells. In the second line, a transgene is introduced in which the *Cre* recombinase gene is placed under the control of a cell type–specific promoter. Both of these parental lines of mice are expected to be phenotypically normal, since the presence of the *loxP* sites in introns of the target gene does not disrupt its expression and Cre recombinase has no effect on the normal mouse genome. However, when these two lines of mice are interbred, Cre mediates recombination of the two *loxP* sites, with concomitant deletion of intervening sequences and inactivation of the targeted gene, but only in the cell types where the *Cre* gene is expressed.

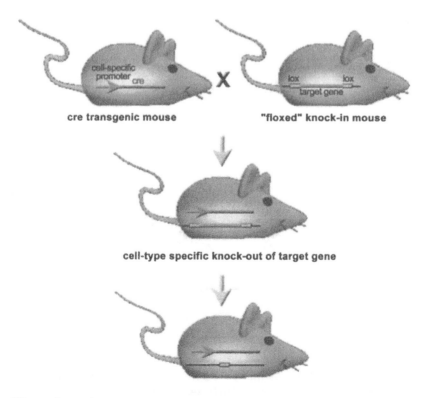

Figure 3 Cell type–specific gene inactivation using the *Cre/loxP* system.

III. TRANSGENIC MOUSE MODELS OF RETINOBLASTOMA

A. LHbeta-Tag Transgenic Mice

The first experimental animal model of hereditary retinoblastoma was the fortuitous result of an attempt to create transgenic mice that develop tumors derived from pituitary gonadotrophs [15]. Several lines of transgenic mice were produced with a transgene (LHbeta-Tag) encoding the simian virus 40 (SV40) T-antigen gene, a potent viral oncogene, under the control of the luteinizing hormone (LH) beta-subunit gene promoter. T antigen is known to transform cells at least in part through its binding to and inactivation of both the pRb and p53 tumor suppressor proteins [16–18]. While mice from the majority of these lines expressed T antigen specifically in the pituitary gland as expected [19], mice from a single line developed bilateral retinal tumors, resulting from high levels of T-antigen expression in the eye [15]. The misexpression of the transgene in this one line of mice is presumed to have resulted from integration of the transgene near the regulatory elements of a retina-specific gene, although this has not been experimentally confirmed.

The LHbeta-Tag mice develop multiple focal retinal tumors with 100% penetrance, beginning at 1 to 2 months of age. The earliest tumors consist of small groups of neoplastic cells located within the inner plexiform layer (Fig. 4A). As the tumors enlarge, they infiltrate adjacent retinal layers and eventually fill the vitreous cavity, leading to total detachment and destruction of the remaining retina (Fig. 4B). Eventually, they invade the retinal pigment epithelium, choroid, optic nerve, and anterior chamber and metastasize to cervical lymph nodes. Histologically and

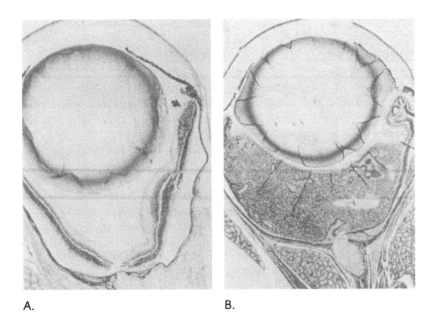

A.   B.

Figure 4   Retinoblastoma in LHbeta-Tag transgenic mice. (A) Early focal tumor arising in inner nuclear layer of peripheral retina (arrow). (H&E, x42.5.) (B) More advanced tumor in older mouse. Tumor has become confluent and involves almost entire retina. (H&E, x42.5.)

ultrastructurally, these tumors display many features of human retinoblastoma, including the presence of Homer-Wright rosettes (Fig. 5), lamelliform nuclear membranes, neurosecretory granules, cytoplasmic microtubules, and cilia with a "9 + 0" pattern of microtubules, (which are observed both in normal human photoreceptors and differentiated human retinoblastoma) [15]. Immunohistochemically, the tumor cells have been shown to express neuron-specific enolase (NSE) and synaptophysin but not vimentin, glial fibrillary acidic protein (GFAP), or S-100, consistent with a neuronal cell type of origin [20]. However, they do not express opsin or other photoreceptor-specific proteins, as do many human retinoblastomas [21–23]. Based on their location in the inner nuclear layer and their ultrastructural and immunohistochemical characteristics, the tumors arising in LHbeta-Tag mice are thought to be of amacrine cell origin, while human retinoblastomas are generally thought to arise from photoreceptor precursors or retinoblasts having the potential to differentiate into photoreceptors [21,23–26].

Interestingly, approximately one-quarter of the LHbeta-Tag transgenic mice also develop midline intracranial tumors arising in the subependymal midbrain adjacent to the cerebral aqueduct [27]. These are generally poorly differentiated tumors that most closely resemble primitive neuroectodermal tumors (PNET) (Fig. 6). The development of primary midline intracranial tumors is also seen in a small subset of retinoblastoma patients and is referred to as trilateral retinoblastoma [28,29]. In most cases, these tumors appear to arise from the pineal gland, and they display many of the differentiated features of retinoblastoma [28,30,31]. However, a subset of the intracranial tumors in patients with trilateral retinoblastoma are undifferentiated suprasellar-parasellar tumors [32] and more closely resemble the tumors seen in the LHbeta-Tag mice.

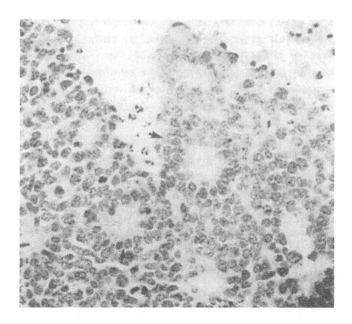

Figure 5 High-power view of LHbeta-Tag retinal tumor. Arrows indicate Homer-Wright rosettes. (H&E, x700.)

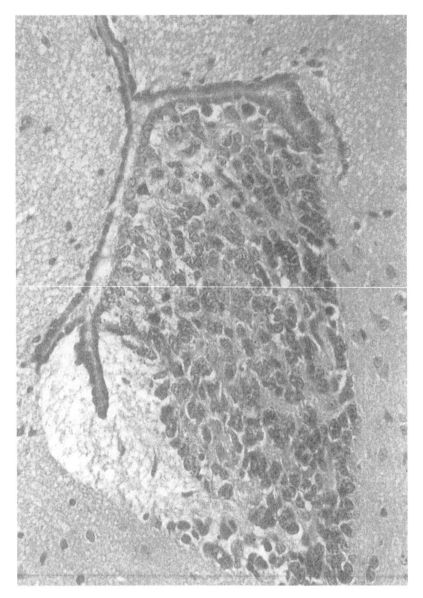

Figure 6 Midbrain primitive neuroectodermal tumor in LHbeta-Tag mouse. Neoplastic cells are adjacent to and appear to replace a portion of the ventral ependymal lining of the cerebral aqueduct. The tumor has not invaded the aqueductal lumen. (H&E, x315.)

B. Opsin-Tag Transgenic Mice

Although the retinal tumors arising in LHbeta-Tag mice share many histological features with human retinoblastoma, they differ from the majority of retinoblastomas in their lack of photoreceptor differentiatio7n. Thus, several attempts have been made to generate transgenic mouse models of retinoblastoma that more closely resemble the human tumor by directing T-antigen expression specifically to photoreceptors or photoreceptor precursor cells. In the first attempt, T-antigen expression was placed under the control of an opsin gene promoter, which normally initiates expression as photoreceptor cells terminally differentiate and become postmitotic [33]. However, rather than developing retinal tumors, opsin-Tag transgenic mice undergo rapid photoreceptor degeneration during the early postnatal period [34]. The retinal cell death is accompanied by continued cell proliferation as late as postnatal day 16 [35], a stage when normal photoreceptors are entirely postmitotic. These results indicate that T antigen–induced proliferation in postmitotic cells triggers an apoptotic response, and that in order for T antigen to promote tumorigenesis, its expression must initiate prior to terminal differentiation, while cells are still mitotically active.

C. IRBP-Tag Transgenic Mice

In subsequent efforts to model retinoblastoma in transgenic mice, T antigen was placed under the control of the interphotoreceptor retinoid-binding protein (IRBP) gene promoter [36,37]. In contrast to opsin, IRBP is expressed during early retinal development (as early as day E12), while retinal precursors are still mitotically active [33]. IRBP-Tag transgenic mice develop intraocular tumors with 100% penetrance that are histologically detectable shortly after birth. Importantly, the tumors arising in these mice are not focal but involve the entire developing photoreceptor cell layer (Fig. 7A). Thus, a laminar retina with normal differentiated photoreceptors never forms. By 6–8 weeks of age, the tumors replace the bipolar cell layer (Fig. 7B) and subsequently invade the optic nerve, ciliary body, iris and vitreous. Tumors in these mice resemble undifferentiated retinoblastomas and generally do not form rosettes (Fig. 7C). They express several neuronal markers including NSE and synaptophysin and also express IRBP but not opsin, suggesting that they are derived from a photoreceptor cell precursor that has not yet activated opsin expression [37].

All IRBP-Tag mice also develop early midline intracranial tumors, which in this model are derived from the pineal gland. By 2 weeks of age, these tumors fill the transverse fissure of the cerebrum (Fig. 8A); by 9–12 weeks, they extend diffusely throughout large portions of the brain. In contrast to the retinal tumors arising in these mice, the pineal tumors resemble highly differentiated retinoblastoma, consisting almost entirely of Homer-Wright rosettes (Fig. 8B). The development of pineal tumors in these mice likely reflects the fact that the IRBP gene is expressed in the pineal as well as the retina; thus T-antigen expression is directed to both tissues in IRBP-Tag transgenic mice.

D. IRBP-E7 and IRBP-*E7/p53*–/– Mice

The fact that retinal tumors in the IRBP-Tag transgenic mice are nonfocal and involve the entire photoreceptor cell layer suggests that expression of T antigen is sufficient to cause oncogenic transformation of photoreceptor precursor cells. In addition to inactivating pRb, T antigen associates with a number of other cellular proteins, most notably the p53 tumor suppressor protein [17,18]. However, the contribution of *p53* inactivation to the development of human retinoblastoma is uncertain, since it is not found to be mutated in retinoblastoma tumors (see Chap. 10

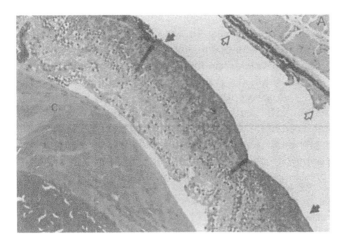

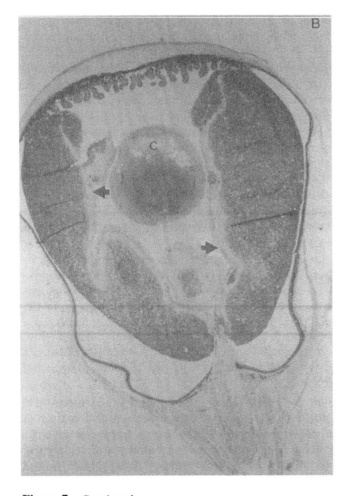

Figure 7 Continued.

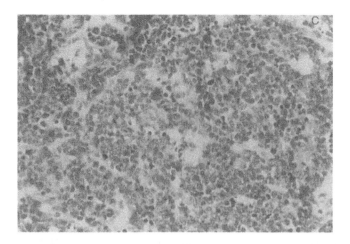

Figure 7   Retinoblastoma in IRBP-Tag transgenic mice. (A) Eye from 4-week-old IRBP-Tag mouse showing replacement of photoreceptor cell layer by tumor cells (solid arrows). In some areas, these have reached the level of the bipolar cells. The retina shows detachment from the pigment epithelium and choroid (empty arrows) and is in contact with the cataractous lens (C). (H&E, x325.) (B) Eye from 8-week-old IRBP-Tag mouse. Inner and middle layers of retina have been replaced by tumor (arrows). Ganglion cells are mostly unaffected. The tumor has not invaded the optic nerve. The lens is cataractous (C). (H&E, x46.) (C) Higher magnification showing absence of rosettes and fleurettes. Numerous small, dark, pycnotic cells are present. (H&E, x650.)

in this volume). Therefore, to test whether inactivation of pRb is sufficient to induce retinoblastoma, transgenic mice were produced in which another viral oncogene that inactivates pRb but not p53 was expressed in the retina [38]. Human papilloma-viruses (HPV) encode two separate oncoproteins, E6 and E7, that together possess many of the transforming functions of T antigen; the E7 protein binds to and

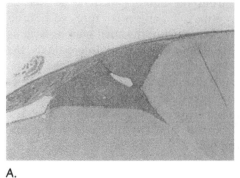

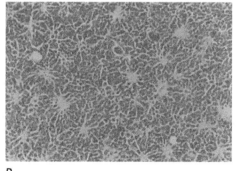

A.   B.

Figure 8   Pineal tumor in 2-week-old IRBP-Tag transgenic mouse. (A) Tumor cells have completely replaced the normal pineal but remain within the confines of the gland. (H&E, x65.) (B) Higher magnification showing abundant Homer-Wright rosettes. Large atypical cells are circled (H&E, x650.)

inactivates pRb [39,40] but not p53, while the E6 protein binds and promotes the degradation of p53 [41] but does not interact with pRb. Thus, if pRb inactivation were sufficient to promote retinal tumorigenesis, transgenic mice expressing HPV E7 in the retina would be expected to develop retinoblastomas much like the IRBP-Tag mice. However, rather than developing tumors, IRBP-E7 mice undergo rapid and dramatic retinal degeneration resulting from apoptosis of photoreceptor precursors in the first few days after birth, when photoreceptors would normally be undergoing terminal differentiation [38]. This finding suggested that inactivation of pRb promotes a p53-dependent form of apoptosis rather than transformation and that simultaneous inactivation of both pRb and p53 may be required for oncogenic transformation of photoreceptor precursors. To test this hypothesis, IRBP-E7 transgenic mice were bred to *p53* knockout mice, in which both alleles of the *p53* gene have been inactivated by homologous recombination [42]. As the hypothesis would predict, IRBP-E7/*p53*−/− mice were found to develop retinal tumors similar to those seen in the IRBP-Tag transgenic mice [38]. However, when eyes from IRBP-E7/*p53*−/− mice were examined histologically in the early postnatal period, before the development of large ocular tumors, it was found that retinal apoptosis was still occurring at a rate only slightly delayed from that seen in IRBP-E7 mice, but that occasional proliferating lesions could be observed arising from the degenerating retina. Thus, the retinal apoptosis induced by E7 expression is largely *p53*-independent, and *p53* loss must be contributing to tumorigenesis in this model by some mechanism other than the abrogation of apoptosis. Additional mouse models that have been created to investigate the sufficiency of *Rb* inactivation in the genesis of retinoblastoma are discussed in Sec. IV.

E. PNMT-Tag Transgenic Mice

While the IRBP-Tag and IRBP-E7 mice were created with the goal of specifically transforming photoreceptor precursors, T antigen or HPV E6/E7 has been directed to other ocular cell types as well. The phenylethanolamine *N*-methyltransferase (PNMT) gene is normally expressed in the adrenal medulla and retina [43], and transgenic mice expressing T antigen under the control of the PNMT promoter develop both pheochromocytomas arising from the adrenal medulla as well as retinoblastomas [44]. Within the transgenic retinas, T antigen is expressed both in amacrine cells in the ganglion cell layer and the inner tier of the inner nuclear layer as well as in horizontal cells in the outer tier of the inner nuclear layer. Interestingly, the majority of the horizontal cells disappear in these mice between 2 and 6 weeks of age, with accompanying thinning of the outer plexiform layer. Focal retinal tumors subsequently arise, primarily in the peripheral inner nuclear and ganglion cell layers, between 9 and 16 weeks of age [45]. These tumors express various neuronal markers, such as synaptophysin and neurofilament proteins, and resemble undifferentiated retinoblastomas, lacking rosettes or fleurettes [44].

F. AlphaA-Crystalline-E6/E7 Transgenic Mice

One additional transgenic mouse model for retinoblastoma is a line of mice that express both the HPV E6 and E7 oncogenes under the control of the alphaA-crystalline gene promoter [46]. These mice were originally developed with the goal of investigating the effects of the E6 and E7 expression in lens epithelial cells, and they display aberrant lens development, with 100% penetrance of bilateral microphthalmia and cataract formation. In addition, a subset of the mice also develop lens tumors at a relatively late age. Unexpectedly, alphaA-crystalline-E6/E7 mice were also found to develop retinoblastomas originating from the bipolar cell layer, resulting from ectopic expression of the transgene in retinal cells. These tumors resemble differentiated human retinoblastomas, with prominent Homer-Wright rosettes. They spread through the optic nerve to the brain, and also metastasize to cervical lymph nodes [46]. Interestingly, the incidence and age of onset of retinoblastomas in this line of transgenic mice is highly dependent on the genetic background of the mice, indicating that other genetic factors in addition to the transgene modulate tumor susceptibility in this model [47].

IV. *Rb* GENE INACTIVATION IN GENETICALLY ENGINEERED MICE

A. *Rb* Heterozygous and Homozygous Knockout Mice

Each of the transgenic mouse models described above involves the expression of a viral oncoprotein that binds and inactivates pRb, and thus these models at least in part molecularly mimic human retinoblastoma, in which no functional pRb protein is produced. However, a caveat to this approach is that each of these viral proteins potentially interacts with a number of other cellular proteins, and these interactions may contribute to the resulting phenotype [48]. A more genetically accurate model for hereditary retinoblastoma would be one in which one copy of the *Rb* gene is inactivated in the mouse germline using a gene targeting approach, and several groups have generated such mice [49–51]. Surprisingly, retinoblastomas are never observed in the heterozygous *Rb* knockout (*Rb* + /−) mice; instead, 100% of these mice develop intermediate lobe pituitary tumors at a mean age of approximately 6–9 months [52–55]. As with human retinoblastomas, the pituitary tumors in these mice invariably show loss of expression of the wild-type *Rb* allele. Thus, although these mice model the human disease in that loss of one *Rb* allele creates a marked tumor susceptibility, the tumor spectrum is distinctly different.

When *Rb* heterozygotes are interbred to generate homozygous knockouts, the *Rb*−/− embryos die in midgestation (days E12–15), displaying defects in liver hematopoiesis, neurogenesis, and lens development [49–51,56]. The hematopoietic defect appears to result from an impairment in end-stage differentiation of red blood cells, as *Rb*−/− embryos have severely reduced numbers of mature (enucleated) erythrocytes, both in circulation and in the liver [49–51], the major site of erythropoiesis at this stage of mouse development. In addition, *Rb*−/− embryos show several areas of massive apoptosis in both the central and peripheral nervous system, associated with inappropriate cell cycle entry in cells that would normally be exiting the cell cycle at this stage of development [57,58]. Similarly, abnormalities are seen in the lens of *Rb*−/− embryos, resulting from inappropriate proliferation and accompanying apoptosis [56]. However, there are no obvious abnormalities in retinal development in *Rb*−/− embryos.

Because pRb is a key regulator of the cell cycle, directly controlling transcription of genes required for entry of cells into S-phase, one might have expected that homozygous inactivation of the *Rb* gene in mice would result in an early embryonic lethal phenotype. The fact that embryos survive as long as they do, approximately two-thirds of the way through gestation, suggests that pRb is not central to the control of every cell cycle. Rather, its major role during development appears to be in the initiation of terminal differentiation, and *Rb*-deficient cells that fail to exit the cell cycle in response to differentiation signals are rapidly eliminated by apoptosis.

B.   *Rb*-Deficient Chimeric Mice

The early embryonic lethality caused by *Rb* deficiency precludes the analysis of its role in later stages of development or the role of *Rb* mutation in tumorigenesis. One strategy that has been employed to circumvent the embryonic lethality is to create chimeric mice by introducing *Rb*−/− ES cells into wild-type blastocysts [53,54,59]. Interestingly, such chimeras are readily obtained and display relatively few pathological abnormalities, despite sometimes extensive contribution of *Rb*−/− cells to most tissue types, including mature erythrocytes, the liver, and the central nervous system (CNS). The fact that *Rb*−/− cells can contribute to tissues in the chimeric mice that show profound defects in fully *Rb*-deficient embryos suggests that wild-type cells can "rescue" the *Rb*−/− cells, either by direct cell-cell contact or by paracrine mechanisms, thereby enabling them to undergo normal terminal differentiation. Thus, the central defect in hematopoiesis, for example, may not lie entirely in the erythroid cells themselves but also in cells contributing to the liver microenvironment necessary to support erythrocyte maturation. This is not the case for all cell types, however, as the lens of chimeric mice exhibits the same defects as in the *Rb* knockout mice, with abnormal proliferation and apoptosis of *Rb*−/− lens fiber cells. The inner retinas of E16.5- to E18.5-day chimeric mice also display regions of ectopic mitosis and apoptosis, and there is a reduced contribution of *Rb*−/− cells to the adult retina as compared to other tissues [54]. Nevertheless, the retinas of adult chimeric mice are grossly normal in appearance [53] and retinoblastomas are never observed. Instead, nearly all chimeras develop inter- mediate lobe pituitary tumors, at significantly earlier ages than the *Rb* heterozygous knockout mice, consistent with the lack of requirement for somatic loss of the second *Rb* allele [53,54].

C.   The Role of *p107* Inactivation in Murine Retinoblastoma

These results indicate that inactivation of *Rb* is insufficient to induce retinoblastoma, at least in the mouse, and that additional genetic alterations are required. One possibility is that other members of the *Rb* gene family, *p107* or *p130*, might share functional overlap with *Rb* and would therefore also need to be inactivated to generate retinoblastoma. This possibility has been explored by creating *p107* knockout mice and mice with mutations in both the *Rb* and *p107* genes [60]. *p107*−/− mice are viable and display no obvious abnormalities. However, *p107* deficiency exacerbates the defects seen in *Rb* heterozygous and homozygous knockouts. *Rb*−/−:*p107*−/− embryos die approximately 2 days earlier in gestation than *Rb*−/− embryos, with accelerated apoptosis in both the liver and the CNS. *Rb*+/−:*p107*−/− mice show pronounced growth retardation and increased mortality in the first 3 weeks of life. Of the mice that survive to adulthood, the majority develop intermediate lobe tumors like the $Rb+/-$ mice; no additional tumor types are observed. The $Rb+/-:p107-/-$ mice do develop multiple focal retinal lesions characterized as retinal dysplasias or degeneration of the photoreceptor cell layer, but retinoblastomas are not observed [60]. These studies demonstrate that there is functional overlap between p107 and pRb in several tissues of the developing and adult mouse, including the retina, but Rb heterozygous mutants nevertheless fail to develop retinoblastoma even in the complete absence of p107.

Because retinal development could not be assessed in the $Rb-/-:p107-/-$ mice due to embryonic lethality, chimeric mice have been generated with ES cells that are deficient in both Rb and $p107$ ($Rb-/-:p107-/-$) in a wild-type background [61]. In contrast to each of the previous knockout approaches described, $Rb-/-:p107-/-$ chimeric mice develop retinoblastomas, and lesions can be observed as early as day E17.5. Although these tumors are often located between the photoreceptor cell layer and the RPE, they express markers consistent with amacrine rather than photoreceptor cell differentiation. $Rb-/-:p107-/-$ retinoblasts expressing IRBP are detectable at day E17.5 but are completely absent by postnatal day 15, indicating that $Rb-/-:p107-/-$ retinoblasts committed to photoreceptor cell differentiation are eliminated during this developmental window. This cell loss is not $p53$-dependent, since the same fate is also observed when chimeras are generated with $Rb-/-:p107-/-$ ES cells also expressing a dominant-negative $p53$ gene under the control of the IRBP promoter [61]. Thus, simultaneous inactivation of both Rb and $p107$ strongly predisposes mice to the development of retinoblastomas of amacrine cell origin, but even the additional inactivation of $p53$ does not contribute to tumorigenesis of photoreceptor precursors.

D. Conditional *Rb* Knockout Mice

One additional approach that has been employed to address the effect of Rb inactivation in the mouse retina is the creation of cell type–specific Rb knockout mice using the $Cre/loxP$ system. Conditional Rb knockout mice with two $loxP$ sites flanking exon 19 (Rb^{F19}) were generated and interbred to IRBP-Cre transgenic mice, to create mice in which the Rb gene is inactivated only in IRBP-expressing cell types [62]. As noted above, the IRBP gene is expressed both in photoreceptor cells and the pineal gland, beginning at approximately day E12 [33]. As expected from the results of the previous studies, the IRBP-Cre:$Rb^{F19/F19}$ mice display completely normal retinal development and fail to develop either retinoblastomas or pinealomas, despite the presence of large numbers of Rb-deficient cells in these cell types. Rather, like the Rb heterozygous knockout mice, they develop pituitary tumors, although in this case the tumors are of both intermediate and anterior lobe origin [62]. The development of pituitary tumors in this model is particularly surprising, since Cre is not expected to be expressed in this cell type. However, the pituitary tumor cells show exon 19 deletion of the Rb gene, indicating that Cre recombinase must be ectopically expressed in the pituitary of the IRBP-Cre mice. The IRBP-Cre:$Rb^{F19/F19}$ mice were also bred to $p107-/-$ mice to generate IRBP-Cre:$Rb^{F19/F19}:p107-/-$ mice, and these mice also displayed normal retinal development. Although this might seem surprising in light of the fact that $Rb-/-:p107-/-$ chimeras develop retinoblastomas, it should be recalled that the $Rb-/-:p107-/-$ cells gave rise only to tumors of amacrine cell origin and not photoreceptor origin in the chimeras, while Rb inactivation in this model is restricted to photoreceptor cell precursors. Finally, IRBP-Cre:$Rb^{F19/F19}$ mice were also bred to $p53$ knockout mice to generate both IRBP-Cre:$Rb^{F19/F19}$:$p53+/-$ and IRBP-Cre:$Rb^{F19/F19}$:$p53-/-$ mice, and a small number of IRBP-Cre:$Rb^{F19/F19}$:$p107+/-$:$p53-/-$ and IRBP-Cre:$Rb^{F19/F19}$:$p107-/-$:$p53-/-$ mice were also generated. Remarkably, none of these mice developed retinoblastoma; rather, they displayed accelerated pineal and pituitary tumorigenesis [62]. Thus, it must be concluded that inactivation of Rb in the mouse is insufficient to induce tumors of photoreceptor origin, and neither $p107$ nor $p53$ inactivation can cooperate with Rb loss to induce tumors of this cell type.

E.   Implications from the *Rb* Knockout Mice

An obvious question arises from these studies: Why does germline Rb mutation cause retinoblastoma in humans but pituitary tumors in mice? The intermediate lobe of the pituitary gland is present in only vestigial form in humans, which could account for the failure of patients with germline Rb mutations to develop tumors arising in this cell type. However, it is less clear why Rb heterozygous mice fail to develop retinoblastomas [63–66]. One possibility is that somatic loss of the remaining normal Rb allele (or acquisition of other required mutations) in developing retinoblasts has a much lower probability of occurring in mice, since they presumably have a significantly smaller population of susceptible cells and a much shorter developmental time frame during which this event can occur. The fact that $Rb-/-$ cells in chimeric mice fail to form retinoblastomas argues against this explanation if loss of the second Rb allele is the only rate-limiting step in retinoblastoma development. However, if additional genetic events are required, then the number of target cells and timing of susceptibility may still be contributing factors. This leads to a second possibility, which is that retinoblasts of mice and humans may differ subtly in the mechanisms controling cell growth, differentiation, and apoptosis, such that mouse retinoblasts have additional genetic safeguards against oncogenic transformation that are lacking in human retinoblasts. For example, the fact that $Rb-/-$:$p107-/-$ cells but not $Rb-/-$ cells can give rise to retinal tumors in mouse chimeras suggests a degree of redundancy between pRb and $p107$ in mice, such that functional $p107$ can protect against transformation of Rb-deficient retinoblasts. In contrast, there is no evidence for mutation of the $p107$ gene in human retinoblastoma [67]. It should be noted, however, that loss of both pRb and $p107$ function is still not sufficient to transform mouse retinoblasts, since not all $Rb-/-$:$p107-/-$ chimeric retinas develop retinoblastomas. It seems likely that an additional mutational event required for full transformation would be one that suppresses apoptosis, since the normal fate of Rb-deficient cells in the developing retina and in many other cell types is apoptosis. Although the $p53$ gene might seem to be an obvious candidate, there is little evidence from the mouse models that $p53$ mutation contributes significantly to retinoblastoma development. It has similarly been suggested that the development of retinoblastoma in humans requires not only loss of both Rb alleles but also at least one other genetic event, which could potentially alter the apoptotic susceptibility of the tumor cells (see this volume, Chapters 7 and 10). Therefore, identification of additional mutations that contribute to retinoblastoma in the mouse may have direct implications for a better molecular understanding of human retinoblastoma.

V. TRANSGENIC MOUSE MODELS OF RETINOBLASTOMA IN THERAPEUTIC STUDIES

In addition to their applications in the study of the molecular genetics of cancer, genetically engineered mouse models of cancer are increasingly being used for the in vivo evalution of novel therapeutic approaches. The LHbeta-Tag mice in particular have been extensively used for evaluating a wide range of therapeutic approaches for the treatment of retinoblastoma, including local delivery of standard chemotherapeutic agents, external-beam radiation, a variety of combined modality approaches, and several novel anticancer agents.

A. Chemotherapeutic Agents

Chemotherapy is the most widely used modality for the treatment of invasive and metastatic retinoblastoma and is also an important component in the primary treatment of intraocular tumors [68,69]. However, systemic administration of cytotoxic agents at the doses required to achieve a sufficient intraocular drug concentration for effective tumor control is often associated with significant toxicity. Local delivery of carboplatin directly to the eye, either by intravitreal or subconjunctival injection, has therefore been explored in the LHbeta-Tag mice [70,71]. These studies demonstrated effective tumor growth inhibition in a dose-dependent manner, but with a relatively narrow therapeutic window and dose-dependent retinal toxicity. Local carboplatin administration has also been evaluated in combination with external-beam radiation therapy (EBRT) or cryotherapy. Although no benefit was gained with the addition of cryotherapy in this model [72], significant enhancement of tumor control was achieved by the addition of radiation therapy [73].

B. External Beam Radiation Therapy

In addition to its combination with carboplatin, EBRT has been explored as a single modality and in combination with hyperthermia in the LHbeta-Tag transgenic mice. In a study evaluating dose and schedule of EBRT administration, hyperfractionated EBRT (administered twice daily) was compared to standard daily EBRT and was found to significantly increase tumor control, allowing for a reduction in the total radiation delivered dose [73]. EBRT was also evaluated in combination with ferromagnetic hyperthermia in this model. Significant synergy was observed with this combination, suggesting that hyperthermia may reduce the total radiation dose necessary for tumor control [74].

C. Vitamin D Analogues

The presence of calcification as a consistent feature of retinoblastoma has led to the suggestion that vitamin D analogues may have activity as chemotherapeutic agents in this tumor type. Systemic administration of vitamin D3 to LHbeta-Tag mice inhibited the growth and local extension of tumors in a dose-dependent manner [75] and was further shown to inhibit tumor angiogenesis in this model [76]. However, vitamin D3 treatment was associated with significant toxicity, including hypercalcemia, weight loss, and death [75]. A number of vitamin D analogues have been developed in recent years, several of which appear to have greater antitumor activity with reduced toxicity [77]. One such analogue, 1,25-dihydroxy-16-ene-23-yne-vitamin D_3, has also been evaluated in the LHbeta-Tag mice, and this compound showed comparable antitumor activity with significantly reduced systemic toxicity [78,79] compared to vitamin D_3. The evaluation of novel vitamin D analogs in LHbeta-Tag transgenic mice is described in greater detail in Chapter 14.

D. Attenuated Herpes Simplex Virus

A number of strategies are currently being developed to employ cytolytic viruses as anticancer agents [80]. Of particular interest are naturally occurring or experimentally modified viruses that retain their ability lyse rapidly growing cells, including tumor cells, but are attenuated in their ability to replicate in normal cells. Herpes simplex virus (HSV) has a natural tropism for neuronal cells, and several attenuated mutant viruses have been characterized, making HSV an attractive virus for the treatment of neuronal malignancies [81]. One such HSV mutant, RE6, was evaluated in the LHbeta-Tag mouse model and was shown to significantly reduce tumor growth following intravitreal injection, although complete tumor control was not obtained [82].

VI. CONCLUDING REMARKS

The development of methodologies for introducing defined genetic alterations into the mouse genome have allowed for the creation of a number of mouse models of retinoblastoma that, like human retinoblastoma, involve loss of pRb function and to varying degrees resemble the human tumor histologically and ultrastructurally. It is somewhat ironic that the majority of these models are transgenic mouse lines that express dominantly acting oncogenes (SV40 T antigen or HPV E7), rather than knockout mice in which the *Rb* gene has been inactivated, since the latter approach would be expected to yield more genetically accurate models of human tumor types originating from loss of tumor suppressor genes. Although none of the approaches that have been employed for inactivating the *Rb* gene in the mouse have yielded mouse models of retinoblastoma (with the exception of the *Rb*−/−:*p107*−/− chimeras), these experiments have raised important questions relating to the molecular genetics of retinoblastoma that are likely to contribute to a better understanding of the human disease. On the other hand, the transgenic mouse models of retinoblastoma have been particularly useful for the evaluation of novel therapeutic strategies, many of which have significant clinical potential, and it is hoped that these studies will lead to improved treatment strategies for retinoblastoma.

REFERENCES

1. Syed NA, Nork TM, Poulsen GL, Riis RC, George C, Albert DM. Retinoblastoma in a dog. Arch Ophthalmol 1997; 115:758–763.
2. Sabet SJ, Darjatmoko SR, Lindstrom MJ, Albert DM. Antineoplastic effect and toxicity of 1,25-dihydroxy-16-ene-23-yne-vitamin D_3 in athymic mice with Y-79 human retinoblastoma tumors. Arch Ophthalmol 1999; 117:365–370.
3. Gallie BL, Albert DM, Wong JJ, Buyukmihci N, Pullafito CA. Heterotransplantation of retinoblastoma into the athymic "nude" mouse. Invest Ophthalmol Vis Sci 1977; 16:256–259.
4. del Cerro M, Seigel GM, Lazar E, Grover D, del Cerro C, Brooks DH, DiLoreto DJ, Chader G. Transplantation of Y79 cells into rat eyes: an in vivo model of human retinoblastomas. Invest Ophthalmol Vis Sci 1993; 34:3336–3346.
5. Chevez-Barrios P, Hurwitz MY, Louie K, Marcus KT, Holcombe VN, Schafer P, Aguilar-Cordova CE, Hurwitz RL. Metastatic and nonmetastatic models of retino-blastoma. Am J Pathol 2000; 157:1405–1412.
6. Klausner R. Studying cancer in the mouse. Oncogene 1999; 18:5249–5252.
7. Kobayashi S, Mukai N. Retinoblastoma-like tumors induced in rats by human adenovirus. Invest Ophthalmol Vis Sci 1973; 12:853–855.
8. Mukai N, Kalter SS, Cummins LB, Matthews VA, Nishida T, Nakajima T. Retinal tumor induced in the baboon by human adenovirus 12. Science 1980; 210:1023–1025.
9. Hogan B, Beddington R, Costantini F, Lacy E. Manipulating the mouse embryo: A laboratory manual. Cold Spring Harbor, NY: Cold Spring Harbor Laboratory Press, 1994.
10. Wassarman PM, DePamphilis ML. Guide to techniques in mouse development. In: Abelson JN, Simon MI, eds. Methods in Enzymology. Vol. 225. San Diego, CA: Academic Press, 1993.
11. Schwenk F, Kuhn R, Angrand PO, Rajewsky K, Stewart AF. Temporally and spatially regulated somatic mutagenesis in mice. Nucleic Acids Res 1998; 26:1427–1432.
12. Lewandowski M. Conditional control of gene expression in the mouse. Nat Rev Genet 2001; 2:743–755.
13. Robertson EJ. Teratocarcinomas and embryonic stem cells: A practical approach. In: Rickwood D, Hames BD, eds. Practical Approach Series. Oxford, UK: IRL Press, 1987.
14. Sauer B. Inducible gene targeting in mice using the Cre/lox system. Methods: A Companion to Methods in Enzymology 1998; 14:381–392.
15. Windle JJ, Albert DM, O'Brien JM, Marcus DM, Disteche CM, Bernards R, Mellon PL. Retinoblastoma in transgenic mice. Nature 1990; 343:665–669.
16. DeCaprio JA, Ludlow JW, Figge J, Shew J-Y, Huang C-M, Lee W-H, Marsilio E, Paucha E, Livingston DM. SV40 large tumor antigen forms a specific complex with the product of the retinoblastoma susceptibility gene. Cell 1988; 54:275–283.
17. Lane DP, Crawford LV. T antigen is bound to a host protein in SV40-transformed cells. Nature 1979; 278:261–263.
18. Linzer DIH, Levine AJ. Characterization of a 54 K dalton cellular SV40 tumor antigen present in SV40-transformed cells and uninfected embryonal carcinoma cells. Cell 1979; 17:43–52.
19. Alarid ET, Windle JJ, Whyte DB, Mellon PL. Immortalization of pituitary cells at discrete stages of development by directed oncogenesis in transgenic mice. Development 1996; 122:3319–3329.
20. Kivela T, Virtanen I, Marcus DM, O'Brien JM, Carpenter JL, Brauner E, Tarkkanen A, Albert DM. Neuronal and glial properties of a murine transgenic retinoblastoma model. Am J Pathol 1991; 138:1135–1148.

21. Bogenmann E, Lochrie MA, Simon MI. Cone cell-specific genes expressed in retinoblastoma. Science 1988; 240:76–78.
22. Vrabec T, Arbizo V, Adamus G, McDowell JH, Hargrave PA, Donoso LA. Rod cell–specific antigens in retinoblastoma. Arch Ophthalmol 1989; 107:1061–1063.
23. Hurwitz RL, Bogenmann E, Font RL, Halcombe V, Clark D. Expression of the functional cone phototransduction cascade in retinoblastoma. J Clin Invest 1990; 85:1872–1878.
24. Gonzalez-Fernandez F, Lopes MB, Garcia-Fernandez JM, Foster RG, De Grip WJ, Rosemberg S, Newman SA, VandenBerg SR. Expression of developmentally defined retinal phenotypes in the histogenesis of retinoblastoma. Am J Pathol 1992; 141:363–375.
25. Nork TM, Schwartz TL, Doshi HM, Millecchia LL. Retinoblastoma—Cell of origin Arch Ophthalmol 1995; 113:791–802.
26. Tsuji M, Goto M, Uehara F, Kaneko A, Sawai J, Yonezawa S, Ohba N. Photoreceptor cell differentiation in retinoblastoma demonstrated by a new immunohistochemical marker mucin-like glycoprotein associated with photoreceptor cells (MLGAPC). Histopathology 2002; 40:180–186.
27. Marcus DM, Carpenter JL, O'Brien JM, Kivela T, Brauner E, Tarkkanen A, Virtanen I, Albert DM. Primitive neuroectodermal tumor of the midbrain in a murine model of retinoblastoma. Invest Ophthalmol Vis Sci 1991; 32:293–301.
28. Jakobiec FA, Tso MOM, Zimmerman LE, Danis P. Retinoblastoma and intracranial malignancy. Cancer 1977; 39:2048–2058.
29. Bader JL, Miller RW, Meadows AT, Zimmerman LE, Champion LAA, Voute PA. Trilateral retinoblastoma. Lancet 1980; 2:582–583.
30. Brownstein S, de Chadarevian JP, Little JM. Trilateral retinoblastoma. Report of two cases. Arch Ophthalmol 1984; 102:257–262.
31. Bullitt E, Crain BJ. Retinoblastoma as a possible primary intracranial tumor. Neurosurgery 1981:706–709.
32. Pesin SR, Shields JA. Seven cases of trilateral retinoblastoma. Am J Ophthalmol 1989; 107:121–126.
33. Liou GI, Wang M, Matragoon S. Timing of interphotoreceptor retinoid-binding protein (IRBP) gene expression and hypomethylation in developing mouse retina. Dev Biol 1994; 161:345–356.
34. Al-Ubaidi MR, Hollyfield JG, Overbeek PA, Baehr W. Photoreceptor degeneration induced by the expression of simian virus 40 large tumor antigen in the retina of transgenic mice. Proc Natl Acad Sci USA 1992; 89:1194–1198.
35. al-Ubaidi MR, Mangini NJ, Quiambao AB, Myers KM, Abler AS, Chang C-J, Tso MOM, Butel JS, Hollyfield JG. Unscheduled DNA replication precedes apoptosis of photoreceptors expressing SV40 T antigen. Exp Eye Res 1997; 64:573–585.
36. Al-Ubaidi MR, Font RL, Quiambao AB, Keener MJ, Liou GI, Overbeek PA, Boeher W. Bilateral retinal and brain tumors in transgenic mice expressing simian virus 40 large T antigen under control of the human interphotoreceptor retinoid-binding protein promoter. J Cell Biol 1992; 119:1681–1687.
37. Howes KA, Lasudry JGH, Albert DM, Windle JJ. Photoreceptor cell tumors in transgenic mice. Invest Opthalmol Vis Sci 1994; 35:342–351.
38. Howes KA, Ransom N, Papermaster DS, Lasudry JGH, Albert DM, Windle JJ. Apoptosis or retinoblastoma: Alternative fates of photoreceptors expressing the HPV-16 E7 gene in the presence or absence of p53. Genes Dev 1994; 8:1300–1310.
39. Dyson N, Howley PM, Munger K, Harlow E. The human papilloma virus-16 E7 oncoprotein is able to bind to the retinoblastoma gene product. Science 1989; 243:934–937.

40. Munger K, Werness BA, Dyson N, Phelps WC, Harlow E, Howley PM. Complex formation of human papillomavirus E7 proteins with the retinoblastoma tumor suppressor gene product. EMBO J. 1989; 8:4099–4105.

41. Scheffner M, Werness BA, Huibregtse JM, Levine AJ, Howley PM. The E6 oncoprotein encoded by human papillomavirus types 16 and 18 promotes the degradation of p53. Cell 1990; 63:1129–1136.

42. Donehower LA, Harvey M, Slagle BL, McArthur MJ, Montgomery CAJ, Butel JS, Bradley A. Mice deficient for p53 are developmentally normal but susceptible to spontaneous tumours. Nature 1992; 356:215–221.

43. Baetge EE, Behringer RR, Messing A, Brinster RL, Palmiter RD. Transgenic mice express the human phenylethanolamine N-methyltransferase gene in adrenal medulla and retina. Proc Natl Acad Sci USA 1988; 85:3648–3652.

44. Fung K-M, Chikaraishi DM, Suri C, Theuring F, Messing A, Albert DM, Lee VM-Y, Trojanowski JQ. Molecular phenotype of simian virus 40 large T antigen-induced primitive neuroectodermal tumors in four different lines of transgenic mice. Lab Invest 1994; 70:114–124.

45. Hammang JP, Behringer RR, Baetge EE, Palmiter RD, Brinster RL, Messing A. Oncogene expression in retinal horizontal cells of transgenic mice results in a cascade of neurodegeneration. Neuron 1993; 10:1197–1209.

46. Griep AE, Herber R, Jeon S, Lohse JK, Dubielzig RR, Lambert PF. Tumorigenicity by human papillomavirus type 16 E6 and E7 in transgenic mice correlates with alterations in epithelial cell growth and differentiation. J Virol 1993; 67:1373–1384.

47. Griep AE, Krawcek J, Lee D, Liem A, Albert DM, Carabeo R, Drinkwater N, McCall M, Sattler C, Lasudry JG, Lambert PF. Multiple genetic loci modify risk for retinoblastoma in transgenic mice. Invest Ophthalmol Vis Sci 1998; 39:2723–2732.

48. Van Dyke TA. Analysis of viral-host protein interactions and tumorigenesis in transgenic mice. Semin Cancer Biol 1994; 5:47–60.

49. Lee EY-HP, Chang C-Y, Hu N, Wang Y-CJ, Lai C-C, Herrup K, Lee W-H, Bradley A. Mice deficient for Rb are nonviable and show defects in neurogenesis and haematopoiesis. Nature 1992; 359:288–294.

50. Jacks T, Fazeli A, Schmitt EM, Bronson RT, Goodell MA, Weinberg RA. Effects of an Rb mutation in the mouse. Nature 1992; 359:295–300.

51. Clarke AR, Maandag ER, van Roon M, van der Lugt NMT, van der Valk M, Hooper ML, Berns A, te Riele H. Requirement for a functional Rb-1 gene in murine development. Nature 1992; 359:328–330.

52. Hu N, Gutsmann A, Herbert DC, Bradley A, Lee WH, Lee EY. Heterozygous Rb-1 delta 20/ + mice are predisposed to tumors of the pituitary gland with a nearly complete penetrance. Oncogene 1994; 9:1021–1027.

53. Williams BO, Schmitt EM, Remington L, Bronson RT, Albert DM, Weinberg RA, Jacks T. Extensive contribution of Rb-deficient cells to adult chimeric mice with limited histopathological consequences. EMBO J 1994; 13:4251–4259.

54. Robanus-Maandag EC, van der valk M, Vlaar M, Feltkamp C, O'Brien J, van Roon M, van der Lugt N, Berns A, te Riele H. Developmental rescue of an embryonic-lethal mutation in the retinoblastoma gene in chimeric mice. EMBO J 1994; 13:4260–4268.

55. Harrison DJ, Hooper ML, Armstrong JF, Clarke AR. Effects of heterozygosity for the Rb-1t19neo allele in the mouse. Oncogene 1995; 10:1615–1620.

56. Morgenbesser SD, Williams BO, Jacks T, DePinho RA. p53-dependent apoptosis porduced by Rb-deficiency in the developing mouse lens. Nature 1994; 371:72–74.

57. Lee EY-HP, Hu N, Yuan SF, Cox LA, Bradley A, Lee W, Herrup K. Dual roles of the retinoblastoma protein in cell cycle regulation and neuron differentiation. Gene Dev 1994; 8:2008–2021.

58. Macleod KF, Hu Y, Jacks T. Loss of Rb activates both p53-dependent and independent cell death pathways in the developing mouse nervous system. EMBO J 1996; 15:6178–6188.

59. Lipinski MM, Macleod KF, Williams BO, Mullaney TL, Crowley D, Jacks T. Cell-autonomous and non-cell-autonomous functions of the Rb tumor suppressor in developing central nervous system. EMBO J 2001; 20:3401–3413.

60. Lee M-H, Williams BO, Mulligan G, Mukai S, Bronson RT, Dyson N, Harlow E, Jacks T. Targeted disruption of p107: Functional overlap between p107 and Rb Genes Dev 1996; 10:1621–1632.

61. Robanus-Maandag E, Dekker M, van der Valk M, Carrozza M-L, Jeanny J-C, Dannenberg J-H, Berns A, te Riele H. p107 is a suppressor of retinoblastoma development in pRb-deficient mice. Genes Dev 1998; 12:1599–1609.

62. Vooijs M, te Riele H, van der Valk M, Berns A. Tumor formation in mice with somatic inactivation of the retinoblastoma gene in interphotoreceptor retinol binding protein–expressing cells. Oncogene 2002; 21:4635–4645.

63. Harlow E. Retinoblastoma. For our eyes only. Nature 1992; 359:270–271.

64. Jacks T. Tumor suppressor gene mutations in mice. Annu Rev Genet 1996; 30:603–636.

65. Hooper ML. Tumour suppressor gene mutations in humans and mice: Parallels and contrasts. EMBO J 1998; 17:6783–6789.

66. Vooijs M, Berns A. Developmental defects and tumor predisposition in Rb mutant mice. Oncogene 1999; 18:5293–5303.

67. Mulligan G, Jacks T. The retinoblastoma gene family: Cousins with overlapping interests. Trends Genet 1998; 14:223–229.

68. Gallie BL, Budning A, DeBoer G, Thiessen JJ, Koren G, Verjee Z, Ling V, Chan HS. Chemotherapy with focal therapy can cure intraocular retinoblastoma without radiotherapy. Arch Ophthalmol 1996; 114:1321–1328.

69. Murphree AL, Villablanca JG, Deegan WF, 3rd, Sato JK, Malogolowkin M, Fisher A, Parker R, Reed E, Gomer CJ. Chemotherapy plus local treatment in the management of intraocular retinoblastoma. Arch Ophthalmol 1996; 114:1348–1356.

70. Harbour JW, Murray TG, Hamasaki D, Cicciarelli N, Hernandez E, Smith B, Windle J, O'Brien JM. Local carboplatin therapy in transgenic murine retinoblastoma. Invest Ophthalmol Vis Sci 1996; 37:1892–1898.

71. Hayden BH, Murray TG, Scott IU, Cicciarelli N, Hernandez E, Feuer W, Fulton, O'Brien JM. Subconjunctival carboplatin in retinoblastoma: Impact of tumor burden and dose schedule. Arch Ophthalmol 2000; 118:1549–1554.

72. Murray TG, Cicciarelli N, O'Brien JM, Hernandez E, Mueller RL, Smith BJ, Feuer W. Subconjunctival carboplatin therapy and cryotherapy in the treatment of transgenic murine retinoblastoma. Arch Ophthalmol 1997; 115:1286–1290.

73. Hayden BC, Murray TG, Cicciarelli N, Scott IU, Alexandridou A, Hernandez E, Wu X, Markoe AM, Feuer W, Fulton L, O'Brien JM. Hyperfractionated external beam radiation therapy in the treatment of murine transgenic retinoblastoma. Arch Ophthalmol 2002; 120:353–359.

74. Murray TG, O'Brien JM, Steeves RA, Smith BJ, Albert DM, Cicciarelli N, Markoe AM, Tompkins DT, Windle JJ. Radiation therapy and ferromagnetic hyperthermia in the treatment of murine transgenic retinoblastoma. Arch Ophthalmol 1996; 114:1376–1381.

75. Albert DM, Marcus DM, Gallo JP, O'Brien JM. The antineoplastic effect of vitamin D in transgenic mice with retinoblastoma. Invest Ophthalmol Vis Sci 1992; 33:2354–2364.

76. Shokravi MT, Marcus DM, Alroy J, Egan K, Saornil MA, Albert DM. Vitamin D inhibits angiogenesis in transgenic murine retinoblastoma. Invest Ophthalmol Vis Sci 1995; 36:83–87.

77. van den Bemd GJ, Chang GT. Vitamin D and vitamin D analogs in cancer treatment. Curr Drug Targets 2002; 3:85–94.

78. Shternfeld IS, Lasudry JG, Chappell RJ, Darjatmoko SR, Albert DM. Antineoplastic effect of 1,25-dihydroxy-16-ene-23-yne-vitamin D_3 analogue in transgenic mice with retinoblastoma. Arch Ophthalmol 1996; 114:1396–1401.

79. Wilkerson CL, Darjatmoko SR, Lindstrom MJ, Albert DM. Toxicity and dose-response studies of 1,25-(OH)2–16-ene-23-yne vitamin D_3 in transgenic mice. Clin Cancer Res 1998; 4:2253–2256.

80. Ring CJ. Cytolytic viruses as potential anti-cancer agents. J Gen Virol 2002; 83:491–502.

81. Markert JM, Parker JN, Gillespie GY, Whitley RJ. Genetically engineered human herpes simplex virus in the treatment of brain tumours. Herpes 2001; 8:17–22.

82. Brandt CR, Imesch PD, Robinson NL, Syed NA, Untawale S, Darjatmoko SR, Chappell RJ, Heinzelman P, Albert DM. Treatment of spontaneously arising retinoblastoma tumors in transgenic mice with an attenuated herpes simplex virus mutant. Virology 1997; 229:283–291.

23

Treatment of Extraocular Retinoblastoma

DIANE PUCCETTI

University of Wisconsin Children's Hospital, Madison, Wisconsin, U.S.A.

I. SCOPE OF THE PROBLEM

Retinoblastoma is the most common primary ocular malignancy of childhood, occurring in about 1 in 18,000 live births in the United States. It is estimated that 200 new cases are diagnosed every year in the United States [1]. There is evidence that retinoblastoma may be more frequent in some developing nations, such as India [2] and in Latin America [3]. The survival of patients in developed nations diagnosed with retinoblastoma has improved over the last century, likely due to earlier diagnosis and improved treatment [1]. Most of these patients present with intraocular disease, while delayed diagnosis has been associated with an advanced stage of disease and a poorer prognosis [2,3]. The previous chapters in this book thoroughly discuss retinoblastoma, primarily intraocular. Therefore, this chapter focuses on extraocular disease.

By definition, extraocular retinoblastoma is disease that has extended beyond the globe. There is currently no standard staging system for this situation. The three most common systems include the Abramson Staging System for Retinoblastoma, the St. Jude Children's Research Hospital Clinical Staging System, and the Reese-Ellsworth Classification. The first divides extraocular disease into orbital, optic nerve, intracranial, metastasis, and hematogenous metastasis [4], while the second distinguishes tumor confined to the retina, the globe, extraocular (regional) extension, and distant metastases [5]. The Reese-Ellsworth Classification is a method to predict prognosis of eyes treated to preserve vision when disease is limited to the globe of the eye. To allow comparison of therapeutic modalities, most individuals divide stages into intraocular tumor, involvement of optic nerve, orbital extension, and finally, distant metastases. There is a new proposed clinical and pathological staging classification for retinoblastoma from the American Joint Committee on Cancer.

A. Incidence of Extension and Metastatic Disease

Previous studies have reported that approximately 10% of patients will develop metastatic disease at a mean age of about 3 years, averaging 12 months from time of diagnosis [7–9]. A retrospective study of 261 patient's treatment in Saudi Arabia found that 14.9% had metastatic disease, with an average age of 3.1 years [10]. A prospective study in Argentina found that 48% of the 101 eligible patients had extraocular disease, including 9 patients with intracranial or hematogenous metastases [11]. Two studies in the United States reported an incidence of extraocular disease at diagnosis of 3% [12] and 9% [5] respectively.

B. Mechanism of Disease Extension and Metastatic Spread

Invasion of the optic nerve accounts for the most common route of spread, with the potential to involve the optic chiasm or infiltrate into the subarachnoid space to perhaps involve the cerebrospinal fluid and subsequently the brain and spinal cord. Tumor spread from the choroid into the orbit accounts for the second route of dissemination [13]. Once the tumor extension is extraocular, the chances of hematogenous and lymphatic spread increase. The four routes for metastatic spread include the following [14,15]:

1. Direct infiltration into brain or orbit
2. Subarachnoid spread into brain, spinal cord, or the other optic nerve
3. Orbital or lymph node invasion, which may lead to hematogenous dissemination
4. Lymphatic dissemination if the eyelid, conjunctiva, or extraocular tissues are involved

C. Risk Factors and Ancillary Testing

Information regarding sites of metastatic disease in the past has relied on data obtained from autopsy studies, indicating that orbital and cranial bones are the most common sites, with tumor also involving long bones, lymph nodes, and liver and kidney [9,16,17].

Over the past 20 years, many studies have reported the results of ancillary testing for presence of metastatic disease at time of diagnosis. Earlier reports had recommended routine examinations of cerebrospinal fluid and bone marrow in all newly diagnosed patients [18,19], but several large studies have shown that incidence of metastasis at diagnosis or development of metastatic disease can be correlated with certain histopathological risk factors. A multivariate analysis of risk factors found that tumor invasion into the sclera, optic nerve, and orbit were most highly predictive of metastatic disease [20]. Three other studies looked specifically at correlation of invasion of optic nerve and choroid [21], optic nerve invasion [22], and choroidal involvement of disease [23] with risk of metastatic disease. Conclusions from the two more recent studies are that choroidal invasion alone is not a significant risk factor for development of metastasis [23], while optic nerve invasion beyond the lamina cribrosa is associated with a greater metastatic risk [22].

Three studies have reported incidence of bone marrow involvement of disease from zero to 1.7% [12,24,25], while Karcioglu [10] reported 10% of patients had evidence of disease metastatic to the marrow, all with extraocular disease. Involvement of cerebrospinal fluid in these four studies ranged from zero [12,24] to 1% [25] with 4% of patients in Karcioglu's study [10].

Current recommendations are magnetic resonance imaging (MRI) of the brain and lumbar puncture be performed in patients with optic nerve extension or choroidal invasion. In addition, bone marrow examination or bone scan reserved for those with clinical signs/symptoms referred to these areas [1].

II. TREATMENT OF EXTRAOCULAR RETINOBLASTOMA WITH STANDARD CHEMOTHERAPY

The previous chapters in this book discuss in detail the treatment options for retinoblastoma. This section focuses on treatment modalities for the patient with extraocular retinoblastoma. The management of patients with trilateral retinoblastoma is discussed separately further on in this chapter.

The goals of therapy for any child diagnosed with cancer is to provide curative treatment with the least possible toxicity, both acute and long-term. Preservation of life, protection of vision, limitation of serious side effects, and not adding unnecessarily to the risk of a second malignancy is the "gold standard" in treating children with retinoblastoma. This becomes more of a challenge with the patients who have extraocular disease, because their survival rates are lower than that of patients with intraocular disease [1,7,11,13,19,20].

Like patients with intraocular disease, the treatment plan for a patient with extraocular retinoblastoma must be individualized and take into account the patient's age, metastatic risk, likelihood of second malignancy, disease laterality, and size and location of tumor.

Children with extraocular retinoblastoma are not a homogenous group. The survival rate and ideal treatment for each subgroup may vary and, for some situations, there is no clear-cut "best" treatment approach. The therapies utilized for this diverse group of patients have included systemic and intrathecal chemotherapy, external-beam radiation therapy, high-dose chemotherapy with peripheral stem rescue, and combinations of two or more of the above [1,7,11,13,19,26–28].

The effectiveness of chemotherapy in treating retinoblastoma in the setting of extraocular and metastatic disease has previously been reported [7,11,16,19]. The responses of single chemotherapy agents and combination chemotherapeutic agents in patients with measurable extraocular disease treated at St. Jude Children's Research Hospital included cyclophosphamide and ifosfamide, demonstrating measurable effects as single agents, while the two- or three-drug combinations did show complete responses in some instances [7]. Grabowski and colleagues treated patients with extraocular disease with the combination of cyclophosphamide and doxorubicin and reported a survival of 10 of 12 patients [19].

A phase II study of etoposide and carboplatin administered to 20 patients with extraocular retinoblastoma reported a response rate of 85%, with 9 patients experiencing complete responses [29]. In addition, regimens of carboplatin and etoposide with or without vincristine have been employed in the setting of both intraocular and extraocular disease [1,30].

A. Extraretinal Intraocular Disease

With that background information, the role of standard dose chemotherapy can be explored in various subgroups of patients with extraretinal intraocular and extraocular disease. The first group of patients comprises those with extraretinal spread (choroids, extension to sclera, or disease beyond the lamina cribrosa but not extending to the cut end of the nerve). What appears clear is that extensive invasion of the choroid in the setting of optic nerve invasion beyond the lamina cribrosa warrants prophylactic therapy [1,23,27].

A less obvious subgroup includes those with significant choroidal involvement in the absence of optic nerve invasion in whom prophylactic adjuvant therapy should be considered [1,9,13,23,27,30]. Patients with significant deep involvement of the choroid, optic nerve, ciliary body, or iris have received treatment with chemotherapy including doxorubicin and cyclophosphamide as well as the three-drug combination of vincristine, etoposide, and carboplatin [27,30]. There have been reports suggesting that prophylactic chemotherapy in patients with these high-risk features may lessen the risk of metastases, although the absence of randomized trials to select the best regimen and, as well, no randomized study to prove the benefit of chemoprophylaxis in this group of patients with extraretinal disease makes it difficult to give a definitive recommendation [31].

B. Extraocular Disease—Optic Nerve

For patients with extraocular disease, previous studies have reported results utilizing a combined treatment approach with chemotherapy and radiotherapy [19,26,27,29,32]. The chemotherapeutic agents employed include etoposide, carboplatin, cisplatin, doxorubicin, cyclophosphamide, and vincristine. The overall survival rates ranged from 60–80%. Within this group of patients, there were subsets of patients who had lower survival rates and shared common histopathological features. Invasion of the optic nerve beyond the cut end is a major prognostic factor for relapse and in retrospective studies those patients have fared poorly with a relapse rate of nearly 80% [21,22,33]. Several prospective studies that examined the impact of tumor involving the cut end of the optic nerve have conflicting outcomes with survival rates ranging from 41–80% [29,32]. More recently, chemoprophylaxis appeared to be of benefit in preventing metastasis in patients with optic nerve involvement to the cut end or beyond the lamina cribrosa [34].

Invasion of the optic nerve beyond the lamina cribrosa is not as strong a predictor of relapse, and previous studies have not addressed the question of necessity of adjuvant therapy [11]. It has been suggested that chemotherapy without radiation therapy is sufficient, and Schvartzman and colleagues successfully treated 11 of 12 patients with chemotherapy alone [11,35].

C. Orbital Disease

Radiotherapy and chemotherapy have been successful in the treatment of overt orbital retinoblastoma [29,36].

D. Hematogenous Disease

The group with the poorest prognosis includes patients with hematogenous or central nervous system metastasis [1,19]. Patients with hematogenous spread of disease have responded to different chemotherapeutic agents, but this has not always been long-lasting [7,11,19,26,29,37]. Schvartzman and colleagues reported a 50% survival rate for their patients with hematogenous metastasis who received chemotherapy with vincristine, cyclophosphamide, doxorubicin, cisplatin, and etoposide as well as radiotherapy [11].

E. Central Nervous System Disease

Finally, the patients with metastatic disease involving the central nervous system fare the worst [1,11,19,38]. There are few long-term survivals among patients who present with central nervous system metastasis or develop it. The treatment regimens previously studied have included combination chemotherapy and radiotherapy and intrathecal administration of chemotherapy [7,11,19,26,27,29]. The external-beam radiation therapy given to these patients included focal brain, whole-brain, and craniospinal treatment [7,11,19,26,28,29].

    Consensus has not be achieved as to the optimal radiation therapy approach to the patients with evidence of central nervous system metastasis. The morbidity of whole-brain and/or craniospinal irradiation is significant for these patients, who are usually young at the time of their presentation [39,40]. Intrathecal chemotherapy has included methotrexate, hydrocortisone, and cytarabine, with disappointing results [27]. Newer agents under evaluation include topotecan and melphalan [27].

III. TREATMENT OF EXTRAOCULAR RETINOBLASTOMA WITH INTENSIVE CHEMOTHERAPY AND AUTOLOGOUS RESCUE

Because of the poor prognosis for patients with metastatic retinoblastoma treated with conventional therapy, there has been interest in intensifying chemotherapy with autologous stem cell or bone marrow rescue. This approach has been successful in other childhood cancers, especially in neuroblastoma [41]. Earlier published work suggests that this intensive approach may be beneficial for this poor-risk population [42,43].

    Investigators at the Institut Curie treated 25 high-risk retinoblastoma patients (extraocular disease at diagnosis or relapse, or invasion of cut end of optic nerve) with high-dose carboplatin, etoposide, and cyclophosphamide followed by autologous hematopoietic stem cell rescue (ASCR). The 3-year disease free survival was 67%, and 5 of the 8 patients with metastatic disease (no central nervous system involvement) were event-free survivors with this approach. Central nervous system disease recurrence developed in 3 patients, who died within 20 months of their high-dose chemotherapy, and 3 patients experienced progressive disease during the conventional chemotherapy given during induction and never received the high-dose chemotherapy. For the group of patients with metastatic disease (not initially involving the central nervous system), 5 of the 11 were event-free survivors [28].

Recent reports have described the use of thiotepa, carboplatin, and etoposide with ASCR for patients with metastatic retinoblastoma. Thiotepa was chosen because it penetrates the central nervous system, and the toxicity profile lends it to dose escalation [44]. The five patients treated in this manner are event-free survivors 46–80 months after their diagnosis. The sites of disease included bone, lymph nodes, bone marrow, and liver, but none of the patients had central nervous system disease [45,46].

Radiation therapy was administered to sites of original bulky disease in one study, but in the other two reports no radiation therapy was given to sites of bony metastases; 5 of the 6 patients were event-free survivors in the group not irradiated [28,45,46].

The predominant acute toxicities included myelosuppression and mucositis, with long-term ototoxity related to carboplatin [28,45,46]. These chemotherapy agents are mutagenic and may increase the risk of second cancers. The same can be said for external-beam irradiation [47,48].

IV. TRILATERAL RETINOBLASTOMA

Jakobiec and associates were the first to describe the association of bilateral retinoblastoma with intracranial malignancy, later termed trilateral retinoblastoma by Bader and colleagues [49,50]. Over the decades, more information has become available regarding this entity.

The incidence of trilateral retinoblastoma is approximately eight cases per year in the United States. In nearly all cases, it develops in a subset of retinoblastoma patients harboring germline mutations with the inheritable form of retinoblastoma (bilateral or multifocal, or positive family history). Clinical variants of this presentation have been reported, including lack of ocular involvement or unilateral retinoblastoma [51–53]. The pineal gland is the most common location, but tumors occur in the suprasellar region and typically present earlier than pineal lesions. The histopathological features can be variable, with the majority of tumors undifferentiated and the rest demonstrating degrees of neuronal or photoreceptor differentiation [53,54]. The mean age at diagnosis is 30 months, with signs and symptoms of increased intracranial pressure in the majority of patients [15,53,54].

The vast majority of patients will succumb to their disease, despite multimodality treatment, with a median survival of 6 months. There are reports of long-term survivors who received a variety of treatments, including systemic chemotherapy and intrathecal chemotherapy in some instances. Patients who received treatment experienced a longer median survival than those who received only palliative care. The main pattern of failure was spread to the neural axis [15,53,54]. A comprehensive metanalyses concluded that neuroimaging could improve the cure rate if trilateral retinoblastoma was diagnosed while patients were asymptomatic and tumors were less than 15 mm [15,53]. Because the majority of patients can be detected within 1 year of the diagnosis of retinoblastoma, screening with brain imaging should be considered in children with bilateral or familial retinoblastoma [15,53,54].

Shields and colleagues performed a retrospective study to evaluate whether neoadjuvant intravenous chemotherapy (vincristine, etoposide, and carboplatin) reduced the risk of development of trilateral retinoblastoma. Comparison was made between the group receiving neoadjuvant chemotherapy versus the nonchemotherapy control group and the development of trilateral retinoblastoma. Based on recent analyses of the prevalence of this disorder, 5–15 patients (in the chemotherapy group) would be projected to develop an intracranial tumor of the 99 children at risk secondary to bilateral and/or family disease. No intracranial tumors were diagnosed in the group receiving chemotherapy, while one patient in the nonchemotherapy control group experienced intracranial development consistent with the expected frequency for that group. Longer follow-up will be necessary to fully appreciate the effect of chemoreduction [55].

REFERENCES

1. Hurwitz RL, Shields CL, Shields JA, Chévez-Barrios P, Hurwitz MY, Chintagumpala MM. Retinoblastoma. In: Pizzo PA, Poplack DG, eds. Principles and Practice of Pediatric Oncology. 4th ed. Philadelphia: Lippincott, Williams & Wilkins, 2002, pp 825–846.

2. Sahu S, Banavali SD, Pai SK, Nair CN, Kurkure PA, Motwani SA, Advani SH. Retinoblastoma: Problems and perspectives from India. Pediatr Hematol Oncol 1998; 15:501–508.

3. Pérez C, Travezan R, Salem E. Delayed diagnosis and treatment in retinoblastoma (RB): Peruvian reality (abstr). Proc Am Soc Clin Oncol 1994; 13:417.

4. Abramson DH, Dunkel I, McCormick BM. Neoplasms of the eye. In: Holland JF, Bast RC Jr, Morton DL. eds. Cancer Medicine, 4th ed. Amsterdam: Lippincott, Williams & Wilkins, 1996, pp 1517–1536.

5. Pratt CB. Management of malignant solid tumors in children. Pediatr Clin North Am 1972; 19:1141–1155.

6. Reese AB, Ellsworth RM. Management of retinoblastoma. Ann NY Acad Sci 1964; 114:958–962.

7. Pratt CB, Crom DB, Howarth C. The use of chemotherapy for extraocular retinoblastoma. Med Pediatr Oncol 1985; 13:330–333.

8. de Sutter E, Havers W, Höpping W, Zeller G, Albert W. The prognosis of retinoblastoma in terms of survival. A computer assisted study. Part II. Ophthalmic Paediatr Genet 1987; 8:85–88.

9. Messmer EP, Heinrich T, Höpping W, de Sutter E, Havers W, Sauerwein W. Risk factors for metastases in patients with retinoblastoma. Ophthalmology 1991; 98:136–141.

10. Karcioglu ZA, Al-Mesfer SA, Abboud E, Jabak MH, Mullaney PB. Work up for metastatic retinoblastoma: A review of 261 patients. Ophthalmology 1997; 104:307–312.

11. Schvartzman E, Chantada G, Fandiño A, de Dávila MT, Raslawski E, Manzitti J. Results of a stage-based protocol for the treatment of retinoblastoma. J Clin Oncol 1996; 14:1532–1536.

12. Moscinski LC, Pendergrass TW, Weiss A, Hvizdala E, Buckley KS, Kalina RE. Recommendations for the use of routine bone marrow aspiration and lumbar punctures in the follow-up of patients with retinoblastoma. J Pediatr Hematol Oncol 1996; 18:130–134.

13. Khelfaoui F, Validire P, Auperin A, Quintana E, Michon J, Pacquement H, Desjardins L, Asselain B, Schlienger P, Vielh P, Dufier J-L, Zucker J-M, Doz F. Histopathologic risk factors in retinoblastoma: A retrospective study of 172 patients treated in a single institution. Cancer 1996; 77:1206–1213.

14. McLean I, Burnier M, Zimmerman L, Jakobiec F. Tumors of the retina. In: McLean IW, Burnier MN, Zimmerman LE, FA J, eds. Atlas of Tumor Pathology. Tumors of the Eye and Ocular Adnexa. Washington, DC: Armed Forces Institute of Pathology, 1994, pp 100–135.

15. Kivelä T. Trilateral retinoblastoma: A meta-analysis of hereditary retinoblastoma associated with primary ectopic intracranial retinoblastoma. J Clin Oncol 1999; 17:1829–1837.

16. Carbajal UM. Metastasis in retinoblastoma. Am J Ophthalmol 1959; 48:47–69.

17. Merriam GR Jr. Retinoblastoma: Analysis of seventeen autopsies. Arch Ophthalmol 1950; 4:71–108.

18. Reese AB, Ellsworth RM. The evaluation and current concept of retinoblastoma therapy. Trans Am Acad Ophthalmol Otolaryngol 1963; 67:164–172.

19. Grabowski EF, Abramson DH. Intraocular and extraocular retinoblastoma. Hematol Oncol Clin North Am 1987; 1:721–735.

20. Kopelman JE, McLean IW, Rosenberg SH. Multivariate analysis of risk factors for metastasis in retinoblastoma treated by enucleation. Ophthalmology 1987; 94:371–377.

21. Stannard C, Lipper S, Sealy R, Sevel D. Retinoblastoma: Correlation of invasion of the optic nerve and choroid with prognosis and metastases. Br J Ophthalmol 1979; 63:560–570.

22. Shields CL, Shields JA, Baez K, Cater JR, De Potter P. Optic nerve invasion of retinoblastoma. Cancer 1994; 73:692–698.

23. Shields CL, Shields JA, Baez KA, Cater J, DePotter PV. Choroidal invasion of retinoblastoma: Metastatic potential and clinical risk factors. Br J Ophthalmol 1993; 77:544–548.

24. Mohney BG, Robertson DM. Ancillary testing for metastasis in patients with newly diagnosed retinoblastoma. Am J Ophthalmol 1994; 118:707–711.

25. Pratt CB, Meyer D, Chenaille P, Crom DB. The use of bone marrow aspirations and lumbar punctures at the time of diagnosis of retinoblastoma. J Clin Oncol 1989; 7:140–143.

26. Pratt CB, Fontanesi J, Chenaille P, Kun LE, Jenkins JJ III, Langston JW, Mounce KG, Meyer D. Chemotherapy for extraocular retinoblastoma. Pediatr Hematol Oncol 1994; 11:301–309.

27. Pratt CB. Use of chemotherapy for retinoblastoma. Med Pediatr Oncol 1998; 31:531–533.

28. Namouni F, Doz F, Tanguy ML, Quintana E, Michon J, Pacquement H, Douffet E, Gentet JC, Plantaz D, Lutz P, Vannier JP, Validire P, Neuenschwander S, Desjardins L, Zucker JM. High-dose chemotherapy with carboplatin, etoposide, and cyclophosphamide followed by a haematopoietic stem cell rescue in patients with high risk retinoblastoma: A SFOP and SFGM study. Eur J Cancer 1997; 33:2368–2375.

29. Doz F, Neuenschwander S, Plantaz D, Courbon B, Gentet JC, Bouffet E, Mosseri V, Vannier JP, Mechinaud F, Desjardins L, Vielh P, Zucker JM. Etoposide and carboplatin in extraocular retinoblastoma: A study by the Société Française d'Oncologie Pédiatrique. J Clin Oncol 1995; 13:902–909.

30. Friedman DL, Himelstein B, Shields CL, Shields JA, Needle M, Miller D, Bunin GR, Meadows AT. Chemoreduction and local ophthalmic therapy for intraocular retinoblastoma. J Clin Oncol 2000; 18:12–17.

31. Honavar SG, Singh AO, Shields CL. Does post-enucleation prophylactic chemotherapy in high risk retinoblastoma prevent metastasis? (abstr.) Invest Ophthalmol Vis Sci 2000; 41(4):5953.

32. Mustafa MM, Jamshed A, Khafaga Y, Mourad WA, Al-Mesfer S, Kofide A, El-Husseiny G, Gray A. Adjuvant chemotherapy with vincristine, doxorubicin, and cyclophosphamide in the treatment of postenucleation high risk retinoblastoma. J Pediatr Hematol Oncol 1999; 21:364–369.

33. Magramm I, Abramson DH, Ellsworth RM. Optic nerve involvement in retinoblastoma. Ophthalmology 1989; 96:217–222.

34. O'Brien JM, Uusitalo M, Van Quill K, Scott I, Murray T. Chemoprophylaxis for high risk factors on histopathologic examination of retinoblastoma eyes. Poster Presentation, 1999.

35. Grabowski EF, McCormick B, Abramson DH. Management of optic nerve extension in retinoblastoma (abstr). Proceedings of the VI International Symposium on Retinoblastoma. Siena Italy, June 1992.

36. Goble R, McKenzie J, Kingston J. Orbital recurrence of retinoblastoma successfully treated by combined therapy. Br J Ophthalmol 1990; 74:97–98.

37. Chantada GL, Fandiño A, Mato G, Casak S. Phase II window of idarubicin in children with extraocular retinoblastoma. J Clin Oncol 1999; 17:1847–1850.

38. White L. Chemotherapy in retinoblastoma: Current status and future directions. Am J Pediatr Hematol Oncol 1991; 13:189–201.

39. Moore BD 3rd, Atre JL, Copeland DR. Improved neuropsychological outcome in children with brain tumors diagnosed during infancy and treated without cranial irradiation. J Child Neurol 1992; 7:281–290.

40. Ambrosino MM, Hernanz-Schulman M, Genieser NB, Wisoff J, Epstein F. Brain tumors in infants less than a year of age. Pediatr Radiol 1988; 19:6–8.

41. Stram DO, Matthay KK, O'Leary M, Reynolds CP, Haase GM, Atkinson JB, Brodeur GM, Seeger RC. Consolidation chemoradiotherapy and autologous bone marrow transplantation versus continued chemotherapy for metastatic neuroblastoma: A report of two concurrent Children's Cancer Group studies. J Clin Oncol 1996; 14:2417–2426.

42. Saleh RA, Gross S, Cassano W, Gee A. Metastatic retinoblastoma successfully treated with immunomagnetic purged autologous bone marrow transplantation. Cancer 1988; 62:2301–2303.

43. Saarinen UM, Sariola H, Hovi L. Recurrent disseminated retinoblastoma treated by high-dose chemotherapy, total body irradiation, and autologous bone marrow rescue. Am J Pediatr Hematol Oncol 1991; 13:315–319.

44. Heideman RL, Cole DE, Balis F, Sato J, Reaman GH, Packer RJ, Singher LJ, Ettinger LJ, Gillespie A, Sam J. Phase I and pharmacokinetic evaluation of thiotepa in the cerebrospinal fluid and plasma of pediatric patients: Evidence for dose-dependent plasma clearance of thiotepa. Cancer Res 1989; 49:736–741.

45. Dunkel IJ, Aledo A, Kernan NA, Kushner B, Bayer L, Gollamudi SV, Finlay JL, Abramson DH. Successful treatment of metastatic retinoblastoma. Cancer 2000; 89:2117–2121.

46. Hertzberg H, Kremens B, Velten I, Beck JD, Greil J. Recurrent disseminated retinoblastoma in a 7-year-old girl treated successfully by high-dose chemotherapy and CD34-selected autologous peripheral blood stem cell transplantation. Bone Marrow Transplant 2001; 27:653–655.

47. Messmer EP, Fritze H, Mohr C, Heinrich T, Sauerwein W, Havers W, Horsthemke B, Hopping W. Long-term treatment effects in patients with bilateral retinoblastoma: Ocular and mid-facial findings. Graefes Arch Clin Exp Ophthalmol 1991; 229:309–314.

48. Eng C, Li FP, Abramson DH, Ellsworth RM, Wong FL, Goldman MB, Seddon J, Tarbell N, Boice JD Jr. Mortality from second tumor among long-term survivors of retinoblastoma. J Natl Cancer Inst 1993; 85:1121–1128.

49. Jakobiec FA, Tso MO, Zimmerman LE, Danis P. Retinoblastoma and intracranial malignancy. Cancer 1977; 39:2048–2058.

50. Bader JL, Miller RW, Meadows AT, Zimmerman LE, Champion LA, Voute PA. Trilateral retinoblastoma. Lancet 1980; 2:582–583.

51. Guyer B, Strobino DM, Ventura SJ, MacDorman M, Martin JA. Annual summary of vital statistics—1995. Pediatrics 1996; 98:1007–1019.

52. DePotter P, Shields CL, Shields JA. Clinical variations of trilateral retinoblastoma: A report of 13 cases. J Pediatr Ophthalmol Strabismus 1994; 31:26–31.

53. Marcus DM, Brooks SE, Leff G, McCormick R, Thompson T, Anfinson S, Lasudry J, Albert DM. Trilateral retinoblastoma: Insights into histogenesis and management. Surv Ophthalmol 1998; 43:59–70.

54. Paulino AC. Trilateral retinoblastoma. Is the location of the intracranial tumor important? Cancer 1999; 86:135–141.

55. Shields CL, Meadows AT, Shields JA, Carvalho C, Smith AF. Chemoreduction for retinoblastoma may prevent intracranial neuroblastic malignancy (trilateral retinoblastoma). Arch Ophthalmol 2001; 119:1269–1272.

Index

Printed and bound by CPI Group (UK) Ltd, Croydon, CR0 4YY

23/10/2024

01778246-0003